1997
YEAR BOOK OF
ANESTHESIOLOGY AND PAIN MANAGEMENT®

Statement of Purpose

The YEAR BOOK Service

The YEAR BOOK series was devised in 1901 by practicing health professionals who observed that the literature of medicine and related disciplines had become so voluminous that no one individual could read and place in perspective every potential advance in a major specialty. In the final decade of the 20th century, this recognition is more acutely true than it was in 1901.

More than merely a series of books, YEAR BOOK volumes are the tangible results of a unique service designed to accomplish the following:

- to *survey* a wide range of journals of proven value
- to *select* from those journals papers representing significant advances and statements of important clinical principles
- to provide *abstracts* of those articles that are readable, convenient summaries of their key points
- to provide *commentary* about those articles to place them in perspective

These publications grow out of a unique process that calls on the talents of outstanding authorities in clinical and fundamental disciplines, trained literature specialists, and professional writers, all supported by the resources of Mosby, the world's preeminent publisher for the health professions.

The Literature Base

Mosby and its editors survey more than 1,000 journals published worldwide, covering the full range of the health professions. On an annual basis, the publisher examines usage patterns and polls its expert authorities to add new journals to the literature base and to delete journals that are no longer useful as potential YEAR BOOK sources.

The Literature Survey

The publisher's team of literature specialists, all of whom are trained and experienced health professionals, examines every original, peer-reviewed article in each journal issue. More than 250,000 articles per year are scanned systematically, including title, text, illustrations, tables, and references. Each scan is compared, article by article, to the search strategies that the publisher has developed in consultation with the 270 outside experts who form the pool of YEAR BOOK editors. A given article may be reviewed by any number of editors, from one to a dozen or more, regardless of the discipline for which the paper was originally published. In turn, each editor who receives the article reviews it to determine whether or not the article should be included in the YEAR BOOK. This decision is based on the article's inherent quality, its probable usefulness to readers of that YEAR BOOK, and the editor's goal to represent a balanced picture of a given field in each volume of the YEAR BOOK. In addition, the editor indicates when to include figures and tables from the article to help the YEAR BOOK reader better understand the information.

Of the quarter million articles scanned each year, only 5% are selected for detailed analysis within the YEAR BOOK series, thereby assuring readers of the high value of every selection.

The Abstract

The publisher's abstracting staff is headed by a seasoned medical professional and includes individuals with training in the life sciences, medicine, and other areas, plus extensive experience in writing for the health professions and related industries. Each selected article is assigned to a specific writer on this abstracting staff. The abstracter, guided in many cases by notations supplied by the expert editor, writes a structured, condensed summary designed so that the reader can rapidly acquire the essential information contained in the article.

The Commentary

The YEAR BOOK editorial boards, sometimes assisted by guest commentators, write comments that place each article in perspective for the reader. This provides the reader with the equivalent of a personal consultation with a leading international authority—an opportunity to better understand the value of the article and to benefit from the authority's thought processes in assessing the article.

Additional Editorial Features

The editorial boards of each YEAR BOOK organize the abstracts and comments to provide a logical and satisfying sequence of information. To enhance the organization, editors also provide introductions to sections or individual chapters, comments linking a number of abstracts, citations to additional literature, and other features.

The published YEAR BOOK contains enhanced bibliographic citations for each selected article, including extended listings of multiple authors and identification of author affiliations. Each YEAR BOOK contains a Table of Contents specific to that year's volume. From year to year, the Table of Contents for a given YEAR BOOK will vary depending on developments within the field.

Every YEAR BOOK contains a list of the journals from which papers have been selected. This list represents a subset of the more than 1,000 journals surveyed by the publisher and occasionally reflects a particularly pertinent article from a journal that is not surveyed on a routine basis.

Finally, each volume contains a comprehensive subject index and an index to authors of each selected paper.

The 1997 Year Book Series

Year Book of Allergy, Asthma, and Clinical Immunology: Drs. Rosenwasser, Borish, Gelfand, Leung, Nelson, and Szefler

Year Book of Anesthesiology and Pain Management®: Drs. Tinker, Abram, Chestnut, Roizen, Rothenberg, and Wood

Year Book of Cardiology®: Drs. Schlant, Collins, Gersh, Graham, Kaplan, and Waldo

Year Book of Chiropractic®: Dr. Lawrence

Year Book of Critical Care Medicine®: Drs. Parrillo, Balk, Calvin, Franklin, and Shapiro

Year Book of Dentistry®: Drs. Meskin, Berry, Kennedy, Leinfelder, Roser, Summitt, and Zakariasen

Year Book of Dermatologic Surgery®: Drs. Greenway, Papadopoulos, and Whitaker

Year Book of Dermatology®: Drs. Sober and Fitzpatrick

Year Book of Diagnostic Radiology®: Drs. Federle, Gross, Dalinka, Maynard, Rebner, Smirniotopolous, and Young

Year Book of Digestive Diseases®: Drs. Greenberger and Moody

Year Book of Drug Therapy®: Drs. Lasagna and Weintraub

Year Book of Emergency Medicine®: Drs. Wagner, Dronen, Davidson, King, Niemann, and Roberts

Year Book of Endocrinology®: Drs. Bagdade, Braverman, Horton, Kannan, Landsberg, Molitch, Morley, Nathan, Odell, Poehlman, Rogol, and Ryan

Year Book of Family Practice®: Drs. Berg, Bowman, Davidson, Dexter, and Scherger

Year Book of Geriatrics and Gerontology®: Drs. Beck, Burton, Ostwald, Rabins, Reuben, Roth, Shapiro, and Whitehouse

Year Book of Hand Surgery®: Drs. Amadio and Hentz

Year Book of Hematology®: Drs. Spivak, Bell, Ness, Quesenberry, Wiernik, and Blume

Year Book of Infectious Diseases®: Drs. Keusch, Barza, Bennish, Poutsiaka, Skolnik, and Snydman

Year Book of Medicine®: Drs. Klahr, Cline, Petty, Frishman, Greenberger, Malawista, Mandell, and Utiger

Year Book of Neonatal and Perinatal Medicine®: Drs. Fanaroff, Maisels, and Stevenson

Year Book of Nephrology, Hypertension, and Mineral Metabolism: Drs. Schwab, Bennett, Emmett, Hostetter, Kumar, and Toto

Year Book of Neurology and Neurosurgery®: Drs. Bradley and Wilkins

Year Book of Nuclear Medicine®: Drs. Gottschalk, Blaufox, Neumann, Strauss, and Zubal

Year Book of Obstetrics, Gynecology, and Women's Health: Drs. Mishell, Herbst, and Kirschbaum

Year Book of Occupational and Environmental Medicine®: Drs. Emmett, Frank, Gochfeld, and Hessl

Year Book of Oncology®: Drs. Ozols, Cohen, Glatstein, Loehrer, Tallman, and Wiersma

Year Book of Ophthalmology®: Drs. Wilson, Augsburger, Cohen, Eagle, Flanagan, Grossman, Laibson, Maguire, Nelson, Penne, Rapuano, Sergott, Spaeth, Tipperman, Ms. Gosfield, and Ms. Salmon

Year Book of Orthopedics®: Drs. Sledge, Poss, Cofield, Dobyns, Griffin, Springfield, Swiontkowski, Wiesel, and Wilson

Year Book of Otolaryngology–Head and Neck Surgery®: Drs. Paparella and Holt

Year Book of Pathology and Laboratory Medicine: Drs. Mills, Bruns, Gaffey, and Stoler

Year Book of Pediatrics®: Dr. Stockman

Year Book of Plastic, Reconstructive, and Aesthetic Surgery®: Drs. Miller, Cohen, McKinney, Robson, Ruberg, Smith, and Whitaker

Year Book of Podiatric Medicine and Surgery®: Dr. Kominsky

Year Book of Psychiatry and Applied Mental Health®: Drs. Talbott, Ballenger, Breier, Frances, Meltzer, Schowalter, and Tasman

Year Book of Pulmonary Disease®: Dr. Petty

Year Book of Rheumatology®: Drs. Sergent, LeRoy, Meenan, Panush, and Reichlin

Year Book of Sports Medicine®: Drs. Shephard, Alexander, Drinkwater, Eichner, George, and Torg

Year Book of Surgery®: Drs. Copeland, Bland, Deitch, Eberlein, Howard, Luce, Seeger, Souba, and Sugarbaker

Year Book of Thoracic and Cardiovascular Surgery®: Drs. Ginsberg, Wechsler, and Williams

Year Book of Urology®: Drs. Andriole and Coplin

Year Book of Vascular Surgery®: Dr. Porter

1997

The Year Book of ANESTHESIOLOGY AND PAIN MANAGEMENT®

Editor in Chief

John H. Tinker, M.D.

Professor, Department of Anesthesia, University of Iowa College of Medicine, Iowa City, Iowa

Editors

Stephen E. Abram, M.D.

Professor, Department of Anesthesiology, University of New Mexico School of Medicine, Albuquerque, New Mexico

David H. Chestnut, M.D.

Alfred Habeeb Professor and Chairman, Department of Anesthesiology; Professor of Obstetrics and Gynecology, The University of Alabama at Birmingham, Birmingham, Alabama

Michael F. Roizen, M.D.

Professor and Chair, Department of Anesthesia and Critical Care; Professor of Medicine, University of Chicago, Chicago, Illinois

David M. Rothenberg, M.D.

Associate Professor of Anesthesiology; Director, Division of Anesthesia–Critical Care, Assistant Dean, Rush Medical College, Rush-Presbyterian/St. Luke's Medical Center, Chicago, Illinois

Margaret Wood, M.D.

E.M. Papper Professor and Chairman, Department of Anesthesiology, College of Physicians and Surgeons of Columbia University, New York, New York

Mosby

St. Louis Baltimore Boston Carlsbad Chicago Naples New York Philadelphia Portland
London Madrid Mexico City Singapore Sydney Tokyo Toronto Wiesbaden

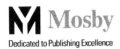

Mosby
Dedicated to Publishing Excellence

A Times Mirror
Company

Vice President and Publisher, Continuity Publishing: Kenneth H. Killion
Director, Editorial Development: Gretchen C. Murphy
Developmental Editor: Bernadette Buchholz
Acquisitions Editor: Linda M. Sheehan
Project Specialist, Editing: Denise M. Dungey
Senior Project Manager, Production: Max F. Perez
Freelance Staff Supervisor: Barbara M. Kelly
Illustrations and Permissions Coordinator: Steven J. Ramay
Director, Editorial Services: Edith M. Podrazik, B.S.N., R.N.
Information Specialist: Terri Santo, R.N.
Information Specialist: Margery Marble, B.S., R.N.
Circulation Manager: Lynn D. Stevenson

1997 EDITION

Printed in the United States of America
Composition by Reed Technology and Information Services, Inc.
Printing/binding by Maple-Vail

Mosby–Year Book, Inc.
11830 Westline Industrial Drive
St. Louis, MO 63146
Customer Service: customer.support@mosby.com
www.mosby.com/Mosby/CustomerSupport/index.html

Editorial Office:
Mosby–Year Book, Inc.
161 North Clark Street
Chicago, IL 60601
series.editorial@mosby.com

International Standard Serial Number: 1073-5437
International Standard Book Number: 0-8151-8780-7

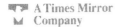

Table of Contents

Journals Represented

Mosby and its editors survey more than 1,000 journals for its abstract and commentary publications. From these journals, the editors select the articles to be abstracted. Journals represented in this YEAR BOOK are listed below.

Acta Anaesthesiologica Scandinavica
Acta Neurochirurgica
Acta Neurologica Scandinavica
Acta Obstetricia et Gynecologica Scandinavica
American Journal of Cardiology
American Journal of Obstetrics and Gynecology
American Journal of Orthopedics
American Surgeon
Anaesthesia
Anaesthesia and Intensive Care
Anesthesia and Analgesia
Anesthesiology
Annals of Internal Medicine
Annals of Surgery
Annals of Thoracic Surgery
Archives of Internal Medicine
Archives of Pathology and Laboratory Medicine
Archives of Surgery
British Journal of Anaesthesia
British Journal of Surgery
British Medical Journal
Canadian Journal of Anaesthesia
Chest
Clinical Journal of Pain
Clinical Pharmacology and Therapeutics
Critical Care Medicine
European Journal of Anaesthesiology
Gynecologic and Obstetric Investigation
Intensive Care Medicine
International Journal of Epidemiology
International Journal of Obstetric Anesthesia
JOGNN: Journal of Obstetric, Gynecologic, and Neonatal Nursing
Journal of Bone and Joint Surgery (American Volume)
Journal of Cardiothoracic and Vascular Anesthesia
Journal of Clinical Anesthesia
Journal of Clinical Investigation
Journal of Family Practice
Journal of Heart and Lung Transplantation
Journal of Neurosurgery
Journal of Pain and Symptom Management
Journal of Pediatric Surgery
Journal of Physiology
Journal of Thoracic and Cardiovascular Surgery
Journal of Vascular Surgery
Journal of the American Medical Association
Lancet
Neuroradiology

Neurosurgery
New England Journal of Medicine
Obstetrics and Gynecology
Pain
Regional Anesthesia
Scandinavian Journal of Thoracic and Cardiovascular Surgery
Science
Southern Medical Journal
Stroke
Transfusion
World Journal of Surgery

STANDARD ABBREVIATIONS

The following terms are abbreviated in this edition: acquired immunodeficiency syndrome (AIDS), cardiopulmonary resuscitation (CPR), central nervous system (CNS), cerebrospinal fluid (CSF), computed tomography (CT), deoxyribonucleic acid (DNA), electrocardiography (ECG), health maintenance organization (HMO), human immunodeficiency virus (HIV), intensive care unit (ICU), intramuscular (IM), intravenous (IV), magnetic resonance (MR) imaging (MRI), and ribonucleic acid (RNA).

NOTE

The YEAR BOOK OF ANESTHESIOLOGY AND PAIN MANAGEMENT® is a literature survey service providing abstracts of articles published in the professional literature. Every effort is made to ensure the accuracy of the information presented in these pages. Neither the editors nor the publisher of the YEAR BOOK OF ANESTHESIOLOGY AND PAIN MANAGEMENT® can be responsible for errors in the original materials. The editors' comments are their own opinions. Mention of specific products within this publication does not constitute endorsement.

To facilitate the use of the YEAR BOOK OF ANESTHESIOLOGY AND PAIN MANAGEMENT® as a reference tool, all illustrations and tables included in this publication are now identified as they appear in the original article. This change is meant to help the reader recognize that any illustration or table appearing in the YEAR BOOK OF ANESTHESIOLOGY AND PAIN MANAGEMENT®may be only one of many in the original article. For this reason, figure and table numbers will often appear to be out of sequence within the YEAR BOOK OF ANESTHESIOLOGY AND PAIN MANAGEMENT®.

Introduction

It is with a considerable degree of renewed enthusiasm that I report that science, both clinical and basic, seems to be undergoing a solid resurgence in our specialty. This YEAR BOOK, to be sure, still contains numerous cost-efficacy–type studies, as it did last year, and I do not mean to belittle their importance in today's semichaotic market.

Nonetheless, as I had hoped, our basic interests in patient care, pharmacology, physiology, mechanisms of actions of drugs, understanding adverse events and their causation, and other genuinely clinical attributes of our specialty have indeed regained their rightful place at the forefront of this year's literature.

I want to give special notice of the first paper I included in this YEAR BOOK (Abstract 1–1). It is a continuation of the long-term anesthesia risk and outcome studies of the New South Wales, Australia, group originally founded by Dr. Ross Holland. This is, by far, the longest running and most consistently based anesthesia risk and outcome study in our specialty. I find it encouraging that anesthesia-related risks are indeed improving, over time, at least in Australia. I think every anesthesiologist and nonphysician anesthesia care provider knows, intuitively, that our efforts do make a difference, and that improvements in our skills, monitoring, pharmacology, and anesthetic techniques really do have positive effects; it is comforting to have at least some objective evidence of that. I hope that Dr. Holland and his stalwart colleagues will accept our heartiest congratulations for their latest continuation efforts. We should encourage them to continue these great studies well into the 21st century. As I have opined before, it would be a real benefit to American patients to have some sort of an anesthesia risk registry, protected by law from medical-legal discovery, so that studies of low (but not zero) incidence events, such as anesthesia risk, could be done with very large populations of patients to analyze. I have not seen any evidence of legislative or governmental interest in this kind of protection and, unfortunately, without it, I do not believe we can gather appropriately large databases in this country to really answer important questions about the relative contributions of various anesthetic techniques, drugs, monitoring systems, etc., to overall perioperative risk.

Last year's hottest topic was the newly introduced (but old) volatile fluorocarbon anesthetic sevoflurane, and the possibility that its relatively high metabolic breakdown via hepatic mixed function oxidasis (approximately 5% of an inhaled dose) might release sufficient fluoride to result in nephrotoxicity and/or might produce hepatic toxicity via fluoroformaldehyde or formaldehyde formation. During this past year, several million more anesthetics have been given with sevoflurane. This YEAR BOOK contains five studies regarding fluorides with respect to renal function. There is, for example, a paper in which sevoflurane was given as a bronchodilator treatment for a long period to several patients who were in status asthmaticus. Although the fluoride release was not measured at ideal times throughout the therapy, the patients did not seem to have suffered renally. On the other hand, there is indication in several studies that renal function is at least temporarily affected after sevoflurane anesthesia. Last year's flurry of interest in compound A, which is released from the slow breakdown of sevoflurane by soda lime, does not seem to have been repeated this year, i.e., the editors chose only one paper on the subject for this YEAR BOOK. An indication of the growing clinical acceptance and interest in sevoflurane is the fact that there are eight papers regarding the clinical characteristics of the drug, including one paper that discusses that it is possible to do a single-breath induction with sevoflurane! We have not seen single-breath inductions since cyclopropane (may that awful drug rest permanently in our history).

As usual, there still is considerable interest in preoperative cardiovascular evaluation. It is my view, at least, that despite the fact that coronary artery disease is still the most common cause of death in the United States, there has not been dramatic progress made in its preoperative diagnosis in asymptomatic patients.

This year we are including a considerable number of studies about epidural anesthesia and analgesia, most in the obstetric arena. It is obvious that everything "from soup to nuts" is being or has been introduced into the epidural or intrathecal spaces. It is also obvious that, despite the natural childbirth movement, there is enormous interest in pain relief during labor and delivery. By their demands for pain relief during this critical time, many women are clearly siding with Queen Victoria, who, the reader may recall, in 1848, was told by the Archbishop of Canterbury that it was sinful to ask for pain relief (with chloroform) during labor and delivery. Having had seven previous children (there is some debate as to the exact number), Queen Victoria asked James Y. Simpson to administer chloroform for her eighth delivery. Advised by the Archbishop that the Bible contended that the bearing of children should be done in pain, Queen Victoria is alleged to have said something to this effect: "*We* are having this child, and *we* will have chloroform." Based on the volume and variety of this year's papers, pain relief during labor and delivery is still a challenge for us.

There is an important experimental paper buried in all the clinical obstetric anesthesia papers that comes from Dr. Chestnut's group; it casts grave concern about the use of magnesium sulfate. The authors report that magnesium sulfate adversely affects fetal survival in pregnant ewes (Abstract 9–14). That paper may prove to be one of the most significant of the year.

I was surprised at the dearth of studies of remifentanil in this YEAR BOOK, but I suppose with its introduction this year (1997), the 1998 YEAR BOOK will remedy that deficit. There also is apparently only minimal interest, these days, in the newer neuromuscular blockers, e.g., cisatracurium and mivacurium. Most clinical anesthesiologists I know have become pretty well saturated with the seemingly endless introduction of new neuromuscular blockers.

As I have stated before in past YEAR BOOK introductions, I continue to be underwhelmed by anesthesiologists' interest in prevention and treatment of nausea and vomiting after general anesthesia. This YEAR BOOK does contain a study of a new nausea preventor, tropisetron, but there is little discussion about mechanisms of this continuing problem.

With respect to monitoring, I have been fascinated by the very real possibility that we do now have a useful awareness monitor, namely bispectral analysis. Yet despite that interest on my part, there is only one paper about that new mode of analysis of the electroencephalogram in this YEAR BOOK. We will hear considerably more about this in the future.

Our section about complications, mishaps, and other troubles, as usual, contains a spate of papers wherein things happen during and after regional anesthesia. Those who continually extol the wonders of that type of (antique? now I am in real trouble ...) anesthesia will certainly opine that our editors are simply biased against it, but I doubt that this is the case. At its core, regional anesthesia is the injection of an aqueous substance somewhere near a fatty-sheathed nerve. Is it any wonder that it does not always work? Is it any wonder that there is, sometimes, toxicity? I think this is an area of our practice that could use some new exciting developments. We need agents that penetrate nerves faster, without neurotoxicity. We need ways to monitor the onset and offset of blocks, especially if general anesthesia is to be combined with them. We need local anesthetics that do not cause seizures or cardiotoxicity. We need ways to turn regional anesthesia on and off rapidly in outpatients. Based on this year's YEAR BOOK, we have a long way to go.

As always, recently there has been enormous interest in both acute and chronic pain management. This year, acute pain management studies chosen by the editors outnumber the papers regarding chronic pain management. The new local anesthetics ropivacaine, clonidine, and ketorolac, and the new opioid remifentanil and other agents are being used in our pain armamentarium in various new ways. There also is considerable interest in various chronic infusion methodologies.

There may be an exciting new development in critical care medicine, namely liquid ventilation with advanced fluorocarbon materials. In the past, fluorocarbons have been problematic because of their uptake by the reticuloendothelial system and the fact that, from there, the body did not seem to know what to do with them. These new fluorocarbons may not be any better in that regard, but it is exciting to see our intensivists working with something this radically different, after decades of peak end-expiratory pressure, continuous positive airway pressure, BIPAP, and the various other methods of applying pressure fluctuations to the trachea. We need to get beyond those into more specific therapies. There are also surprisingly few papers about various aspects of nitric oxide in this volume. Clearly it is a pulmonary vasodilator, i.e., it makes the numbers look a lot better at least in the short run. Whether it helps adults survive is, frankly, not obvious to me.

I want to thank the superb editors on our editorial board. We have a truly outstanding pharmacologist in Dr. Margaret Wood; Dr. David Rothenberg, our intensivist editor, is rapidly becoming a guru; all of our readers know Dr. Michael Roizen, who is clearly a world class expert in many areas, including outcome analysis and cost efficacy; Dr. David Chestnut is unequaled as an expert in obstetric anesthesia; and Dr. Stephen Abram is one of the world's best known authorities on pain management. I deliberately listed our authors in reverse alphabetical order, because with a name starting with a "T," I usually stand at the end of the queue! Seriously, this is a wonderful editorial board, and I thank each and every member for their many contributions. I think you will find their commentary enjoyable and valuable.

Finally, I said in the beginning of this introduction, I think clinical and experimental science is alive and well in anesthesiology. I think genuine advances are being made, and I hope that our specialty will again (soon) attract large numbers of bright young medical graduates. Our recent troubles with resident recruitment have been widely attributed to job availability. That might be so, but perhaps the specialty itself was perceived by outsiders to be losing some of its former excitement and verve. I think there is plenty of excitement denoted in the pages of the 1997 YEAR BOOK. It is indeed a pleasure and a privilege to be your editor in chief.

John H. Tinker, M.D.

1 Studies of Outcomes and Costs

Large General Outcome Studies

Deaths Attributed to Anaesthesia in New South Wales, 1984–1990
Warden JC, Horan BF (Royal North Shore Hosp, St Leonards, Australia; St Vincent's Hosp, Darlinghurst, Australia)
Anaesth Intensive Care 24:66–73, 1996 1–1

Objective.—In the Australian state of New South Wales, a special committee investigates deaths occurring during, within 24 hours of, or resulting from anesthesia. Of 1,503 deaths investigated from 1984 to 1990, 172 were classified as being at least partly attributable to anesthesia. These deaths were investigated in detail.

Findings.—The rate of death occurring before complete recovery from anesthesia was 4.4 per 10,000 anesthetics overall, with 6.6 per 10,000 for males and 2.8 per 10,000 for females. One death was caused by anesthesia in every 20,000 operations. In 11 of the 172 deaths attributed to anesthesia, the choice and administration of anesthesia could not be criticized. In the remaining 161 cases, a mean of 1.8 anesthetic errors per death was identified. The most common errors were inadequate preparation for anesthesia, inadequate postoperative care, inappropriately selected or applied anesthetic technique, and overdose, in that order (Table 1). Elderly patients were the age group most likely to die from anesthesia. Men were nearly twice as likely to die of anesthesia than women. Abdominal and orthopedic operations were the most common types of surgery involved. Twenty-six percent of deaths attributable to anesthesia were urgent non-emergency cases, which accounted for 10% of the 1,503 deaths classified.

Conclusions.—In deaths that are caused by anesthesia, errors in patient preparation are the most common category of causes, especially related to the clinical assessment by history, physical examination, and appropriate tests. Airway management and ventilation are potential pitfalls in postoperative care. Some deaths are related to the choice and application of anesthetic technique; greater attention is needed to the contraindications to spinal and epidural anesthesia. Particular care is needed in managing

TABLE 1.—Frequency of Factors Identified as Contributing to Death in 161 Cases

Inadequate Preparation	72
Inadequate Postoperative Care	52
Anaesthetic Technique or Drug	44
Overdose	43
Inadequate Intraoperative Resuscitation	24
Inadequate Reversal	13
Inadequate Observation	12
Inexperience	10
Inadequate Crisis Management	9
Technical Mishap	7
Inhalation Gastric Contents	3
Inadequate Ventilation	1
Incompetence	0
Total errors	290
Mean No. of errors per case	1.8

Note: In a further 11 cases, although the administration of the anesthetic caused the patient's death, the New South Wales Special Committee Investigating Deaths Under Anaesthesia identified no error in the choice of agent, and management of the case could not be criticized.

(Courtesy of Warden JC, Horan BF: Deaths attributed to anaesthesia in New South Wales, 1984–1990. *Anaesth Intensive Care* 24:66–73, 1996.)

elderly patients undergoing emergency abdominal surgery and surgery for fracture of the femoral neck.

► The timely reports by Australia's Dr. Ross Holland, over the past 30 years or so, represent the longest term and some of the most valid, in my opinion, anesthesia risk studies anywhere in the literature. This encouraging report tells me that Dr. Holland's successors are continuing the project.

I said that this was one of the most valid anesthesia risk studies for several reasons. The enormous long-term database adds validity. Also, the considerable legal protection for risk reportage that still exits in Australia allows, indeed mandates, that these deaths be reported and investigated, yet allows reasonable protection to the physicians involved.

I believe that there are 2 groups of factors involved with anesthetic risks. The first can be grouped together under skill, training, and experience, but the second should be considered under a category of human errors and other related inadvertencies. In the latter group, the anesthetist had knowledge, skill, and training, but for one reason or another the job did not get done correctly. If you look at Table 1, you see the dramatic importance of human error. Table 1 is a stark depiction of the reason why provider-based anesthesia risk studies have not shown physician providers, despite greater levels of medical training, skill, and/or experience, to necessarily be safer than supervised nonphysician providers of anesthesia. I think this study is worth considerable attention.

J.H. Tinker, M.D.

Anesthesia Providers, Patient Outcomes, and Costs
Abenstein JP, Warner MA (Mayo Clinic, Rochester, Minn)
Anesth Analg 82:1273–1283, 1996 1–2

Background.—To determine the providers of anesthesia services in the United States, the delivery models used, and the effects of the various delivery models on patient outcomes and cost-effectiveness, the scientific literature was reviewed. These findings were expansions of a report originally compiled in Minnesota on statewide anesthesia services.

Providers and Delivery Models.—Anesthesia services may be administered by anesthesiologists, nurse anesthetists, or anesthesiologists' assistants. There are 4 basic models of anesthesia services delivery. In an anesthesiologist-only practice, all anesthetics are administered by an anesthesiologist. In a nurse-anesthetist-only practice, all anesthetics are administered by a nurse working under the direction of the surgeon. In an anesthesia care team practice, anesthetic is administered by a resident, nurse anesthetist, or anesthesiologists' assistant under the direction of an anesthesiologist, who is present during critical points. In a hybrid practice, anesthetic is administered by any physician or nonphysician member of the anesthesia care team, with physicians always available.

Patient Outcomes.—Patient outcomes have improved significantly since the 1940s. Anesthesiologist-only practices have been associated with better patient outcomes than nurse anesthetist-only practices, but patient outcomes are best with anesthesia care team practices or hybrid practices, in terms of both mortality and morbidity. It is likely that the superior outcomes associated with the anesthesia care team models can be attributed to the dynamics of the model, in which the talents and observational skills of multiple professionals are combined to provide a synergistic benefit.

Cost Implications.—Although the costs of delivering anesthesia care may be greater with the anesthesia care team model, this model is most cost-effective, because it produces the best patient outcomes, which significantly reduces the cost of the entire episode of care. Cost-effectiveness also is related to the dynamics of the model, in which comprehensive perioperative medical and postoperative pain management services are included, as opposed to other practice models, in which the range of services provided is limited.

Conclusions.—The provision of anesthesia services by an anesthesia care team or a hybrid practice is the safest and most cost-effective method of delivering anesthesia care. This information can be used to guide policy decisions on workforce size and composition, quality of care expectations, and costs of anesthesia services.

► The authors are very strong in their conclusion that "the anesthesiologist-led anesthesia care team is the safest and most cost-effective method of delivering anesthesia care." I wish their data were more convincing because that conclusion agrees with my biases. Even though the team concept makes sense, it is exceedingly hard to prove. I think these authors have done as good a job as has been done in a long time in trying to "prove" this case. I do commend this article to our readers.

J.H. Tinker, M.D.

Educational Level of Spouses and Risk of Mortality: The WHO Kaunas-Rotterdam Intervention Study (KRIS)

Bosma H, Appels A, Sturmans F, et al (Univ of Limburg, Maastricht, The Netherlands)

Int J Epidemiol 24:119–126, 1995 1–3

Introduction.—There is increasing evidence of a greater prevalence of premature mortality and coronary heart disease (CHD) among patients with lower socioeconomic status. Recently, studies have also suggested an association between premature mortality or CHD and the spouse's socioeconomic status. This association was investigated in a cohort of men in 2 countries followed up for 9.5 years.

Methods.—The married men participating in a cardiovascular screening program in Kaunas and Rotterdam between 1972 and 1974 were studied. Approximately 9.5 years later, the status of the men was followed up, using death certificates, the morbidity register for the Kaunas population, and a morbidity questionnaire for the Rotterdam population. The educational level of the men's spouses had been determined with a survey at the time of the screening and was classified as elementary education only, intermediate education (including vocational, homemaking, or secondary education), or university education. Associations were estimated between the spouse's education and all-cause mortality, mortality from cardiovascular disease (CVD), mortality from CHD, and the incidence of nonfatal myocardial infarction (MI).

Results.—The level of the wife's education was associated significantly with all-cause mortality in both cohorts, even after adjustment for the men's educational levels. This association was significant also for mortality from CVD, mortality from CHD, and the incidence of nonfatal MI. The influence of the men's educational levels on mortality and morbidity actually became insignificant after adjustment for the wives' educational levels. The independent significance of the wives' educational levels remained after adjustment for other cardiovascular risk factors.

Conclusions.—Men with wives with little education have an increased risk of premature mortality and heart disease. This finding has significance for future research, in that studies examining risk factors for mortality should include the socioeconomic characteristics of significant others.

► This an extremely interesting study because it indicates that if you want to improve your chances of survival, your spouse should be as smart as possible. This study shows that a patient's educational level and a patient's spouse's educational level may be important in determining the patient's physiologic age and chances of surviving an operation. Although the latter is all extrapolation of the data, it is still logical from the data we have indicating perioperative risk relating to your physiologic age. How is it that a spouse with a lower educational level can cause an increase in your physiologic age? It is not clear from the article, but it is an intriguing article that speculates on the etiology of this phenomenon.

M.F. Roizen, M.D.

Risk/Outcome Studies in Obstetrical Anesthesia

Failed Intubation Revisited: 17-Yr Experience in a Teaching Maternity Unit

Hawthorne L, Wilson R, Lyons G, et al (St James's Univ, Leeds, England)
Br J Anaesth 76:680–684, 1996 1–4

Objective.—Although failure to intubate has been associated with anesthesia-related maternal death and injury, changes in clinical practice appear to have reduced maternal morbidity and mortality during obstetric general anesthesia even though the prevalence of failure to intubate has increased since 1978. To assess these changes, a prospective study of failure to intubate in the maternity unit between 1978 and 1994 was conducted.

Methods.—During these years, 5,802 cesarean sections were performed. Patients were divided into 3 groups depending on intubation time: group 1 was intubated between 8 AM and 5 PM by obstetric staff and consulting anesthetists; group 2, between 5 PM and 9 PM by obstetric and medical staff; and group 3, between 9 PM and 8 AM by midwives, operating room assistants, and duty doctors.

Results.—Results showed 23 (0.4%) failures to intubate, defined as inability to intubate with a single dose of suxamethonium. Failed intubations increased from 1 in 300 in 1984 to 1 in 250 in 1994, whereas the use of general anesthesia declined from 83% in 1981 to 23% in 1994. Sixteen failures were found in group 3, 5 in group 1, and 2 in group 2. Twenty of the surgeries were emergency. Before surgery, difficulty in intubation was predicted in only one third of failed intubations. A regional technique was used in 18 of these patients; extradural anesthesia, in 10; spinal, in 5; and combined extradural-spinal, in 3. Although signs of fetal distress were noted in 7 patients, delivery was uneventful for mother and neonate, except for 1 mother whose twins had cerebral damage. Postoperatively, 9 patients were found to have a receding jaw, 7 had a limited mouth opening, and 5 had both.

Conclusion.—The number of intubation failures, cesarean sections, and surgeries performed under regional anesthesia has increased. Maternal mortality has decreased. The laryngeal mask has been increasingly used in patients in whom intubation cannot be done. The high percentage of problems experienced by black and Asian patients resulted from the increased use of general anesthesia in these groups.

▶ Failed intubation remains the leading cause of anesthesia-related mortality in obstetric patients. Every anesthesiologist should have a plan for managing failed intubation. In recent years, I have added the laryngeal mask airway to the algorithm that I teach our residents. I recommend using the laryngeal mask airway in patients in whom both intubation and mask ventilation are impossible. In this series, the laryngeal mask airway was tried in 4 cases of failed intubation/failed ventilation and was used successfully in 3.

If neither mask ventilation nor laryngeal mask airway ventilation is successful, I recommend placement of a large-gauge IV cannula through the cricothyroid membrane, followed by transtracheal oxygenation/ventilation.

D.H. Chestnut, M.D.

Practice Patterns of Anesthesiologists Regarding Situations in Obstetric Anesthesia Where Clinical Management Is Controversial

Beilin Y, Bodian CA, Haddad EM, et al (Mount Sinai School of Medicine, New York)

Anesth Analg 83:735–741, 1996 1–5

Background.—Obstetric anesthesiologists must sometimes make controversial management decisions. Obstetric anesthesiologists in academic and private practice were surveyed to determine the practice patterns of these 2 groups in controversial decision-making situations.

Methods.—One hundred fifty-three directors of obstetric anesthesia in academic practice and 153 anesthesiologists in private practice were mailed a 47-item survey. The physicians were asked about preoperative laboratory testing, pre-eclampsia and possible coagulopathies, epidural catheter placement in women with spinal problems, and the use of epidural opioids and IV supplementation. The response rates were 74% and 61% for the academic and private anesthesiologists, respectively.

Findings.—Overall, the responses of the 2 groups were similar. Univariate analysis showed that responses differed significantly on 14 questions, but these differences remained significant for only 8 after adjustment for the amount of clinical time currently spent on obstetric anesthesia. Before epidural placement in a healthy parturient, 68% of the private practitioners and 45% of the academic physicians said that they would order a complete blood count. Thirty-one percent and 17%, respectively, would order a complete platelet count. More than half of both groups would place an epidural anesthetic in an otherwise healthy parturient with a platelet count of 80,000–100,000/mm^3. Also, three fourths of the academic physicians and two thirds of the private practitioners would remove the catheter if a coagulopathy developed after epidural catheter placement only after the coagulation status has been documented. Most anesthesiologists in both groups said that they would place an epidural anesthetic in women taking 80 or 325 mg of aspirin per day. In women with pre-eclampsia, the number of laboratory tests requested increases with the severity of the condition. Most respondents said that they would place an epidural anesthetic in a woman with a Harrington rod, scoliosis, or a symptomatic or asymptomatic herniated lumbar disk. The drugs most commonly used to supplement a regional anesthetic during cesarean section are ketamine, fentanyl, and midazolam.

Conclusions.—In general, anesthesiologists' approach to situations in which management is controversial appears to be supported by the literature. The use of bleeding test time to assess platelet function may be an exception. Private practitioners tend to be more cautious than academic physicians in that they require more laboratory tests for healthy parturients and for women with pre-eclampsia or possible platelet abnormalities. Private practitioners are also more cautious in their management of women with spinal problems or an increased temperature.

▶ In this study I was most surprised by the responses to questions about use of the bleeding time. Specifically, I was surprised by the number of anesthesiologists who stated that the bleeding time measurement would affect their decision regarding the use of epidural anesthesia in a patient taking aspirin. Likewise, I was equally surprised by the number of anesthesiologists who stated that they would obtain a bleeding time measurement to guide their decision about the use of epidural anesthesia in a woman with pre-eclampsia and a low platelet count. Of interest, in the latter circumstance the bleeding time measurement is used more often by private practitioners than academicians.

I believe that the bleeding time measurement is a test in search of an indication. I am not convinced that it accurately predicts the risk of bleeding elsewhere in the body. Also, anesthesiologists should remember that epidural hematoma is a rare complication of epidural anesthesia in obstetric patients. Measurement of the platelet count, along with clinical assessment, represents an adequate means of assessment for most obstetric patients (unless of course the patient is at increased risk for coagulopathy). I obtain a bleeding time measurement only when other factors might dissuade me from the administration of epidural anesthesia.

D.H. Chestnut, M.D.

Patients' Versus Nurses' Assessments of Pain and Sedation After Cesarean Section

Olden AJ, Jordan ET, Sakima NT, et al (Johns Hopkins Hosp, Baltimore, Md)
J Obstet Gynecol Neonatal Nurs 24:137–141, 1995 1–6

Background.—Patient-controlled analgesia (PCA) is widely used for pain control after cesarean section and is reportedly more effective in relieving postoperative pain than intramuscular opioid injections. The goal of this prospective, randomized study was to compare nurses' and patients' assessments of pain and sedation in patients receiving epidural or IV PCA after cesarean deliveries.

Participants and Methods.—Twenty patients undergoing cesarean delivery and nurses assigned to care for these patients were included in the study. Twelve patients were randomly assigned to receive epidural sufentanil PCA and 8 to receive IV morphine PCA. No differences in age, height, weight, and history of previous cesarean section were noted between patient groups. A 10-cm visual analogue scale (VAS) was used twice daily on the day of surgery and on the first and second postoperative days to evaluate pain and sedation from patients' and nurses' perspectives.

Results.—There were no significant correlations between nurses' VAS pain score assessments and the patients' VAS pain scores. Nurses underestimated and overestimated patients' pain scores 55% and 43% of the time, respectively. The average difference between nurses' assessment and patients' VAS pain score was 20 mm. Similarly, no significant correlation between nurses' VAS sedation assessment and patients' VAS scores were noted. Underestimation of patients' VAS sedation levels was observed 85% of the time when evaluating nurses' assessments. The incidence of underestimated sedation scores did not differ between epidural and IV PCA groups. Ninety-four percent of the nurses indicated that they would recommend PCA for patients and 88% indicated that use of PCA allowed more time for other patient care activities.

Conclusions.—The finding that nurses routinely underestimate patients' subjective sedation scores has clinical implications. Patients using PCA may resume self-care activities more rapidly and with less pain than patients given intramuscular opioids. Because of this, nurses may assume that patients are experiencing less sedation than is literally being felt, and may therefore allow their patients to take on activities that require greater cognitive function and physical coordination before it is actually safe to do so. Although PCA does effectively relieve pain after cesarean section and is widely accepted by health care providers, nurses' and patients' assessments of pain and sedation do differ. For this reason, the routine use of a standardized self-assessment tool (such as the VAS) is encouraged, inasmuch as this will ensure that analgesic treatment is based on patients' subjective perceptions, as opposed to nurses' assessment and judgment alone.

► In the present study of patients receiving epidural or intravenous PCA after cesarean section, the authors observed that nurses' and patients' perceptions of pain and sedation differ. Specifically, the authors observed no significant correlation between the nurses' and patients' pain or sedation scores. Nurses were as likely to overestimate as to underestimate patients' pain. However, the nurses consistently *underestimated* patients' subjective sedation scores. The authors noted that, "The danger in this discrepancy is that patients may receive permission to assume more complex activities that require greater cognitive function and physical coordination than they are ready to perform safely." The authors suggested that a standardized self-assessment tool is preferred to a scheme that depends on the nurses' assessment of pain and sedation.

D.H. Chestnut, M.D.

Infant Survival After Cesarean Section for Trauma

Morris JA Jr, Rosenbower TJ, Jurkovich GJ, et al (Vanderbilt Univ, Nashville, Tenn; Harborview Med Ctr, Seattle; San Diego Med Ctr, Calif; et al)

Ann Surg 223:481–491, 1996 1–7

Background.—Although there have been many studies of trauma and pregnancy, few researchers have reported on trauma in the third trimester. The current multicenter, retrospective cohort study was done to test the hypothesis that emergency cesarean section is not justified in trauma victims in their third trimester of pregnancy.

Methods and Findings.—Thirty-two pregnant women undergoing emergency cesarean section at 9 level I trauma centers between January 1986 and December 1994 were identified. All emergency cesarean sections were performed for fetal distress (defined as bradycardia, deceleration, or lack of fetal heart tones) and/or maternal distress (defined as shock or acute decompensation). Forty-five percent of the fetuses and 72% of the mothers survived. Thirteen of the 33 fetuses delivered had no fetal heart tones and did not survive. Of 20 potential survivors with fetal heart tones and an estimated gestational age of 26 weeks or more, 75% survived. Infant survival was unassociated with maternal distress or maternal injury severity score. Recogition of fetal distress was delayed in the 5 potential survivors who died. Sixty percent of these deaths occurred in the infants of women with mild to moderate injuries.

Conclusions.—The viability of infants of pregnant trauma victims is defined by the presence of fetal heart tones and estimated gestational age of 26 weeks or greater. The survival rate of viable infants after cesarean section is 75%, which is acceptable and disproves the original hypothesis. In the current series, 60% of the infant deaths among potential survivors resulted from delayed recognition of fetal distress and from cesarean section and may thus have been preventable.

▶ To my knowledge, this is the largest published series of pregnant trauma victims who required emergency cesarean section. I disagree with the authors' recommendation that fetal viability in the trauma patient be defined as age 26 weeks. The lack of surviving infants at 23–25 weeks' gestation is likely a function of the small number of patients in that group.

D.H. Chestnut, M.D.

Wearing of Masks for Obstetric Regional Anaesthesia: A Postal Survey

Panikkar KK, Yentis SM (Westminster Hosp, London)

Anaesthesia 51:398–400, 1996 1–8

Background.—The need to wear surgical masks during administration of regional anesthesia is controversial. The proportion of anesthetists who wear such masks is unknown. A survey was mailed to all members of the Obstetric Anaesthetists Association in the United Kingdom and Ireland to determine how many use surgical masks when performing obstetric regional anesthesia.

Methods and Findings.—Eight hundred one anesthetists were sent the postal survey. The response rate was 67.3%. Of the 539 respondents, 41.3% wore masks routinely while performing spinal and epidural anesthetic procedures. Four percent said they wore masks only for epidural procedures, and 3.9% wore masks only for spinal procedures. Thus, about half the respondents did not use surgical face masks. Twenty-one percent of the anesthetists who routinely wore masks did not believe that the use of masks decreased the risk of infection. Only 32% of mask wearers changed their masks between patients.

Conclusions.—Obstetric anesthetists in the United Kingdom and Ireland do not agree on the need to wear surgical face masks when central neural blockade is performed. Because infective events after neuraxial blockade are extremely rare, a randomized, prospective clinical study of the value of mask use is not feasible.

▶ I acknowledge that central nervous system infections (e.g., epidural abscess, meningitis) represent rare complications of epidural and spinal anesthesia. However, the consequences of these infections are devastating. I find it incredible that only 41% of the respondents in the present study routinely wear masks while administering spinal or epidural anesthesia. The authors correctly acknowledged that a randomized, prospective clinical trial is impractical. In my judgment, such a trial would also be unethical. It seems a small inconvenience for the anesthesiologist (and all others in the room) to wear a mask during administration of epidural or spinal anesthesia.

D.H. Chestnut, M.D.

Epidural Anaesthesia and Low Back Pain After Delivery: A Prospective Cohort Study

Macarthur A, Macarthur C, Weeks S (Royal Victoria Hosp, Montreal; McGill Univ, Montreal)

BMJ 311:1336–1339, 1995 1–9

Introduction.—Retrospective studies suggest that women receiving epidural anesthesia for childbirth are twice as likely to develop low back pain as are those who did not receive the anesthesia. These surveys had a low response rate along with the inherent difficulties of recall studies. This project was a prospective design of the relationship of anesthesia and low back pain after childbirth.

Methods.—All women admitted to 1 hospital for a vaginal delivery of a live infant were included in the study. Epidural anesthesia was performed on request by 1 of 6 anesthesiologists. The primary outcome was the occurrence of low back pain and functional impairment as reported from a questionnaire. Women were interviewed 1 day, 1 week, and 6 weeks after delivery. Demographic variables were also collected.

Results.—A total of 164 women had epidural anesthesia and 165 did not. Low back pain was highest 1 day after delivery. The incidence of low back pain was 53% and 43% in the epidural and nonepidural groups, respectively. No between-group differences occurred in incidence or in pain scores. Similar results were also obtained for women with no history of low back pain.

Conclusion.—Low back pain was common and quickly diminished over time. The relationship between low back pain and method of anesthesia was inconsistent. The only noticeable difference was for the first day after delivery.

▶ The present study provides further evidence that epidural analgesia during labor does not increase the incidence of chronic low back pain. It seems appropriate to reassure pregnant women that any increased risk of chronic low back pain after epidural anesthesia during labor—if present at all—is small.

D.H. Chestnut, M.D.

Long Term Backache After Childbirth: Prospective Search for Causative Factors

Russell R, Dundas R, Reynolds F (Guy's/St Thomas's Hosp, London)
BMJ 312:1384–1388, 1996 1–10

Background.—An association between new-onset postdelivery long-term backache and epidural analgesia during labor has been suggested in 2 retrospective studies performed in the United Kingdom. The incidence of long-term backache after childbirth was assessed prospectively, to ascertain its relation to use of epidural analgesia in general and to motor block resulting from high- and low-dose epidural infusions of bupivacaine during labor.

Methods.—Between October 1991 and March 1994, 399 women in labor who requested epidural analgesia were randomly assigned to receive either bupivacaine alone (200 women) or low-dose bupivacaine with opioid (199 women). Two hundred more women laboring during this period who did not receive epidural analgesia were also included. Questionnaires mailed 3 months after childbirth were returned by 75% of the participants. Those women reporting new backache at this time were evaluated again 1 year after childbirth.

Results.—Backache lasting 3 months after delivery was reported by 152 women (33.8% of responders); 33 of these women (7.3%) had not previously had backache. Neither overall incidence of postnatal backache, new backache, nor other postpartum symptoms differed significantly among treatment groups. Of all the demographic, obstetric, and epidural variables examined, only previous backache before and during pregnancy was significantly associated with backache after childbirth. New backache had disappeared by 1 year after delivery in 60% of women; in none was it troublesome enough to warrant further medical attention.

Conclusions.—Women who received epidural analgesia during labor did not show a significantly increased incidence of new long-term backache. Development of backache was not linked with motor block associated with epidural local anesthetic administration.

► Retrospective studies have suggested that there is an association between epidural analgesia for labor and long-term back pain after delivery. In this prospective study, the authors did not observe an increased incidence of long-term backache among women who received epidural analgesia during labor. Also, the occurrence of motor block during the administration of epidural analgesia was not associated with an increased incidence of backache.

D.H. Chestnut, M.D.

Epidural Analgesia in Labour Is Not Compatible With Midwife-led Care

Brighouse D (Southampton Gen Hosp, England)

Int J Obstet Anesth 5:126–129, 1996 1–11

Introduction.—The Cumberlege Report recommends that midwives provide antenatal, intrapartum, and postpartum care for women with predicted normal outcomes and that obstetricians be available for women who have special medical needs or have unexpected complications. The use of epidural analgesia with midwife-led care is a strongly debated issue in the United Kingdom. Views of a proponent and opponent on this issue were reported. Both are anesthetists in the United Kingdom.

Epidural Not Compatible With Midwife-led Care.—Women say they want woman-centered care during childbirth. They want continuity of care that is low tech and considered a physiologic, not a pathologic process, whenever possible. It has been shown that the requirement for analgesia is reduced with 1-on-1 care from a knowledgeable attendant, good antenatal education, and care in a low-tech environment. Even though women may report similar pain ratings with an obstetrician and midwife, a midwife who has given good antenatal education and is well versed in pain control techniques should be able to help a woman cope with the pain of a normal delivery. Normal labor is altered with the administration of an epidural. Uterine tone and contraction is altered, and the pelvic floor musculature is relaxed. Epidural anesthesia may increase the instrumentation delivery rate and precipitate fetal heart rate abnormalities. It is associated with a greater risk of maternal hypotension and urinary retention. With the aforementioned changes and risks, how could a woman receiving epidural analgesia be considered to be at low risk of intervention in delivery? This question is of medicolegal significance.

Epidural Compatible With Midwife Care.—If women under the care of a midwife are in prolonged labor or have an impending fetal or maternal problem that may require operative intervention, they should be referred to an obstetrician. Labors requiring epidural analgesia should occur in a fully equipped maternity unit with competent obstetric staff on immediate standby in the event of an unexpected complication. There is a 30% to 50% chance that women will require assistance with their first delivery. In the United Kingdom, this must presently be performed by an obstetrician. In the developing world, instrumental delivery is commonly performed by midwives. With structured postgraduate education, midwives could extend their role and incorporate low-cavity instrumental delivery into their practice. This would help reduce the long hours of junior medical staff. Why should an obstetrician have to become involved just because a woman wants effective pain relief?

Conclusion.—The issue of continued midwife-led care in the event of an epidural has implications for anesthetists. Safety and legal concerns question the feasibility of continued midwife care when an epidural is administered. These concerns were countered with the suggestion that the role of the midwife be expanded with appropriate education to include low-cavity instrumental delivery. That way, a woman involved in a normal delivery can receive effective pain relief if she requests it without the obstetric staff needing to become involved.

Does Midwifery-led Intrapartum Care Require Anaesthetic Services?

Pickett JA, Oppenheimer CA, May AE (Leicester Royal Infirmary NHS Trust, England)

Int J Obstet Anesth 5:152–155, 1996 1–12

Introduction.—The Cumberlege Report strongly urges major changes in the delivery of maternal services in the United Kingdom. It suggests that women with uncomplicated pregnancies be offered midwifery-led antenatal and intrapartum care and that obstetricians become involved with these patients only in the presence of unexpected obstetric complications. The role of the anesthetist was barely considered. The role of the anesthetist was retrospectively evaluated in a midwifery-led delivery scheme.

Methods.—Women were admitted to a midwifery-led "Home from Home" unit that simulated a home confinement. Immediately adjacent was a traditional style delivery room. Pain relief was provided by intramuscular pethidine, inhalation of nitrous oxide/oxygen, or transcutaneous electrical nerve stimulation. If the need for epidural analgesia was requested or obstetric complications occurred, patients could be easily transferred.

Results.—Of 1,610 patients admitted to the "Home from Home" delivery scheme in labor, 397 (25%) were transferred to the main delivery suite. Of the women transferred, 181 (11% of the total population) received anesthetic intervention. The mean age of patients who remained in "Home from Home" and those who were transferred was similar. The women who did not require transfer were predominantly multiparous, and those who did were predominantly primiparous. Of women who required anesthetic intervention, 59 had normal deliveries, 43 had forceps delivery, 21 had ventouse extraction, 2 had assisted breech delivery, and 53 had lower-segment cesarean delivery. Three patients with major anesthetic risks were not referred antenatally for anesthetic evaluation. One patient had rheumatoid arthritis, one had acute intermittent porphyria, and another was a Jehovah's Witness.

Conclusion.—A number of women who were considered to have uncomplicated pregnancies and were involved in a midwifery-led scheme required anesthetic intervention. Expectant mothers, particularly those who are primiparous, should be made aware of these findings when choosing where to deliver. Guidelines are needed to define which women should be referred antenatally for an anesthetic evaluation.

► The authors are anesthetists in Great Britain, but the issues are similar to those that exist in the United States. During the next decade, it is likely that an increased number of anesthesiologists will be asked to provide epidural analgesia to patients whose accoucheur is a nurse midwife. The American Society of Anesthesiologists' "Guidelines for Regional Anesthesia in Obstetrics" state: "Regional anesthesia should not be administered until: (1) the patient has been examined by a qualified individual; and (2) the maternal and fetal status and progress of labor have been evaluated by a physician with privileges in obstetrics who is readily available to supervise the labor and manage any obstetric complications that may arise."[1] I interpret these guidelines to indicate that an anesthesiologist may administer epidural analgesia to a patient whose accoucheur is a midwife, provided that an obstetrician is readily available to perform an emergency cesarean section or manage other obstetric complications. Anesthesiologists and obstetricians must define "readily available" at the local level.

D.H. Chestnut, M.D.

Reference

1. American Society of Anesthesiologists: Guidelines for Regional Anesthesia in Obstetrics. Park Ridge, Ill, American Society of Anesthesiologists, 1991.

The Anaesthetic Management of Caesarean Section for Placenta Praevia: A Questionnaire Survey

Bonner SM, Haynes SR, Ryall D (South Cleveland Hosp, Middlesbrough, England)

Anaesthesia 50:992–994, 1995 1–13

Background.—Few consistent guidelines are available for choosing anesthesia for cesarean section in relation to differing degrees of placenta previa. Although some authors suggest that regional anesthesia may be appropriate for elective cesarean section, others maintain that general anesthesia should be used for all patients with placenta previa because use of regional anesthesia in the face of severe hemorrhage may exacerbate hypotension. Current practices in the United Kingdom were assessed by questionnaire.

Methods.—All 588 members of the Obstetric Anaesthetists Association were sent a postal questionnaire in July 1993. The questionnaires described a range of clinical situations (Table 1) and asked whether the clinician would consider using regional anesthesia for each. Respondents were also asked to indicate their level of experience and typical anesthetic techniques and to state whether written guidelines existed for trainees in their departments.

Results.—The questionnaire response rate was 68%; 376 usable replies were evaluated. Responses to the various clinical situations described in the questionnaire were reported (Fig 1). Those respondents classified as consultants (324) were further classified into 2 groups: 1 group committing fewer than 2 regular sessions per week to obstetric anesthesia and analgesia (137), and 1 group working 2 or more such sessions per week (187). Consultants in the latter group were significantly more likely to use regional anesthesia in patients with placenta previa than were either consultants in the former group or trainees (52). This tendency held whether the patient was undergoing elective surgery, spotting blood vaginally, or bleeding freely. Only 12 respondents confirmed that written guidelines for trainees were available in their departments.

TABLE 1.—Description of Ultrasound Reports Used in the Questionnaire

(a)	A posterior placenta praevia whose lower border stops short of the os.
(b)	An anterior placenta encroaching onto the lower segment (the surgeon feels that he can incise the uterus under the lower border of the placenta).
(c)	A low lying placenta covering the internal os.
(d)	An anterior placenta encroaching onto the os.
(e)	A low lying posterior placenta whose lower border encroaches onto, but does not cover the os.
(f)	A central placenta completely covering the internal os with anterior extension.

(Reprinted from Bonner SM, Haynes SR, Ryall D: The anaesthetic management of caesarean section for placenta praevia: A questionnaire survey. *Anaesthesia* 50:992–994, 1995 by permission of the publisher, WB Saunders Company, Ltd., London.)

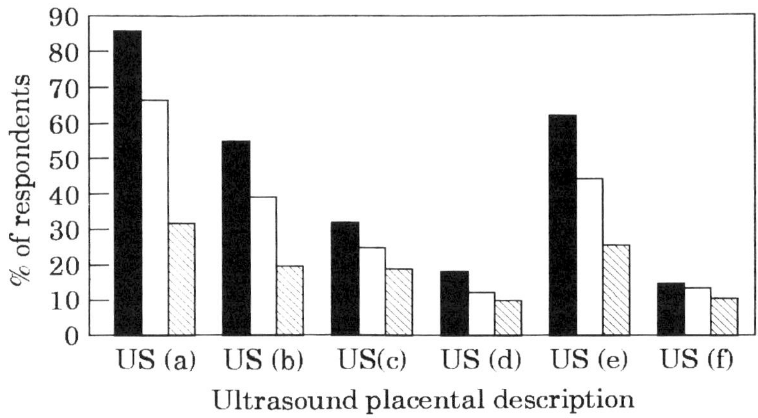

FIGURE 1.—Percentage of respondents prepared to use regional blockade for cesarean section for each case of placenta previa (split according to bleeding status). *Solid bar,* elective; *open bar,* labor; *crosshatched bar,* bleeding. (Reprinted from Bonner SM, Haynes SR, Ryall D: The anaesthetic management of caesarean section for placenta praevia: A questionnaire survey. *Anaesthesia* 50:992–994, 1995 by permission of the publisher, WB Saunders Company, Ltd., London.)

Conclusions.—No consensus exists in the United Kingdom regarding the appropriate use of regional anesthesia in patients with placenta previa. The data do suggest that regional anesthesia is used frequently. Familiarity with techniques in different clinical situations appears relevant in choice of anesthesia. Many consultants surveyed expressed a desire for guidelines on the anesthetic management of placenta previa.

► Women with a history of cesarean section have an increased incidence of placenta previa in subsequent pregnancies. Further, women with a history of cesarean section and current placenta previa have an increased risk of placenta previa. Such patients are at high risk for substantial intraoperative hemorrhage. Few anesthesiologists would administer regional anesthesia for cesarean section to a patient who is actively bleeding. But there remains controversy regarding the anesthetic management of those patients with a history of cesarean section and current placenta previa who are about to have an elective cesarean section. Some anesthesiologists prefer to give general anesthesia to all of these women, to avoid the need to secure the airway during an episode of massive blood loss. However, many women desire to be awake for delivery of their infant, and some anesthesiologists offer regional anesthesia with the understanding that it may be necessary to administer general anesthesia and secure the airway in the event of massive blood loss. I typically favor the latter approach. However, I acknowledge that it is unclear to what extent the administration of regional anesthesia attenuates the patient's compensatory response to hemorrhage and hypovolemia.

D.H. Chestnut, M.D.

Risk/Outcome Studies in Pediatric Anesthesia

The Demographics of Inpatient Pediatric Anesthesia: Implications for Credentialing Policy

Macario A, Hackel A, Gregory GA, et al (Stanford Univ, Calif; Univ of California, San Francisco)
J Clin Anesth 7:507–511, 1995 1–14

Introduction.—Many licensing bodies now require performance-based credentialing of physicians. This credentialing system is based on the provider's training and experience, and on a review of the quality of care provided. For the analysis to take place, a minimum and yet undefined number of cases is required. There is concern that too few procedures are performed to permit credentialing of practitioners who provide anesthesia for infants and children. This question was examined in a review of all hospitals in northern California.

Methods.—Data for the study were obtained from the State of California's Office of Statewide Health Planning and Development. The review sought to include all inpatients younger than 6 years who underwent a surgical procedure requiring anesthesia during 1991. Surgical procedures and date of surgery were linked to create "procedure-days," each of which counted as 1 anesthesia case. Annual hospital procedure-days were recorded for 3 age subgroups (0 to 6 months, 7 to 24 months, and 25 to 72 months), and hospitals were grouped according to number of procedures per year (0, 1 to 20, 21 to 50, 51 to 100, and more than 100). The proximity of hospitals with smaller surgical volumes to those with larger volumes also was recorded.

Results.—Inpatient surgical procedures were reported for 205 hospitals in the study area, and 162 of these hospitals had at least 1 procedure-day for children younger than 6 years. The total number of anesthesia cases (procedure-days) was 14,435. For each of the 3 age subgroups, most hospitals (81% to 90%) fell into the categories of 1 to 50 cases per year. When all 3 age groups were combined, 59% of hospitals had fewer than 20 cases per year, 72% had fewer than 50 cases per year, and 86% had fewer than 100 cases per year. Three fourths of the hospitals with fewer than 100 cases per year were within 50 miles of a hospital with more than 100 cases per year.

Discussion.—If at least 100 cases per year were needed for credentialing based on caseload, few hospitals in northern California would meet this requirement. Even with a required caseload per year of 21 or more, 59% of hospitals would have an inadequate number of cases for effective credentialing. With the current distribution of patients, most hospitals care for a few children and most children are cared for in a few hospitals.

▶ This excellent article stems from the perception of the impending institution of performance-based credentialing. Performance-based credentialing is credentialing based on analysis of the quality of care provided by the physician based on, for instance, 100 cases a year. So, if one wanted to do performance-based credentialing for a pediatric anesthesiologist, or for an anesthesiologist providing care to pediatric patients, one would have to have the outcome of that anesthesiologist providing care to enough patients to be meaningful.

This study examined whether there were enough cases in most hospitals that offered pediatric surgery for this process to occur in a reliable fashion. What Macario and colleagues found was quite the opposite. Eighty-six percent of hospitals in northern California that did pediatric anesthesia had less than 100 cases per year. Thus, even if one had only 1 anesthesiologist providing all pediatric care and that person was on call day and night, every day of the year, less than 86% of the hospitals did enough cases to do performance-based credentialing effectively. Furthermore, you may want to have performance-based credentialing based on caring only for infants 0 to 6 months old. Even if one dropped the case load to 50 and had only 1 anesthesiologist do it, more than 80% of the hospitals in the region would not have enough cases to credential 1 anesthesiologist. The good news, bad news part of this story is that 75% of the hospitals with caseloads of less than 100 per year were within 50 miles of hospitals with caseloads of greater than 100 per year. Because the authors continue to speculate that because most hospitals take care of a few children and most children are taken care of in a few hospitals, political and economic forces will continue to consolidate and merge health care delivery systems, especially among pediatric patients. Clearly, Macario and company have not seen Chicago, where formerly there were 2 large children's hospitals and a third hospital that took care of some children. In the last year, 3 new children's hospitals have emerged. Although these are just "wings" of established hospitals, they further dilute pediatric care so that it will be increasingly difficult to provide individuals who do mainly pediatric anesthesia for all these sites, 24 hours a day, 7 days a week, 365 days a year. Thus, performance-based credentialing and even teaching may be more difficult. The authors are to be congratulated on a provocative and, I think, important article.

M.F. Roizen, M.D.

The Effects of Patient Volume and Level of Care at the Hospital of Birth on Neonatal Mortality

Phibbs CS, Bronstein JM, Buxton E, et al (Veterans Affairs Palo Alto, Calif; Stanford Univ, Calif; Univ of Alabama, Birmingham, et al)

JAMA 276:1054–1059, 1996 1–15

Introduction.—The development of neonatal intensive care units (NICUs) produced significant improvements in neonatal mortality. The concept of regionalization emerged, with formal designation of tertiary (level III) and intermediate (level II) NICUs. In the past, neonatal mortality was consistently better for infants born at hospitals with level III NICUs. More recent experience suggests that the distinction between level II and

III NICUs may have lessened. Experience with the treatment of high-risk infants, regardless of the NICU level, may result in better care. The effects of NICU level and patient volume were assessed using a large data base.

Methods.—Birth certificate data were used to identify all 594,104 singleton births occurring in nonfederal hospitals in California during 1990. Of these births, 473,209 were successfully linked with hospital discharge abstracts, permitting control for major risk factors besides birth weight. These risks were controlled for by logistic regression. A total of 53,229 infants were identified as likely NICU admissions. Each hospital was classified according to the level of NICU care available and the average NICU census. The effects of NICU level and patient volume on risk of death within the first 28 days of life—or within the first year of life for continuously hospitalized infants—were analyzed.

Findings.—Both NICU level and patient volume significantly affected neonatal mortality. Risk-adjusted mortality was significantly lower (odds ratio 0.62) for infants born at a hospital with a level III NICU and an average NICU census of at least 15 patients per day, compared to infants born at hospitals with no NICU. However, risk-adjusted mortality for infants born at hospitals with smaller-volume level III NICUs was not significantly different from that for infants born at hospitals with level II or II+ NICUs, regardless of unit volume. Mortality was higher for infants born at hospitals with low-volume level III NICUs versus high-volume level III NICUs.

Conclusions.—Infants born at hospitals with large-volume level III NICUs have significantly lower mortality than infants born at other hospitals. The costs of care in large level III NICUs are no higher than the costs at other units. Concentrating high-risk deliveries in urban areas with level III NICUs may reduce neonatal mortality with no accompanying increase in cost.

▶ There is a trend toward directing mothers and babies to facilities with a lower level of neonatal intensive care to reduce cost. Patient volume and level of care have statistically significant effects on neonatal mortality, and a plan to concentrate high-risk deliveries in a smaller number of hospitals (this will increase volume) that provide tertiary-level care might improve outcome without an increase in financial risk.

M. Wood, M.D.

Parental Presence During Induction of Anesthesia: A Randomized Controlled Trial

Kain ZN, Mayes LC, Caramico LA, et al (Yale Univ, New Haven, Conn)
Anesthesiology 84:1060–1067, 1996 1–16

Objective.—Whether parental presence during induction of general anesthesia is beneficial is controversial. The relationships between parents, children, and anesthesiologist must be evaluated before a definitive answer can be found. The results of a randomized, controlled trial of relationships between parents, children, and anesthesiologist, anxiety levels in children, long-term behavioral sequelae, and factors predicting which pairs of parents and children will benefit from parental presence are presented.

Methods.—A group of 84 children aged 1–6 years was randomly assigned to parent-absent (control) or parent-present (intervention) groups before undergoing elective outpatient surgery. No premedication was administered and a single anesthesiologist participated. The Anxiety Visual Analog Scale (VAS), EASI Instrument of child temperament (EASI), and State Trait Anxiety Inventory (STAI) were administered 1 week preoperatively to the parents, and the Post Hospitalization Behavior Questionnaire (PHBQ) was administered to the parents after surgery. The VAS, Clinical Anxiety Rating Scale (CARS), and Yale Preoperative Anxiety Scale (YPAS) were administered to trained observers. Blinded observers rated the anxiety of parents and children on the day of surgery. The child's cooperation (VAS) and anxiety (YPAS, CARS) were measured during induction of anesthesia. In the recovery room, parents were asked to rate their helpfulness during anesthesia induction and their satisfaction with the staff and procedure (VAS). Parents filled out and returned the PHBQ at 2 weeks (92.8% response) and 6 months (73.8% response) after surgery. Serum cortisol levels in children were measured.

Results.—No significant behavioral or physiologic differences were found between the control and intervention groups in the preoperative holding area or during induction of anesthesia. Responses at 2 weeks and 6 months did not differ between groups. When serum cortisol levels were used as a measure of the child's anxiety, parental presence, child's age, baseline anxiety of the parent, and baseline temperament were significant predictors of the child's anxiety. Children older than 4, children whose parents had a low anxiety score, and children who had a low baseline temperament score had significantly lower serum cortisol levels.

Conclusion.—Parental presence during induction of anesthesia benefited children older than 4, children whose parents had a low anxiety score, and children who had a low baseline temperament score.

▶ Some pediatric anesthesiologists are great believers in parental presence and involvement during anesthesia induction; others are not. A single anesthesiologist administered all the anesthetics and we do not know that particular individual's views on this subject, although it is of note that the anesthesiologist rated only a minority of parents as helpful (12%). I thought it interesting and important that 98% of the parents would like to be present during induction if their child needed surgery again. In these days of quality improvement, patient satisfaction scores, and the like, parental presence may become (or is now) a factor that affects "customer" satisfaction in this patient group.

M. Wood, M.D.

A Prospective Study of Rectal Methohexital: Efficacy and Side Effects in 648 Cases

Audenaert SM, Montgomery CL, Thompson DE, et al (Univ of Louisville, Ky; Shriners' Hosp for Crippled Children, Lexington, Ky; Univ of Kentucky, Lexington)

Anesth Analg 81:957–961, 1995 1–17

Background.—Rectally administered methohexital has long been used for anesthesia induction in younger children, with reported efficacy rates of 85% to 100% and usually only minor side effects. However, there have been no large, prospective studies detailing its safety and efficacy. A prospective series of 648 pediatric patients treated with rectal methohexital was reported.

Methods.—The study included 648 patients at 1 children's hospital who received rectal methohexital, 30 mg/kg of a 10% solution, for the induction of anesthesia. The patients then were monitored for side effects and complications—including partial or complete airway obstruction, apnea, and seizures—until other anesthetics were given. The sedative and sleep-inducing effects of methohexital at 15 minutes were recorded. The results were analyzed separately for patients with myelomeningocele or cerebral palsy and for those who were receiving phenobarbital or phenytoin for seizure disorders.

Results.—Eighty-five percent of the patients went to sleep after receiving rectal methohexital. The average time to sleep was 6 minutes, and most of the patients who did not fall asleep were at least moderately sedated. Patients with myelomeningocele and those who were taking phenobarbital or phenytoin were less likely to fall asleep. Thirteen percent of patients had hiccups and 10% defecated, but these side effects carried no morbidity. Immediate defecation was common only in children with myelomeningocele. Four percent of patients had partial airway obstruction or an oxygen saturation level of 93% or less, but most of them responded to blow-by oxygen, jaw thrust, or both. Two patients needed aggressive anesthesiologic airway intervention. There were no cases of apnea or seizures.

Conclusions.—Rectal methohexital is a highly efficacious agent for the quick induction of anesthesia in children. Because of variable absorption, the methohexital dose that causes moderate sedation in 1 patient will produce general anesthesia in another. Airway compromise occurs in about 4% of patients and is potentially life-threatening. Rectal methohexital should be used only when adequate monitoring and skilled personnel are present.

▶ Rectal methohexital has been available for many years, and has been disliked because of its unpredictable duration of effect, a feature that was not considered in this study. The authors emphasize that methohexital administration is not without real danger, and careful monitoring by skilled personnel is essential.

M. Wood, M.D.

Operating Room Management/Cost Studies

Desflurane Is Not Associated With Faster Operating Room Exit Times in Outpatients

Patel N, Smith CE, Pinchak AC, et al (Case Western Reserve Univ, Cleveland, Ohio)
J Clin Anesth 8:130–135, 1996 1–18

Background.—Desflurane is identical in structure to isoflurane except for the substitution of a fluorine for a chlorine. The low blood gas solubility of desflurane means that its washin and washout is faster; thus, emergence time should be faster, which may translate into decreased operating room exit time. Operating room exit times after desflurane was added to 1 hospital formulary were investigated.

Methods.—A total of 1,568 outpatients needing anesthesia in an ambulatory surgery unit were included in the prospective study. After desflurane was added to the formulary and desflurane vaporizers were substituted for enflurane vaporizers in the ambulatory surgery unit, data were collected for 6 months.

Findings.—The general anesthetic administered was desflurane in 209 patients, isoflurane in 429, halothane in 192, and propofol in 72. Major conduction was used in 43 patients, peripheral nerve blocks in 90, and IV sedation in 528. Patients receiving general anesthesia had significantly longer exit times than those receiving spinal/epidural anesthesia, nerve blocks, and IV sedation. Among older patients, exit times were longer after

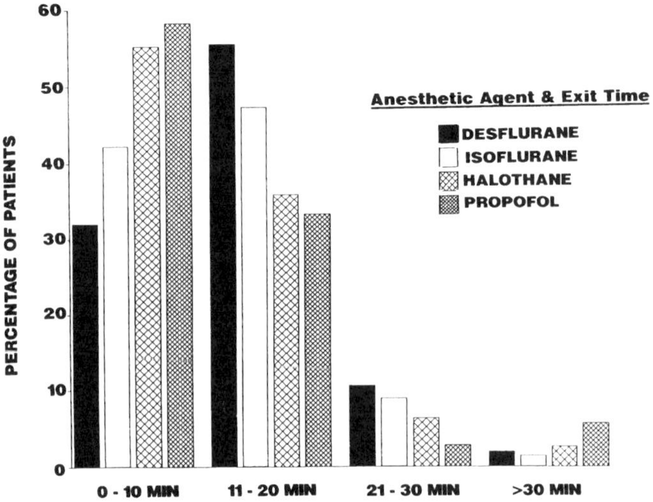

FIGURE 2.—Primary anesthetic drug and distribution of operating room exit times in 907 outpatients receiving general anesthesia. Data are percentage of patients receiving the various anesthetic drugs. (Reprinted by permission of the publisher from Patel N, Smith CE, Pinchak AC, et al: Desflurane is not associated with faster operating room exit times in outpatients. *J Clin Anesth* 8:130–135. Copyright 1996 by Elsevier Science Inc.)

general anesthesia than after IV sedation. Among patients given IV sedation, exit times were shorter as the duration of surgery increased. Exit times were unaffected by primary anesthetic agent (Fig 2).

Conclusions.—Operating room exit times were faster with regional anesthesia and IV sedation than with general anesthesia. The use of desflurane did not shorten exit times, despite its shorter elimination kinetics and recovery characteristics.

▶ These kinds of studies are enormously difficult because recovery rooms have protocols, both written and unwritten. It is hard to know, as a reviewer or commentator, whether the recovery room protocol, either informal or formal, written or unwritten, calls for patients who had general anesthesia to stay more or less a certain length of time. Individual recovery room nurses often have specific times in mind that patients who had particular anesthetic management strategies "need." Exit times are determined by complex interactions, including the abovementioned protocols, long-established practice, individual postanesthesia care unit nurse preference, and, probably last, the duration of anesthetic A vs. anesthetic B. This paper is not surprising. Based on our own mathematical modeling techniques, using our data, we have come to the same conclusions.

J.H. Tinker, M.D.

Decreases in Anesthesia-controlled Time Cannot Permit One Additional Surgical Operation To Be Reliably Scheduled During the Workday

Dexter F, Coffin S, Tinker JH (Univ of Iowa, Iowa City)

Anesth Analg 81:1263–1268, 1995 1–19

Background.—It is generally believed that operating room (OR) costs could be reduced if anesthesiologists would work more quickly. This may be so if the OR personnel are able to do more operations per day, without overtime. The ability of anesthesiologists to reduce OR costs by working faster was evaluated in a quantitative study.

Methods.—The study included a case series of 709 consecutive patients undergoing 1 of 11 elective surgical procedures at a tertiary care hospital. The procedures were selected to reflect a broad range of specialties, case lengths, and complexity. Two time durations were added to determine the anesthesia-controlled time (ACT) for each procedure: the time from the patient's entry to the OR until the start of preparation or surgical positioning and the time from completion of the surgical dressing until the patient's departure from the OR. The data were used to determine whether eliminating ACT could permit surgeons to perform additional scheduled procedures or see more scheduled patients during the workday.

Findings.—Statistical analysis suggested that even if ACT were completely eliminated, there would still be insufficient time for even 1 additional 30-minute procedure. The only way that all cases in an OR could predictably be finished early each day would be if ACT was decreased to zero and all cases took less than 45 minutes to perform.

Conclusions.—Simply having anesthesiologists work faster would not permit scheduling of additional OR cases during the workday. Some of the measures proposed to reduce ACT—such as preoperative IV catheter teams, procedure rooms, and shorter-acting drugs—may actually increase costs. A collective effort by anesthesiology, surgical, and nursing personnel will be needed to achieve real cost reductions in the OR.

▶ Dexter and colleagues have again stimulated us with this article to look at staffing patterns. Much like I believe the flaws in an article on recovery room time, I also believe there are consistent flaws in this study. Nevertheless, I think it is a valuable first attempt at teaching us how a computer model may work to staff an operating room. Obviously, if you had 10 operating rooms and normal variability in those rooms, then quicker turnaround time might yield an extra case in 1 of the 10. Nevertheless, Dexter and colleagues seem to ignore this possibility; maybe I misunderstand their writing. More importantly, however, this study does show that such a case cannot predictably be done in any 1 room and has to go to the first empty room available rather than giving a surgeon a predictable area to go in to schedule the extra room. If this commentary and explanation seem fuzzy, then read the article.

M.F. Roizen, M.D.

Geriatric Anesthesia Risk/Outcome Studies

Factors Associated With Survival to 75 Years of Age in Middle-aged Men and Women

Goldberg RJ, Larson M, Levy D (Univ of Massachusetts, Worcester)

Arch Intern Med 156:505–509, 1996 1–20

Background.—Factors associated with overall and cause-specific morbidity and mortality have been investigated in a variety of epidemiologic studies. However, little is known about the factors associated with longevity, especially those in middle-aged women and men.

Methods.—Data about 973 women and 747 men enrolled in the Framingham Study were analyzed. The research subjects were free of cancer, cardiovascular disease, and diabetes and were 50 years of age at the time of a routine clinical examination performed for the Framingham Study. Variables associated with survival to 75 years of age were determined in a logistic regression analysis.

Findings.—In both sexes, the factors associated with longevity were fewer cigarettes smoked per day, lower systolic blood pressure, and greater forced vital capacity. Lower heart rate was also associated with longevity in men. Among women, parental survival to 75 years of age was also correlated with longevity.

Conclusions.—Increased longevity among middle-aged men and women is associated with several lifestyle factors and 1 familial factor. These findings further support efforts to encourage middle-aged men and women to quit smoking and to control hypertension.

▶ One would hypothesize that physiologic age, rather than calendar age, is related to preoperative risk, and this study shows that fewer cigarettes smoked, lower systolic blood pressure, and higher functional residual capacity are associated with a decreased physiologic age. Similarly, lower resting heart rate in men and parental survival to age 75 years in women are also associated with a decreased physiologic age. I commend this epidemiologic study as one of the Framingham reports that may prove important for assessing perioperative risk.

M.F. Roizen, M.D.

Cost Efficacy Issues

Practical Cost-effective Choices: Ambulatory General Anesthesia
Philip BK (Brigham and Women's Hosp, Boston)
J Clin Anesth 7:606–613, 1995 1–21

Introduction.—An analysis of the cost-effectiveness of anesthetic care must include a definition of effectiveness and consideration of several factors: the price of acquisition, hidden costs, costs due to nonanesthetic factors, and the recovery times and side effects of the anesthetic agents. These factors were examined in a study of the choices available for ambulatory general anesthesia.

Effectiveness and Costs.—An effective anesthetic has a smooth onset and provides good intraoperative conditions. Its effectiveness must continue during the 3 stages of recovery—early, intermediate, and late—providing rapid immediate recovery, minimum postoperative sequelae, and a prompt return to preoperative status. Drug prices are readily obtained, but hidden costs and costs related to nonanesthetic factors also must be identified and estimated. Hidden costs include pharmacy markup, costs of preparations, costs billed to different budgets, the cost of waste resulting from package size versus unit dose, and costs of equipment. Nonanesthetic factors include duration of surgery, operating room time, and preferences of the surgeon, patient, or facility administrator.

Induction and Maintenance of Anesthesia.—The cost of an anesthetic dose can be calculated from the dose used per patient, patient weight, and acquisition price (drug cost per mg): mg/kg × kg × $/mg = $. Thiopental, for example, has a far lower acquisition cost ($0.51) than methohexital ($1.54) and propofol ($7.28), but the significant recovery disadvantages of thiopental may not make it the most cost-effective choice. There have been many studies comparing the benefits and costs of agents used for anesthesia maintenance. These comparisons illustrate the need to balance acquisition costs against recovery time and the likelihood of side effects. Time savings in the operating room or recovery areas, however, will generate cost savings only if staffing actually decreases. And protocols that mandate a specific duration of stay can negate the apparent savings associated with an agent's postoperative advantages.

Conclusions.—Drug prices are easily obtained, but determinations of cost-effectiveness must be based on the value acquired for the price paid. Specific recovery goals should be identified and the hidden costs of each anesthetic method analyzed.

► Dr. Philip reviews the fact that cost includes more than acquisition cost, such as the excess cost and excess recovery time associated with complications, including nausea, vomiting, dizziness, and increased coughing. The article then reviews the acquisition costs of common anesthetics that are used in ambulatory anesthesia and describes how to calculate excess cost for complications.

M.F. Roizen, M.D.

Practical, Cost-effective Regional Anesthesia for Ambulatory Surgery

Greenberg CP (Columbia Presbyterian Med Ctr, New York)

J Clin Anesth 7:614–621, 1995 1–22

Objective.—Regional anesthesia can be a cost-effective choice for patients undergoing ambulatory surgery. The practical and cost-effective aspects of specific techniques were discussed and a model for the analysis of anesthesia costs in the ambulatory setting was presented.

Cost Factors.—Factors to be considered when selecting anesthesia for ambulatory procedures involve direct and indirect costs to be incurred before, during, and after surgery. The area of indirect costs is particularly relevant in ambulatory surgery. In this setting, regional anesthesia usually is associated with reduced intensity of care, minimal side effects, decreased recovery time and time to discharge, and excellent postoperative pain control.

Principles of Selection.—Regional anesthesia and the specific technique used must be appropriate for the surgical procedure, anesthesiologist, surgeon, patient, and facility. The technique selected must be reliable in its effect and duration, and potential complications should be anticipated. Supplemental sedation offers several advantages, but is associated with cost and has inherent risk. It is important to realize that regional anesthesia must follow the same standards of preoperative screening, intraoperative monitoring, restrictions on oral intake, need for escort, and discharge criteria that apply to general anesthesia.

Techniques of Regional Anesthesia.—Numerous techniques suitable for outpatient use are available, including IV regional anesthesia, the "kiddie caudal" block for pediatric patients, and upper and lower extremity nerve blocks. The more complicated techniques of spinal and epidural anesthesia are required in some procedures. Spinal anesthesia has several practical and economic advantages compared to epidural anesthesia: lower cost for supplies, shorter time to perform, and more rapid onset. Epidural anesthesia has extended duration and may be preferable in some cases. Regional and local anesthesia also appear to have an advantage over general anesthesia alone in providing long-term analgesia.

Cost Models.—The model presented breaks down the total cost for each type of anesthetic into 3 components: anesthetic drugs/techniques, supplies, and depreciation of capital equipment. A model for regional anesthesia is categorized by technique (spinal, nerve block, or epidural) and components (local anesthetic, disposable regional kit, block needle, and supplementary sedation). To determine which drugs and techniques are most cost-effective, anesthesia costs must be assessed in relation to the quality and outcome of the ambulatory surgery experience.

▶ This is an excellent article that looks at much of the total cost of anesthetics and compares regional vs. general vs. MAC. As you can guess, regional anesthesia seems to cost considerably less, both for the first hour of anesthesia and for additional hours. You would be wise to read this article if you wish to do this type of cost comparison in your hospital.

M.F. Roizen, M.D.

Understanding Cost Analyses: Part 1. A Practitioner's Guide to Cost Behavior

Lubarsky DA (Duke Univ, Durham, NC)

J Clin Anesth 7:519–521, 1995 1–23

Background.—Because of the growing importance of economic considerations in the area of health care delivery, anesthesiologists must interpret articles on the cost implications of their practice. Yet, few studies in the general medical or surgical literature qualify as thorough economic analyses. A certain knowledge base is required to critique the anesthesiology cost literature. Among the necessary steps in that process are an understanding of terminology and an awareness of the behavior of costs in a medical setting.

Cost Behavior.—The behavior of costs refers to the way that costs change in response to a change in practice. Commonly described cost behaviors are variable, fixed, semi-variable, and semi-fixed. Truly variable costs, like those for drugs and syringes, exhibit a linear and direct correlation with the number of anesthetics administered. Fixed costs remain the same, independent of volume. An example of a fixed cost would be the depreciation of pulse oximeters in the operating room: depreciation cost per year is not affected by the number of cases per day.

Semi-variable costs remain fixed to a point, then vary with the volume of anesthetics after a certain threshold is reached. Under capitated agreements, for example, additional money is paid to the physician for each additional patient anesthetized. Few semi-variable costs now exist for anesthesiologists. The most important cost behavior for anesthesiology is that of semi-fixed costs. Personnel costs act in a semi-fixed way, for doing

1 more case or adding a few minutes to a patient's postanesthesia care unit (PACU) time does not necessarily increase salary costs. An increased use of perioperative resources, however, eventually will require additional personnel. It remains difficult to equate reduced recovery time with reductions in recovery room staffing and to show cost savings from a specific anesthetic drug choice. Actual patient discharge requires a variety of services, and the patient may be unable to leave the unit when medically ready.

Discussion.—Staffing reductions in the PACU often are cited as a means of cost savings, because PACU staffing typically costs 5 to 10 times more than drugs in a routine surgical case. It is important, however, to realize that fewer minutes in the PACU do not necessarily generate savings or recommend 1 anesthetic drug over another, and studies that discuss PACU savings in these terms should be read critically.

▶ This is 1 of a group of articles published together in the *Journal of Clinical Anesthesia* relating to cost analyses, and delivering value in your anesthetic practice. This study reviews the difference between variable, fixed, semi-variable, and semi-fixed costs, and tells of the difficulty in calculating PACU costs as if they are variable, when in fact they are semi-fixed and only change, to any great degree, when you can hire or reassign personnel in a relatively flexible fashion. This is an excellent article to start you learning about cost analysis.

M.F. Roizen, M.D.

A Multicenter Comparison of Maintenance and Recovery With Sevoflurane or Isoflurane for Adult Ambulatory Anesthesia

Philip BK, Kallar SK, Bogetz MS, et al (Harvard Med School, Boston; Med College of Virginia, Richmond; Univ of California, San Francisco; et al)

Anesth Analg 83:314–319, 1996 1–24

Background.—Because of its low blood gas solubility, sevoflurane may be associated with rapid emergence from anesthesia, which would make it

TABLE 3.—Number (%) of Patients Able to Complete Either the Asleep-Wide Awake Component of the VAS or the DSST at Each Time Period After Anesthesia

	VAS		DSST	
Evaluation time (min)	Sevoflurane	Isoflurane	Sevoflurane	Isoflurane
15	102 (68%)	50 (52%)*	83 (56%)	36 (37%)*
30	137 (92%)	79 (82%)*	128 (86%)	73 (75%)*
60	146 (98%)	87 (91%)*	145 (97%)	87 (90%)*
90	145 (97%)	90 (94%)	144 (97%)	89 (92%)
120	144 (97%)	89 (93%)	144 (97%)	89 (92%)

*$P < 0.05$ vs. sevoflurane group.

Abbreviations: VAS, visual analog scale; *DSST*, digit symbol substitution test.

(Courtesy of Philip BK, Kallar SK, Bogetz MS, et al: A multicenter comparison of maintenance and recovery with sevoflurane or isoflurane for adult ambulatory anesthesia. *Anesth Analg* 83:314–319, 1996.)

TABLE 4.—Percentage of Patients With Adverse Experiences During Recovery and at the 24-Hour Follow-up

	During recovery*		At 24 hr	
Symptoms	Sevoflurane	Isoflurane	Sevoflurane	Isoflurane
Nausea	36	51†	9	24†
Vomiting	19	25	7	8
Dizziness	11	14	7	12
Drowsiness	15	26†	12	14
Cough	11	10	13	8

*All adverse experiences after anesthesia and before discharge at least possibly related to the study drug, with an incidence of 5% or greater.

†$P < 0.05$ versus sevoflurane group.

(Courtesy of Philip BK, Kallar SK, Bogetz MS, et al: A multicenter comparison of maintenance and recovery with sevoflurane or isoflurane for adult ambulatory anesthesia. *Anesth Analg* 83:314–319, 1996.)

suitable for ambulatory surgery. Sevoflurane was compared with isoflurane in adults undergoing such procedures.

Methods.—Two hundred forty-six patients with American Society of Anesthesiologists class I to III physical status were enrolled in the multicenter trial. Midazolam, 1 to 2 mg, and fentanyl, 1 µg/kg, were administered, and anesthesia was induced with propofol, 2 mg/kg, and maintained with sevoflurane or isoflurane. These agents were given in 60% nitrous oxide to maintain arterial blood pressure at ± 20% of baseline. During induction and maintenance, fresh gas flows were 10 L/min and 5 L/min, respectively.

Findings.—Sevoflurane was associated with significantly faster time to eye opening, command response, orientation, and ability to sit without nausea or dizziness. Significantly more patients given sevoflurane met phase 1 of postanesthesia care unit (PACU) Aldrete recovery criteria at arrival (95% receiving sevoflurane and 81% receiving isoflurane). In addition, significantly more patients given sevoflurane could complete psychomotor recovery tests in the first 60 minutes after anesthesia. Discharge times in the 2 groups were comparable. Patients receiving sevoflurane had significantly lower incidences of postoperative somnolence and nausea in the PACU and for 24 hours after discharge. Ninety-seven percent of the patients in the sevoflurane group and 93% in the isoflurane group were satisfied with anesthesia (Tables 3 and 4).

Conclusions.—Sevoflurane resulted in faster early recovery and fewer adverse effects than isoflurane. Inhalational sevoflurane may be useful in maintenance of adult ambulatory anesthesia.

► In this multicenter trial comparing isoflurane and sevoflurane, postoperative nausea occurred about twice as often with isoflurane and vomiting occurred about 3 times as often, although these findings were not statistically significant. Drowsiness occurred more than twice as often, again with isoflurane. This paper also tends to support my recent contention that, despite theoretical objections to the contrary, sevoflurane is proving to be user friendly and is "catching on" in various settings, particularly ambulatory anesthesia for adults.

J.H. Tinker, M.D.

The Effect of Managed Care on ICU Length of Stay: Implications for Medicare

Angus DC, Linde-Zwirble WT, Sirio CA, et al (Univ of Pittsburgh, Pa; Health Process Management Inc, Doylestown, Pa)

JAMA 276:1075–1082, 1996 1–25

Introduction.—More U.S. patients are receiving health care under managed care. The question of whether managed care is less costly because the patients require fewer resources has been raised. With managed care, a recent study showed that resource consumption, defined as ICU length of stay, decreased by 35%. A comparison was made of ICU length of stay between patients under a managed care plan and patients not in a managed care plan.

Methods.—Using split-halves validation to adjust for differences in age, sex, severity of illness, diagnosis, discharge status, and payer, ICU length-of-stay regression models were constructed for 88,050 patients who were divided into 4 groups: commercial fee-for-service, younger than 65 years; commercial managed care, younger than 65 years; traditional Medicare, older than 65 years; and Medicare-sponsored managed care, older than 65 years. The state of Massachusetts was chosen because it is one of the most highly penetrated managed care markets in the country.

Results.—Unadjusted ICU length of stay was significantly shorter among those covered by managed care, despite similar age and disease distribution in the younger group (2.9 days for managed care compared to 3.43 days for traditional). However, ICU length of stay was not affected by payer status. Among those admitted for elective surgical procedures, their ICU length of stay was 26% shorter than that of their traditional counterparts. There was no apparent difference in ICU length of stay among the older groups in managed care or under a traditional plan. For those covered by managed care, mortality rates tended to be lower. For those younger than 65 years, managed care patients had a mortality rate of 3.9% compared to 5.1% for traditional patients. For the older group, the mortality rate was 8.7% for the managed care patients compared to 12.1% for the traditional patients. Mortality was influenced by age, severity of principal diagnosis, comorbidity, and reason for admission.

Conclusion.—Cost savings are not apparent in the ICU management of older patients, even though managed care plans appear to be providing health care at lower cost in many arenas. As the managed care case mix changes to include sicker and older patients, one wonders whether managed care organizations will continue to offer health care coverage at a lower cost. The ongoing impact of expanding the proportion of Medicare patients enrolled in managed care programs must be studied carefully.

► This article may worry large managed care plans as more elderly patients enter into their fold. It will be interesting to observe whether these insurance companies raise premiums, as suggested by this article, or whether there will be a greater push to limit the use of this expensive resource.

D.M. Rothenberg, M.D.

Patient Satisfaction

Patient Satisfaction With General Anaesthesia: Too Difficult to Measure?

Whitty PM, Shaw IH, Goodwin DR (Northern and Yorkshire Regional Health Authority, Newcastle Upon Tyne; Newcastle Gen Hosp, Newcastle Upon Tyne, England)

Anaesthesia 51:327–332, 1996 1–26

Purpose.—Despite the general emphasis on patient satisfaction as a health care outcome, there have been few efforts to assess patient satisfaction with general anesthesia. The difficult process of designing patient satisfaction questionnaires may be facilitated through the use of focus groups and other qualitative techniques.

Methods.—Three focus groups—representing patients undergoing general, maxillofacial, and ophthalmologic surgery—were held to help in developing a questionnaire to assess patient satisfaction with general anesthesia. After a pilot study, an audit was performed to validate the final questionnaire. One hundred twenty-six patients participated in the audit study, with a response rate of 73%.

Results.—The focus groups underscored the importance of explaining postanesthetic sequelae. Major factors emerging from the audit study included the lack of information about anesthesia before hospital admission, the long period without food and drink before surgery, and the lack of explanations about postoperative sequelae (Table 4). The patients were more likely to find fault with the anesthetic technique used than with the anesthetists. The overall patient satisfaction level was high.

Conclusions.—Questionnaires can be developed to identify areas of general anesthetic practice in need of further improvement. Such instruments must ask for detailed information about all aspects of the patient's experience, with a comprehensive focus on communication. The survey should include graded response categories and specific questions about having the same anesthesia or anesthetist again.

► Assessment of outcome is topical, and 1 outcome is patient satisfaction. Patient satisfaction is very difficult to measure; often, our patient assessment includes factors that either are out of the anesthesiologist's control or are not the usual topics considered by quality assurance auditing. This questionnaire relating to the process of anesthetic care was designed after interviewing focus groups, and may be of value as a starting point for other

TABLE 4.—Summary of Responses to Questions About the Process of Anesthetic Care (Total Number of Respondents, 126)

Question	Number (%) in partial or full agreement*
Before you came into hospital	
Worried about the anaesthetic	36 (29%)
Enough information about the anaesthetic	57 (45%)
Before you had your operation	
Visited by an anaesthetist	115 (91%)
Able to ask questions of anaesthetist	97 (77%)
Examined by anaesthetist	50 (40%)
Enough privacy for talk with anaesthetist	102 (81%)
Reassured about the anaesthetic after visit	94 (75%)
(Of those not visited) Unhappy about not being visited	2 (out of 6 or 33.3%)
(Of total) Without food for 5 hours or less pre-operatively	7 (6%)
Without food for more than 12 hours pre-operatively	34 (27%)
Without drink for 5 hours or less pre-operatively	23 (18%)
Without drink for more than 12 hours pre-operatively	28 (22%)
Bothered by lack of food	9 (7%)
Bothered by lack of drink	44 (35%)
Received premedication	43 (33.3%)
Unhappy with length of time waited in theatre prior to induction	7 (5%)
The operation	
Anaesthetised by same anaesthetist who visited pre-operatively	90 (71%)
Unhappy if not anaesthetised by pre-operative visiting anaesthetist	1 (0.8%)
Not talked to directly by anaesthetist	2 (1.6%)
Anaesthetic not explained by anaesthetist	3 (2.4%)
Anaesthetist appeared competent	113 (90%)
Anaesthetic an unpleasant experience	12 (9%)
Evidence of awareness	0 (0%)
After your operation	
In recovering room, in pain	34 (27%)
felt sick	21 (17%)
frightened	10 (8%)
shivery	15 (12%)
Received prompt treatment if desired	33 of 34 in pain (97%)
Longer term and sufficient to cause distress	14 of 21 who were sick (67%)
dry mouth	50 (40%)
cut lip/tongue	2 (2%)
teeth damage	2 (2%)
sore throat	36 (28%)
aching jaw	10 (8%)
muscle/joint aches	41 (32%)
numbness	9 (7%)
sickness/vomiting	12 (10%)
sore/itchy eyes	4 (excluding ophthalmic patients)
drip/injection site pain	16 (13%)
Anaesthetic problems explained	24 (out of 88 who had problems; 27%)
At home	
Needed to call GP out for anaesthetic problem	0 (0%)
Looking back	
Did not perceive anaesthetist as doctor	38 (30%)
Had received a patient information leaflet	23 (18%)

*For simplicity, the response categories that agreed with the statement as phrased in the table were combined (e.g., "very reassured" and "quite reassured" were combined to give "number in partial or full agreement").

(Courtesy of Whitty PM, Shaw IH, Goodwin DR: Patient satisfaction with general anesthesia: Too difficult to measure? *Anaesthesia* 51:327–332, 1996. Reprinted by permission of the publisher, WB Saunders Company Limited, London.)

anesthesiologists who wish to design their own survey of patient satisfaction.

M. Wood, M.D.

Emesis After Anesthesia

Twenty-four of Twenty-seven Studies Show a Greater Incidence of Emesis Associated With Nitrous Oxide Than With Alternative Anesthetics

Hartung J (State Univ of New York, Brooklyn)

Anesth Analg 83:114–116, 1996 1–27

Background.—There has been considerable controversy about whether nitrous oxide increases the incidence of vomiting. A meta-analysis of the literature was used to examine this question.

Methods.—Computer and hand searches were done to identify studies comparing the incidence of emesis in patients receiving nitrous oxide and in patients receiving anesthetics or analgesics without nitrous oxide. Only studies differentiating between the incidence of nausea and the incidence of emesis were included. The absolute incidence was compared. Studies without a statistically significant association between nitrous oxide and emesis were evaluated to determine whether there was enough statistical power to detect a 20% difference in incidence.

Results.—Of the 27 identified studies, 24 showed a higher absolute incidence of vomiting in patients who received nitrous oxide than in those treated with anesthetics or analgesics without nitrous oxide. The association between nitrous oxide and an increased incidence of vomiting also was statistically significant in these 24 studies. Only 2 of the other 3 studies had enough statistical power to detect a 20% effect size.

Conclusions.—Nitrous oxide is a ubiquitous drug used in anesthesiology, that induces a significantly greater incidence of emesis. Therefore, further study is needed to identify the context and circumstances under which nitrous oxide causes vomiting.

► This is, in essence, a "meta" analysis and as such is subject to several problems. For a meta-analysis to accurately reflect what is going on in the real world, the published studies need to be unbiased. By unbiased I specifically mean not skewed. With many meta-analyses, this is difficult because many of the studies were done with very real previous biases.

Here, in contrast, most of these studies were not specifically studying nitrous oxide as a putative cause of emesis. Still, because nitrous oxide is nearly universally used, bias may have been introduced in the studies that did not use nitrous oxide. Nonetheless, this article confirms what many have long suspected, namely, that the persistent problem of nausea and/or vomiting after anesthesia may have more to do with nitrous oxide (and maybe thiopental) than anything else.

J.H. Tinker, M.D.

Blood and Fluid Issues

The Risk of Transfusion-transmitted Viral Infections

Schreiber GB, for the Retrovirus Epidemiology Donor Study (Westat Inc, Rockville, Md)

N Engl J Med 334:1685–1690, 1996 1–28

Introduction.—There is ongoing concern regarding the safety of the blood supply. Efforts to monitor the safety of transfused blood and to assess the benefits of new screening tests require accurate information on the risks of transmitting infectious diseases by blood transfusion. Blood donated by seronegative donors during the infectious "window" period, before seroconversion has occurred, poses the main threat to the safety of the blood supply. The risks of transmitting HIV and other viral infections in blood donated during the window period were assessed.

Methods.—The analysis included 586,507 individuals who gave blood on repeated occasions between 1991 and 1993, for a total of 2,318,356 allogeneic blood donations. The incidence of seroconversion was assessed for individuals whose donated blood passed all screening tests. These rates were then adjusted to reflect the estimated window period for each virus under consideration, i.e., HIV, human T-cell lymphotropic virus (HTLV), hepatitis C virus (HCV), and hepatitis B virus (HBV). Further reductions in risk that might accrue from the use of new and more sensitive screening tests were also estimated.

Results.—The adjusted incidence rates of seroconversion were 3.37/100,000 person-years for HIV, 1.12/100,000 for HTLV, 4.32/100,000 for HCV, and 9.80/100,000 for HBV (Table 1). The estimated risks of giving blood during an undetected infection were 1 in 493,000 for HIV, 1 in 202,000 for HTLV, 1 in 641,000 for HCV, and 1 in 63,000 for HBV (Table 2). The overall risk of donating during an infectious window period was 1 in 34,000; HBV and HCV made up 88% of this risk. With new viral antigen or nucleic acid screening tests, it was estimated that the risk could be reduced by 27% to 72%.

Conclusion.—The risk that virus-infected blood will be undetected during the infectious window period is very small and should become smaller still with the introduction of new screening tests. The surveillance program used in this study, which includes data from 5 blood centers across the United States, will be useful in providing essential data on blood safety issues.

► Of the multitude of therapies offered to patients, very few kindle the emotions more than the specter of receiving a blood transfusion. Immediate thoughts of contracting AIDS enter into the mind of the prospective recipient while he or she contemplates whether it would be the appropriate time to convert to the Jehovah's Witness faith. Results of this study, however, should begin to assuage the fears of the general public, with the authors citing an aggregate risk of transmitting any of the 4 viruses (HBV, HCV, HIV

TABLE 1.—Crude and Adjusted Incidence Rates of Seroconversion Associated With Each of Four Major Blood-borne Viruses

Virus	Crude Rate			Adjusted Rate		
	No. of Seroconversions	No. of Person-yr	Incidence Rate per 100,000 Person-yr	No. of Seroconversions	No. of Person-yr	Incidence Rate per 100,000 Person-yr (95% CI)*
HIV	33	822,494	4.01	27	801,571	3.37 (2.22–4.76)
HTLV	9	822,417	1.09	9	801,572	1.12 (0.51–1.98)
HCV†	16	330,924	4.84	14	324,356	4.32 (2.35–6.87)
HBV						
HBsAg	33	822,426	4.01	33	801,553	4.12 (2.83–5.64)
Total HBV‡	—	—	9.54	—	—	9.80 (6.74–13.42)

*Among donors whose prior donations were usable.

†Data are limited to donations screened by the second-generation enzyme immunoassay, the use of which began in March and April 1992.

‡Data were adjusted for transient antigenemia by multiplying the incidence rate of hepatitis B surface antigen (*HBsAg*) seroconversion and the 95% confidence interval (*CI*) by 2.38, on the assumption that 42% of hepatitis B virus (*HBV*) infections are detected by the assay for HBsAg.

Abbreviations: HTLV, human T-cell lymphotropic virus; *HCV*, hepatitis C virus.

(Courtesy of Schreiber GB, for the Retrovirus Epidemiology Donor Study: The risk of transfusion-transmitted viral infections. *N Engl J Med* 334:1685–1690, 1996, by permission of *The New England Journal of Medicine*. Copyright 1996, Massachusetts Medical Society.)

TABLE 2.—Residual Risks to the Blood Supply Associated With Window-period Donations by Seroconverting Donors

Virus	Length of Window Period (days)		Residual Risk (per million donations)	
	Estimate	Range	Estimate*	Range†
HIV	22‡	6–38	2.03	0.36–4.95
HTLV	51§	36–72	1.56	0.50–3.90
HCV	82‖	54–192	9.70	3.47–36.11
HBV				
HBsAg	59¶	37–87	6.65	2.87–13.43
Total HBV**	—	—	15.83	6.82–31.97

*Calculated by multiplying the adjusted incidence rate of seroconversion (Table 1) by the length of the window period.
†The lower and upper bounds of the range were calculated by multiplying the lower and upper limits of the window-period range by the lower and upper limits of the 95% confidence interval for the adjusted incidence rate, respectively.
‡Data were obtained from Busch MP, Lee LL, Satten GA, et al: Time course of detection of viral and serologic markers preceding human immunodeficiency virus type 1 seroconversion: Implications for screening of blood and tissue donors. *Transfusion* 35:91–97, 1995.
§Data were obtained from Manns A, Wilks RJ, Murphy EL, et al: A prospective study of transmission by transfusion of HTLV-I and risk factors associated with seroconversion. *Int J Cancer* 51:886–891, 1992.
‖Data were obtained from Busch MP, Korelitz JJ, Kleinman SH, et al: Declining value of alanine aminotransferase in screening of blood donors to prevent posttransfusion hepatitis B and C virus infection. *Transfusion* 35:903–910, 1995, and Lelie PN, Cuypers HT, Reesink HW, et al: Patterns of serological markers in transfusion-transmitted hepatitis C virus infection using second-generation HCV assays. *J Med Virol* 37:203–209, 1992.
¶Data were obtained from Mimms LT, Mosley JW, Hollinger FB, et al: Effect of concurrent acute infection with hepatitis C virus on acute hepatitis B virus infection. *BMJ* 307:1095–1097, 1993.
**Data were adjusted for transient antigenemia by multiplying the estimated residual risk of hepatitis B surface antigen (*HBsAg*) seroconversion and the range by 2.38, on the assumption that 42% of hepatitis B (*HBV*) infections are detected by the assay for HBsAg.
Abbreviations: HTLV, human T-cell lymphotropic virus; *HCV*, hepatitis C virus.
(Courtesy of Schreiber GB, for the Retrovirus Epidemiology Donor Study: The risk of transfusion-transmitted viral infections. *N Engl J Med* 334:1685–1690, 1996, by permission of *The New England Journal of Medicine*. Copyright 1996, Massachusetts Medical Society.)

or HTLV) as being 1 per 34,000 units donated. It was not too long ago that the risk of contacting HCV infection alone was 1 per 200 units. It is still true, of course, that the maximal use of blood conservation techniques and the judicious use of all blood products are necessary to further minimize the risks of transfusion-related infections.

D.M. Rothenberg, M.D.

Albumin and Nonprotein Colloid Solution Use in US Academic Health Centers

Yim JM, Vermeulen LC, Erstad BL, et al (Univ Hosp Consortium, Oak Brook, Ill; Univ of Wisconsin, Madison; Univ of Arizona, Tucson; et al)
Arch Intern Med 155:2450–2455, 1995 1–29

Objective.—Using crystalloids to increase intravascular volume is considerably less expensive than using nonprotein colloids (NPCs) or albumin. The University Hospital Consortium (UHC), a national alliance of health care centers, developed clinical use guidelines for albumin, NPCs, and crystalloid substances based on an assessment of use patterns. The use of these solutions at member centers was characterized in a prospective, multicenter observational study to evaluate adherence to the guidelines.

Methods.—Use data were collected between April 11 and May 6, 1994, and included patient and prescriber demographics, indications for use, outcome, and adverse events. Costs of therapy were compared.

Results.—A total of 969 reports from 688 patients (42% women), aged 1 to 92 years, were evaluated. Albumin (83%) and NPCs (17%) were administered mainly in ICUs (50%) or operating rooms (31%), and were prescribed most commonly by anesthesiologists (20%) and surgeons (45%). Among other prescribers, the breakdown was house staff (61%), attending physicians (31%), and fellows (8%). Data were estimated to represent 85% of albumin and NPC use. Of the 834 reports analyzed for appropriateness of use, 76% were deemed inappropriate. Costs were estimated at $100 per 500 mL of 5% albumin, $50 per 500 mL of hetastarch, $40 per 500 mL of dextran 40, and less than $5 per 500 mL of crystalloid solutions. Of the $202,655 spent for albumin and NPCs, $124,939 was spent inappropriately and $28,014 was spent for unevaluated indications. In 87% of cases, albumin and NPCs were given to achieve a certain outcome, whereas in 13% of cases, the desired outcome was unknown.

Conclusions.—About $17,518 could have been saved if NPCs rather than albumin had been used. Only one fourth of albumin or NPC solutions were administered according to UHC guidelines. Institutions need to adopt guidelines that concentrate on the cost-effective use of these solutions.

► This article raises important points, and no one would argue the importance of cost-effective use of these solutions in a cost-conscious healthy economy. However, it is important to recognize how these data were generated. It was a multicenter, "observational" study conducted by the UHC, and it is not clear who filled in the case report forms and how the decision to enroll a patient was made. Patient outcome was not addressed. Albumin and NPC solutions were administered to reach a defined end point (77% of use to achieve a target physiologic state or resolve a pathophysiologic condition) in 87% of cases, but we do not know whether this was achieved.

M. Wood, M.D.

Teaching/Outcome/Risk Issues

The Initial Employment Status of Physicians Completing Training in 1994

Miller RS, Jonas HS, Whitcomb ME (American Med Assoc, Chicago; Assoc of American Med Colleges, Washington, DC)

JAMA 275:708–712, 1996 1–30

Background.—The United States soon will have a serious oversupply of physicians. It has been reported that physicians who complete residency in some specialties have problems finding suitable work, and that some established physicians have seen a serious decline in the number of patients they treat. The career status of physicians who completed residency training in the 1993–1994 academic year was studied.

Methods.—A survey was completed by 3,090 directors of residency programs. The survey included questions about total number of graduates, number of physicians working full-time in their specialty, and number of physicians who had trouble finding employment.

Results.—Of nearly 16,000 physicians who completed residency in 1 of 26 specialties, 63% were seeking employment. Of those not seeking employment, 93% were pursuing additional training. The percentage of physicians who did not find a full-time job in their specialty ranged from 0% in urology to almost 11% in pathology, and was 5.5% in rheumatology. The total percentage of physicians who did not find a full-time job in their specialty was 3%. About 70% of graduates seeking employment obtained a position in their specialty. Physicians in more general specialties, such as family practice and internal medicine, had less trouble finding a position in their field. Program directors in nongeneral specialties believed that it will become more difficult to find a full-time position.

Conclusions.—The full-time employment opportunities for physicians in some specialties are becoming more limited in some parts of the United States. These findings may be helpful to medical students and members of the academic medical community who make decisions about the supply of physicians and the relation to graduate medical education.

▶ There is concern that anesthesiology residents may not find positions at the end of their training and that the need for subspecialists has decreased. This has had a marked effect on medical student recruitment into the specialty. However, it is important to recognize that anesthesia is not alone, and it is encouraging to note that critical care medicine graduates are a group that report a low percentage without full-time jobs in their specialty. Over the coming years, it will be increasingly difficult for physicians pursuing generalist careers to find positions as the available positions become saturated. I believe it is important to choose a career not for 1997 or 1998, but for the rest of one's life; so my advice is to choose a career (whether generalist or subspecialist) that provides for individual satisfaction when one goes home at night.

M. Wood, M.D.

The Digital Toolbox for Teaching

Sandroni S, McGee J (Univ of Florida, Jacksonville)

South Med J 88:1199–1203, 1995 1–31

Background.—Advances in computer technology have significantly enhanced clinical teaching. A "digital toolbox," consisting of personally accessible hardware and software products to aid in clinical teaching, was described.

The Digital Toolbox for Teaching.—Many currently available software programs are useful in clinical teaching. The ILIAD program, which makes connections between physical, historical, and other data types, can be used to generate a diagnosis. There also is equipment available that allows the acquisition and display of images in almost any setting. Displaying clinical images greatly enhances medical education. New MacIntosh computers are useful for multimedia. With IBM clones, multimedia efforts require a 486DX processor, at least 8 megabytes of random access memory, Windows 3.1, a color monitor capable of at least 16-bit color display, a hard drive capacity of at least 160 megabytes, and preferably more. The ability to create quality presentations and enhance teaching depends on access to high-quality digitized materials. Another useful tool in the toolbox is decision analysis software. Some authors use TreeAge DATA. Although formal decision analysis is too time-consuming to be used routinely, merely structuring a clinical problem as a decision tree and discussing the various branches are useful.

Conclusions.—A range of practical products is available to enhance many aspects of clinical teaching. The tools described require no programming skill or specialized computer expertise for initial use.

► I believe that this is an important article for those of us who are struggling to make our presentations more meaningful. However, the recent advent of visual images, x-rays, and ECGs on a Netscape version in our hospital is making digital teaching and access at the bedside possible, and slide-making even easier. For the first time in my life as a computerphile and avid user of computers, I can honestly say that I believe that computers are beginning to make my life easier, not just more interesting—they have made my medical care easier, better, and even consistently more efficient.

M.F. Roizen, M.D.

The Regional Anesthesia "Learning Curve": What Is the Minimum Number of Epidural and Spinal Blocks to Reach Consistency?

Kopacz DJ, Neal JM, Pollock JE (Virginia Mason Clinic, Seattle)

Reg Anesth 21:182–190, 1996 1–32

Objective.—Surveys suggest that residents often do not receive exposure adequate to achieve the desired level of competency in the use of regional anesthetic techniques. Seven beginning CA-1 anesthesiology residents were observed for a 6-month period to determine the minimum number of epidural and spinal blocks that must be performed to reach consistency during the learning of these techniques.

Methods.—A data collection sheet was used to track regional anesthetic technique variables and the degree of success attained in placing a needle in its proper location. The usual manner of training residents was followed. Success was defined by objective measures: obtaining CSF during attempted spinal anesthesia, subsequent anesthetic block during epidural placement, and detection of end-tidal CO_2 for endotracheal intubation. A 5-point scale categorized degree of success; 100% indicated that the resident performed the entire procedure alone.

Results.—Each resident attempted a mean of 86 endotracheal intubations, 77 epidural anesthetics, and 44 spinal anesthetics. The group learning curve and individual resident learning curves were similar during the study period. Endotracheal intubation was performed with an overall success rate of 99.2%. Improvement relative to baseline was seen after 20 attempts, but 45 attempts were required for sustained improvement. The overall success rate for location of the epidural space was 98.6%, and the midline approach was significantly more successful than the paramedian approach. Sixty attempts were required to reach and maintain the 90% success rate in locating the epidural space. Location of the subarachnoid space was achieved in 79.3% of cases, for a 99.1% overall success rate. An early peak was followed by a reduction in success for attempts 26 to 30.

Discussion.—To achieve a percentage level of success consistent with competency (90%), a resident should be required to attempt at least 45 spinal and 60 epidural anesthetics. The trough that occurs after early success may be attributed to an increasing difficulty of cases and a decreasing level of staff supervision. With repeated practice, a satisfactory plateau should be reached.

► I find it fascinating that these authors came up with more or less the same numbers that our esteemed Residency Review Committee in anesthesiology decided were the minimal numbers for legitimate Board eligibility. On the other hand, these authors believe that 90% success is not reached until considerably more spinals and epidurals are performed. Luckily, perhaps, the authors do not tell us old folks how fast our skills deteriorate or how many we need to do in a year. I think it is extraordinarily problematic to be arbitrarily setting such numbers and "requiring" such experiential levels for medical technical/mechanical tasks. Mechanical ability varies enormously from one trainee to another. Such abilities have been termed "motor intelligence." All of us have seen residents who are facile after far smaller numbers than these. All of us have seen residents who are decidedly not facile despite experiences way beyond these numbers. Also, these are averages; another problem is that these averages can easily be used by attorneys to attack experience levels in court. Perhaps the "mechanical police" will want to mandate certain motor skill levels, by some test or other, in our potential trainees before allowing them to even try. I am unenthusiastic about this kind of publication, to say the least.

J.H. Tinker, M.D.

Fiberoptic Intubation Using Anesthetized, Paralyzed, Apneic Patients: Results of a Resident Training Program

Cole AFD, Mallon JS, Rolbin SH, et al (Univ of Toronto)
Anesthesiology 84:1101–1106, 1996 1–33

Background.—The potential of fiberoptic intubation is limited not so much by lack of equipment as by lack of expertise, and there is no consensus as to the best way of teaching the technique. A program in which anesthesiology residents were trained to perform fiberoptic tracheal intubation in anesthetized, paralyzed patients was described and evaluated.

Methods.—Eight first-year anesthesiology residents were trained simultaneously in rigid laryngoscopic and fiberoptic intubation techniques in anesthetized patients. Efforts were made to simulate the upper airway of conscious patients during fiberoptic intubation training. The residents performed a total of 743 laryngoscopic and 223 fiberoptic intubations. After training, their ability to perform both techniques was assessed in a prospective, single-blind, randomized trial of 131 patients. In this study, 71 fiberoptic and 57 laryngoscopic intubations were compared for intubation times, SpO_2, $ETCO_2$, hemodynamic changes associated with intubation, and complications.

Results.—Intubation could not be achieved within 180 seconds for 2 patients in the laryngoscopic group and 1 in the fiberoptic group. In these cases, mask ventilation was performed and the alternative technique was implemented successfully. There were no instances of hypoxemia or hypercarbia. The hemodynamic parameters were similar with the 2 techniques, as was the incidence of sore throat or hoarseness. Fiberoptic intubation took a mean of 56 seconds, compared to 34 seconds for laryngoscopic intubation. However, there were no differences in average lowest SpO_2 or highest postintubation $ETCO_2$ (Table 2). For individual residents, mean intubation times were unrelated to the number of practice or study intubations performed.

TABLE 2.—Intubation Times and Respiratory Variables

	Group 1 (Rigid Laryngoscopic)	Group 2 (Fiberoptic)
n	57	71
Intubation times (s)	34 ± 10	56 ± 24*
	(19–68)	(23–147)
Lowest O_2 saturation (%)	98 ± 1.0	98 ± 1.0
	(95–100)	(94–100)
Highest postintubation $ETCO_2$ (mmHg)	35 ± 5	36 ± 4
	(21–46)	(26–43)

Note: Values are mean ± SD (range).
**P* < 0.001 vs. group 1.
(Courtesy of Cole AFD, Mallon JS, Rolbin SH, et al: Fiberoptic intubation using anesthetized, paralyzed, apneic patients: Results of a resident training program. *Anesthesiology* 84:1101–1106, 1996.)

Conclusions.—When fiberoptic and laryngoscopic intubation are taught under similar conditions to anesthesiology residents, the residents learn them equally well. The training program described seems to be safe and effective for use in anesthesiology residency programs. Training in fiberoptic intubation should be a routine part of any residency program and should not be reserved for senior residents.

► Informed consent was obtained from the patients. If fiberoptic intubation is learned as a technique in the same way as conventional tracheal intubation at the very beginning of a residency program, then it is assumed to be routine and is easy to learn. Outcome studies for resident training are important, and we need more of them.

M. Wood, M.D.

Forum: The Accuracy of References in *Anaesthesia*

Asano M, Mikawa K, Nishina K, et al (Kobe Univ, Japan)

Anaesthesia 50:1080–1082, 1995 1–34

Background.—McLellan and colleagues have reported various citation errors in these anesthetic journals: *Anesthesiology*, *Anesthesia and Analgesia*, *British Journal of Anaesthesia*, and *Canadian Journal of Anaesthesia*. There are no reports of the accuracy of citations from the journal *Anaesthesia*. The occurrence of reference errors in the journal *Anaesthesia* from 2 calendar years was investigated.

Methods.—All issues of *Anaesthesia* from 1990 and 1994 were studied. From each year, 100 references were selected at random. Nonjournal references were omitted, leaving 197 citations that were carefully examined. The authors, article title, journal, volume number, page number, and year were all compared with the original publication. References were classified as correct if there were no errors. Errors that made it difficult to retrieve the original report were classified as major and included errors in volume, year, and first page of the reference.

Results.—Of the 197 citations examined, 32% from 1990 and 41% from 1994 contained at least 1 error. Most errors were minor. Major errors were found in 4 articles from 1990 and 2 articles from 1994. These major errors were in journal title, volume, and page numbers. The most common errors were in article title, authors, page number, journal title, and volume number.

Discussion.—The rate of errors in *Anaesthesia* did not improve from 1990 to 1994. The error rates for this journal were lower than the rates reported by McLellan and colleagues for 4 other anesthetic journals. It is the authors' responsibility to cite references accurately. Inaccurate references damage the credibility of the journal and frustrate those who search for the articles.

► This article is from the British journal after other reviews showed a 20% to 50% inaccuracy rate of references in *Anesthesiology, Anesthesia and Analgesia*, the *British Journal of Anaesthesia*, and the *Canadian Journal of Anaesthesia*. It should be remembered that very few of these are what we would call major problems—most of them are misspellings, or typographical errors such as substituting the word "people" for the word "individuals." Few of them are different page numbers or missing page numbers, an inappropriate journal name or a different volume. In fact, a total of less than 3% were this type of serious error. Nevertheless, it does seem incumbent on authors, editors, and reviewers to validate the references better.

M.F. Roizen, M.D.

Screening Cost/Efficacy Issues

Controversies in Prostate Cancer Screening: Analogies to the Early Lung Cancer Screening Debate

Collins MM, Barry MJ (Massachusetts Gen Hosp, Boston)

JAMA 276:1976–1979, 1996 1–35

Introduction.—There is ongoing controversy regarding the early detection and aggressive treatment of prostate cancer. Some authors maintain that screening for prostate cancer by digital rectal examination and prostate-specific antigen will reduce mortality, just as screening for breast cancer does. Others cite the example of lung cancer screening by chest radiography and sputum cytology, which has proven ineffective. The results of clinical trials of prostate cancer screening will not be available for another 10 to 15 years. Some lessons from the lung cancer screening debate were reviewed.

Lung Cancer Screening.—The concept of lung cancer screening arose from the detection of silent, curable lung cancers in the course of tuberculosis screening. The idea was that earlier referral to surgery would increase the chances of successfully fighting lung cancer. Chest radiography was considered an inexpensive screening procedure, and primary care physicians were pressured to take an active role in lung cancer detection. When randomized controlled studies of this issue were initiated in 1971, recommendations called for an annual chest radiograph and sputum cytologic studies in male smokers aged 45 years and older. The widespread use of screening threatened the validity of trials designed to test the efficacy of screening. Early results showed that screening was associated with a shift toward postsurgical stage I lung cancer; however, the final results found no reduction in lung cancer mortality with screening. By 1980, screening was no longer recommended.

Lessons for Prostate Cancer Screening.—As in the lung cancer screening debate, proponents of prostate cancer screening point to a stage shift among screened subjects. The proportion of early-stage, potentially curable prostate cancers is 30% to 40% in screened subjects versus 70% to 85% among unscreened subjects. However, this shift will not necessarily translate into better outcomes. In both situations, 2 screening modalities are used to increase sensitivity at the expense of specificity. There also are other parallels, including the active promotion and recommendation of screening in the absence of trial results. In addition, like lung cancer screening, prostate cancer screening actually may cause harm in the form of worry about abnormal test results, discomfort from prostate biopsy, and the risks associated with aggressive treatment.

Discussion.—The current controversy over the use of early prostate cancer screening recalls the previous debate over lung cancer screening. Prostate cancer screening eventually may prove effective. Until it does, experience suggests that the trend toward widespread prostate cancer screening should be tempered by the lack of experimental evidence supporting its use.

► Retropubic prostatectomy with nerve-sparing is becoming a very common operation in 50- to 60-year-old men. Prostate cancer is present in 50% of autopsied men older than 85 years and, although it is 1 of the top 5 lethal cancers among men in the United States, it is present in the same percentage of men and is much less often deadly in Asian countries. A current controversy exists as to whether early detection and radical prostate removal would lead to increased survival, as in breast cancer, or just to more morbidity, as in lung cancer. Of course, other strategies, such as prevention by changing to a diet with less fat and more green tea, have been recommended. Nevertheless, the controversy in prostate cancer screening is an important one for us to follow because more than 40,000 retropubic prostatectomies were done in the United States in 1994, and this appears to be 1 of the fastest-growing major operations done in this country. Collins and Barry seem to indicate that the controversy in prostate cancer screening, and the data collected to date, more closely follow the lung cancer scenario than the breast cancer scenario. If you are a man aged 45 years or older, should you wait before screening until the results of randomized controlled trials are completed in 15 years, or get screened and face the possibility of radical retropubic prostatectomy with nerve-sparing? The protagonists in this article are very careful to lay out the scenarios meticulously. It is clear that reading this article probably will not change your mind, and we all must wait 10 to 15 years for the results of the randomized clinical trials.

M.F. Roizen, M.D.

Screening for Problem Drinking in Older Primary Care Patients

Adams WL, Barry KL, Fleming MF (Med College of Wisconsin, Milwaukee; Univ of Wisconsin, Madison)

JAMA 276:1964–1967, 1996 1–36

Background.—Heavy use of alcohol contributes to morbidity and mortality among the elderly. In the general population older than 65 years, the incidence of alcohol abuse is 2% to 4%, and the incidence of less severe alcohol-related problems is as high as 10%. In the United States, even if the current incidence remains the same, the number of elderly individuals with alcohol problems will increase because the population is aging. Alcohol consumption can exacerbate or increase the risk of other health problems. Screening tools for problem drinking in the elderly should be able to identify those who may be at risk for medical problems related to alcohol abuse. The ability of the CAGE questionnaire (Cut down, Annoyed by criticism, Guilty about drinking, Eye-opener drinks) to identify heavy and binge drinking was evaluated in a cross-sectional study.

Methods.—A survey was conducted of 5,065 individuals older than 60 years who were enrolled from the offices of 88 primary care physicians. The Health Screening Survey was distributed to patients on arrival at their physician's office and asks about drinking, smoking, exercise, and diet. The CAGE questionnaire was also completed by patients. Demographic data were obtained.

Results.—Of the 5,065 individuals who completed the questionnaire, 56% were women, 84% were aged 60–75 years, 16% were older than 75 years, and 23% lived alone. Regular drinking exceeding the limits recommended by the National Institute of Alcohol Abuse and Alcoholism was reported by 15% of men and 12% of women (more than 7 drinks per week for women and more than 14 drinks per week for men). Also, 9% of men and 2% of women reported consuming more than 21 drinks per week on a regular basis. The CAGE questionnaire identified 9% of men and 3% of women positive for alcohol abuse within 3 months. The CAGE questionnaire was poor at detecting individuals who drank heavily or who were binge drinkers.

Discussion.—These findings indicate that the CAGE questionnaire cannot adequately identify problem drinking in an elderly, primary care population. It is recommended that various screening tools be combined when screening for problem drinking. This and other studies have shown that men, college graduates, and married individuals are more likely to drink heavily. Consuming 2–3 alcoholic drinks per day raises the risk of hypertension and possibly diabetes, breast cancer, head and neck cancers, and hip fracture.

► This study is important for us in anesthesia because problem drinkers and older drinkers often have cognitive deficits after surgery. Whether weaning drinkers of alcohol before hand is effective at reducing cognitive deficits after surgery is not known, nor is whether other anesthetic techniques are better for such patients. Nevertheless, such should be known so that their risks of having an operation can be properly conveyed to them and properly informed risk benefit choices can be made. These authors point out that the CAGE questionnaire, which is the classic questionnaire used to detect drinking, may not be most effective and that 2 other questions have proved effective in other questionnaires—have you had a drink in the last 72 hours, and have you ever had a problem with drinking? These authors point out that it is also easy to ask the following question, "Have you consumed alcohol in any of the previous 3 months?" Those who respond "yes" are then asked more detailed questions about consumption of 3 categories of beverages, beer, wine, or liquor. Examples are cited and respondents are asked to indicate on an average the number of days per week the beverage was consumed and the number of glasses in the case of wine, bottles or cans in the case of beer, or shots in the case of liquor consumed on 1 day by marking the appropriate category. Alcohol consumption is tabulated as the average number of drinks per week of all 3 types of alcohol consumed. The second area of use, the number of episodes of binge drinking, is determined by a question about the number of times the patient has had 6 or more drinks on 1 occasion in the past 3 months. It turned out that among individuals between 61 and 65 years, 11.2% had greater than 21 drinks per week among the men and 2.5% of the women had that. Similarly, numbers were obtained for those whose calendar age was 66–75 years and older than 75 years.

What this study shows is that the commonly recommended CAGE questionnaire is insufficient to detect the full spectrum of problem drinking seen in primary care patients. Because moderately heavy drinking, such as 3 drinks per day, clearly increases the risk of high blood pressure and several other conditions such as diabetes, breast cancer, head and neck cancers, and hip fractures, it is important to look for these conditions. In addition, men, college graduates, and married people are more likely to drink heavily than others. I suppose we need to be alert to this in the preoperative clinics, so as to search for these problems and at least document them and give appropriate informed consent before they end up causing surprising deficits in cognition postoperatively.

M.F. Roizen, M.D.

Preoperative Anxiety Scale

The Amsterdam Preoperative Anxiety and Information Scale (APAIS)
Moerman N, van Dam FSAM, Muller MJ, et al (Univ of Amsterdam, The Netherlands; Netherlands Cancer Inst, Amsterdam, The Netherlands)
Anesth Analg 82:445–451, 1996 1–37

Introduction.—That anxious patients respond differently to anesthesia than do nonanxious patients is well known. Several investigations have also indicated that recovery from surgery may be enhanced in patients who have been given information about their operation. Patient anxiety and information requirements were assessed using a newly developed 6-item questionnaire that could be completed within 2 minutes: the Amsterdam Preoperative Anxiety and Information Scale (APAIS).

Methods.—Four items in the APAIS questioned fear of the anesthesia/surgical procedure and 2 inquired about the need for information. A total of 320 consecutive patients visiting the anesthesiology outpatient department were asked to complete the APAIS. For comparison, the last 200 patients were also asked to complete the State version of Spielberger's Anxiety Inventory (STAI-State).

Results.—The correlation between the anxiety items on the APAIS and the STAI-State was high. The correlation between the information items on the APAIS and the STAI-State was low. Women had significantly higher anxiety scores than did men on the anxiety questions. Men with prior surgery(s) had a lower score on the anxiety scale than did those with no prior surgery. In women, no difference existed in anxiety score between those who had and had not undergone previous surgery. Patients with the highest information requirements were the same ones who were the most anxious. Patients with high anxiety scores were less likely to have had previous surgery, compared to those with lower education requirements. The prevalence of patients with high anxiety scores was 32%.

Conclusion.—Findings indicate that anesthesiologists should consider patients' preoperative fears and anxieties with utmost regard. The usefulness of the APAIS must be further tested.

► This study indicates that you can assess preoperative anxiety readily. I would guess that it is the starting point for many other studies that say whether assessing preoperative anxiety actually makes a difference to perioperative treatment and consequently to better outcome or satisfaction. It should be noted that this is only a starting point, as this study answers none of the definitive questions.

M.F. Roizen, M.D.

Placebo Effect in Analgesic Trials

Variation in the Placebo Effect in Randomised Controlled Trials of Analgesics: All Is as Blind as It Seems

McQuay H, Carroll D, Moore A (Univ of Oxford, England)

Pain 64:331–335, 1995 1–38

Background.—The placebo response has often been misunderstood to involve both a fixed fraction of the population and a fixed extent of reaction. However, data have shown a varying proportion of the population to be affected across studies and an effect that can vary systematically with the efficacy of the active agent. These findings have brought into question the possibility of both selection bias and observer bias in randomized, double-blind, placebo-controlled trials. To examine this possibility, the variations in placebo responses were examined in 5 randomized, double-blind, parallel-group trials of analgesic agents.

Methods.—Individual patient data from 5 placebo-controlled, double-blind, randomized trials of analgesic agents were analyzed. Each of the trials used 3 scales to determine pain intensity and 2 scales to determine pain relief. The relationship between pain relief and time was calculated for each patient and was compared with the maximum possible pain relief in relation to time.

Results.—Of the 525 patients in the 5 trials, 130 received placebo. These patients had 0% to 100% of the maximum possible pain relief, whereas the patients receiving active agents had 0% to 97% of the maximum

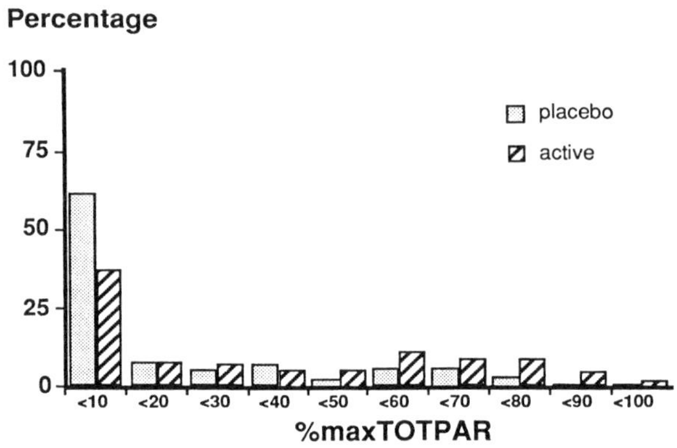

FIGURE 1.—Distribution of percentage of the maximum possible pain relief (*%maxTOTPAR*) scores for the 130 patients given placebo and for the 395 patients given active drugs. (Reprinted from McQuay H, Carroll D, Moore A: Variation in the placebo effect in randomised controlled trials of analgesics: All is as blind as it seems. *Pain* 64:331–335. Copyright 1995 with kind permission of Elsevier Science–NL, Sara Burgerhartstraat 25, 1055 KV Amsterdam, The Netherlands.)

possible pain relief (Fig 1). When the patients in the placebo groups who had less than 50% of the maximum possible pain relief were compared with those with more than 50% of the maximum possible pain relief, they differed only in age, with no differences in gender, height, weight, initial pain intensity, or mood. The mean percentage of maximum possible pain relief varied from 11% to 29% in the placebo study arms and from 12% to 49% in the active study arms. There was a significant relationship between the mean values in the placebo and the active study arms of each study, with the mean placebo results averaging 54% of the mean active results. However, there was no significant relationship between the median

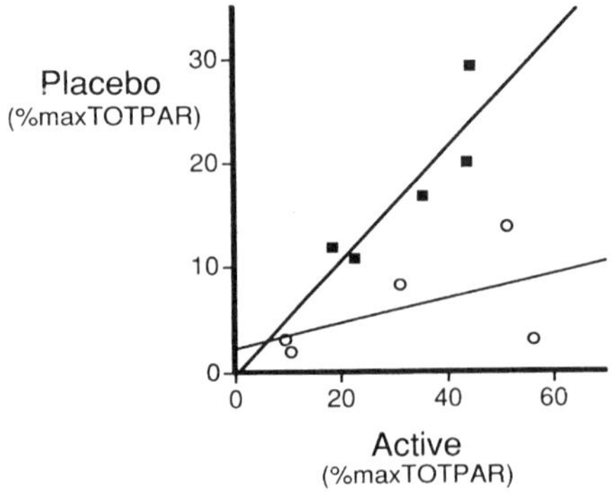

FIGURE 2.—Percentage of the maximum possible pain relief (*%maxTOTPAR*) placebo and active scores for the 5 trials. Linear regressions: mean: $y = 0.543x - 0.139$, $r^2 = 0.765$. *Open circles*, median; *closed squares*, mean: $y = 0.120x - 2.300$, $r^2 = 0.278$. (Reprinted from McQuay H, Carroll D, Moore A: Variation in the placebo effect in randomised controlled trials of analgesics: All is as blind as it seems. *Pain* 64:331–335. Copyright 1995 with kind permission of Elsevier Science–NL, Sara Burgerhartstraat 25, 1055 KV Amsterdam, The Netherlands.)

active and placebo responses, with the median placebo response averaging less than 10% of the median active response (Fig 2).

Conclusions.—Using inappropriate statistical methods has led to the recognition of a constant relationship between active analgesic and placebo response. Median responses, and not mean responses, should be used to evaluate the efficacy of analgesic agents in clinical trials.

▶ It is important to note that mean scores may be similar for placebo and active drugs in a study in which there are substantial differences between active drug and placebo. As shown in Figure 1, the most obvious difference is often the discrepancy between active drug and placebo in the number of nonresponders. As shown in Figure 2, it is the median scores that provide a better measure of the differences between groups when the distribution is not normal.

S.E. Abram, M.D.

Smoking Cessation via Intraoperative Suggestion

Double-blind, Randomized Trial of Cessation of Smoking After Audiotape Suggestion During Anaesthesia
Myles PS, Hendrata M, Layher Y, et al (Alfred Hosp, Victoria, Australia)
Br J Anaesth 76:694–698, 1996 1–39

Introduction.—Smoking is the cause of death in almost 20% of all deaths in developed countries. Patients may be able to reassess their smoking behavior after surgery with the use of audiotape suggestion during anesthesia. A beneficial effect on postoperative recovery has been demonstrated with audiotape suggestion. During general anesthesia, patients having elective surgery listened to a tape to determine whether tape suggestion could promote cessation of smoking.

Methods.—There were 363 smokers who wanted to stop smoking and had smoked an average of 21 cigarettes a day for 19 years. The smokers were randomized into either a treatment group to receive the suggestion tape or a control group, which received a blank tape. The suggestion tape had 3 minutes of explanation, reassurance, and positive encouragement to give up smoking. Before surgery, patients used a 100-mm visual analogue scale to rate their motivation to give up smoking. After surgery, they were asked to remember the words spoken during the operation. At 2 and at 6 months, their smoking level was determined.

Results.—At 2 months, 56 patients, or 15.4%, claimed to have stopped smoking. At 6 months, 29 patients, or 8%, claimed to have stopped smoking. At 2 or 6 months, there was no difference between the groups. There was no difference between groups in the preoperative/postoperative ratio of a visual analogue scale measuring the patient's motivation to stop smoking.

Conclusion.—Intraoperative tape suggestion does not change smoking behavior.

▶ I believe there is a thorny ethical issue here. If general anesthesia is a time during which the patient might be "suggestive" and I am presenting "therapeutic advertising" during that time, 2 ethical questions arise. Why not use that vulnerable time to present commercial advertising? Worse, what if the anesthesiologist were biased in the direction of "light" anesthesia? Did the authors do anything to minimize this potential in this study? The more I think about it, the angrier I become that our anesthetized patients could even be considered potential subjects for "behavior modification" during this critical time in their lives when they place their very lives in our hands. No matter how valid the "therapeutic" motive might be, namely, smoking cessation in this case, the whole concept leaves me with revulsion. It is also a leap of faith to contend as a hypothesis that complex behavior could be changed via such a "therapy."

J.H. Tinker, M.D.

Identification of Adverse Effects

Identifying Adverse Events Caused by Medical Care: Degree of Physician Agreement in a Retrospective Chart Review

Localio AR, Weaver SL, Landis JR, et al (Pennsylvania State Univ, Hershey; Harvard School of Public Health, Boston; Rush Univ, Chicago; et al)

Ann Intern Med 125:457–464, 1996 1–40

Objective.—Problems with retrospective case review include failure to agree on which outcomes are adverse and on the appropriateness and effectiveness of treatments. The degree of agreement of physicians on the cause of adverse patient outcomes and the implications for quality assurance, performance evaluation, and proposals for no-fault patient compensation were assessed.

Methods.—A random sampling of 7,533 patients' cases were examined for adverse events by 127 paired physicians in 51 inpatient facilities in New York state. Agreements and disagreements, and rates at which reviewers found patient injuries caused at least in part by medical personnel, were tallied.

Results.—There were more cases of strong disagreement on the existence of an adverse event (12.9%) than there were cases in which reviewers agreed on the existence of an adverse event (10%). Wound infection had the highest rate of agreement and failure to diagnose and omission of therapy had the lowest rates. Experienced reviewers agreed significantly more often than did inexperienced reviewers. The rates at which physicians found adverse events were significantly dependent on the facility from which the records came, the age of the patient, whether the patient died in the hospital, the duration of the hospital stay, and the 4 diagnosis-related groups.

Conclusion.—There was marked disagreement among reviewers regarding the existence and cause of adverse patient outcomes. Methods for disagreement resolution must be developed before quality assurance systems, performance evaluations, and no-fault patient compensation mechanisms will be effective.

► Quality assurance/improvement and auditing have become important as demands are made on hospitals to provide physician- and hospital-specific mortality and morbidity rates. How are these data that are often widely disseminated derived? From a black box? This study shows the degree of physician disagreement on the cause of adverse patient outcomes.

M. Wood, M.D

2 Perioperative Cardiovascular Evaluation, Outcomes, and Risk Management

Neurologic Complications After Cardiovascular Surgery

Adverse Cerebral Outcomes After Coronary Bypass Surgery
Roach GW, for the Multicenter Study of Perioperative Ischemia Research Group and the Ischemia Research and Education Foundation Investigators (Kaiser Permanente Med Ctr, San Francisco; New York Univ; Stanford Univ, Calif; et al)
N Engl J Med 335:1857–1863, 1996 2–1

Purpose.—Around the world, more than 800,000 myocardial revascularization procedures are performed annually. Cerebral complications are a frequent source of perioperative death among these patients. However, the reported incidence of perioperative stroke varies from 0.4% to 5.4%, and the frequency of in-hospital neuropsychological dysfunction from 25% to 79%. The incidence and predictors of adverse neurologic events associated with coronary artery bypass grafting (CABG) were evaluated.

Methods.—The prospective, multicenter study included 2,108 patients undergoing elective CABG. A panel of 6 investigators reviewed information on all new neurologic findings during the perioperative period. Each case was classified as type I (e.g., fatal stroke or hypoxic encephalopathy or nonfatal stroke or transient ischemic attack) or type II (e.g., new neurologic abnormalities without evidence of focal injury). Within each type, the diagnoses were ranked by severity.

Findings.—About one third of the patients were aged 70 years or older. Histories of hypertension, unstable angina, heart failure, or diabetes were common, and 8% of patients had had previous stroke or transient ischemic attack. About 3% of patients had type I outcomes and another 3% had type II outcomes. Proximal aortic atherosclerosis was an independent predictive factor, carrying more than a 4-fold increase in the risk of type I outcomes. Other independent predictors included history of neurologic disease, age 70 years or older, and history of pulmonary disease. Perioperative hypotension and ventricular venting procedures were not significant predictors, although they were clinically relevant. Certain factors were unique predictors for type II outcomes, including excessive alcohol consumption and previous CABG surgery. Conservative cost estimates suggested that type I outcomes caused an additional $10,266 per patient in in-hospital costs, and type II outcomes an additional $6,150.

Conclusions.—The incidence of adverse perioperative cerebral outcomes in patients undergoing elective CABG was found to be 6%. These outcomes are associated with higher mortality, higher costs, and greater need for prolonged care. Risk factors for focal and diffuse cerebral injury were identified, which should aid in risk stratification.

► This is 1 of 2 studies, within a 2-week period, from the anesthesia community, specifically the McSpi group, that was published in *The New England Journal of Medicine* and grabbed a lot of public media attention. This article grabbed attention because it had a higher than expected (by the general public) rate of adverse cerebral outcomes after coronary bypass surgery. These data were collected from 24 U.S. institutions, each of which contributed 100 or more unselected cases of coronary artery bypass surgery and prospectively collected data. The higher than expected rate of type I neurologic outcomes, which essentially were stroke or the consequences of stroke but also included 2 transient ischemic attacks among the about 2,400 cases, was 3.1%, whereas the rate of type II events, or cognitive dysfunction without focal neurologic change, was an additional 3%. The correlates of these outcomes were important. For the stroke outcomes, they were proximal aortic atherosclerosis, history of neurologic disease, diabetes, history of hypertension, and age. For the type II cerebral outcomes, they were history of pulmonary disease, history of hypertension, history of excessive alcohol consumption, requirement of a CABG in the past, history of hypotension, and congestive heart failure on the day of surgery. Thus, these are changes that preoperatively contribute to rapid arterial aging and, consequently, the development of emboli.

What can be done to prevent these? Well, clearly if one could segregate patients so that one did not operate on the physiologically older, that is, those who have had diabetes, hypertension, proximal aortic atherosclerosis, or excessive alcohol consumption, one could lessen the stroke rate. But would this improve patient outcome? Maybe those patients should be segregated for medical therapy, or at least an alteration in surgical technique, so that aortic cannulation is not done in an area that could possibly "throw" emboli. That brings up the other major alteration: surgical technique may be altered to use fem-fem bypass or some other way if that is shown prospectively to decrease the rate of type I or focal neurologic deficits. The authors have another interesting way of looking at this, in that they looked at the excessive hospital stay and mortality of such patients. If you estimate charges of $890 for a day in an ICU and $370 for a day in a ward, then a type

I neurologic outcome costs $10,000 more per patient and a type II or cognitive deficit results in an additional $6,150 per patient.

If you do engage in a practice of cardiovascular anesthesia, or if you are about to do something that might be unhealthy, like not get therapy for your hypertension, not tightly treat your diabetes, excessively consume alcohol, or do any of the other things that each of us knows stimulates atherosclerosis, then you are commended to read this article. For me, immediately after reading the article, I decided to exercise so that I could decrease my risk of atherosclerosis and increase the possibility of avoiding both coronary artery bypass surgery and its potential consequences.

M.F. Roizen, M.D.

The Effect of Temperature Management During Cardiopulmonary Bypass on Neurologic and Neuropsychologic Outcomes in Patients Undergoing Coronary Revascularization

Mora CT, Henson MB, Weintraub WS, et al (Emory Univ, Atlanta, Ga; Univ of Western Ontario, London, Canada)

J Thorac Cardiovasc Surg 112:514–522, 1996 2–2

Background.—Hypothermia is the basis of organ protection during cardiopulmonary bypass surgery, especially for the heart and brain. In the 1990s, studies suggested that normothermic cardioplegia may improve myocardial protection. Since then, normothermic techniques have been widely used and evaluated in several studies. Findings indicate that normothermic cardioplegia provides acceptable myocardial protection, but there are conflicting results regarding associated neurologic outcomes. A study was undertaken to determine whether there is a higher rate of perioperative CNS complications in patients undergoing coronary revascularization with a systemic temperature maintained between 35°C and 37°C than in patients treated with hypothermic perfusion.

Methods.—There were 138 patients undergoing coronary revascularization who were randomly assigned to a normothermia (35°C or higher) or hypothermia (less than 28°C) treatment group. Neurologic and neuropsycholgical outcomes were used to determine CNS morbidity. Follow-up was 4 to 6 weeks.

Results.—Patients given normothermic treatment were older, had a lower incidence of pre-existing cerebrovascular disease, and had higher values for bypass blood glucose. Of the 68 patients in the normothermic group, 7 had a central neurologic deficit. Of the 70 patients in the hypothermic group, none had a central neurologic deficit. In more than 50% of all patients, neuropsychological test performance deteriorated immediately postoperatively. About 1 month postoperatively, this performance returned to preoperative levels in 85% of patients. This was unrelated to the method of temperature management.

Conclusion.—Normothermic temperature management of patients during coronary revascularization increases the risk of neurologic deficits.

Factors that may have contributed to these results include age, inclusion and risk criteria, and the strictly controlled study protocol. Patients undergoing cardiopulmonary bypass surgery should not be actively warmed to between 35°C and 37°C. The optimal temperature management technique for protecting the heart and the brain needs to be established.

▶ We went to hypothermic cardiopulmonary bypass to try to reduce the risk of neurologic dysfunction and also to try to give the surgeons a little more time if a mechanical disaster occurred in the operating room. Recent pressure to speed things up has pushed us back in the direction of normothermic operations. This paper concludes that our premise, namely, a moderate degree of cerebral protection with moderate hypothermia is probably still valid.

J.H. Tinker, M.D.

Neurological Outcome in Coronary Artery Surgery With and Without Cardiopulmonary Bypass

Malheiros SMF, Brucki SMD, Gabai AA, et al (Statistics Escola Paulista de Medicina, São Paulo, Brazil)

Acta Neurol Scand 92:256–260, 1995 2–3

Background.—Although CNS complications of coronary artery bypass graft (CABG) surgery have been attributed to the adverse effects of cardiopulmonary bypass (CPB), patients requiring CABG may have an intrinsically greater risk of neurologic injury. The frequency of neurologic and neuropsychological complications after CABG were compared in patients with and without CPB. In addition, the effects of preoperative, operative, and postoperative factors on these complications were analyzed.

Methods.—Eighty-one patients who underwent elective CABG, including 48 operated with CPB and 33 operated without CPB, were studied prospectively. Data on demographic features, risk factors for cerebrovascular disease, and pre-existent neurologic abnormalities were collected 3 days before surgery. Neuropsychological evaluation was repeated 5–7 days after surgery. The relationships between new neurologic and neuropsychological complications and demographic features, risk factors, and surgical factors were analyzed.

Results.—There were no differences between the CPB and no-CPB groups in sex, race, education, or potential risk factors for cerebral vascular disease. The 2 groups differed only in the median number of grafts (3 with CPB, 2 without CPB) and median total duration of surgery (300 minutes with CPB and 100.5 minutes without CPB). There were 5 perioperative deaths, 3 in the CPB group and 2 in the no-CPB group. Of the 76 patients with postoperative neurologic examinations, new abnormalities were observed in 35.6% of the CPB group and 38.7% of the no-CPB group, a nonsignificant difference. There were no correlations between neurologic abnormalities and the number of grafts or total surgical duration.

Conclusions.—Cardiopulmonary bypass does not appear to be the single cause of neurologic morbidity after CABG. It is likely that general and hemodynamic aspects of the surgery are more significant causes of postoperative neurologic and neuropsychological deficits.

► Coronary bypass can be done without cardiopulmonary bypass, even though it is a bit of a tour de force. The authors studied neurologic outcome, but the operation they used was, of necessity, a closed heart operation. Since the incidence of neurologic dysfunction is lower after closed heart surgery anyway, I am not sure what their results mean. I included the paper, if for no other reason, to inform our readers that coronary bypass can be done without cardiopulmonary bypass, however interesting that might be.

J.H. Tinker, M.D.

Stroke Rate Is Markedly Reduced After Carotid Endarterectomy by Avoidance of Protamine

Mauney MC, Buchanan SA, Lawrence WA, et al (Univ of Virginia, Charlottesville)

J Vasc Surg 22:264–270, 1995 2–4

Background.—Carotid endarterectomy (CEA) is now the most common peripheral vascular operation done in the United States. However, neurologic injury continues to be a significant risk associated with this procedure. Such injury results from embolization of debris and formation of thrombis on the newly endarterectomized surface. The risk of postoperative neurologic injury may be lower in patients not receiving protamine for heparin anticoagulation reversal.

Methods.—Three hundred forty-eight consecutive primary CEAs performed since 1986 were reviewed. Protamine had been given to 193 patients after surgery was completed.

Findings.—All patients survived to hospital discharge. The stroke rate among patients given protamine was 2.6%, compared with 0 in the patients receiving no protamine. One percent of the patients in the protamine group and 1.9% in the no-protamine group had hematoma requiring re-exploration. Intraoperative shunting was done in 84% of the patients not receiving protamine and in 67% of those receiving it. Patch angioplasty was done in 35% of the patients given protamine and in 15% of those not given it. However, stroke rates were not influenced significantly by shunting or patching.

Conclusions.—Carotid endarterectomy without reversal of heparin anticoagulation appears to be associated with a decreased stroke rate after surgery with no significant increase in morbidity. However, additional research involving greater numbers of patients from multiple centers is needed to verify these findings.

▶ For a long time, I was privileged to work with surgeons who were good enough to avoid protamine and who were also fast enough to have incredibly short carotid occlusion times. Out of the 2,000 carotid endarterectomies I gave anesthesia for, and looked for gross changes in CNS function, we only had 3 strokes. This remarkable record continued when I moved from UCSF to U of C. I always attributed the low stroke rate, of course, to great anesthesia, coupled of course with wonderful surgery. But now the truth comes out; both sets of surgeons I worked with avoided protamine. The difference of a 0% vs. 2.6% stroke rate in the protamine vs. nonprotamine group was just significant. Based on back-of-the-envelope power analysis, the difference between groups could be as small as 0.8% or as great as 7.5% (by my rough estimation of the 95% confidence intervals). In any case, this is an impressive difference that I hope gets tested in perhaps another study where there is random allocation. Is it ethical to do random allocation for such a study now? I believe so, as this was clearly an anecdotal study without random allocation and protamine may have been used for reasons that were associated with stroke and not causally related to stroke. In any case, I commend the authors for bringing up a potentially very important issue. It is clear now that the hypocoagulable state exists after surgery, and that a way of decreasing myocardial infarctions, deep vein thrombosis, and pulmonary emboli may be to begin low-dose low molecular weight heparin in the perioperative period. Thus, it has always made no sense to me to use protamine reversal of heparin toward the end of operations, just to start heparin 30 minutes later.

M.F. Roizen, M.D.

Atherosclerotic Disease of the Aortic Arch as a Risk Factor for Recurrent Ischemic Stroke

The French Study of Aortic Plaques in Stroke Group (Hôpital Saint-Antoine, Paris; Marie Curie Univ, Paris; Universitaire de Grenoble, Paris; et al)

N Engl J Med 334:1216–1221, 1996 2–5

Background.—Recent evidence indicates that atherosclerotic disease of the aortic arch may be a source of cerebral emboli. The risk for recurrent brain infarction and vascular events in patients with aortic arch plaques 4 mm thick or more was compared with the risk in patients with smaller or no plaques.

Methods.—A cohort of 331 patients aged 60 years or older was followed for 2 to 4 years. All patients had been hospitalized with brain infarction and had transesophageal echocardiography to search for atherosclerotic plaques in the aortic arch proximal to the ostium of the left subclavian artery. Three groups of patients were formed on the basis of the

TABLE 3.—Incidence of Events According to Plaque Thickness in the Aortic Arch Proximal to the Ostium of the Left Subclavian Artery

Plaque Thickness (mm)	Recurrent Brain Infarction			Any Vascular Event*		
	Person-Years of Follow-Up†	No. of Events	Incidence per 100 Person-Years of Follow-Up	Person-Years of Follow-Up†	No. of Events	Incidence per 100 Person-Years of Follow-Up
<1	359.3	10	2.8	354.0	21	5.9
1–3.9	312.6	11	3.5	308.2	28	9.1
≥4	92.4	11	11.9	88.4	23	26.0

*Includes brain infarction, myocardial infarction, peripheral embolism, and death from vascular causes.

†Differences between the total person-years of follow-up in each category of plaque thickness are due to censored data at the time of the first event.

(Courtesy of The French Study of Aortic Plaques in Stroke Group: Atherosclerotic disease of the aortic arch as a risk factor for recurrent ischemic stroke. *N Engl J Med* 334:1216–1221, 1996. Reprinted by permission of *The New England Journal of Medicine*. Copyright 1996, Massachusetts Medical Society.)

thickness of the aortic arch wall: less than 1 mm (group 1), 1 to 3.9 mm (group 2), and 4 mm or greater (group 3).

Findings.—Group 1 consisted of 143 patients; group 2, 143 patients; and group 3, 45 patients. The incidence of recurrent brain infarction was 2.8 per 100 person-years of follow-up in group 1, 3.5 per 100 person-years

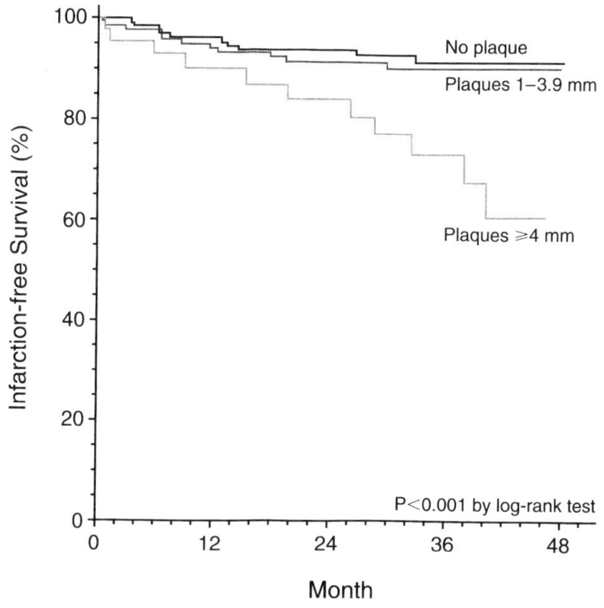

FIGURE 1.—Kaplan-Meier analysis of survival with recurrent brain infarction, according to plaque thickness in the aortic arch proximal to the ostium of the left subclavian artery. (Courtesy of The French Study of Aortic Plaques in Stroke Group: Atherosclerotic disease of the aortic arch as a risk factor for recurrent ischemic stroke. *N Engl J Med* 334:1216–1221, 1996. Reprinted by permission of *The New England Journal of Medicine*. Copyright 1996, Massachusetts Medical Society.)

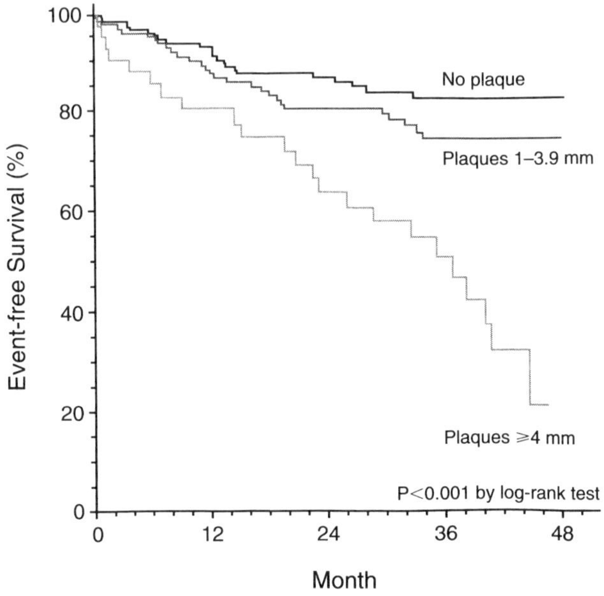

FIGURE 2.—Kaplan-Meier analysis of survival without vascular events (brain infarction, myocardial infarction, peripheral embolism, or death from vascular causes), according to plaque thickness in the aortic arch proximal to the ostium of the left subclavian artery. (Courtesy of The French Study of Aortic Plaques in Stroke Group: Atherosclerotic disease of the aortic arch as a risk factor for recurrent ischemic stroke. *N Engl J Med* 334:1216–1221, 1996. Reprinted by permission of *The New England Journal of Medicine*. Copyright 1996, Massachusetts Medical Society.)

of follow-up in group 2, and 11.9 per 100 person-years of follow-up in group 3. The overall incidence of vascular events in the 3 groups was 5.9, 9.1, and 26 per 100 person-years of follow-up, respectively. The presence of aortic plaques 4 mm thick or more independently predicted recurrent brain infarction and all vascular events after adjustment for carotid stenosis, atrial fibrillation, peripheral arterial disease, and other risk factors (Table 3; Figs 1 and 2).

Conclusions.—In patients who had had brain infarction and had plaques 4 mm thick or more in the aortic arch, the recurrence rate was 11.9 per 100 person-years of follow-up, and the incidence of all vascular events was 26 per 100 person-years of follow-up. These rates are among the highest in patients who had had ischemic stroke and were treated with antiplatelet drugs. The high risk for vascular events in the current series may have important implications for preventive treatment in patients 60 years of age or older who have plaques of 4 mm thick or greater in the aortic arch. The risks and benefits of treatment in such patients should be reassessed.

▶ The data presented in this article are intriguing and reaffirm the belief that most perioperative strokes that follow cardiopulmonary bypass are related to embolic phenomena. As our sophistication with transesophageal echocardiography improves, it may be quite possible for anesthesiologists to detect patients at risk for perioperative stroke before aortic cross-clamping. (This information might influence the surgical decision to perform coronary artery bypass grafting with an internal mammary artery so that aortic cross-clamping is avoided.)

D.M. Rothenberg, M.D.

Pulmonary Risks of Cardiovascular Surgery

Risk of Pulmonary Complications After Elective Abdominal Surgery
Lawrence VA, Dhanda R, Hilsenbeck SG, et al (Univ of Texas, San Antonio)
Chest 110:744–750, 1996 2–6

Objective.—Pulmonary complications are common after intra-abdominal operations but have not been as well studied as cardiac complications. Preoperative indicators of pulmonary risk were studied in a large cohort of patients undergoing elective abdominal operations using a nested case-control design.

Methods.—Between 1982 and 1991, 2,291 patients underwent elective abdominal operations. After validating the patients' charts, 82 patients with pulmonary complications and 82 control subjects remained. Of the 82 patients with pulmonary complications, 27 also had cardiac complications. Risk indicators for postoperative pulmonary complications were identified.

Results.—Pulmonary complications included respiratory failure (30%), pneumonia or possible pneumonia (47%), effusion (12%), tracheobronchitis (9%), and bronchospasm (2%). Eighteen patients with complications died. Eleven of those had both pulmonary and cardiac complications. Twenty of 37 patients with respiratory failure also had cardiac complications. Patients with complications had worse morbidity and smoking scores than control patients. Variables significantly associated with pulmonary complications included Charlson comorbidity index (odds ratio [OR] 2.0), abnormal lung examination results (OR 4.6), abnormal chest radiography (OR 23.2), and Goldman cardiac risk index (OR 1.5). There was no correlation between spirometry results, including obstructive lung disease, and postoperative pulmonary complications.

Conclusion.—Pulmonary and cardiac comorbidity, abnormal chest radiography, and abnormal lung examination results were preoperative risk factors for pulmonary complications after intra-abdominal surgery. Spirometry was not useful in predicting patients at risk. Additional research should prospectively address the incidence, outcomes, and risk factors for pulmonary and cardiac complications after intra-abdominal surgery.

▶ This is an interesting paper that suggests that spirometry is not helpful in the assessment of risk for pulmonary complications after elective abdominal surgery. Preoperative Assessment Clinic functions are presently undergoing reevaluation, and studies such as these help to define perioperative management strategies.

M. Wood, M.D.

The Association of Tracheal Anomalies and Tetralogy of Fallot

Kazim R, Quaegebeur JM, Sun LS (Columbia Univ, New York)
J Cardiothorac Vasc Anesth 10:589–592, 1996 2–7

Background.—Tetralogy of Fallot is the second most common congenital heart defect, and affected children also may have cyanosis. There are reports of congenital tracheal abnormalities in children with heart defects, including isolated cases of children with tetralogy of Fallot. Because of an experience with a pediatric patient who had tetralogy of Fallot with no preoperative evidence of airway pathology, but who had perioperative complications resulting from tracheal abnormalities, the incidence of tracheal anomalies in all children with tetralogy of Fallot at 1 institution was examined.

Methods.—The medical records of all children with tetralogy of Fallot who had primary or palliative cardiac surgery during a 3-year period were reviewed. Tracheal abnormalities were identified by direct laryngoscopic evidence, radiographic evidence, or inability to intubate the trachea with an endotracheal tube.

Results.—The records of 44 children were reviewed. Of these, 5 (11%) had tracheal anomalies. These were divided into 2 categories: isolated upper airway pathology (glottic or subglottic stenosis) and lower tracheal

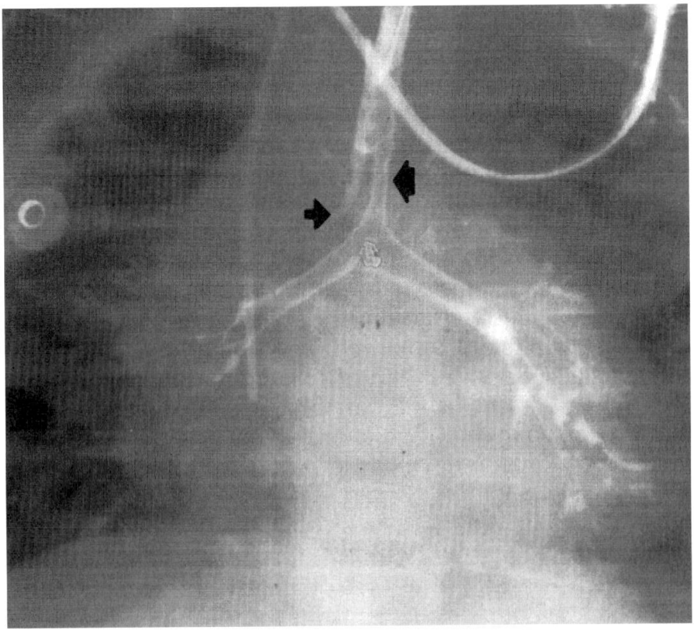

FIGURE 1.—*Case 1.* Tracheobronchogram through an endotracheal tube showing long segment tracheal stenosis (*bold arrow*) and accessory bronchus (*small arrow*). (Courtesy of Kazim R, Quaegebeur JM, Sun LS: The association of tracheal anomalies and tetralogy of Fallot. *J Cardiothorac Vasc Anesth* 10:589–592, 1996.)

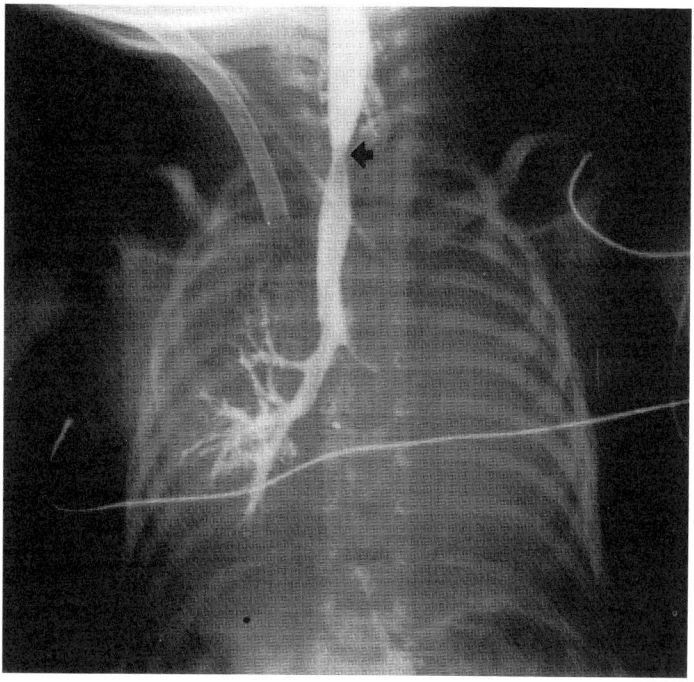

FIGURE 2.—*Case 2.* Unilateral tracheobronchogram showing a complete circular ring (*arrow*). (Courtesy of Kazim R, Quaegebeur JM, Sun LS: The association of tracheal anomalies and tetralogy of Fallot. *J Cardiothorac Vasc Anesth* 10:589–592, 1996.)

pathology. Of these 5 children, none had preoperative signs of airway problems. Four of the 5 children had significant perioperative complications from the underlying tracheal pathology. One patient had an accessory right bronchus and a long segment tracheal stenosis with complete circular rings (Fig 1). Another patient had become increasingly difficult to ventilate during postoperative intubation; tracheobronchography revealed 1 complete circular ring (Fig 2). The morbidity rate for patients with tetralogy of Fallot was 9%.

Conclusions.—There is a significant number of children with tetralogy of Fallot who have tracheal anomalies. Clinicians may have to use smaller endotracheal tubes when intubating these patients. If perioperative ventilation becomes difficult, CT scanning and rigid bronchoscopy should be used before extubation to evaluate for underlying tracheal pathology.

► I selected this article because, a few years ago, I encountered a few patients with tetralogy of Fallot who either had airway obstruction or required a smaller endotracheal tube for intubation of the trachea than we had anticipated. This review of children with tetralogy of Fallot provides an explanation.

M. Wood, M.D.

Value of Transesophageal Echocardiographic Evaluation

High Reproducibility in the Interpretation of Intraoperative Transesophageal Echocardiographic Evaluation of Aortic Atheromatous Disease

Hartman GS, Peterson J, Konstadt SN; et al (Cornell Univ, New York; Mount Sinai School of Medicine, New York)

Anesth Analg 82:539–543, 1996 2–8

Introduction.—Intraoperative treatment strategies are frequently based on the interpretation of transesophageal echocardiography (TEE) results. Determining interobserver variability of TEE findings is important. Interobserver variability for the interpretation of TEE results was evaluated in 3 experienced blinded observers.

Methods.—A total of 189 patients undergoing coronary artery bypass grafting had TEE examinations. A subset of 40 segments of TEE videotapes considered representative of a complete spectrum of aortic atheromatous disease were evaluated by the 3 blinded observers in real time. Freeze-frame and slow-motion review were not available to the observers. The observers were 2 anesthesiologists and 1 cardiologist from 2 separate institutions. Observers graded aortic atheromatous disease for the ascending aorta, aortic arch, and descending thoracic aorta.

Results.—Interobserver agreement was excellent for all 3 aortic segments.

Conclusion.—The high agreement in interpretation of TEE videotapes shows excellent reproducibility of TEE grading of aortic atheroma, particularly in the setting of 3 observers with different educational backgrounds. Findings suggest that TEE is an excellent tool for evaluating the thoracic aorta.

▶ This is a superb study that appears to be very well done. Those interested in aortic atheromata and echocardiographic detection of atheromatous disease should read this study.

M.F. Roizen, M.D.

Echocardiography for Assessing Cardiac Risk in Patients Having Noncardiac Surgery

Halm EA, for the Study of Perioperative Ischemia Research Group (Massachusetts Gen Hosp, Boston; Univ of California, San Francisco)

Ann Intern Med 125:433–441, 1996 2–9

Introduction.—Patients undergoing noncardiac operations sometimes have serious and potentially fatal cardiac complications. Several diagnostic tests have been proposed to assess cardiac risk before noncardiac surgery, including transthoracic echocardiography. However, the role of this preoperative test is still unclear. The prognostic value of echocardiography to assess cardiac risk in patients undergoing noncardiac surgery was evaluated.

Methods.—The prospective cohort study included 339 consecutive men at a VA medical center who were scheduled for major noncardiac surgery. All had known or suspected coronary artery disease. History, physical examination, ECG, and laboratory data were available on each patient. The echocardiograms were analyzed to determine the left ventricular systolic ejection fraction, any regional wall motion abnormalities, and left ventricular hypertrophy. After surgery, the patients were followed up for the occurrence of ischemic events, including cardiac death, nonfatal myocardial infarction, and unstable angina; congestive heart failure; and ventricular tachycardia. The prognostic value and operating characteristics of preoperative echocardiography were assessed.

Results.—Ischemic events occurred in 3% of patients, congestive heart failure in 8%, and ventricular tachycardia in 8%. None of the echocardiographic variables were significantly associated with ischemic events. Univariate analysis suggested that an ejection fraction of less than 40% increased the risk of all cardiac outcomes, of congestive heart failure, and of ventricular tachycardia. After multivariate analyses to adjust for clinical risk factors, ejection fraction still predicted all cardiac outcomes (odds ratio 2.5) but was not significantly associated with congestive heart failure or ventricular tachycardia. Wall motion score was also a risk factor for all cardiac events combined (odds ratio 1.3). An ejection fraction of less than 40% was 28% to 31% sensitive and 87% to 89% specific in predicting all types of adverse outcomes. However, its operating characteristics were poor. Echocardiography did not provide any clinically useful predictive information in addition to that supplied by clinical risk factors.

Conclusions.—Echocardiography is not useful in assessing the risk of cardiac complications in patients undergoing noncardiac surgery. It adds no predictive information to that provided by clinical risk models, and it performs poorly as a diagnostic test. Echocardiography should not be included in the cost-effective approach to cardiac risk assessment.

► The evaluation of cardiac risk in patients scheduled for surgery is difficult and screening can be costly.[1, 2]

If transesophageal echocardiography (TEE) is performed before surgery, how are the results going to alter the anesthesiologist's management of the patient, and if they do alter management, should they have altered management, and did that alteration improve outcome? A very simple question, but the strategy of diagnostic testing before elective surgery to assess cardiac risk has still not been clearly defined. Dennis Mangano and his group, who have performed extensive work in this area, determined in this cohort study that TEE has limited prognostic value in the setting of noncardiac surgery.

M. Wood, M.D.

References

1. Fleisher LA, Eagle KA: Screening for cardiac disease in patients having noncardiac surgery. *Ann Intern Med* 124:767–772, 1996.
2. Bodenheimer MM: Noncardiac surgery in the cardiac patient: What is the question? *Ann Intern Med* 124:763–766, 1996.

Risks/Outcome Issues in Cardiovascular Anesthesia/Surgery

Survival in Thoracic or Thoracoabdominal Aortic Aneurysm

Myrmel T, Robertsen S, Almdahl SM, et al (Univ Clinic, Tromsø, Norway)
Scand J Thorac Cardiovasc Surg 29:105–109, 1995 2–10

Background.—Practice guidelines for surgical treatment of thoracic aortic disease have been specified by the 4 principal cardiothoracic surgical societies in the United States. These guidelines address acceptable morbidity and mortality rates and relative contraindications to surgical therapy. The relative contraindication for surgical repair of thoracic aortic aneurysm is that the patient will not be able to recover from the procedure. At the study institution, the decision to operate is based on the surgeon's estimation of this risk. Morbidity and survival of patients who were treated by surgery and of those who were rejected for surgery were compared.

Methods.—The medical records of 69 patients with thoracic or thoracoabdominal aortic aneurysm were reviewed for extent of aortic disease, symptoms, treatment, outcome, and follow-up information. Patients were between 21 and 86 years of age. Patients were grouped according to site of aneurysm: ascending aorta, descending or thoracoabdominal aorta, or arch or complete aorta.

Results.—Surgery was performed in 22 patients and 47 patients were treated without surgery. In patients with ascending aortic aneurysm, surgical mortality was low. Surgical mortality was higher in patients with descending or thoracoabdominal aortic aneurysm. Of 20 patients with descending or thoracoabdominal aortic aneurysm who were treated without surgery, 15 died after a mean of 1.1 year. The only patient who had surgery for aortic arch aneurysm died of cerebral ischemia 2 days after the procedure. Most of the 19 patients with aneurysm of the arch or total aorta who did not have surgery were never considered for surgical treatment; the mean age of these patients was 76 years.

Discussion.—These findings support an aggressive approach in the treatment of ascending, descending, or thoracoabdominal aortic aneurysms. This is based on the low surgical mortality associated with ascending aortic aneurysm and the very poor prognosis for nonsurgical treatment of descending or thoracoabdominal aortic aneurysms. High-risk surgical intervention of aneurysm of the aortic arch or total aorta in older patients with complicating diseases is seldom indicated.

► This hospital study compared outcome of thoracic or thoracoabdominal aortic aneurysms with medical vs. surgical management. It should be noted that the majority of the 20 nonsurgically managed patients were not offered surgical repair. It is not clear why these offers were not made, other than perhaps the surgeons judged them too sick to undergo surgery. On average, they were approximately 20 years older than those operated upon. Thus, the high mortality of the nonoperated group may be because they had a high risk of dying of other diseases, not just their aneurysms. Fifteen of the 20 died during the follow-up of a little over 1 year, with 2 having malignant disease at presentation, and 10 being judged to be inoperable candidates. Perhaps the other interesting thing in this paper is the discussion of the practice guidelines in thoracic surgery by the 4 main cardiothoracic surgical societies. In those guidelines, one of the relative contraindications for thoracic aortic aneurysm repair is, "in the surgeon's judgment the patient is unable to recover from the surgical procedure." Furthermore, the guidelines specify that for this type of operation a 15% to 20% or lower mortality rate must be maintained to reveal a quality practice for nonruptured descending and thoracoabdominal aortic aneurysms.

Thus, this study is informative in teaching us something about the natural history of the disease, and in discussing the practice guidelines as they pertain to one hospital's practice of surgery.

M.F. Roizen, M.D.

Small, Oral Dose of Clonidine Reduces the Incidence of Intraoperative Myocardial Ischemia in Patients Having Vascular Surgery

Stühmeier K-D, Mainzer B, Cierpka J, et al (Institut für Klinische Anaesthesiologie, Düsseldorf, Germany)
Anesthesiology 85:706–712, 1996 2–11

Objective.—The ability of α-$_2$-adrenoceptor agonists to dilate coronary vessels and reduce the incidence of hypertension and tachycardia may make them an effective preventive of perioperative ischemic episodes in patients undergoing major noncoronary vascular surgery. The effect of a small oral dose of clonidine (2 µg/kg) in patients undergoing noncoronary vascular surgery in reducing the incidence of new intraoperative myocardial ischemic events without affecting hemodynamic stability was tested in a randomized, double-blind study.

Methods.—A total of 297 patients, aged 28 to 82, undergoing elective vascular surgery received either 2 µg/kg of oral clonidine (n=145, 44 women) or placebo (n=152, 47 women). There were 250 patients who completed the study. ST segment trends were monitored from pre-anesthetic preparation through surgery and were correlated. Arterial blood pressure, central venous pressure, and pulmonary artery pressure (in 34 patients) were recorded continuously. The incidence of perioperative myocardial ischemic episodes, myocardial infarction, and death were recorded. Hemodynamic patterns during ischemic events were analyzed and

TABLE 3.—Episodes of New Perioperative Myocardial Ischemia

Perioperative Period during Which Ischemic Episodes Were Observed	Clonidine (n = 145)	Placebo (n = 152)	P Value
No. of ischemic episodes	51	96	
Arrival	4 (3%)	11 (7%)	0.08
Anesthetic induction	2 (1%)	7 (5%)	0.1
Surgical stimulation	30 (21%)	48 (32%)	0.01
No. of episodes*	36	68	
Tracheal extubation	9 (6%)	10 (7%)	0.88

*During surgical stimulation.

(Courtesy of Stühmeier, K-D, Mainzer B, Cierpka, J, et al: Small, oral dose of clonidine reduces the incidence of intraoperative myocardial ischemia in patients having vascular surgery. *Anesthesiology* 85:706–712, 1996.)

correlated. Dose requirements for vasoactive and anti-ischemic drugs and amount of presurgical fluid volume were recorded.

Results.—There were 152 placebo patients and 145 clonidine patients. There were nonfatal myocardial infarctions in 4 placebo and 0 clonidine patients and cardiac deaths in 2 placebo and 1 clonidine patients. There were no differences in hemodynamic patterns, duration of ischemic episodes, or number of ischemic episodes. There was no difference between groups in the doses of vasoactive or anti-ischemic drugs required. Significantly fewer clonidine than placebo patients had new episodes of myocardial ischemia (Table 3). Clonidine patients received more preoperative fluid volume than did placebo patients (951 versus 867 mL). The incidence of myocardial ischemia for placebo patients was 41% for supra-aortic, 35% for aortic, and 41% for infra-aortic procedures, compared with 24%, 20%, and 29%, respectively, for clonidine patients.

Conclusion.—A small oral dose of clonidine administered during surgery to patients undergoing vascular surgery significantly reduces the incidence of perioperative myocardial ischemia without affecting hemodynamic variables.

▶ The incidence of intraoperative myocardial ischemia seems high in patients receiving placebo and not clonidine, but it must be recognized that patients who undergo vascular surgical procedures do experience a high incidence of perioperative ischemia. It is not clear whether an analysis was performed to determine how many patients should be studied to reliably achieve statistical significance. Studies such as this provide the impetus for large multicenter trials.

M. Wood, M.D.

Operative Mortality Rates After Elective Infrarenal Aortic Reconstructions

Huber TS, Harward TRS, Flynn TC, et al (Univ of Florida, Gainesville)
J Vasc Surg 22:287–294, 1995 2–12

Objective.—To determine the leading cause of death after elective infrarenal aortic reconstruction.

Background.—Previous studies of abdominal aortic reconstructions have reported that the leading cause of postoperative death was complications of coronary artery disease. Since then, cardiac testing has become an important preoperative procedure before aortic reconstruction. Recent reports have shown low cardiac mortality rates after elective vascular reconstruction, and suggestion has been made that these low rates may result from limited preoperative cardiac testing. Other reports have indicated mortality rates of 3% to 6%.

Methods.—Medical records were reviewed of all patients who had elective infrarenal aortic reconstructions between 1982 and 1994. The causes of perioperative death were determined. Findings were compared to findings from 266 survivors to identify risk factors for death.

Results.—Of 722 patients who had aortic reconstruction for aneurysmal or occlusive disease, 44 patients died. Mortality after aortic reconstruction alone was 4.9%, but increased to 8.9% after including renal procedures and to 15.8% after including lower extremity vascular procedures. The cause of death was multisystem organ failure in 56.8% of patients and cardiac events in 25% of patients. The most common cause of multisystem organ failure was visceral organ dysfunction in 56% of patients and postoperative pneumonia in 36% of patients. Risk factors associated with increased operative mortality were patient age, history of myocardial infarction or congestive heart failure, ejection fraction less than 50%, length of operation, and additional surgical procedures.

Conclusions.—The leading cause of death in these patients was multisystem organ failure, largely from visceral organ dysfunction. More complex procedures and a higher number of comorbid conditions are associated with increased risk of multisystem organ failure and operative death.

▶ The discussion appended to this paper is particularly enlightening. While the authors have maintained that with better perioperative care, the incidence of cardiac mortality is declining, Hollier points out in the discussion that this paper has similar incidence of cardiac death to those of many series, 1.5% to 2%. What is different in this series is the 4+% incidence of multisystem organ failure, which is usually around 0.5% in most other series. Hollier states that these must be much sicker populations or more difficult cases compared to the usual. I believe the answer is that either patients with serious comorbidities or poor quality of surgery makes multisystem organ failure more likely than cardiac to be the cause of death. Why, for instance, did these elective infrarenal aortic reconstructions average over 6.5 hours? Why was the cross clamp more than 1 hour? I think one has to be careful in interpreting surgical series like these to understand that the risk factors patients bring and the quality of surgery may not be similar between all series.

M.F. Roizen, M.D.

Predicting Respiratory Complications After Surgery on the Abdominal Aorta

Durand M, Combes P, Briot R, et al (CHU de Grenoble, France)
Can J Anaesth 42:1101–1107, 1995 2–13

Background.—Pulmonary function testing (PFT) and arterial blood gas (ABG) measurement often are done in patients scheduled for elective abdominal aortic reconstruction. However, the usefulness of these tests for assessing the risk of postoperative respiratory complications has not been shown. To further examine whether there is a link between preoperative pulmonary function and the risk of postoperative respiratory complications, a group of high-risk patients undergoing elective AA reconstruction were studied.

Patients.—The study population consisted of 195 patients (93.8% men) with a mean age of 65 years who had undergone PFT and ABG measurement in the month before operation. For each variable of PFT and ABG, receiver operating characteristic curves were constructed and the Youden index for each measured variable was calculated. All patients were operated on under general anesthesia and received mechanical ventilation until rewarming was complete and their hemodynamic status had stabilized.

Results.—Six patients (3%) died in the hospital. Surgical complications occurred in 8% of the patients, renal complications in 14%, cardiac complications in 13%, and respiratory complications in 15%. There was a weak but significant correlation between low vital capacity (VC) or low forced expiratory volume in 1 sec (FEV_1) values and length of stay in the cardiac ICU or length of stay in the hospital. The risk of respiratory complications was significantly increased in patients older than 75 years, but not in obese patients and not in smokers. Among patients with restrictive syndromes, the respiratory complication rate increased from 12% for a vital capacity of 77% or more of the predicted value to 35% for a vital capacity of less than 77%. Among those with obstructive syndromes, the respiratory complication rate increased from 10% for a FEV_1 76% or more of predicted value to 34% for a FEV_1 less than 76%. However, the sensitivity of the different variables in this analysis was low.

Conclusions.—Routine preoperative PFT and ABG measurement is not useful for predicting which patients are at increased risk of respiratory complications after an abdominal aortic repair.

► I wish I read French—the data tables from this article are still important and show many things: (1) more patients with low vital capacity and low FEV_1 have complications than if those are normal; (2) the partial pressure of carbon dioxide, arterial, and partial pressure of oxygen, arterial, are not useful predictors, and (3) the receiver operating characteristic curves were so bad as to render all tests useless. I only wish the authors had done a test such as pulse rate on 2-block walking, or something simple like that. Maybe they did, and we will have to wait for another report for it, or at least for someone who can translate French better than I can.

M.F. Roizen, M.D.

Meta-analysis of Randomised Trials Comparing Coronary Angioplasty With Bypass Surgery

Pocock SJ, Henderson RA, Rickards AF, et al (Wythenshawe Hosp, Manchester, England; Royal Brompton Hosp, London; Univ Hosp, Nottingham, England; et al)

Lancet 346:1184–1189, 1995 2–14

Background.—Interventional strategies based on an initial percutaneous coronary angioplasty (PTCA) or an initial coronary artery bypass graft (CABG) are clinically feasible for many patients with severe angina. The relative value of these 2 strategies has not been established. A meta-analysis of randomized trials comparing PTCA and CABG was performed.

Methods and Findings.—Eight published randomized studies were analyzed. A total of 3,371 patients, followed up for a mean of 2.7 years, were included in these studies. Seventy-three patients who underwent CABG died, compared with 79 who underwent PTCA. The relative risk was 1.08. Cardiac death and nonfatal myocardial infarction occurred in 169 patients who had PTCA and 154 who had CABG. Eighteen percent of the patients who were randomly assigned to PTCA needed CABG within 1 year. In subsequent years, the need for additional CABG procedures was about 2% a year. Additional interventions in the first year of follow-up also were needed in 33.7% of the patients who received PTCA and 3.3% of those who received CABG. After 1 year, patients who underwent PTCA had a substantially greater prevalence of angina than those who underwent CABG, but this difference had attenuated at 3 years. Overall, the outcomes in all 8 trials were very similar. When the 732 patients with single-vessel disease and the 2,639 with multivessel disease were analyzed separately, the results were largely consistent, although mortality, additional intervention rates, and prevalence of angina were slightly lower in patients with single-vessel disease.

Conclusions.—Intermediate-term risks of death and myocardial infarction were comparable in patients randomly assigned to undergo PTCA or CABG. However, the requirement for additional revascularization procedures and symptomatic relief during 3 years differed significantly. Further research is needed to determine the longer-term effects of these 2 strategies on clinical outcome.

▶ Anesthesiologists frequently treat patients requiring emergency cardiac surgery who have undergone coronary angioplasty. What should a patient with severe angina choose, angioplasty or bypass revascularization? The CABRI trial is 1 of several studies comparing PTCA and CABG in the treatment of multivessel coronary artery disease; 2 are from the United States. Preliminary findings suggest that symptomatic relief and a reduced incidence of subsequent events is improved when patients are treated with primary surgery. The CABRI trial results show that for symptomatic patients with multivessel coronary disease, both surgery and angioplasty relieve angina at an equivalent risk of death or myocardial infarction. However, patients undergoing PTCA are more likely to require repeated intervention and are more likely to have clinically important angina at 1 year. Females appear to be at higher risk for 1-year mortality and, when randomly assigned to undergo PTCA, are more likely to have angina at 1 year than are males randomly assigned to undergo CABG or PTCA.

The meta-analysis of randomized trials attempts to define the relative merits of PTCA versus CABG based on an analysis of published findings from 9 randomized trials. It is important to recognize that these trials have published only early findings; of interest are mortality, myocardial infarction, additional interventions, and symptoms of angina during follow-up. Do these results apply to all patients equally? What about subgroups such as females, the elderly, or diabetics? Diabetic patients may have a higher mortality rate with PTCA than CABG, and may be more likely to show recurrent stenosis after angioplasty. Other factors not considered in these trials are complications of CABG, such as stroke, cerebral microemboli, and possible need for blood transfusions. Many of these trials were started more than 5 years ago, and we would like to think that anesthetic techniques have improved, so that the results may not be applicable to 1997. In addition, angioplasty has changed, and we have seen rapid advances in stent technology. These trials will influence the future choice of CABG or PTCA, and in the long term will have a major influence on anesthetic practice.

M. Wood, M.D.

Association Between Prior Cytomegalovirus Infection and the Risk of Restenosis After Coronary Atherectomy

Zhou YF, Leon MB, Waclawiw MA, et al (Natl Heart, Lung and Blood Inst, Bethesda, Md; Washington Hosp, Washington, DC)
N Engl J Med 335:624–630, 1996 2–15

Purpose.—As many as 50% of patients undergoing coronary angioplasty experience restenosis. The mechanisms by which restenosis develops are unclear. A recent study found cytomegalovirus (CMV) DNA in restenotic lesions from atherectomy specimens, suggesting that CMV might play a role in the development of restenosis. Latent CMV may be locally reactivated in response to vascular injury in some patients undergoing coronary angioplasty. The possible link between CMV and restenosis was assessed in a prospective study.

Methods.—Seventy-five consecutive patients with symptomatic coronary artery disease who were scheduled for direction coronary atherectomy were studied. Anti-CMV IgG antibodies were measured before atherectomy in all patients. Six months later, coronary angiography was performed to determine whether restenosis had occurred.

Results.—The results of CMV antibody testing were positive in 49 patients and negative in 26. The mean minimal luminal diameter in the treated vessel was 3.18 mm in seropositive patients vs. 2.89 mm in seronegative patients. Six months later, the reduction in luminal diameter was 1.24 mm in the seropositive group and 0.68 mm in the seronegative group. The restenosis rates were 43% in the seropositive group and 8% in the negative group. Multivariate analysis showed that CMV seropositivity and CMV titer were independently associated with restenosis, with odds ratios of 12.9 and 8.1, respectively. Neither group of patients had evidence of acute CMV infection.

Conclusions.—Previous exposure to CMV is a major risk factor for the development of restenosis after coronary atherectomy. If the results are confirmed by further studies, CMV antibody testing may become a useful method of predicting patients' risk of restenosis. This knowledge may be useful in deciding whether to perform atherectomy or coronary artery bypass grafting. If CMV proves to be a cause of restenosis, then preventive antiviral treatment strategies could be developed.

▶ This article brings up that old clever editorial question, "Are all diseases infectious?" Well, clearly we are learning about slow viruses and "Prions" and other causes of neurologic and other dysfunctions that are relatively infectious. But, restenosis after coronary artery bypass grafting or after angioplasty? Yes, it appears so from the study.

Perhaps most dramatic is the quote, "Of the 49 patients with prior exposure to CMV, 21 (43%) had restenosis at 6 months, as compared with only 2 of the 26 patients (8%) without prior exposure to the virus." Thus, the mechanism by which angioplasty physicians may try to decrease their restenosis rate in the future may be to exclude patients who have had prior CMV infection. How can CMV cause this? Again, the present study does not answer that issue, but CMV (DNA sequences) include expression of IE84, one of the virus' immediate early proteins. IE84 binds to and inhibits p53 tumor-suppressor gene products. These effects may enhance the proliferation of smooth muscle cells or inhibit apoptosis, either of which can contribute to restenosis. The present work provides evidence that prior exposure to CMV as indicated by the presence of long-standing CMV antibodies is a strong independent risk factor for restenosis. Should we be routinely measuring such an infection, or such past infection because 1 of 3 or more patients have had this infection in their life? Or if the patient is about to have a vascular anastomosis as in coronary artery bypass grafting or vascular procedures? Well, clearly, if this study is borne out, with knowledge based on results of a simple standard blood test (given that patients have less than a 10% of restenosis if they are seronegative or a 40% chance if they are seropositive), such patients might undergo different procedures or be maintained by medical management.

M.F. Roizen, M.D.

Atrial Fibrillation Following Coronary Artery Bypass Graft Surgery: Predictors, Outcomes, and Resource Utilization

Mathew JP, Parks R, Savino JS, et al (Yale Univ, New Haven, Conn; Ischemia Research and Education Found, San Francisco; Univ of Pennsylvania, Philadelphia; et al)

JAMA 276:300–306, 1996 2–16

Background.—Atrial fibrillation and flutter are common after CABG surgery. Postoperative AFIB results in greater use of resources by extending the patient's hospital stay. Atrial fibrillation and flutter after CABG surgery is associated with a higher rate of postoperative stroke, ventricular arrhythmias, and need for a pacemaker. A prospective, observational study was done to determine the incidence and predictors of postoperative atrial fibrillation and flutter (AFIB) in patients who have had coronary artery bypass graft (CABG) surgery, and to study the effects of postoperative AFIB on outcome and use of resources.

Methods.—During a 2-year period, 2,417 patients participated, with a minimum of 100 patients from each of 24 hospitals. Data on each patient were obtained before, during, and after CABG surgery, with or without valvular surgery. Predictors of AFIB were calculated, and outcomes were assessed.

Results.—The overall rate of postoperative AFIB was 27%. Independent predictors of postoperative AFIB included older age, male sex, history of AFIB, history of congestive heart failure, and a precardiopulmonary bypass heart rate of more than 100 beats per minute. Prebypass use of β-blocking agents was independently associated with a lower rate of postoperative AFIB. Surgical practices that were independent predictors of postoperative AFIB were pulmonary vein venting, bicaval venous cannulation, postoperative atrial pacing, and longer cross-clamp times. Patients with postoperative AFIB were in the ICU 13 hours longer and in the hospital 2.6 days longer than those without postoperative AFIB. Those with postoperative AFIB had a higher risk of having postoperative congestive heart failure, renal insufficiency, infection, and minor and major neurologic injury develop.

Conclusions.—Patients at higher risk of postoperative AFIB included those with a history of postoperative AFIB and patients who had concurrent valvular surgery. Certain surgical practices also were associated with a higher risk. Because use of resources is greater in patients with postoperative AFIB and its complications, it should be determined whether changing these surgical practices would lower the risk of postoperative AFIB.

► In identifying risk factors for AFIB after CABG surgery, the task of appropriately preventing this complication must be addressed. Better preoperative management either with more judicious use of β-adrenergic blockade or with elective cardioversion may be indicated. Closer attention to perioperative magnesium levels and the more frequent use of magnesium replacement may also aid in limiting postoperative AFIB. Bringing back the old-fashioned premedicant, scopolamine, to augment perioperative amnesia may also be of benefit. Although this may delay the "fast track" approach to postoperative recovery, perhaps 1 additional day in the ICU may negate the 2 additional days spent in the hospital from AFIB.

I also am curious as to the nature of the anesthetic techniques used at the 24 various institutions (my own notwithstanding) and question whether lower intraoperative doses of opiates may have contributed to higher catecholamine states postoperatively. Finally, it would be interesting to assess whether the preoperative use of the central α-adrenergic antagonist clonidine (an agent that has been effective in treating AFIB) minimized the occurrence of this dysrhythmia.

D.M. Rothenberg, M.D.

Risks/Outcome Issues in Imaging/Screening

Adenosine Radionuclide Perfusion Imaging in the Preoperative Evaluation of Patients Undergoing Peripheral Vascular Surgery

Marshall ES, Raichlen JS, Forman S, et al (Thomas Jefferson Univ, Philadelphia)

Am J Cardiol 76:817–821, 1995 2–17

Background.—Risk of acute myocardial infarction (AMI) is increased in patients undergoing peripheral vascular surgery, partly because of the high incidence of coronary artery disease in this population. Adenosine radionuclide perfusion (ARP) imaging is a sensitive and specific indicator of coronary artery disease; its utility in determining cardiac risk in patients requiring peripheral vascular surgery was studied.

Findings.—In 122 patients, ARP imaging was done before elective peripheral vascular surgery. Coronary revascularization was done in 5 patients before the peripheral vascular surgery. Among the other 117 patients, 19 instances of pulmonary edema, 10 of AMI, and 2 deaths occurred after surgery. Only history of congestive heart failure was predictive for perioperative pulmonary edema, and no clinical variables were predictive for AMI or death. With multivariate analysis, the only adenosine variable predictive of ischemic events was the number of reversible perfusion defects (increased frequency of ischemic events was associated with the presence of more than 1 reversible defect). By univariate analysis, the number of coronary artery distributions with a radionuclide perfusion defect was also a predictor of AMI and death.

Conclusions.—According to these data, (1) perioperative pulmonary edema may be predicted by a history of congestive heart failure, and (2) identification of patients at risk for a perioperative ischemic event can be aided by noting the presence or absence of multiple reversible defects on ARP imaging.

▶ This study provides further evidence that congestive heart failure and the number of reversible perfusion defects are useful information to find out preoperatively in patients with vascular problems who have 1 or more of the classic 5 problems preoperatively—diabetes, previous history of an AMI, congestive heart failure, angina, or Q waves on ECG. Although there are no new data in this article, it is another piece of information that confirms what we thought we knew.

M.F. Roizen, M.D.

Risk/Outcome Issues with Various Therapies

Multicenter Study of Target-controlled Infusion of Propofol-Sufentanil or Sufentanil-Midazolam for Coronary Artery Bypass Graft Surgery

Jain U, for the Multicenter Study of Perioperative Ischemia (McSPI) Research Group (Univ of California, San Francisco; Harvard Med School, Boston; Med College of Virginia, Richmond; et al)

Anesthesiology 85:522–535, 1996 2–18

Introduction.—Target-controlled infusion of anesthesia in coronary artery bypass graft (CABG) surgery has not been investigated extensively. The cardiovascular responses of 2 anesthetic regimens using target-controlled infusions of propofol or sufentanil with supplementation of sufentanil or midazolam infusion, respectively, were evaluated.

Methods.—A total of 329 patients at 14 clinical sites were given a target-controlled infusion of either propofol-sufentanil or sufentanil-midazolam. Heart rate and blood pressure were assessed at every minute throughout. A 3-lead continuous Holter ECG was used perioperatively and transesophageal echocardiography was used during surgery to assess myocardial ischemia.

Results.—The measured cardiovascular parameters were similarly satisfactory in both patient groups. There was no between-group difference in the percentage of patients with intraoperative ST segment deviation. The incidence of left ventricular wall motion abnormality detected by transesophageal echocardiography before and after cardiopulmonary bypass did not differ significantly between groups. In the propofol-sufentanil anesthetic group, the changes in intraoperative target concentration were more frequent, compared to the sufentanil-midazolam group. The incidence of intraoperative hypotension and use of inotropic/vasopressor medications and administration of crystalloids was significantly higher in the propofol-sufentanil group. The incidence of intraoperative hypertension and use of antihypertensive/vasodilator medications was significantly less in the propofol-sufentanil group, compared to the sufentanil-midazolam group.

Conclusions.—Target-controlled infusions of propofol or sufentanil, supplemented by infusions of sufentanil or midazolam, respectively, were appropriate for CABG surgery. The occurrence of systolic hypertension, hypotension, tachycardia, and bradycardia was common. Hypotension occurred more frequently in the propofol-sufentanil group and hypertension was more common in the sufentanil-midazolam group. There was no significant between-group difference for the primary end point, which was the percentage of patients having intraoperative ST segment depression or elevation.

► Cardiac anesthesia traditionally used a "high-dose" opioid (originally morphine and then fentanyl) technique. When propofol was introduced into clinical anesthetic practice, the cardiovascular effects were considered equivalent to thiopental and, therefore, propofol initially was not administered to patients with severe cardiovascular disease. How our philosophy has changed! Fast-track cardiac anesthesia is now in vogue. This is a fascinating study and compares what have become 2 standard anesthetic regimens for CABG surgery. The results are not surprising, but they are important.

M. Wood, M.D.

Effect of Diuretic-based Antihypertensive Treatment on Cardiovascular Disease Risk in Older Diabetic Patients With Isolated Systolic Hypertension

Curb JD, for the Systolic Hypertension in the Elderly Program Cooperative Research Group (John A Burns School of Medicine, Honolulu, Hawaii; Univ of Texas, Houston; Natl Heart, Lung and Blood Inst, Bethesda, Md; et al)

JAMA 276:1886–1892, 1996 2–19

Introduction.—Oral diuretics given to control elevated blood pressure (BP) reduce cardiovascular morbidity and mortality, but also cause adverse effects. Among the undesirable effects of diuretic treatment are increases in blood glucose, total cholesterol, and low-density lipoprotein cholesterol levels. The effect of low-dose, diuretic-based antihypertensive treatment on cardiovascular disease (CVD) risk in older, non–insulin-treated diabetic patients with isolated systolic hypertension (ISH) was assessed in a multicenter, randomized trial.

Methods.—The double-blind trial, the Systolic Hypertension in the Elderly Program (SHEP), enrolled men and women aged 60 and older who had ISH at baseline. The study group included 583 patients with non–insulin-dependent diabetes and 4,149 patients without diabetes. Those randomly assigned to active treatment received a low dose of chlorthalidone (12.5 to 25.0 mg/day) with a step-up to atenolol (25.0 to 50.0 mg/day) or reserpine (0.05 to 0.10 mg/day) if needed. Patients in the placebo group took placebo and any active antihypertensive drugs prescribed by their private physicians for persistently high BP. The primary end point in SHEP was nonfatal plus fatal stroke. Also recorded were 5-year rates of major CVD events, nonfatal myocardial infarction, fatal coronary heart disease (CHD), major CHD events, and all-cause mortality.

Results.—The 4 patient subgroups (active treatment, placebo, diabetic, and nondiabetic) were generally comparable in baseline characteristics and adherence to the study regimen. Both diabetic and nondiabetic patients had BP lowered with the SHEP antihypertensive drug regimen, and all outcome rates were lower for the active treatment group than for the placebo group. The 5-year major CVD rate was 34% lower for active treatment compared with placebo, and this effect was seen in both diabetic and nondiabetic patients. Reflecting the higher CVD risk of diabetic patients, the absolute risk reduction with active treatment was twice as great for diabetic patients as for nondiabetic patients. No adverse effects were associated with the antihypertensive regimen.

Discussion.—The SHEP low-dose antihypertensive treatment, with chlorthalidone as the step-1 drug, substantially reduced the 5-year relative risk and absolute risk of nonfatal and fatal CVD events in older, diabetic and nondiabetic men and women with ISH. These positive effects were not negated by any adverse effects of treatment, a finding that contrasts with a recent report suggesting an excess mortality among diabetic patients who received diuretic therapy for hypertension.

► This article reports on studies examining the benefits and risks of treating systolic hypertension in the elderly. Perhaps one of the most important things to come out of all the recent epidemiologic studies on hypertension and the massive Intersalt Trial across many countries is that systolic hypertension is as great a risk as diastolic hypertension for the development of arterial aging or arterial disease. These data reveal that a systolic BP elevation of 6 mm Hg is equivalent to a 4-mm Hg diastolic rise in terms of the rate of development of arterial disease. Thus, a systolic BP of 145 mm Hg is as risky as a diastolic BP of 96 mm Hg. In the excellent Veterans Administration (VA) studies, and 10 other studies that have studied men aged 53 at the start of the trials, diastolic BPs in the range of 95 to 100 mm Hg, if left untreated, resulted in greater than 55% rate of morbidity within 5 years that was reduced by two thirds with treatment to normalize diastolic pressures. Of course, the systolic pressures also were normalized by treatment in that regimen.

This study of systolic hypertension in the elderly tries to do the same type of research, but with ISH. The average diastolic BP of patients in this study was below 80 mm Hg; in fact, it was near the ideal for longevity at the start of the study, around 75 to 77 mm Hg. However, the systolic pressures were around 170 mm Hg in all 4 groups, which included persons with diabetes in active treatment and placebo groups, and persons without diabetes in active treatment and placebo groups. The treatment with a diuretic in these patients was randomized and well followed. For example, after 4 years, 91% of both diabetic and nondiabetic participants randomized to the intervention group were still receiving the active antihypertensive drug, chlorthalidone. On the other hand, of those randomized to the placebo group, 54% of diabetic patients and 39% of nondiabetic patients were receiving no active antihypertensive drug at year 4. The other medication that was added tended to be atenolol in both groups. The authors summarize the significant findings into 4 areas for older, non–insulin-treated diabetics and nondiabetic men and women with ISH: the reduction in risk over a 5-year period went from 3.5% for cardiovascular events in the placebo group of diabetics vs. 21.4% in the active treatment group and 18.4% in the placebo nondiabetic treatment group vs. 13.3%. Although this still shows that there is a sizable benefit to the treatment of ISH, it is only 20% of the risk or benefit in 5 years of treatment of both systolic and diastolic hypertension combined in the DVA studies. Part of that failing may clearly be the lack of success in treatment; the average reduction in systolic hypertension under treatment was 9.8 mm Hg in systolic pressure and 2.2 mm Hg in diastolic pressure for diabetic patients, compared to 12.5 and 4.1 mm Hg, respectively, for nondiabetics. This is obviously considerably less than the degree of reduction in the VA studies of treatment of moderate systolic and diastolic hypertension. Thus, in preoperative visits with such patients, it is important to consider consultation with the patients and their primary care physicians about more aggressive treatment, not only in the perioperative period but life long, because their morbidity and mortality rates without treatment are considerably greater than the benefits of most surgical interventions. That is, the benefits of treatment of their systolic hypertension may be greater than the benefits of treatment of their surgical interventions. As anesthesiologists, we have this high-risk time in the perioperative period and heightened concentration on health care to influence them positively, and I think we should take that opportunity.

M.F. Roizen, M.D.

Catecholamine and Cortisol Responses to Lower Extremity Revascularization: Correlation With Outcome Variables

Parker SD, Breslow MJ, Frank SM, et al (Johns Hopkins Med Insts, Baltimore, Md; Med College of Wisconsin-St Luke's Med Ctr, Milwaukee)

Crit Care Med 23:1954–1961, 1995 — 2–20

Introduction.—It has been hypothesized that regional anesthetic techniques reduce perioperative complications. Proof of this does not exist. The inclusion of postoperative physiologic data in the analysis of this question may provide the answer. Epidural anesthesia/epidural fentanyl analgesia and general anesthesia/intravenous morphine analgesia were compared in patients undergoing lower extremity revascularization to evaluate the relationships between perioperative hormonal responses and postoperative complications.

Methods.—Sixty patients were randomly allocated to receive either epidural or general anesthesia. Increases or decreases in heart rate and blood pressure were first treated conservatively before more aggressive hemodynamic drugs were used. Blood was drawn for plasma epinephrine, norepinephrine, and plasminogen activator inhibitor-1 concentrations, and urine was collected for free cortisol concentrations at appropriate intervals in the intraoperative and postoperative periods. Nonfatal myocardial infarction, cardiac death, and graft occlusion were the outcomes analyzed.

Results.—Complete data was available on 57 of 60 patients. Epinephrine and norepinephrine remained at preinduction concentrations intraoperatively until skin closure. At this time, these levels increased to twice basal concentrations in the general anesthesia group, but not the epidural group. Postoperatively, norepinephrine remained higher in the general anesthesia group than in the epidural group. During emergence from anesthesia, epinephrine was higher in the general anesthesia group. Positive correlation existed between plasma norepinephrine concentration and arterial pressure during emergence from anesthesia. Patients with postoperative hypertension had higher plasma catecholamine concentrations. Plasma norepinephrine was significantly higher in patients undergoing reoperation for graft revision, thromboectomy, or amputation. Emergence norepinephrine was associated with reoperation for graft occlusion. Anesthetic regimen was not associated with reoperation for graft occlusion. Seventeen patients with increased preoperative plasminogen activator inhibitor-1 concentrations had markedly higher secretion of intraoperative cortisol. In the postoperative period, norephinephrine concentrations were higher in patients with increasing plasminogen activator inhibitor-1 concentrations than in patients in whom plasminogen activator inhibitor-1 concentrations did not increase. Three patients were lost to early cardiac morbidity. These patients had markedly increased epinephrine and norepinephrine concentrations throughout the perioperative period.

Conclusion.—Findings suggest that increases in plasma catecholamine values are related to postoperative hypertension, vascular graft occlusion, alterations in fibrinolysis, and morbid cardiac events. Reduced frequency of hypertension occurred in the early postoperative period in patients with epidural anesthesia. Further investigation should consider whether modulation of the hormonal response to surgery would be able to alter the frequency of perioperative complications.

▶ This is an important study, if only because it confirms the later reports of ours, for example Benefiel et al.[1] that are not quoted in this paper. Even if you are not quoted, it is nice to find out the defined confirmation of your earlier hypothesis and study results.

M.F. Roizen, M.D.

Reference

1. Benefiel, et al: Anesthesiology 1987.

3 Perioperative Patient Care Issues

Obstetrical Anesthesia Issues

Comparison of a Trial of Labor With an Elective Second Cesarean Section

McMahon MJ, Luther ER, Bowes WA Jr, et al (Univ of North Carolina, Chapel Hill; Dalhousie Univ, Halifax, NS, Canada)

N Engl J Med 335:689–695, 1996 3–1

Background.—Approximately 50% of cesarean section deliveries in the United States and Canada are performed only to avoid labor after a previous cesarean section. Several conferences have concluded, however, that vaginal delivery can be safe for women who have had a previous low-transverse cesarean section. A population-based, longitudinal study determined how morbidity and mortality associated with a trial of labor compared with that of an elective cesarean section.

Methods.—Study data were obtained from records of the Reproductive Care Program of Nova Scotia, Canada. From 1986 through 1992, a total of 6,457 women who delivered a live singleton infant had previously undergone 1 cesarean section; 6,138 met eligibility requirements. Of these women, 3,249 attempted vaginal delivery after a previous low-transverse cesarean section and 2,889 elected to undergo a second cesarean section. These 2 groups were compared for demographic and maternal characteristics and the type and incidence of complications.

Results.—Women more likely to attempt a trial of labor were either 19 years of age or younger or 30 years or older, had a previous vaginal delivery in addition to a cesarean section, and had attended prenatal classes. The perinatal mortality rate was 5 per 1,000 live births in the elective cesarean section group and 9 per 1,000 in the trial of labor group. There were no maternal deaths. Complications occurred in 8.1% of women and were major in 1.3%. The trial of labor group was 1.8 times more likely to have major complications but 20% less likely to have minor complications. Risk of puerperal fever was 25% higher in the elective cesarean group. Of those who underwent a trial of labor, vaginal delivery was accomplished in 60.4%; women 35 years or older were less likely than younger women to have a successful trial of labor.

Discussion.—Major maternal complications are almost twice as likely among women who undergo a trial of labor after a previous cesarean section than among those who have a second cesarean section. Morbidity is greatest when the trial is unsuccessful and a second cesarean section is required. Apgar scores, admissions to the neonatal ICU, and perinatal mortality were similar among infants in the trial of labor and second cesarean section groups.

▶ During the last 2 decades, many obstetricians have strongly encouraged women with a history of previous low transverse cesarean section to undergo a trial of labor in a subsequent pregnancy. Some third-party payers have withheld reimbursement for patients who did not attempt vaginal birth after cesarean section. The present study brings some balance to this discussion. Surprisingly, only 60% of the women who underwent a trial of labor had a vaginal delivery. This is a lower success rate than that reported in previous studies, and it likely affected the results in the present study. The authors correctly noted that "the way to decrease the overall risk entailed by a trial of labor. . . is by selecting women who have a high probability (perhaps more than 80%) of delivering their babies vaginally." Unfortunately, there is no proven method of identifying those women who are most likely to have a successful trial of labor.

D.H. Chestnut, M.D.

Toward Fewer Cesarean Sections: The Role of a Trial of Labor
Paul RH (Univ of Southern California, Los Angeles)
N Engl J Med 335:735–736, 1996 3–2

Background.—Reducing the high rate of cesarean section requires decreasing the number of elective operations performed by increasing the frequency of a trial of labor. New information about the risks and benefits of a trial of labor in women who have had a cesarean section was provided in a recent study by McMahon et al.

Editorial.—In the study by McMahon et al., a large number of pregnant women who had previously had 1 cesarean section chose a trial of labor or elective cesarean section. Outcomes were compared in the 2 groups. In both groups, complications were rare and none of the mothers died. However, the overall rate of major complications (1.3%), defined as the need for hysterectomy, uterine rupture, or operative injury, was twice as high in the trial-of-labor group than in the elective cesarean group. On the other hand, the authors' definition of major complications could be challenged. Perinatal outcomes were also similar in the 2 groups. However, 2 of the perinatal deaths occurred after uterine rupture in women in the trial-of-labor group and thus were associated with the trial of labor. Whether the rates of major and minor maternal complications and perinatal mortality varied according to hospital type would be interesting to know.

Conclusions.—Reducing the rate of cesarean section is a worthwhile goal. Ultimately, this reduction must be achieved by decreasing the rate of both first and subsequent elective cesarean sections.

► I have heard anecdotal reports that some third-party payers now require all pregnant women with a history of a low-transverse cesarean section to undergo a trial of labor in a subsequent pregnancy. The present study reminds us that although a trial of labor after previous cesarean section is safe for most patients, it may not be the best choice for all patients. Hopefully, obstetricians will develop methods to identify those patients who are most likely to have a successful vaginal birth after cesarean section. It is also important that obstetricians identify those patients for whom elective repeat cesarean section is the best choice.

D.H. Chestnut, M.D.

Alkalinization of Lidocaine 2% Does Not Influence the Quality of Epidural Anaesthesia for Elective Caesarean Section

Gaggero G, Meyer O, van Gessel E, et al (Univ Hosp of Geneva)

Can J Anaesth 42:1080–1084, 1995 3–3

Background.—Several factors have been shown to affect onset, duration, and quality of epidural anesthesia, including local anesthetic dose, volume and concentration of solutions, and additives. Some researchers have reported that alkalinization of local anesthetic solutions are associated with a faster onset and better quality of sensory and motor blocks, whereas other studies have found no advantage of alkalinization over plain solutions. Because the timing of alkalinization of the local anesthetic had not been addressed, a double-blind randomized trial compared the effects of an epidural injection of lidocaine hydrochloride 2% (HCl) and alkalinized lidocaine 2% injected immediately or 1 hour after preparation.

Methods.—Forty-five parturients scheduled for elective cesarean section were included. Fifteen were injected with HCl 2% (group 1); 15 with alkalinized lidocaine 2%, 1 mL $NaHCO_3$ per 10 mL of solution, immediately after preparation (group 2); and 15 with alkalinized lidocaine 2%, 1 mL $NaHCO_3$ per 10 mL of solution 1 hour after preparation (group 3). The total dose was 16 mL in each patient.

Findings.—Mean pH values measured just before epidural injection were 6.77, 7.34, and 7.35 in groups 1, 2, and 3, respectively. Median maximal sensory level was T_3 in group 1, obtained at 19 minutes; T_4 in group 2, obtained at 18 minutes; and T_4 in group 3, obtained at 16 minutes. Eleven group 1 patients, 10 group 2 patients, and 14 group 3 patients achieved a motor block of grade 2 or 3 on the Bromage scale. There were no failures, but 3 patients in group 1, 5 in group 2, and 2 in group 3 needed a supplementary bolus 20 minutes after the initial injection because of inadequate sensory level or pain at the surgical site.

Conclusions.—In women undergoing elective cesarean section, neither onset nor quality of epidural anesthesia are influenced by the timing of lidocaine 2% alkalinization. Findings were comparable in women receiving solutions alkalinized immediately or 1 hour before injection.

▶ The title of this study is curious, given that the authors did not specifically evaluate quality of analgesia. Rather, they reported sensory levels over time, and they also reported the number of patients who required supplemental bolus injections of local anesthetic.

The authors did not explain why they administered solutions of lidocaine *without* epinephrine. In my experience, the addition of epinephrine to the lidocaine enhances the quality of analgesia, increases the likelihood of success, and decreases the risk of systemic local anesthetic toxicity. Unlike other local anesthetics, the addition of epinephrine to lidocaine enhances analgesia quality and patient safety.

D.H. Chestnut, M.D.

Prospective Examination of Epidural Catheter Insertion

D'Angelo R, Berkebile BL, Gerancher JC (Forsyth Mem Hosp, Winston-Salem, NC)

Anesthesiology 84:88–93, 1996 3–4

Background.—Epidural catheter insertion-related complications reportedly are reduced when catheters are inserted 3 to 4 cm into the epidural space. Prospective, randomized studies investigating epidural insertion lengths have not, however, been conducted. The effects of catheter insertion length on insertion-related complications and the efficacy of epidural catheter manipulation in providing analgesia for labor and delivery were prospectively evaluated in this randomized study.

Patients and Methods.—Eight hundred women in active labor who had requested epidural anesthesia were included in the study. Two hundred patients each were randomly assigned to epidural catheter insertion lengths of 2, 4, 6, or 8 cm. Any occurrences of IV cannulation, unilateral sensory analgesia, and catheter dislodgment were documented. To evaluate the efficacy of catheter manipulation, insertions that resulted in IV cannulation or unilateral analgesia were incrementally withdrawn and retested with subsequently administered local anesthetic.

Results.—Intravenous cannulation was more likely to occur in patients who had epidural catheters inserted 8 cm within the epidural space. In patients with catheters inserted 2 cm within the epidural space, unilateral sensory analgesia was less likely to occur, although catheters tended to become dislodged more often. Of the catheters inserted more than 2 cm within the epidural space, 23% required manipulation. Catheter replacement was required more often in patients who had catheters inserted 2 to 4 cm, compared with those whose catheters were inserted 6 or 8 cm. Of the catheter insertions that resulted in unilateral sensory analgesia and IV

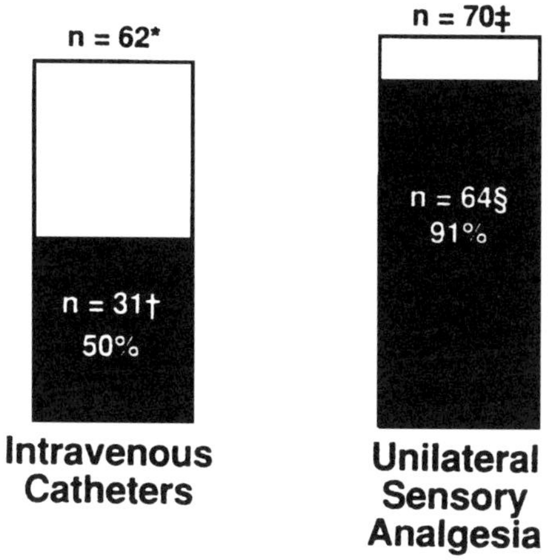

FIGURE 1.—Epidural catheters associated with intravenous cannulation or unilateral sensory analgesia. *Total number of intravenous catheters. †Intravenous catheters that functioned well after manipulation. ‡Total number of epidural catheters inserted more than 2 cm associated with unilateral sensory analgesia. §Epidural catheters associated with unilateral sensory analgesia that functioned well after manipulation. (Courtesy of D'Angelo R, Berkebile BL, Gerancher JC: Prospective examination of epidural catheter insertion. *Anesthesiology* 84:88–93, 1996.)

cannulation, 91% and 50% provided analgesia for labor and delivery after incremental withdrawal (Fig 1).

Conclusions.—Although no optimal insertion length was identified in this study, epidural catheters inserted 2 cm within the epidural space reduce the risk of IV cannulation and unilateral sensory analgesia. These catheters do, however, dislodge significantly more often than those inserted more than 2 cm, particularly during prolonged labor. Therefore, 2 cm insertions may provide better results during rapid labor. Conversely, 6 cm catheter insertions may be best used during prolonged labor, or in patients at increased risk for cesarean delivery. The 6-cm insertion length does reduce the risk of IV cannulation, although unilateral sensory analgesia may be experienced more frequently, and catheter manipulation and replacement may be necessary. Catheter insertions that do result in IV cannulation or unilateral sensory analgesia can, however, be manipulated effectively to provide analgesia for labor and delivery.

▶ I recommend this excellent clinical study to all anesthesiologists who provide care for obstetric patients. The authors evaluated outcome in a large population of patients. The conclusions are sound, and the recommendations are practical. In my practice, I remain reluctant to insert an epidural catheter only 2 cm, even when rapid labor is anticipated. I insert the catheter approximately 3 cm when rapid labor is anticipated. I insert the epidural catheter approximately 5 cm in patients in whom prolonged labor is expected or cesarean section is likely. Finally, I insert the epidural catheter approximately 5 to 6 cm in obese patients.

D.H. Chestnut, M.D.

Epidural Infusion of Low-dose Bupivacaine and Opioid In Labour: Does Reducing Motor Block Increase the Spontaneous Delivery Rate?

Russell R, Reynolds F (St Thomas' Hosp, London)
Anaesthesia 51:266–273, 1996 3–5

Background.—Epidural infusions of plain local anesthetic provide good pain relief during labor but result in unacceptably dense motor blockade and poor rates of spontaneous delivery. Adding opioids to the infusions reduces the concentration of local anesthetic needed and subsequent motor block. Such infusions can be continued throughout the second stage of labor with no increase in instrumental deliveries. Epidural infusions containing plain 0.125% bupivacaine were compared with those of a less concentrated bupivacaine solution supplemented with opioids in a controlled, randomized trial.

Methods.—Three hundred ninety-nine women in labor were randomly assigned to epidural infusions of plain bupivacaine or to 0.0625% bupivacaine combined with 2.5 $\mu g \cdot ml^{-1}$ fentanyl or 0.25 $\mu g \cdot ml^{-1}$ sufentanil, initially at 12 $mL \cdot h^{-i}$ and adjusted as needed to maintain analgesia. Hourly and total doses of bupivacaine were significantly lower in patients given the combination infusions.

Findings.—Patients receiving combination infusions had a significantly lower incidence of motor block. Motor block was also significantly less severe in this group. These decreases did not result in a significant increase of spontaneous deliveries. Women given the combination infusions were significantly more satisfied with first and second stage analgesia than those given plain bupivacaine. However, the addition of opioid to the infusion did not decrease the incidence of perineal pain. The 2 groups had similar neonatal outcomes and incidences of early postnatal symptoms.

Conclusions.—Low-dose bupivacaine combined with fentanyl or sufentanil epidural infusions during labor appear to be as effective as more concentrated solutions of bupivacaine only. Combination infusion is associated with reductions in the incidence and severity of motor block. In addition, maternal satisfaction with analgesia is greater with the combination infusion, and the number of spontaneous deliveries is not reduced.

▶ In an earlier study done at the University of Iowa, we observed that the continuous epidural infusion of 0.0625% bupivacaine/0.0002% fentanyl resulted in less motor block, but did not result in an increased incidence of spontaneous vaginal delivery, when compared with the continuous epidural infusion of 0.125% bupivacaine alone.[1] Decreased motor block is itself a desirable outcome, and this result may provide sufficient justification for the epidural administration of more dilute solutions of local anesthetic during labor. However, anesthesiologists and obstetricians should not automatically conclude that this will result in an increased likelihood of spontaneous vaginal delivery.

D.H. Chestnut, M.D.

Reference

1. Chestnut DH, Owen CL, Bates JN, et al: Continuous infusion epidural analgesia during labor: A randomized double blind comparison of 0.0625% bupivacaine/ 0.0002% fentanyl versus 0.125% bupivacaine. *Anesthesiology* 68:754–759, 1988.

Epidural Morphine vs Hydromorphone in Post–Caesarean Section Patients

Halpern SH, Arellano R, Preston R, et al (Women's College Hosp, Toronto; Univ of Toronto)

Can J Anaesth 43:595–598, 1996 3–6

Background.—Epidural morphine provides excellent analgesia for pain after cesarean section, but it also causes troubling side effects such as pruritis, nausea, and vomiting. Epidural hydromorphone appears to be an equally effective analgesic with a similar duration of action in nonobstetric patients, and may have fewer side effects. The analgesic effectiveness and side effects of epidural morphine and hydromorphone after cesarean section were compared.

Methods.—Participating in the double-blind study were 46 women undergoing elective cesarean section and receiving epidural anesthesia with incremental doses of carbonated lidocaine 2% with 1:200,000 epinephrine and 50 μg of fentanyl. After the infants were delivered, patients were randomly assigned to receive either 0.6 mg of hydromorphone (group 1,

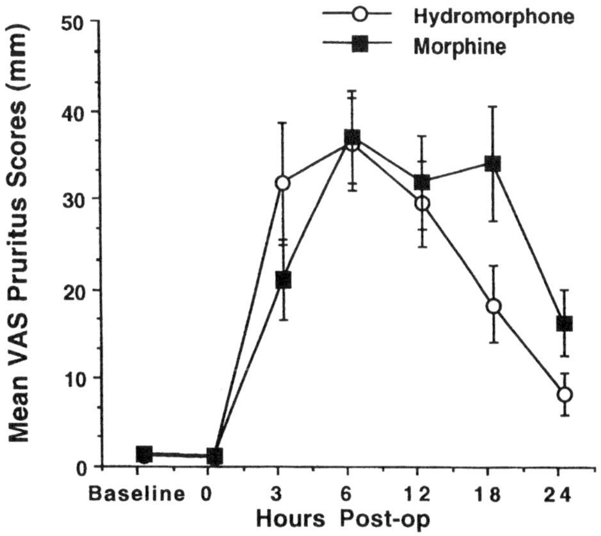

FIGURE 1.—Visual analogue scale (*VAS*) scores for pruritis. Values expressed as mean ± SEM. (Courtesy of Halpern SH, Arellano R, Preston R, et al: Epidural morphine vs. hydromorphone in post-caesarean section patients. *Can J Anaesth* 42:595–598, 1996.)

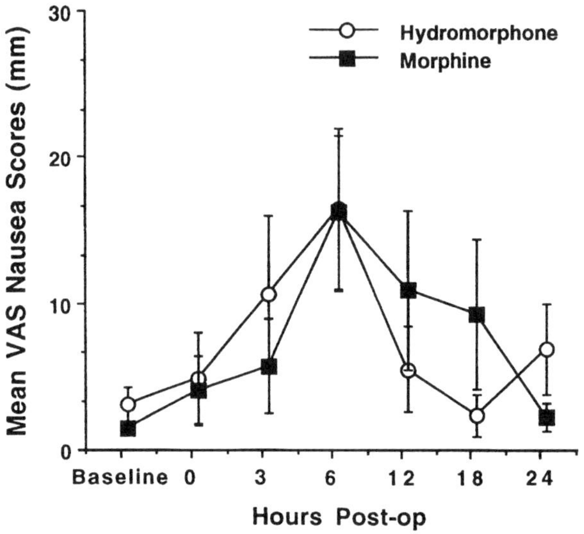

FIGURE 2.—Visual analogue scale (*VAS*) scores for nausea. Values expressed as mean ± SEM. (Courtesy of Halpern SH, Arellano R, Preston R, et al: Epidural morphine vs. hydromorphone in post-caesarean section patients. *Can J Anaesth* 42:595–598, 1996.)

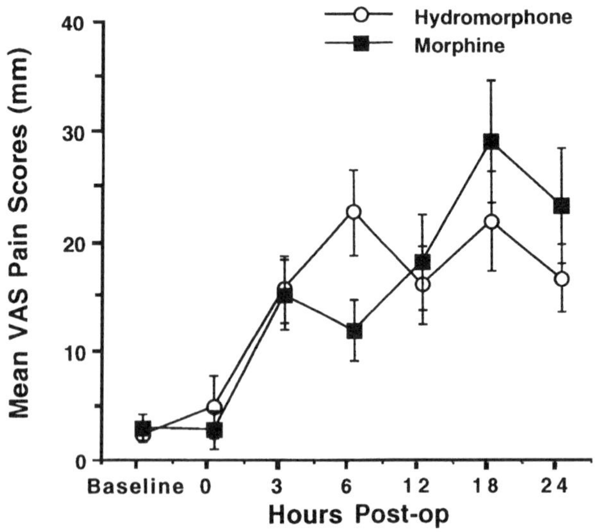

FIGURE 3.—Visual analogue scale (*VAS*) scores for pain. Values expressed as mean ± SEM. (Courtesy of Halpern SH, Arellano R, Preston R, et al: Epidural morphine vs. hydromorphone in post-caesarean section patients. *Can J Anaesth* 42:595–598, 1996.)

24 patients) or 3 mg of morphine (group 2, 22 patients). Pain, pruritis, and nausea were measured by visual analogue score, requests for additional medication, and overall satisfaction score.

Results.—Visual analogue scores for pruritis (Fig 1), nausea (Fig 2), and pain (Fig 3) did not differ significantly between groups. No significant differences between groups were found for pain relief or side-effect severity. Within the first group, pruritis was most pronounced within the first 6 hours, whereas within the second group it was most pronounced at 18 hours.

Conclusions.—After cesarean section, substitution of epidural hydromorphone for epidural morphine does not affect the incidence and severity of pruritis, nor does it affect the severity of nausea or the level of analgesia. Hence, hydromorphone appears to offer no clinical benefit over morphine for epidural postoperative analgesia after cesarean section.

► A decade ago, we evaluated the epidural administration of 1.0 mg of hydromorphone for postcesarean analgesia.[1] In that study, we did not compare the efficacy and side effects of epidural hydromorphone vs. epidural morphine. However, it was our clinical impression that epidural hydromorphone resulted in fewer side effects than an equipotent dose of epidural morphine. In this study, there was no difference between groups in the incidence or severity of side effects. This suggests that our clinical impression was incorrect. The doses used in this study (i.e., 0.6 mg of hydromorphone and 3.0 mg of morphine) reflect the trend toward smaller doses of epidural opioids administered for postcesarean analgesia.

D.H. Chestnut, M.D.

Reference

1. Chestnut DH, Choi WW, Isbell TJ: Epidural hydromorphone for postcesarean analgesia. *Obstet Gynecol* 68:65, 1986.

Patient-controlled Extradural Analgesia With Bupivacaine, Fentanyl, or a Mixture of Both, After Caesarean Section

Cooper DW, Ryall DM, McHardy FE, et al (South Cleveland Hosp, Middlesbrough, England)

Br J Anaesth 76:611–615, 1996 3–7

Background.—It is unclear whether adding bupivacaine to fentanyl is beneficial in postoperative extradural analgesia. The efficacy of combining extradural bupivacaine with extradural fentanyl in patient-controlled extradural analgesia (PCEA) after cesarean delivery was investigated.

Methods.—Sixty women scheduled for elective cesarean section while receiving extradural analgesia were included in the study. All had American Society of Anesthesiologists Status I to II. By random assignment, patients received 0.1% bupivacaine (group B), fentanyl 4 μg mL^{-1} (group F), or combined 0.05% bupivacaine and fentanyl 2 μg mL^{-1} (group BF).

Findings.—Adding fentanyl to bupivacaine decreased the dose of bupivacaine by as much as 68%. Analgesia at rest was also improved, and PCEA use was reduced. Motor and sensory block were also lessened in the combination group, but more pruritus occurred. Patient satisfaction was improved. The addition of bupivacaine decreased the fentanyl dose by as much as 57% without changing pain scores or PCEA use. There was an increase in sensory block but no reduction in pruritis. In 3 patients, bupivacaine 0.05% was associated with clinically significant leg weakness. Overall, patient satisfaction was unaffected.

Conclusions.—An additive analgesic effect exists between extradural 0.05% bupivacaine and fentanyl. However, the combination of these drugs was no more beneficial clinically than fentanyl alone. The clinical benefits of this combination may be more evident in patients who do not ambulate early.

► In this study, the addition of 0.05% bupivacaine to fentanyl resulted in inability to walk in 53% of the patients in that group, without enhancing analgesia. Parturients are at increased risk for deep vein thrombosis and pulmonary thromboembolism during the postpartum period. Also, because women need to provide care for their newborn infants, it is important that epidural analgesia not interfere with early ambulation during the puerperium.

D.H. Chestnut, M.D.

Pulmonary Function Changes During Epidural Anesthesia for Cesarean Delivery

Yun E, Topulos GP, Body SC, et al (Harvard Med School, Boston)

Anesth Analg 82:750–753, 1996 3–8

Background.—The pulmonary function changes that occur during pregnancy have been well documented, but the superimposed effects of regional anesthesia on these changes have not been studied. Changes in results of pulmonary function tests in parturients undergoing elective cesarean delivery with 0.5% bupivacaine or 2% lidocaine with epinephrine were investigated.

Methods.—Nineteen women of American Society of Anesthesiologists physical status I were included in the randomized, double-blind trial. A calibrated spirometer with computer-recorded flow volume loops was used to measure pulmonary function test results. Several variables were measured before epidural placement and at the T-10 and T-4 levels.

Findings.—Neither group showed changes from baseline peak inspiratory pressure, forced expiratory volume in 1 s (FEV_1)/forced vital capacity, FEV_1, forced vital capacity, peak expiratory flow rate, or peak inspiratory flow rate. Patients given lidocaine had a significantly greater reduction in peak expiratory pressure at the T-10 and T-4 levels.

Conclusions.—Peak expiratory pressure was not affected by bupivacaine in these patients, possibly because this agent provides a less dense motor block. Thus, bupivacaine may be a better choice for women with preexisting pulmonary disease undergoing cesarean delivery.

▶ When administering epidural anesthesia for elective cesarean section, I prefer to use 2% lidocaine with epinephrine for most patients. Heretofore, I have used 0.5% bupivacaine only for patients in whom a slower onset of block is desired (e.g., women with preeclampsia). The present study suggests another possible indication for use of 0.5% bupivacaine—namely, for parturients with preexisting pulmonary disease.

D.H. Chestnut, M.D.

A Double-blind Comparison of 0.25% Ropivacaine and 0.25% Bupivacaine for Extradural Analgesia in Labour

Eddleston JM, Holland JJ, Griffin RP, et al (Manchester Royal Infirmary, Oxford, England; St Thomas' Hosp, London; Freeman Hosp, Newcastle Upon Tyne, England; et al)

Br J Anaesth 76:66–71, 1996 3–9

Background.—Ropivacaine, a new aminoamide local anesthetic, has a greater threshold for systemic toxicity than bupivacaine. It also has a high selectivity for sensory fibers. Thus, ropivacaine was hypothesized to be superior to bupivacaine in obstetric analgesia.

Methods and Findings.—By random assignment, 104 parturients requesting extradural analgesia received ropivacaine or bupivacaine, 0.25%. More top-up doses of bupivacaine were needed to maintain analgesia. However, the 2 groups were similar in onset of sensory block, quality of analgesia, ultimate level of maximum sensory block, and patient satisfaction. Women receiving ropivacaine had a slightly, nonsignificantly increased incidence, intensity, and duration of motor block. The incidence of spontaneous vaginal delivery was greater in the patients given ropivacaine. Neonatal outcomes were similar in both groups.

Conclusions.—Ropivacaine and bupivacaine in concentrations of 0.25% were equally effective in relieving pain during labor. Neither anesthetic adversely affected neonatal outcomes.

▶ These authors found similar analgesia in the 2 groups. They noted 2 benefits in the ropivacaine group. First, the ropivacaine group required fewer top-up doses to maintain analgesia. Second, women in the ropivacaine group were more likely to have spontaneous vaginal delivery. It is unclear whether or not these results can be extrapolated to current clinical practice in the United States. Most anesthesiologists administer analgesia by giving a more diluted solution of bupivacaine through continuous epidural infusion. It has been a long time since I maintained epidural analgesia during labor using only bolus doses of 0.25% bupivacaine.

D.H. Chestnut, M.D.

Effect of Epidural Analgesia on Fundal Dominance During Spontaneous Active-phase Nulliparous Labor

Nielsen PE, Abouleish E, Meyer BA, et al (Univ of Texas, Houston; State Univ of New York, Stony Brook)

Anesthesiology 84:540–544, 1996 3–10

Background.—The effects of epidural analgesia on the physiologic mechanisms of labor have not been investigated thoroughly. The question of whether epidural anesthesia established during active labor eliminates or reverses fundal dominance was studied.

Methods.—Eleven nulliparous women in spontaneous active labor were enrolled in the prospective study. Upper and lower uterine segment intrauterine pressures were assessed for 50 minutes before and 50 minutes after the epidural administration of 0.25% bupivacaine. Data on 958 contractions were analyzed.

Findings.—The number of contractions before epidural analgesia did not significantly differ from the number after epidural analgesia. Pressure readings in the upper segment were significantly greater than in the lower segment, consistent with fundal dominance, before and after analgesia. Fundal dominance after epidural analgesia was increased compared with the preanalgesia period.

Conclusions.—Patients in spontaneous active labor apparently have no elimination or reversal of intrauterine pressure 50 minutes after epidural analgesia. Evidence of fundal dominance was seen before and after analgesia in this study. Immediately after analgesia administration, fundal dominance was increased.

▶ Fundal dominance was first described by Reynolds and colleagues as "a gradient of diminishing physiologic uterine contractile activity from the fundus to the lower uterine segment."[1] The authors of this article observed significantly greater intrauterine pressure measurements in the upper uterine segment than in the lower uterine segment before and after administration of epidural analgesia in 11 nulliparous women. Further, the authors observed a significant increase in fundal dominance after administration of epidural analgesia. This increase resulted from a greater increase in upper uterine segment pressures—compared to lower uterine segment pressures—after administration of epidural analgesia. No patient "lost" fundal dominance during the 50 minutes after administration of epidural analgesia.

Unfortunately, the authors did not assess obstetric outcome, and they evaluated intrauterine pressures in a small group of patients. Further, they did not include a control group of women who did not receive epidural analgesia. Is it possible that women not exposed to epidural analgesia may experience an even greater increase in fundal dominance than that observed in the present study? Finally, the authors limited their study to women in active-phase labor. In the present study, the mean cervical dilation at the time of administration of epidural analgesia was 5.6 cm. Most of the current debate relates to the effect of epidural analgesia administered during latent-phase.

D.H. Chestnut, M.D.

Reference

1. Reynolds SRM, Hellman LM, Bruns P: Patterns of uterine contractility in women during pregnancy. *Obstet Gynecol Surv* 3:629–645, 1948.

Single Bolus Compared With a Fractionated Dose Injection Technique of Bupivacaine for Extradural Caesarean Section: Effect on Uteroplacental and Fetal Haemodynamic State

Karinen J, Mäkäräinen L, Alahuhta S, et al (Oulu Univ Hosp, Finland)
Br J Anaesth 77:140–144, 1996 3–11

Background.—Bupivacaine in fractionated doses is routinely used to induce extradural block in patients undergoing cesarean section, but onset of surgical anesthesia is slow. Delivery of a single bolus dose via either needle or catheter may speed up the onset of sensory block for use in emergency situations. Using a color Doppler technique, the effects of a single bolus vs. a fractionated dose of bupivacaine on maternal uterine and fetal umbilical artery blood flow velocity waveforms were assessed in a randomized, double-blind fashion.

Methods.—Twenty-six healthy parturients undergoing elective cesarean section at term participated. The women received extradural block with 0.5% plain bupivacaine: first a 3-mL test dose, then 20 mL given as either a single bolus (over 5 minutes) or a fractionated dose (over 25 minutes). Pulsed color Doppler was used to measure blood flow velocities in the maternal placenta and nonplacental uterine and fetal umbilical arteries before extradural block and 4 times during its establishment.

Results.—In the bolus group, median sensory block reached T3; in the fractionated-dose group, T4. Intravenous ephedrine was required to correct a systolic arterial pressure below 90 mm Hg in 2 patients in each group. No significant difference between groups was noted in blood flow velocity waveform indices of the uterine and umbilical arteries. Neonatal outcome, as assessed by umbilical artery pH values and Apgar scores, also did not differ significantly between groups.

Conclusions.—Administration of a single-bolus dose of bupivacaine did not result in deterioration of the uteroplacental circulation. Local anesthetics must be given with care; accidental intravascular or intrathecal injection of local anesthetic may result in toxic maternal and fetal plasma concentrations or total spinal anesthesia.

► The title of this article is misleading. The authors did not administer a single-bolus dose of bupivacaine. In the single-dose group, the authors administered 20 mL of 0.5% bupivacaine over 5 minutes. (This occurred 4 minutes after administration of a 3-mL test dose.) Regardless, it is unclear why anyone would want to establish epidural anesthesia in this manner. Unintentional IV injection of a large dose of bupivacaine may result in disaster. If one wants to establish epidural anesthesia quickly, it is preferable to use 2-chloroprocaine, which has a faster onset and is less likely to result in systemic toxicity.

D.H. Chestnut, M.D.

Epidural Opioids in Labour Introduce More Problems Than They Solve

Reynolds F (St Thomas' Hosp, London)

Int J Obstet Anesth 5:54–58, 1996 3–12

Introduction.—When opiate receptors were discovered in the substania gelatinosa of the spinal cord and brain, it was hoped that intrathecal and epidural administration of opioids would produce long-lasting analgesia without side effects because the agonist would be placed close to its receptor. This was not true. The problems and advantages of epidural opioids in labor were reviewed.

Problems.—Administration of epidural and intrathecal morphine for postoperative pain relief is accompanied by significant side effects, such as itching, nausea, somnolence, urinary retention, and respiratory depression. The occurrence of respiratory depression is of particular concern during labor. Intrathecal surentanil has provided significant analgesia at a dose of 10 μg. A bolus of fentanyl, 80–150 μg epidurally, in combination with local anesthetic produces analgesia in labor, but provides analgesia that lasts only marginally longer than bupivacaine alone. Patients may have nausea, vomiting, leg weakness, hypotension, pruritis, and drowsiness with fentanyl and bupivacaine. The use of pethidine can delay gastric emptying. Opiate infusions have been correlated with episodes of maternal hemoglobin desaturation. Epidural opioids in labor have introduced a new side effect, pruritis, and may include the risks of neurotoxicity and neonatal depression.

Controversies.—The addition of opioids to epidural infusions of bupivacaine provides better analgesia. The dose of bupivacaine can be reduced by half when fentanyl or sufentanil are added and can thus decrease the incidence of motor block. Yet, there has not been a reduction in the instrumental delivery rate as a result of this approach. Some investigations suggest that reduced motor power contributes to postnatal backache. A prospective randomized trial found that the incidence of postpartum backache is not significantly different between groups of women receiving epidural or no epidural anesthesia.

Advantages.—Epidural opioids can give a better quality of analgesia, including faster onset, longer duration, and alleviation of perineal pain. They can also be used to lower the dose of local anesthetics, which decrease the risk of systemic toxicity and lower the degree of motor block. In theory, lowering the degree of motor blockage reduces the need for instrumental delivery. The addition of opioids may also decrease the incidence and severity of shivering precipitated by epidural local anesthetics.

Conclusion.—Epidural opioids in labor are associated with significant side effects. Their use, in theory, may help reduce the problems caused by motor blockage when local anesthetics are used alone, but this has not been proved. The maternal and neonatal problems associated with epidural opioids may not justify their use.

▶ Some anesthesiologists believe that successful epidural analgesia during labor requires the addition of an opioid to the solution of local anesthetic. I disagree. Dr. Reynolds has provided a succinct discussion of the disadvantages of epidural opioids during labor. I should like to add another disadvantage not included in her review; namely, epidural opioids may confound the anesthesiologist's efforts to confirm the optimal placement of the epidural catheter within the epidural space. Systemic absorption of fentanyl will provide some analgesia, even in those cases where the epidural catheter is not positioned correctly within the epidural space. In contrast, bupivacaine will not provide pain relief unless the epidural catheter is positioned within the neuraxis. I avoid epidural opioids in those patients in whom I want to be absolutely certain of the position of the epidural catheter.

D.H. Chestnut, M.D.

Epidurals Redefined in Analgesia and Anesthesia: A Distinction With a Difference

Youngstrom PC, Baker SW, Miller JL (Kaiser Found Health Plan, Cleveland, Ohio; Ohio State Univ, Columbus)

J Obstet Gynecol Neonatal Nurs 25(4):350–354, 1996 3–13

Background.—An improved understanding of pain has led to a new, meaningful distinction between epidural analgesia and anesthesia. The principles underlying this distinction in the management of labor pain were discussed.

Epidural Anesthesia.—Collateral effects on motor and autonomic transmission, which account for the adverse effects of epidural anesthesia in the management of labor pain, cannot be avoided when intense sensory input is blocked at the spinal level with local anesthetic alone. Sacral spinal segment blockade becomes progressively more dense with time, and repeated doses from lumbar epidural anesthesia, which results in pelvic autonomic transmission interruption and subsequently interferes with normal bladder function, makes catheterization necessary in many women. Furthermore, normal progress in labor relies on the conveyance of sensory inputs along pelvic parasympathetic afferents. The blockade of pelvic autonomics also interrupts the automatic intensification of uterine expulsive activity. Stopping epidural anesthesia late in labor may help restore the bearing down reflex, but this also results in a return of severe pain.

Epidural Analgesia.—With epidural analgesia, the neural pain stimuli processing mechanisms are tempered, mainly through manipulation of spinal opiate and α-adrenergic receptors. Potent analgesia can be provided by this method while minimizing the indiscriminate motor and autonomic effects of local anesthetics. Usually, the local anesthetic component in epidural analgesic regimens is bupivacaine. Doses can be reduced significantly through the use of an ultra–low-dose regimen in which fentanyl and epinephrine replace much of the bupivacaine. This combination results in spinally mediated analgesia of better quality and duration than that resulting from either agent alone.

Conclusions.—An appreciation of the analgesia/anesthesia distinction in epidural therapy allows new opportunities and flexibility in labor pain management. The need for anesthesia is based on the need for surgical intervention; it is not the preceding choice of labor analgesia.

► For many years I have argued that epidural analgesia is not a generic procedure. These authors correctly call attention to the analgesia/anesthesia distinction in epidural therapy. Unfortunately, it is unclear that ultra–low-dose epidural analgesia provides satisfactory pain relief during labor in all parturients.

D.H. Chestnut, M.D.

Epidural Analgesia for Labour and Delivery: Fentanyl or Sufentanil?

Cohen S, Amar D, Pantuck CB, et al (Albert Einstein College of Medicine, Bronx, NY; Mem Sloan-Kettering Cancer Ctr, New York; Columbia Univ, New York)

Can J Anaesth 43:341–346, 1996 3–14

Objective.—Both epidurally infused fentanyl and sufentanil, combined with other drugs, provide satisfactory analgesia during labor and delivery, although patients experience lower extremity sensory loss. Fentanyl and sufentanil were compared with regard to effectiveness of analgesia during labor and delivery, neonatal outcome, and opioid accumulation in blood of mother and neonate.

Methods.—In a double-blind random study, women received either 2 $Mg \cdot mL^{-1}$ fentanyl (50 patients, group 1) or 1 $Mg \cdot mL^{-1}$ sufentanil (50 patients, group 2) in combination with bupivacaine 0.015% and epinephrine 2 $Mg \cdot mL^{-1}$. Patients assessed pain intensity on a 0–10 (no pain to worst pain) scale, satisfaction on a 0–10 (no satisfaction to best satisfaction) scale, and side effects (pruritus, sedation, nausea, and vomiting) on a 1–3 (mild to severe) scale every hour. Infusion rates were adjusted as needed. Plasma opioid concentrations were obtained from selected patients in each group at the end of the infusions.

Results.—Patients in group 1 reported significantly higher pain scores in both the first and second stages of labor than did group 2 patients. Additional bupivacaine was requested by significantly more patients in group 1

(42%) than in group 2 (6%). Group 1 required significantly more bupivacaine than did group 2. There was no difference between groups with respect to lower sensory levels, time from discontinuation of infusion to delivery, durations of first and second stages of labor, or incidence of side effects. Maternal concentration of fentanyl was 0.28 ng·mL^{-1}, umbilical vein plasma concentrations of fentanyl was 0.18 ng·mL^{-1}, maternal concentration of sufentanil was 0.11 ng·mL^{-1} and umbilical vein plasma concentration was 0.09 ng·mL^{-1}. Neonatal outcomes were uneventful.

Conclusion.—Patients receiving fentanyl reported less pain and required less bupivacaine rescue. No serious maternal or fetal side effects occurred.

► Recently, some anesthesiologists have reported that the epidural administration of very dilute solutions of local anesthetic with opioid is compatible with ambulation during labor. In this study, the authors did not indicate whether any of the patients were able to ambulate. The high cesarean section rate in this study—20% in the fentanyl group and 28% in the sufentanil group—is bothersome.

D.H. Chestnut, M.D.

Epidural Bupivacaine/Fentanyl Infusions vs. Intermittent Top-ups: A Retrospective Study of the Effects on Mode of Delivery in Primiparous Women

Driver I, Popham P, Glazebrook C, et al (Addenbrooke's Hosp, Cambridge, England; Univ of Cambridge, England)

Eur J Anaesthesiol 13:515–520, 1996 3–15

Background.—The use of epidural infusions containing bupivacaine plus fentanyl was introduced at the authors' hospital in 1991. The choice of infusion or intermittent "top-up" technique has remained with the anesthetist. The possible effect of this practice on the mode of delivery in primiparous women was investigated.

Methods.—The records of 4,362 consecutive primiparous women were reviewed. All were expected to deliver vaginally. Data were analyzed in a logistic regression analysis adjusting for age, weight, gestation, cervical dilation at epidural insertion, use of oxytocin, year of entry into the study, and type of epidural block.

Findings.—Among the 1,534 women given an epidural block at 3–6 cm of dilation, those receiving infusions were significantly less likely to need emergent cesarean section than were women receiving intermittent top-ups. Also, in this patient subgroup the cesarean section rate specifically for failure to progress showed the same trend, although it did not reach statistical significance.

Conclusions.—The use of an epidural infusion of bupivacaine plus fentanyl was associated with a significant reduction in cesarean delivery when compared with intermittent top-ups in nulliparous women. Additional research is needed to determine the effect of the different epidural techniques on delivery outcome, especially in women requesting or needing an epidural block very early in the first stage of labor.

► In this retrospective study, the authors observed an increased incidence of cesarean section in those patients who received epidural analgesia with a cervical dilation of less than 3 cm. Our 2 studies at the University of Iowa demonstrated that administration of epidural analgesia in nulliparous women with a cervical dilation of 3–5 cm did not increase the cesarean section rate when compared with the administration of epidural analgesia in women with a cervical dilation greater than 5 cm.[1, 2] We did not evaluate the effect of epidural analgesia administered before 3-cm cervical dilation. I hope that someone will perform a prospective study that evaluates the effect of very early epidural analgesia (i.e., before 3-cm cervical dilation) on the progress of labor and method of delivery.

D.H. Chestnut, M.D.

References

1. Chestnut DH, McGrath JM, Vincent RC Jr, et al: Does early administration of epidural analgesia affect obstetric outcome in nulliparous women who are in spontaneous labor? *Anesthesiology* 80:1201–1208, 1994.
2. Chestnut DH, Vincent RD Jr, McGrath JM, et al: Does early administration of epidural analgesia affect obstetric outcome in nulliparous women who are receiving intravenous oxytocin? *Anesthesiology* 80:1193–1200, 1994.

The Effect of Postoperative Analgesia With Continuous Epidural Bupivacaine After Cesarean Section on the Amount of Breast Feeding and Infant Weight Gain

Hirose M, Hara Y, Hosokawa T, et al (Kyoto Prefectural Univ, Japan)
Anesth Analg 82:1166–1169, 1996 3–16

Background.—Research has shown that pain suppresses breast milk production after delivery and that narcotics and sedatives can interfere with breast-feeding. Postoperative analgesia with epidural bupivacaine may enhance breast-feeding and infant growth after cesarean delivery.

Methods.—By random assignment, 15 parturients undergoing elective cesarean section with spinal anesthesia received epidural bupivacaine postoperatively, and 15 did not. A continuous 3-day epidural infusion of 0.25% bupivacaine, 0.7 mL/hr, was delivered epidurally. All patients were given diclofenac on demand.

Findings.—Women receiving epidural bupivacaine had a significantly lower visual analogue pain score after surgery. Also, the weight of the milk fed by breast and infant weight were significantly greater than in the control group. Women in the control group needed a greater dose of diclofenac postoperatively than those receiving epidural analgesia.

Conclusions.—Satisfactory pain relief provided by 3 days of postoperative epidural bupivacaine improved the amount of infant feeding and infant weight gain for 11 days after cesarean delivery. The mechanism underlying this effect is not known.

▶ Third-party payers are demanding evidence that postoperative epidural analgesia improves outcome. This welcome study suggests that effective epidural bupivacaine analgesia improves the amount of breast-feeding and infant weight gain after cesarean section when compared with ineffective analgesia provided by diclofenac. Unfortunately, this study has several limitations. First, the authors placed the epidural catheter at either the T12-L1 or the L1-2 interspace, which does not represent standard practice for the administration of epidural analgesia in obstetric patients in the United States. As a result, the authors were able to provide effective analgesia by giving only 0.7 mL/hr of 0.25% bupivacaine. That is remarkable. (The authors did not state whether the continuous epidural infusion of bupivacaine interfered with maternal ambulation. Impaired mobility would be an undesirable outcome in postcesarean patients, who are at increased risk for deep vein thrombosis and pulmonary embolism.) Second, it appears that the authors deliberately provided ineffective analgesia in the diclofenac group. Few thoughtful physicians would deny access to adequate doses of effective analgesics, including parenteral opioids, after cesarean section. Third, if anyone doubts that the authors' method of practice differs from that in the United States, they should read the methods section. The authors stated that all patients were discharged from the hospital on the 12th or 13th day after cesarean section.

D.H. Chestnut, M.D.

The Effect of Epidural Anesthesia on the Length of Labor

Johnson S, Rosenfeld JA (East Tennessee State Univ, Bristol)

J Fam Pract 40:244–247, 1995 3–17

Background.—Epidural anesthesia is widely used during labor despite reports that it prolongs the labor process. Its use has been linked to an increase in the number of cesarean sections performed. The effect of epidural anesthesia on the course of labor was evaluated in a large group of patients in Tennessee.

Method.—Demographic, labor, and delivery data were collected on 180 women through retrospective chart review. Data were interpreted using chi-square and *t* test analysis.

Results.—The rate of epidural anesthesia dropped significantly from the first half of the study year to the second half when Tenncare, a state-funded insurance plan, was instituted. In primiparas, second-stage labor lasted 84 minutes with epidural anesthesia compared to 46 minutes without epidural anesthesia. The second-stage averaged 40 minutes with and 17 minutes without epidural anesthesia in multiparas.

Discussion.—Epidural anesthesia significantly increased the second-stage of labor in both primiparas and multiparas. The effect of prolonged labor on maternal and child well-being requires more study.

► Other studies have noted that the introduction of an epidural analgesia service in a hospital did not result in an increased incidence of cesarean section in that hospital. To my knowledge, this is the first study that observed the effect of a sharp reduction in the use of epidural analgesia on the cesarean section rate. A decrease in the epidural analgesia rate from 71% to 27% did not result in a decreased incidence of cesarean section. This study casts further doubt on the existence of a causal relationship between epidural analgesia during labor and cesarean section for dystocia.

D.H. Chestnut, M.D.

Effect of Second-stage 0.25% Epidural Bupivacaine on the Outcome of Labor

Luxman D, Wolman I, Niv D, et al (Tel Aviv Univ, Israel)

Gynecol Obstet Invest 42:167–170, 1996 3–18

Introduction.—Some authors contend that epidural analgesia prolongs the second stage of labor and increases the chances of instrumental delivery. Others suggest that the higher rate of instrumental delivery stems from the greater use of epidural analgesia in complicated labors. Various techniques have been proposed to lower the rate of instrumental deliveries. The effects of giving epidural bupivacaine during the second stage of labor were evaluated.

Methods.—The randomized study included 70 patients at term with uncomplicated pregnancies and in spontaneous labor. All the patients received epidural 0.25% bupivacaine without adrenaline. Half the patients received continuous "top-ups" of epidural bupivacaine throughout labor. The other half received no further bupivacaine after the cervix was dilated to 8 cm. The 2 groups were compared for duration of the second stage of labor, instrumental delivery rate, and Apgar scores.

Results.—There were no differences in premature rupture of the membranes, oxytocin augmentation, or cesarean section rate. Mean duration of the second stage of labor was 43 minutes in group 1 and 38.5 minutes in group 2. The rates of mechanical assisted delivery were 14% and 17%, respectively. Neither of these differences was significant. The 1- and 5-minute Apgar scores also were similar.

Conclusions.—Giving continuous epidural 0.25% bupivacaine throughout labor and delivery appears to have no adverse effect on the outcome of labor. Continuous epidural analgesia provides the laboring mother with good analgesia when she needs it most. Active management of labor may improve the chances of good progress despite continuous epidural block.

► The present study suffers from a limitation common to other studies of epidural analgesia during the second stage of labor. Namely, the authors did not assess pain scores or the quality of analgesia during the second stage. Thus, it is unclear whether women in group 1 had analgesia that was clearly superior to that experienced by women in group 2.

D.H. Chestnut, M.D.

The Efficacy of Intrathecal Injection of Sufentanil Using a Microspinal Catheter for Labor Analgesia

Abboud TK, Zhu J, Sharp R, et al (Univ of Southern Calif, Los Angeles)
Acta Anaesthesiol Scand 40:210–215, 1996 3–19

Background.—Patients in active labor reportedly experience profound analgesia of 1- to 3-hour durations with delivery of intrathecal sufentanil. For most patients, however, a single injection is not adequate for the duration of labor. The recently introduced microspinal catheter permits repeated injections, thereby prolonging analgesic duration. The effects of multiple intrathecal sufentanil injections on labor analgesia, as well as on maternal and neonatal outcomes, were evaluated.

Patients and Methods.—Seventeen healthy women in active labor were included in the study. All women received multiple injections of 5 μg intrathecal sufentanil through microspinal catheters. A 10-cm visual analogue scale was used to evaluate overall maternal satisfaction with analgesia. Maternal side effects and neonatal outcomes also were assessed.

Results.—After the first injection was delivered, onset of analgesia was less than 5 minutes and lasted for about 148 minutes. With each successive injection, increased tolerance was noted. After the second and third injections were given, mean onset was 12.9 and 20.1 minutes and analgesic duration was 76.6 and 33.9 minutes, respectively (Fig 1). None of the

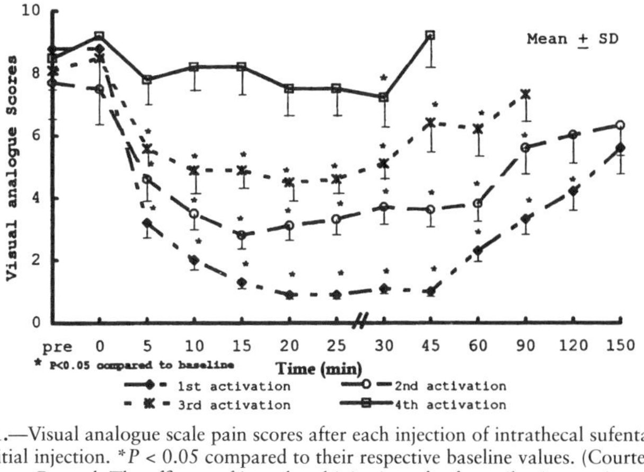

FIGURE 1.—Visual analogue scale pain scores after each injection of intrathecal sufentanil. Time 0 is the time of initial injection. *$P < 0.05$ compared to their respective baseline values. (Courtesy of Abboud TK, Zhu J, Sharp R, et al: The efficacy of intrathecal injection of sufentanil using a microspinal catheter for labor analgesia. *Acta Anaesthesiol Scand* 40:210–215, 1996.)

patients achieved sufficient pain relief after the fourth injection. Motor blockage did not occur in any of the patients, although 88% experienced mild or moderate pruritus. After the first injection, mean systolic blood pressure decreased by a maximum of 11.3% at 30 minutes, and ephedrine therapy was needed in 3 patients. Significant hemodynamic changes were not observed with additional injections. A temporary sensory decrease was noted in 5 patients. Neonatal Apgar scores, Neurologic Adaptive Capacity Scores, fetal heart rate, and umbilical cord acid-base status were grossly normal.

Conclusions.—Tolerance of intrathecal sufentanil was noted after multiple injections were administered to patients in active labor. This analgesic strategy, therefore, may best be suited for parturients with short durations of labor. Mild or moderate pruritus was commonly noted, although no significant maternal or neonatal side effects occurred. Patients with hemodynamic instability will require careful assessment when applying this technique.

▶ Several years ago, the FDA withdrew approval for the use of spinal microcatheters in clinical practice because of a concern that those catheters might predispose the patient to the occurrence of neurologic deficits.

In the present study, the authors observed a progressive decrease in efficacy with the second, third, and fourth doses of intrathecal sufentanil. They concluded that acute tolerance was the reason for the failure to obtain analgesia after the fourth injection of sufentanil in all patients. It is unclear whether this phenomenon resulted from tachyphylaxis or the increasing intensity of pain that occurs during advanced labor.

D.H. Chestnut, M.D.

Hemodynamic Effects of Intrathecal Sufentanil Compared With Epidural Bupivacaine in Laboring Parturients

Pham LH, Camann WR, Smith MP, et al (Brigham and Women's Hosp, Boston; Harvard Med School, Boston)

J Clin Anesth 8:497–501, 1996 3–20

Background.—Intrathecal opioids are commonly used for women in labor. It was initially believed that intrathecal sufentanil did not produce any hemodynamic side effects, but there are reports of hypotension after its use. In previous studies, only maternal blood pressure has been measured, and there is no information comparing central hemodynamic changes after intrathecal sufentanil and epidural bupivacaine. Also in these studies, the amount of IV fluid given before sufentanil or bupivacaine was not standardized. The central hemodynamic effects and adverse effects of IV sufentanil after a standard IV preload and of epidural bupivacaine were compared.

Methods.—A group of 40 patients classed as American Society of Anesthesiologists physical status I were randomized to receive 2 mL of 10 µg intrathecal sufentanil or 12 mL of 0.25% epidural bupivacaine. Saline was given to all patients through the opposite route to ensure that the drugs were administered via a blind protocol. Noninvasive thoracic impedance monitoring was used to evaluate heart rate, blood pressure, cardiac index, stroke index, and systemic vascular resistance index.

Results.—In patients given bupivacaine, the mean arterial pressure was lower at 10 minutes and 20 minutes after onset of analgesia (Fig 1). There were no significant changes in cardiac index, stroke index, or systemic vascular resistance index (Fig 2). In patients given sufentanil, the mean heart rate was lower at 20 minutes and 30 minutes after onset of analgesia. Hypotension occurred in 2 patients given sufentanil and in 4 patients given bupivacaine; these patients required treatment with ephedrine. In patients given sufentanil, pain scores were lower at 10 minutes, but after this, pain scores and the duration of analgesia were similar for both groups. Itching occurred in 14 patients given sufentanil.

Discussion.—There were no significant changes in central hemodynamic parameters, which indicates that decreased blood pressure after intrathecal opioids may result from the onset of analgesia and not from decreases in the preload. The changes in most hemodynamic parameters were small, but several patients had decreased blood pressure and required treatment with ephedrine. Maternal blood pressure must be carefully monitored when using either sufentanil or bupivacaine.

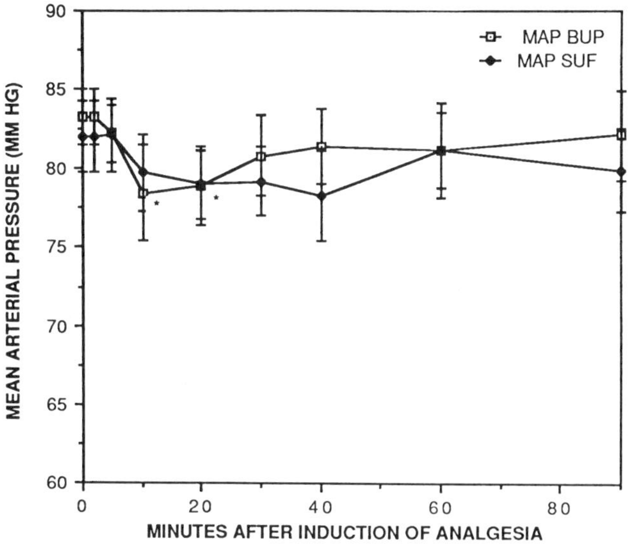

FIGURE 1.—Mean arterial pressure (mm Hg) vs. minutes after induction of analgesia. *Asterisks* indicate statistically significant difference from baseline ($P < 0.05$) in patients given bupivacaine. *Abbreviations*: *BUP*, bupivacaine; *MAP*, mean arterial pressure; *SUF*, sufentanil. (Reprinted by permission of the publisher from Pham LH, Camann WR, Smith MP, et al: Hemodynamic effects of intrathecal sufentanil compared with epidural bupivacaine in laboring parturients. *J Clin Anesth* 8:497–501. Copyright 1996 by Elsevier Science Inc.)

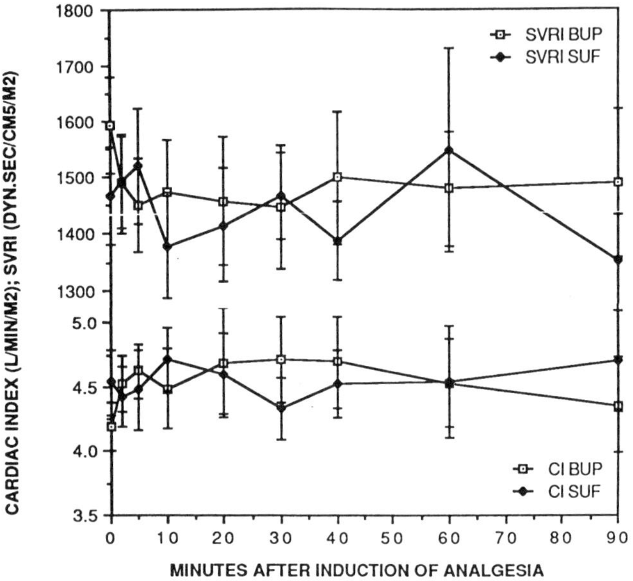

FIGURE 2.—Cardiac index (L/min/m²) and systemic vascular resistance index (dynes·sec/cm⁻⁵/m²) vs. minutes after induction of analgesia. No significant differences were seen. *Abbreviations*: *BUP*, bupivacaine; *SUF*, sufentanil; *SVRI*, systemic vascular resistance index; *CI*, cardiac index. (Reprinted by permission of the publisher from Pham LH, Camann WR, Smith MP, et al: Hemodynamic effects of intrathecal sufentanil compared with epidural bupivacaine in laboring parturients. *J Clin Anesth* 8:497–501. Copyright 1996 by Elsevier Science Inc.)

▶ In the present study, all women received 1 L of Ringer's lactate within a 15-minute period before administration of analgesia. Nonetheless, 2 women in the sufentanil group and 4 in the bupivacaine group required ephedrine for treatment of hypotension. The authors concluded that the absence of changes in central hemodynamic measurements implies that the decreased blood pressure observed after intrathecal sufentanil administration results from the onset of profound analgesia rather than from a decrease in preload.

D.H. Chestnut, M.D.

Hemodynamic Effects of Intrathecal Fentanyl in Nonlaboring Term Parturients

Grant GJ, Susser L, Cascio M, et al (New York Univ)
J Clin Anesth 8:99–103, 1996 3–21

Background.—Intrathecal opioids have been used as anesthetics for patients in labor since 1981. Intrathecal opioids act at spinal opioid receptors, but conduction in motor or autonomic nerves should not be affected. This selective nociceptive block is appropriate for patients in labor and should not reduce blood pressure. However, it has been suggested that various opioids may reduce maternal blood pressure. Previous research of the hemodynamic effects of intrathecal opioids has studied women in labor, which can significantly affect hemodynamics and potentially skew the study results. The effect of intrathecal fentanyl on maternal hemodynamics in patients at term gestation but not in labor was evaluated.

Methods.—In 23 patients scheduled for elective cesarean section who were classed at American Society of Anesthesiologists physical status I, 25 μg fentanyl was administered intrathecally. Patients in group 1 had previously received 1,200 mL of IV Ringer's lactate solution. Patients in group 2 were given no IV fluid. Hemodynamic measurements were recorded.

Results.—Noninvasive blood pressure monitoring and impedance cardiography were used to obtain baseline hemodynamic information. Systolic and diastolic blood pressure, mean arterial pressure, heart rate, stroke volume, cardiac output, end-diastolic volume, and ejection fraction were recorded. Hemodynamic measurements were recorded every 3 minutes for 30 minutes after fentanyl was administered. In group 1, fentanyl did not affect any maternal hemodynamic measurements. In group 2, fentanyl resulted in a few changes in hemodynamics that were not statistically significant. In all patients throughout the study, systolic blood pressure was always greater than 100 mm Hg.

Conclusions.—Intrathecal fentanyl does not affect maternal hemodynamics. Maternal hemodynamic measurements may be affected by other opioids. These patients were not in labor, and it is possible that intrathecal opioids may affect the hemodynamics of women in labor. These findings may be relevant for women at term gestation with cardiovascular disease.

▶ Other studies have evaluated the hemodynamic effects of intrathecal fentanyl or sufentanil in women in labor. The present study differs from earlier studies in that the authors evaluated the hemodynamic effects of intrathecal fentanyl in nonlaboring pregnant women scheduled for elective cesarean section. Thus, the authors eliminated the confounding effects of uterine contractions, increased maternal blood concentrations of catecholamines, and maternal pain. The authors correctly acknowledged that the present study does not exclude the possibility that intrathecal administration of other opioids may produce maternal hemodynamic effects.

D.H. Chestnut, M.D.

Intrathecal Administration of Morphine for Elective Caesarean Section

Milner AR, Bogod DG, Harwood RJ (Nottingham City Hosp, England; Norfolk/Norwich Healthcare NHS Trust, England)

Anaesthesia 51:871–873, 1996 3–22

Background.—Small doses of intrathecal opioids can provide effective analgesia in women scheduled for cesarean section. However, adverse effects, such as nausea and itching, can occur. Respiratory depression can also occur in obese women. It has been suggested that lower doses of intrathecal morphine can provide adequate analgesia with fewer adverse effects. However, the quality of analgesia from higher and lower doses has not been examined; therefore, the quality of analgesia and side effects of 2 doses of morphine in women undergoing cesarean section were evaluated.

Methods.—Morphine (0.1 or 0.2 mg) was administered to 50 patients before elective cesarean section. Morphine was given in addition to 2.5 mL of 0.5% bupivacaine in 8% dextrose. Pain scores and the incidence of adverse effects were recorded postoperatively.

Results.—The quality of analgesia was similar in both groups of patients. The incidence and severity of itching were also similar for both groups. Patients given 0.1 mg morphine had significantly less nausea and vomiting than patients given 0.2 mg morphine. At 24 hours, patient satisfaction with anesthetic care was similar for both groups. No patient experienced respiratory depression.

Conclusions.—In these patients, the quality and duration of analgesia provided by 0.1 and 0.2 mg intrathecal morphine were similar. Less nausea and vomiting occurred when 0.1 mg morphine was administered. Further research is needed with larger patient populations.

► Intrathecal administration of morphine remains an excellent method for providing postcesarean analgesia. The present study supports earlier studies that suggest that there is no advantage to the administration of larger doses of intrathecal morphine. Fewer patients in the 0.1-mg group experienced postoperative nausea and vomiting than did patients in the 0.2-mg group. Surprisingly, there was no difference between the 2 groups in the incidence or severity of itching. Nonetheless, it seems intuitive that delayed respiratory depression is less likely to occur in patients who receive a smaller dose (i.e., 0.1 mg) than in patients who receive a larger dose of intrathecal morphine.

D.H. Chestnut, M.D.

Analgesic Efficacy and Side Effects of Subarachnoid Sufentanil–Bupivacaine Administered to Women in Advanced Labor

Viscomi CM, Rathmell JP, Mason SB, et al (Univ of Vermont, Burlington)
Reg Anesth 21:424–429, 1996 3–23

Background.—Subarachnoid sufentanil is used as an analgesic for women in labor. Most studies have focused on women with cervical dilations of 2–5 cm. Pain at this stage is poorly localized. At the transitional stage of labor when cervical dilation is 7 cm or more, somatic pain also begins. Subarachnoid sufentanil administered early in the first stage of labor provides analgesia for 77–120 minutes. Adding 2.5 mg bupivacaine to 10 μg sufentanil increases the length of analgesia to 150 minutes. The effectiveness and side effects of subarachnoid sufentanil–bupivacaine were determined in women with cervical dilations of 7 cm or more in an open-label, nonrandomized trial.

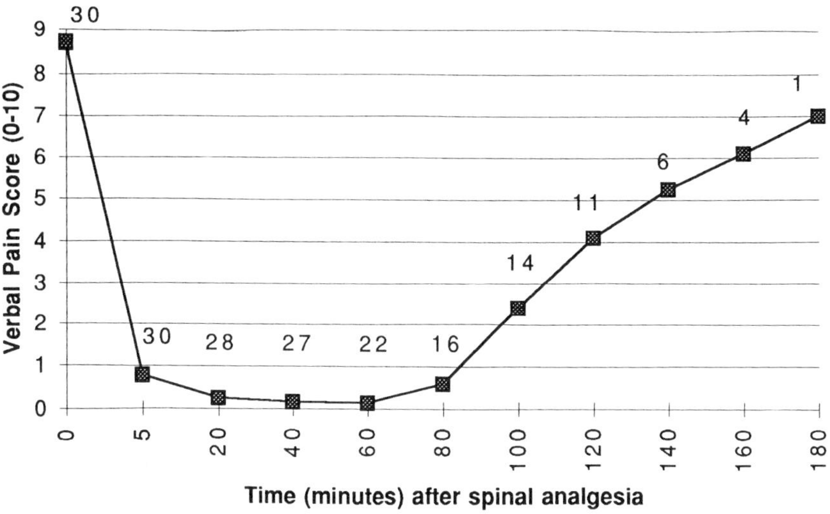

FIGURE 1.—Pain scores after subarachnoid sufentanil–bupivacaine administration. Only undelivered parturients without supplemental analgesics are included. The number of parturients forming each data point is indicated above that data point. (Courtesy of Viscomi CM, Rathmell JP, Mason SB, et al: Analgesic efficacy and side effects of subarachnoid sufentanil–bupivacaine administered to women in advanced labor. *Reg Anesth* 21:424–429, 1996.)

Methods.—Subarachnoid sufentanil (10 µg in 1 mL volume plus 0.25% bupivacaine in 1 mL volume) was given to 32 women whose American Society of Anesthesiologists physical status was I and II and who had cervical dilations of 7 cm or more. Pain scores were recorded, as well as blood pressure, pruritus, Bromage motor block scores, mode of delivery, and need for further anesthesia.

Results.—In 30 of the 32 patients, lumbar puncture was successful. Pain scores were 8.7 before spinal injection and 0.7 five minutes after injection (Fig 1). Pain scores were less than 5 for 130 minutes after injection. There were 24 unassisted vaginal deliveries, 4 instrumental vaginal deliveries, and 2 cesarean deliveries. Nineteen of the 28 patients who delivered vaginally did not require further analgesic and had pain scores of 5 or less. After spinal injection, blood pressure dropped, and 3 patients required treatment. In 26 patients, the Bromage motor block scores were 0; in 4 patients, the scores were 1. In 22 patients, pruritus occurred.

Discussion.—In these patients, subarachnoid sufentanil–bupivacaine provided rapid analgesia for 130 minutes, although pruritus, motor block, and hypotension occurred. Most of these patients had adequate analgesia and were able to delivery vaginally. There may be a correlation between the length of analgesia provided by subarachnoid sufentanil–bupivacaine and the stage of labor at which it is given. Further research of drugs or techniques that provide analgesia should involve patients at similar stages of labor.

► Most studies of intrathecal opioid administration during labor have evaluated the onset, quality, and duration of analgesia in patients in early labor.

In the present study, the authors assessed the efficacy and side effects of intrathecal sufentanil–bupivacaine analgesia only in women with cervical dilations of at least 7 cm. Remarkably, among the 28 women who delivered vaginally, 19 did not require supplemental analgesia and maintained a pain score of 5 or less through the time of delivery.

D.H. Chestnut, M.D.

Advance Prediction of Hypotension at Cesarean Delivery Under Spinal Anesthesia

Kinsella SM, Norris MC (St Michael's Hosp, Bristol, England; Jefferson Med College, Philadelphia)

Int J Obstet Anesth 5:3–7, 1996 3–24

Introduction.—A recent report indicated that pregnant women with a positive "tilt test" are likely to have hypotension more often and require more ephedrine at the time of cesarean delivery, compared with women who have a negative test. These findings were tested in 27 women before surgery for cesarean section.

Methods.—Blood pressure, maternal heart rate, fetal heart rate, and uterine contractions were measured after patients spent 5 minutes in each of the following positions: supine, left lateral, and sitting. Patients were instructed to turn to the left lateral position if they had severe symptoms while supine. Hypotension was defined as a systolic arterial pressure (SAP) of less than 100 mm Hg or a SAP decrease from baseline of greater than 25%. Hypotension was treated using ephedrine. A supine stress test (SST) was considered to be either an increase in heart rate of greater than 10 beats/min while supine, during maternal leg flexion, or both.

Results.—All patients were able to tolerate the supine period for a full 5 minutes. No women or fetuses had severe symptoms during the supine position. Patients with severe hypotension below 70% of baseline were more likely to have a positive SST than women whose blood pressure did not drop similarly. Sensitivity, specificity, positive predictive value, and negative predictive value were 75%, 82%, 86%, and 69%, respectively. A positive SST was significantly correlated with a lower systolic nadir, higher vasopressor dose, and higher hypotension-vasopressor score. The Apgar scores and umbilical blood gases were significantly worse in women with a positive SST, compared with women with a negative SST. Avoidance of the supine position during sleep, maternal symptom history, symptom intolerance of the supine test, and fetal position were not predictive of hypotension.

Conclusion.—A positive preoperative SST was predictive of risk for severe hypotension at cesarean delivery with spinal analgesia. A larger investigation is needed to confirm these findings.

▶ The authors performed this study in healthy women with healthy fetuses whose heart rates were monitored continuously during the time that the mothers were asked to lie supine. The authors stated: "We feel that the disadvantage of deliberately using the supine position for a short time was minor compared to that which already occurs in other clinical areas." This is weak support for a test that may incur risk to the fetus. I have no enthusiasm for a test that requires a pregnant woman at term to lie supine — with its attendant aortocaval compression — for 5 minutes, especially when such a test has limited utility and is unlikely to affect my anesthetic management significantly.

D.H. Chestnut, M.D.

Active Management of Labour Does Not Reduce the Rate of Caesarean Section

Thornton JG (Univ of Leeds, England)

BMJ 313:378, 1996 3–25

Introduction.—Active management is a package of care that was introduced in Dublin in the late 1960s to meet the challenge of rising numbers of hospital deliveries and staff shortages. It consists of special classes to prepare women for labor, strict criteria for determining the onset of labor, psychological support, and regular supervision of the delivery area by senior staff. It also includes revolutionary changes such as routine amniotomy and early recourse to high doses of oxytocin under the supervision of a midwife to speed up slow labors. The goal was to keep labor from lasting more than 12 hours. This was controversial, particularly because it was thought that amniotomy and oxytocin would increase the likelihood of cesarean section. What happened instead was that in the 1970s, the rates of cesarean sections rose everywhere else and remained relatively low in Dublin. Investigations were done, but none were rigorous enough to be convincing. The results of a randomized prospective trial comparing active management and usual care during labor were reported.

Active Management Trial.—Almost 2,000 women were randomly assigned before 30 weeks' gestation to either active management or usual care. Women in the active management group underwent customized childbirth classes, strict criteria for the diagnosis of labor, routine amniotomy, early use of high-dose oxytocin, and 1-to-1 nursing in a separate labor unit. Women in the other group received usual care with the selective use of amniotomy and oxytocin (at lower doses and later than the active management group). Women in the active management group had shorter labor, compared with women in the usual care group. This difference can probably be attributed to a later diagnosis of onset of labor in the active management group. The cesarean rate for the active management and usual care groups was 19.5% and 19.4%, respectively.

Belgium Trial.—A much smaller prospective, randomized trial with 306 women also showed no significant differences in cesarean section rates for active management and usual care groups.

Conclusion.—The argument can no longer be made that active management is associated with lower cesarean rates. Because women prefer natural childbirth and are likely to decline interventions to speed delivery, routine use of active management may disappear.

Active Management of Labor

Peaceman AM, Socol ML (Northwestern Univ, Chicago)

Am J Obstet Gynecol 175:363–368, 1996 3–26

Introduction.—Active management of labor was first introduced in Dublin in the the 1960s. It has been associated with a lower cesarean rate, although findings of recent reports have disagreed. Active management has been suggested as a means to decrease the incidence of cesarean section for dystocia. Active management was described and evaluated as a strategy for lowering the rate of cesarean section for dystocia.

Components of Active Management.—Active management was instituted to shorten what was considered a prolonged experience in nulliparous labor that produced unnecessary fear, pain, and anxiety. Active management was promoted as emphasizing maternal expulsion of the fetus and not delivery by traction. The organizational component of active management consists of prenatal education classes, diagnosis of labor made by the senior labor attendant, constant attendance of the patient during labor (with staffing unaffected by time of day so women could be attended on all shifts), and peer review of all cesarean sections. The medical management consists of patients being encouraged not to come to the hospital until contractions are regular and painful; a diagnosis of labor based on quality of contractions (in conjunction with 1 or more of the following: complete cervical effacement, membrane rupture, and bloody show); amniotomy if membranes are still intact after diagnosis of labor, and use of oxytocin if inadequate progress of labor is determined.

Efficacy.—Data from Dublin indicate that there is a continuing low rate of cesarean section for dystocia since the program began. Of all nulliparous patients admitted in spontaneous labor in 1980, 63% and 98% of patients were delivered within 6 and 12 hours of admission, respectively. Few physicians outside of Ireland were immediately willing to adopt this approach. When active management was evaluated in trials elsewhere, most reported it lowered cesarean rates. Two recent randomized prospective trials have reported that active management does not lower cesarean section rates but that it is associated with shorter labor and reduced infectious morbidity.

Safety Concerns.—The safety of oxytocin use has been questioned. Comparisons of several trials indicate that maternal and fetal morbidity and mortality is not significantly different between women who do and do not receive oxytocin. The risk of uterine rupture seems to be exclusively confined to the parous uterus.

Rationale for Active Management.—One of the most overlooked but important components of the success of the active management program is the establishment of active labor. It recognizes the differences between nulliparous and parous labors, and that spontaneous delivery is more efficient than induced labor. It also discourages the diagnosis of labor until contractions are regular and painful. Infection rates are not increased with the use of amniotomy. Oxytocin dose is higher and intervals between infusions are shorter in active management of labor. Recent reports indicate that cesarean section rates are not significantly different with active management; however, patients with labor abnormalities can be detected sooner and thus dystocia rates may be lowered before fatigue or infection makes the uterus less likely to respond to oxytocin efficiently. The educational and support components lower anxiety. Constant companionship during labor has been associated with lower cesarean rates. Peer review is an educational opportunity and creates a disincentive for deviating from common practice.

Conclusion.—Reports conflict about whether active management decreases the cesarean rate. Active management of labor strongly encourages vaginal delivery as long as the mother and fetus are not compromised. Any approach that advocates vaginal birth deserves support. Some institutions may consider active management as an approach to decreasing operative deliveries for dystocia.

▶ Active management of labor (i.e., a management strategy to decrease the incidence of cesarean section for dystocia) was introduced 3 decades ago at the National Maternity Hospital in Dublin. Obstetricians at this hospital have successfully used this strategy to maintain a low cesarean section rate. Others have used active management of labor with varying success. The authors of these reviews have correctly noted that active management of labor is not a panacea. Peaceman and Socol concluded that "any approach that emphasizes advocacy for vaginal birth is likely to find some success and should receive support."

D.H. Chestnut, M.D.

The Intensity of Labor Pain in Grand Multiparas

Ranta P, Jouppila P, Jouppila R (Oulu Univ Hosp, Finland)

Acta Obstet Gynecol Scand 75:250–254, 1996 3–27

Background.—Current obstetric analgesic management protocols reflect the assumption that labor in multiparas is relatively painless until the end of the first stage. The intensity of pain reported by grand multiparous women (having delivered a minimum of 5 times before) was compared with that of primiparous and II–V parous (having delivered between 2 and 5 times before) women.

Methods.—Participating were 70 consecutive grand multiparas, 70 primiparas, and 70 II–V paras. Using a pain intensity scale of 0–10, pain was

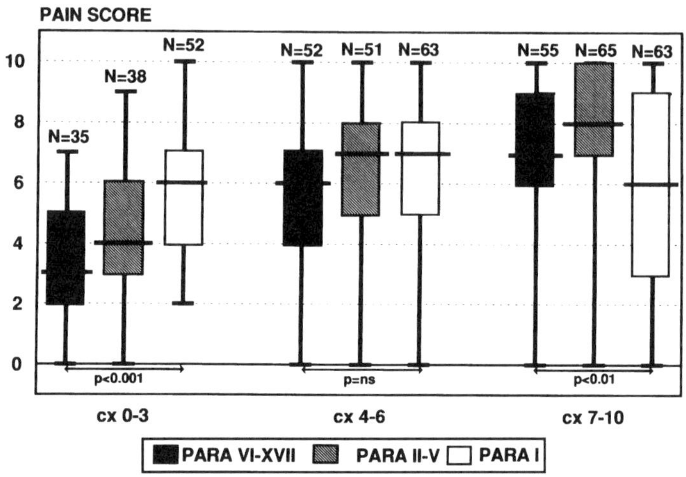

FIGURE 1.—Pain intensity scores (0–10) in grand multiparas (VI–XVII paras), II–V paras, and primiparas in relation to cervical dilatation (*cx*). Minimum, lower (25%) quartile, median, upper (75%) quartile, maximum. (Courtesy of Ranta P, Jouppila P, Jouppila R: The intensity of labor pain in grand multiparas. *Acta Obstet Gynecol Scand* 75:250–254. Copyright 1996, Munksgaard International Publishers Ltd., Copenhagen, Denmark.)

repeatedly assessed according to progress in cervical dilatation at the first and second stage of labor.

Results.—During the latent phase of cervical dilatation, grand multiparas showed a lower median pain score than did primiparas or II–V paras (Fig 1). However, median intensity of pain was significantly higher among grand multiparas than among primiparas at the end of the first stage and during the second stage of labor. Forty percent of primiparas, 3% of II–V paras, and 0% of grand multiparas received epidural blocks. Second-stage pain was rated as "intolerable" (score of 9 or 10) by 21% of grand multiparas and 10% of primiparas. Analgesia was considered insufficient by 47% of grand multiparas on the third day after delivery.

Conclusions.—Great misconceptions exist among health care professionals regarding the nature of labor pain and the need for its relief. The amount of analgesia given during labor depends on the staff's perception of the degree of pain experienced by the parturient. These data suggest that intense labor pain is a common part of childbirth even for experienced parturients. A large proportion of grand multiparas considered their analgesic medication inadequate. Administration of analgesia should be more flexible and more individualized for better effectiveness.

► I remain amazed at the number of individuals who believe that parous patients are unlikely to need or desire pain relief during labor. In this study, approximately half of the parous women rated their pain as severe or intolerable. The timing of epidural analgesia administration in these women is somewhat problematic. With the onset of active phase labor, these patients tend to labor rapidly. The rapid dilation of the cervix and the precipitous descent of the fetal head often result in excruciating pain. I have found that a combined spinal-epidural approach (i.e., intrathecal sufentanil followed by epidural bupivacaine) is a useful technique in some of these patients.

D.H. Chestnut, M.D.

Autonomic Hyperreflexia During Labour
Kobayashi A, Mizobe T, Tojo H, et al (Kyoto Prefectural Univ, Japan)
Can J Anaesth 42:1134–1136, 1995 3–28

Background.—In women with spinal cord injuries, autonomic hyperreflexia (AH) during pregnancy, labor, and delivery is a serious complication.

Case Reports.—Woman, 33, with quadriplegia was hospitalized at 37 weeks' gestation with facial flushing, sweating, and piloerection during abdominal distension or vaginal examination, signs suggesting AH. An epidural catheter was placed at that time in the L_2–L_3 epidural space and kept in situ until after delivery. Lidocaine 1%, 5–10 mL, was injected epidurally before each vaginal examination, and no AH was observed. At 40 weeks' gestation, AH symptoms (pounding headache, hypertension, marked diaphoresis with piloerection, and flushing above the the cord lesion level in the absence of epidural block) heralded labor onset. The epidural injection of 10 mL lidocaine 2% and meperidine 15 mg immediately reduced arterial blood pressure from 160/110 to 110/62 mm Hg, relieving AH symptoms. A girl, weighing 2,704 g and with an Apgar score of 10, was born spontaneously. After delivery, lidocaine 2%, 10 mL, was administered epidurally twice for the management of mild AH. The catheter was removed 48 hours later, and AH symptoms did not return.

Woman, 42, with paraplegia was hospitalized in labor at 37 weeks' gestation. Her uterine contractions caused headache, sweating, facial flushing, and hypertension. An epidural catheter was placed in the L_{1-2} epidural space, and 10 minutes after 5 mL of lidocaine 1% was injected, her blood pressure decreased from 145/83 to 120/77 mm Hg, and AH symptoms were relieved. A cesarean section was scheduled, as the patient's uterine contractions were too weak. Anesthesia was induced with thiopentone, and tracheal intubation was facilitated with succinylcholine chloride. Anesthesia was maintained with sevoflurane and nitrous oxide, and nicardipine was administered to reduce blood pressure. A girl, weighing 2,880 g and with an Apgar score of 8, was delivered, and the mother was taken to the ICU. Nicardipine was given again in an attempt to control her hypertension. Although her blood pressure decreased, sweating and flushing persisted. Three hours after extubation on the following day, the patient reported discomfort and gradually became incoherent, nonresponsive, and apneic. After 48 hours of controlled ventilation and other supportive measures, including glucose administration, the patient recovered fully.

Conclusions.—Epidural anesthesia is effective in controlling AH in labor in patients with spinal cord damage. This approach reduces blood pressure, blocks the noxious stimuli, and relieves AH symptoms.

▶ In the first case, the authors placed the epidural catheter at 37 weeks' gestation—3 weeks before delivery. The authors concluded: "Our experience [one case] suggests that the epidural catheter can be placed 2 to 3 weeks before the date of predicted childbirth . . . ." I think that this is a bad idea. Pre-labor placement of the epidural catheter will not save enough time to justify the risks of catheter malposition and infection.

In the second case, the epidural catheter was dislodged when the patient was moved from the labor room to the operating room. Given the risks of catheter dislodgment and infection, why would anyone want to place an epidural catheter 2 to 3 weeks before delivery?

D.H. Chestnut, M.D.

Effect of Crystalloid and Colloid Preloading on Uteroplacental and Maternal Haemodynamic State During Spinal Anaesthesia for Caesarean Section

Karinen J, Räsänen J, Alahuhta S, et al (Oulu Univ, Finland)
Br J Anaesth 75:531–535, 1995 3–29

Background.—Prophylactic administration of crystalloid preload or reduced colloid preload with ephedrine infusion is commonly used to combat hypotension during spinal anesthesia for cesarean section. Although these techniques may prevent the most severe forms of hypotension, their use has been questioned by studies revealing that the incidence of hypotension during anesthesia is not decreased. Using pulsed color Doppler, the effects of crystalloid and colloid preloading on uteroplacental hemodynamics were compared during the first 20 minutes of spinal anesthesia for cesarean section.

Methods.—Twenty-six healthy parturients undergoing spinal anesthesia for elective cesarean section were studied. Patients were randomly assigned to receive either 1 L of lactated Ringer's solution or 0.5 L of 6% hydroxyethyl starch solution over 10 minutes. Maternal hemodynamics and maternal placental uterine artery circulation were monitored simultaneously.

Results.—Women receiving crystalloid showed a higher incidence of hypotension during anesthesia (62%) than did women receiving colloid (38%). Both groups had an elevation in central venous pressure upon preloading that diminished to baseline after induction of spinal anesthesia. Uterine artery mean pulsatility index (PI) did not change during preload or spinal block. However, uterine artery PI after spinal anesthesia showed wide variation and some high values; individual increases were transient and returned to baseline within 2 minutes.

Conclusions.—The incidence of maternal hypotension was high in both groups; volume preloading with either crystalloid or colloid appears ineffective in preventing maternal hypotension during spinal anesthesia for cesarean section. The transient changes in individual uterine artery PI may reflect responses to external factors and sensitive and rapid hemodynamic regulation of the uteroplacental circulation. Individual high PI values did not correlate with maternal heart rate, systolic arterial pressure, or central venous pressure. If corrected promptly, transient maternal hypotension does not seem to harm the fetus or newborn.

▶ No method of volume expansion will prevent all cases of hypotension during administration of spinal anesthesia for cesarean section. For elective cases, I prefer to give a bolus of approximately 1,500 mL of Ringer's lactate before administration of spinal anesthesia. I typically give a 5- to 10-mg IV bolus of ephedrine immediately after injection of spinal bupivacaine, and I then add 25 mg of ephedrine to the 500 mL remaining in the second bag of Ringer's lactate.

D.H. Chestnut, M.D.

Randomized Trial of Bolus Phenylephrine or Ephedrine for Maintenance of Arterial Pressure During Spinal Anaesthesia for Caesarean Section

Thomas DG, Robson SC, Redfern N, et al (Univ of Newcastle-Upon-Tyne, England)

Br J Anaesth 76:61–65, 1996 3–30

Background.—Women who undergo spinal anesthesia for cesarean section may develop hypotension, which carries the risk of fetal acidemia. The vasopressor of choice for this condition is ephedrine, though prophylactic ephedrine infusion does not reliably prevent maternal hypotension. Alpha-adrenergic agonists are an effective treatment, but there are concerns about their effects on uteroplacental blood flow. The maternal and fetal hemodynamic changes that occur with phenylephrine or ephedrine treatment for hypotension with spinal anesthesia for a cesarean section were assessed.

Methods.—The study included 38 healthy women with uncomplicated singleton term pregnancies who underwent elective cesarean section with spinal anesthesia. They were randomized to receive either phenylephrine 100 μg or ephedrine 5 mg for maintenance of arterial blood pressure. Boluses of vasopressor were given when the systolic pressure declined to 90% or less of baseline values. Automated oscillometry was used to monitor the women's blood pressure and heart rate (HR). Cross-sectional and Doppler echocardiography were performed to measure cardiac output (CO) before and after 1,500 mL of Ringer lactate solution was preloaded and every 2 min after bupivacaine administration. Before and after spinal

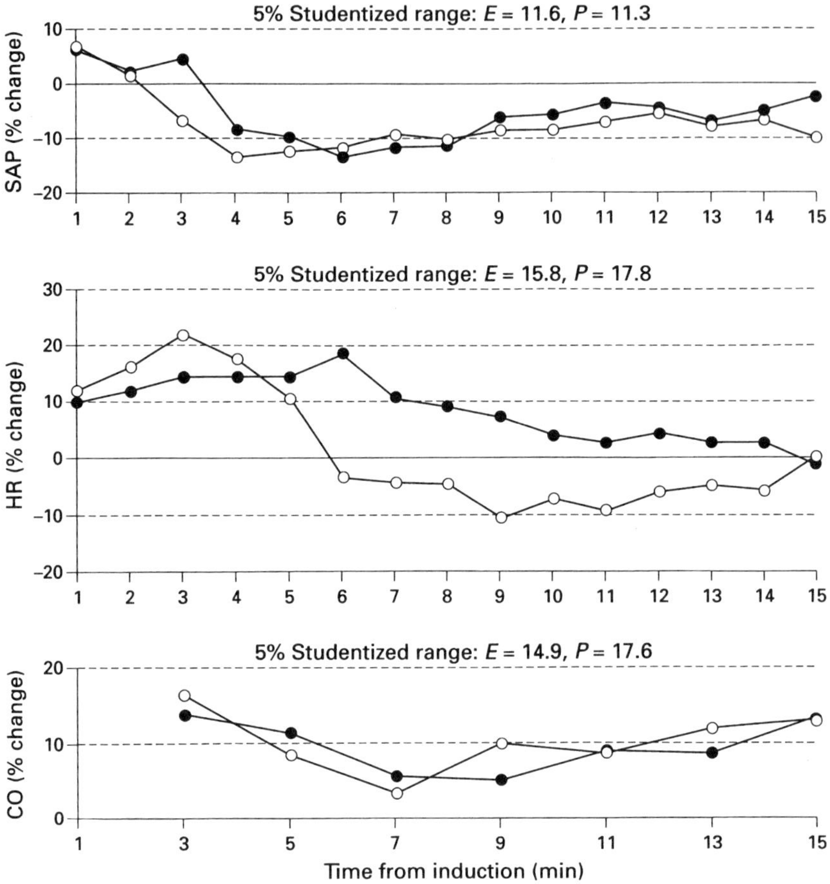

FIGURE 1.—Mean percentage changes in systolic arterial pressure (SAP), heart rate (HR), and cardiac output (CO) from baseline values after induction of spinal anesthesia in the ephedrine (*closed circle*) and phenylephrine (*open circle*) groups, together with the respective Studentized ranges. (Courtesy of Thomas DG, Robson SC, Redfern N, et al: Randomized trial of bolus phenylephrine or ephedrine for maintenance of arterial pressure during spinal anaesthesia for Cesarean section. *Br J Anaesth* 76:61–65, 1996.)

anesthesia, Doppler measurements of umbilical artery pulsatility were obtained.

Results.—There was no significant difference in the median number of vasopressor boluses administered; 6 in the phenylephrine group, and 4 in the ephedrine group. The 2 groups were also similar in terms of maternal systolic blood pressure and CO changes. However, the phenylephrine group had a mean maximal 28.5% decline in maternal HR, compared with 14.4% in the ephedrine group (Fig 1). Because of these HR changes, 58% of patients in the phenylephrine group required atropine, compared with 11% of those in the ephedrine group. The phenylephrine group had a mean umbilical artery pH of 7.29, compared with 7.27 in the ephedrine group.

Conclusions.—Phenylephrine appears to be just as effective as ephedrine in the maintenance of maternal arterial blood pressure during spinal anesthesia for elective cesarean section. In addition, phenylephrine has no adverse effects on fetal hemodynamics or umbilical artery pH. Phenylephrine is associated with a higher incidence of maternal bradycardia, although maternal CO is similar with phenylephrine and ephedrine.

► The more we learn, the more we recognize how much we do not know. This study represents another reevaluation of the safety of small bolus doses of phenylephrine for maintenance of arterial blood pressure during administration of spinal anesthesia for cesarean section. Phenylephrine seems safe provided the anesthesiologist titrates small doses to restore maternal blood pressure toward baseline in healthy parturients.

I am not yet ready to abandon ephedrine as the vasopressor of choice in obstetric patients. However, it seems reasonable to use phenylephrine in patients for whom a reduction in heart rate is desirable. Interestingly, in this study women in the ephedrine group also experienced a small—albeit lesser—decrease in heart rate.

D.H. Chestnut, M.D.

Epinephrine-induced Tachycardia Is Different From Contraction-associated Tachycardia in Laboring Patients

Colonna-Romano P, Salvage R, Lingaraju N, et al (Hahnemann Univ, Philadelphia)

Anesth Analg 82:294–296, 1996 3–31

Background.—In the administration of epidural analgesia, test doses containing epinephrine are used to ensure that there is no unintentional cannulation of an epidural vessel. Tachycardic response has a 100% sensitivity for intravascular cannulation. In women in labor, however, a maternal tachycardic response is often caused by labor pain. The current study determined whether epinephrine-induced tachycardic responses can be distinguished from tachycardic responses induced by labor pain.

Methods.—Fifteen women in active labor were included in the double-blind, prospective study. Each patient served as her own control. Maternal heart rate was recorded continuously after an epidural catheter was placed. In uterine diastole, 2 injections of epinephrine 15 µg plus 45 mg of lidocaine were administered every 2 to 4 minutes, 1 through the epidural catheter and 1 intravenously.

Findings.—The acceleratory phase of epinephrine-induced tachycardic responses (EITRs) was 1.85 bpm and of contraction-associated tachycardic responses (CATRs), 0.69. The 99% confidence interval upper bound was 1.17 bpm. All EITRs could be identified correctly using this value to discriminate between EITRs and CATRs.

Conclusions.—On-line analysis of maternal tachycardic responses may be useful in distinguishing between EITRs and CATRs in women in labor.

Such analysis may further improve the accuracy of an epinephrine test dose during the administration of epidural analgesia.

▶ Several years ago, we published a study in which we observed that painful uterine contractions result in maternal heart rate accelerations similar to those that occur after intravenous injection of 15 μg of epinephrine.[1] In the present study, the authors concluded that EITRs are different from CATRs. They suggested that "on-line analysis of the ascending slope of a maternal tachycardic response...might be used in laboring women to discriminate between EITRs and CATRs...." Is this really necessary? A simpler solution is to administer the epinephrine-containing test dose immediately *after* a uterine contraction. If the anesthesiologist is unable to distinguish between an EITR and a CATR, it seems prudent to repeat the epinephrine-containing test dose.

D.H. Chestnut, M.D.

Reference

1. Chestnut DH, Owen CL, Brown CK, et al: Does labor affect the variability of maternal heart rate during induction of epidural anesthesia? *Anesthesiology* 68:622–625, 1988.

Recent Developments in the Pathophysiology and Management of Preeclampsia

Mushambi MC, Halligan AW, Williamson K (Leicester Royal Infirmary, England)

Br J Anaesth 76:133–148, 1996 3–32

Introduction.—Preeclampsia is a progressive multisystem disorder occurring only in pregnant women after 20 weeks of gestation. The etiology is unknown. The varying presentation most likely includes hypertension, proteinuria, excessive weight gain, and edema. There are no specific diagnostic procedures or specific treatments. Therefore, management is designed to control symptoms.

Pathophysiology.—The underlying pathophysiology is unclear but is most likely related to vascular endothelial damage and dysfunction. In affected mothers, an abnormal placenta may release factors causing damage to vascular endothelial cells throughout the vascular system, which results in vasoconstriction and ischemia, altered fluid compartments, and abnormal immune responses. Increased sensitivity to angiotensin II in patients with preeclampsia can cause severe vasospasms, which may result in hypertension. Increased intravascular hydrostatic pressure, resulting in decreased colloid osmotic pressure, and increased capillary permeability can cause pulmonary edema. Eclamptic convulsions may be caused by cerebral vasospasms or cerebral edema, hemorrhages, and infarcts. These conditions may also cause visual disturbances. The nonselective proteinuria may be caused by increased permeability of the glomerular endothelial cells and glomerular swelling or acute tubular necrosis. Thrombocytopenia may be related to an autoimmune mechanism or an imbalance between prostacyclin and thromboxane.

Management.—The recommended maintenance blood pressure should be less than 170/110 and greater than 130/90 to prevent intracerebral hemorrhage without affecting renal function and uteroplacental blood flow. Methyldopa, β-blockers, and nifedipine can be used to control hypertension, but angiotensin-converting enzyme inhibitors are contraindicated. Hydrazaline is the most common agent for the acute control of hypertension. Vasodilation should be preceded by volume expansion. Oliguria should be treated initially with 500–1,000 mL of crystalloid. Magnesium sulfate is currently the most effective treatment of eclamptic convulsions. The HELLP syndrome (hemolysis, elevated liver enzymes, and low platelets) should be treated aggressively, with immediate delivery, platelet transfusion, and/or a transfusion of fresh whole blood.

Anesthesia and Analgesia.—Extradural analgesia is recommended for pain relief. Because of the possibility of laryngeal edema, variably sized tracheal tubes should be available, and extubation should be performed carefully to avoid exacerbating the edema. Drugs for intubation and extubation should be chosen to attenuate pressor responses.

Conclusions.—Current information on the pathophysiology and management of preeclampsia has not clearly defined the causes of this multisystem disorder. Therefore, its managment is based on response to its varying symptoms.

► The authors made 2 categorical statements that deserve further scrutiny. First, they stated: "Provided that the patient has been preloaded with fluid...and that supine hypotension is avoided, extradural analgesia has been found to increase intervillous blood flow." This statement suggests that epidural analgesia consistently results in improved uteroplacental perfusion in preeclamptic women. Epidural analgesia may improve uteroplacental perfusion in some preeclamptic women, but existing data did not allow us to conclude that this is a consistent occurrence.

Second, the authors stated: "When extradural analgesia is used for pain relief during labour a mixture of an opioid and a local anesthetic administered as an infusion is preferred as this gives continuous pain relief and less hypotension compared with intermittent boluses of local anesthetic." I agree that a continuous epidural infusion is preferred over the intermittent epidural bolus technique. However, the authors did not consider a third option: the continuous epidural infusion of local anesthetic alone. I prefer the third option in preeclamptic women. This allows me to remain certain that the epidural catheter is functioning satisfactorily, and it allows me to remain confident that the epidural catheter may be used successfully for an emergency cesarean section. The disadvantage of epidural administration of both local anesthetic and opioid is that, in some cases, the systemic absorption of opioid delays the recognition of a malfunctioning—or misplaced—epidural catheter.

D.H. Chestnut, M.D.

Laparoscopy During Pregnancy

Curet MJ, Allen D, Josloff RK, et al (Univ of New Mexico, Albuquerque)

Arch Surg 131:546–551, 1996 3–33

Background.—Laparoscopic surgery offers many advantages, but in the pregnant patient, concerns have been raised about fetal acidosis caused by carbon dioxide absorption, fetal hypotension caused by decreased maternal cardiac output, and decreased uterine blood flow caused by increased intra-abdominal pressure. Whether pregnant patients experience advantages in undergoing laparoscopic nongynecologic surgery compared with conventional open surgery, and whether differences in mortality and morbidity occur between patients undergoing these different methods were examined.

Methods.—The population-based study sample consisted of 16 patients undergoing laparoscopic surgery and 18 patients undergoing open laparotomy, each during their first or second trimester of pregnancy. Data were collected during a 5-year period; follow-up ranged from 1 month to 6 years. Surgeries performed included appendectomies and cholecystectomies.

Results.—No difference was found between groups in age, trimester, oxygenation, end-tidal carbon dioxide, Apgar scores, gestational age at delivery, or birth weight. Complications occurred in 4 patients in the laparotomy group and in 6 in the laparoscopy group; only 1 complication (trocar fascial hernia in a patient who underwent laparoscopic cholecystectomy) was clearly related to type of surgery. Incidence of obstetric complications was within the range expected for pregnant patients not undergoing surgery. Operative times were longer (82 vs. 49 minutes), hospital stays were shorter, regular diet was resumed earlier, and duration of IV or IM narcotics was shorter for patients undergoing laparoscopy vs. laparotomy.

Conclusions.—Laparoscopic surgery offers several advantages over open laparotomy for pregnant women. Increased duration of surgery among women who underwent laparoscopy is likely related to a higher percentage of cholecystectomies (as opposed to appendectomies) within that group, and to the initial learning curve associated with the procedure. Perioperative morbidity and mortality did not differ between groups; hence, the data suggest that first- or second-trimester therapeutic laparoscopy is safe.

▶ The authors of this present study concluded that a gestational age of 26–28 weeks seems to be the limit for successful completion of laparoscopic surgery (during pregnancy). The authors also recommended routine use of intraoperative fetal heart rate monitoring in these patients. They recommended the intraoperative use of transvaginal ultrasound fetal heart rate monitoring, although they did not use that technique in this study.

Instead, the authors used transabdominal fetal heart rate monitoring, but they noted that the signal was lost during abdominal insufflation.

D.H. Chestnut, M.D.

Effects of Fetal pH on Local Anesthetic Transfer Across the Human Placenta

Johnson RF, Herman NL, Johnson HV, et al (Vanderbilt Univ, Nashville, Tenn; New York Hosp–Cornell Univ)

Anesthesiology 85:608–615, 1996 3–34

Background.—Fetal acidemia has been found to increase concentrations of umbilical venous bupivacaine in an in situ rabbit model. The effects of declining fetal pH on the rate of maternal-to-fetal clearance of lidocaine, bupivacaine, 2-chloroprocaine, and antipyrine across the isolated, dual-perfused, human placental cotyledon were investigated.

Methods and Findings.—Clearances were determined at fetal pH, during progressive fetal acidemia, and after recovery to fetal pH 7.4 in experiments with a low protein state and with in vivo maternal and fetal protein-binding potentials. Placental transfer of bupivacaine, lidocaine, and 2-chloroprocaine increased linearly as fetal pH declined. There was no effect on antipyrine transfer. Lidocaine and bupivacaine clearance returned to baseline when fetal pH was restored to 7.4. Increasing maternal and fetal protein-binding potentials significantly reduced bupivacaine clearance at fetal pH 7.4. The transfer of bupivacaine and lidocaine increased during fetal acidemia, although to a lesser degree than at low protein concentrations.

Conclusions.—When the pH difference between maternal and fetal perfusates is increased, maternal-to-fetal passage of nonionized lidocaine, bupivacaine, and 2-chloroprocaine is enhanced, probably because of an increased proportion of ionized local anesthetic in the acidemic fetal perfusate and consequent widening of the maternal-to-fetal concentration gradient of the nonionized form. Maternal protein binding limited transfer of lidocaine and bupivacaine.

► The authors suggested that the use of epidural bupivacaine might be preferred to the use of epidural lidocaine in cases where the preterm fetus is likely to be acidemic because of bupivacaine's high degree of maternal protein binding. I am troubled by this recommendation because it considers only one part of the clinical picture. In cases where fetal acidemia is suspected, it is likely that the anesthesiologist will be asked to provide epidural anesthesia quickly. Bupivacaine is a poor choice in such cases, not only because of its slow onset but also because of the increased risk of maternal systemic toxicity.

D.H. Chestnut, M.D.

Maternal Position During Labor: Effects on Fetal Oxygen Saturation Measured by Pulse Oximetry

Carbonne B, Benachi A, Lévèque M-L, et al (Université René Descartes, Paris; Nellcor-France, Jouy-en-Josas)

Obstet Gynecol 88:797–800, 1996 3–35

Objective.—Previous reports have suggested that late decelerations of the fetal heartbeat occur when the mother lies in the supine position. These decelerations, which resolve when the mother shifts to the left lateral position, have been attributed to aortocaval compression. Pulse oximetry can detect changes in fetal oxygen saturation under varying conditions, such as maternal oxygen administration or uterine contractions. This tool was used to assess the effects of maternal position during labor on fetal oxygenation.

Methods.—The study included 15 women in uncomplicated labor. Fetal arterial oxygen saturation was measured by placing a sensor through the cervix and against the side of the fetus' head. Measurements of fetal oxygen saturation were made as the mothers lay in the left lateral, supine, and right lateral positions for 10 minutes each, in random order. The results were analyzed by repeated measures of analysis of variance.

Results.—Successful readings were obtained during all 3 positions in 12 women. Fetal oxygen saturation was significantly lower when the mother was in the supine position than in the left lateral position. It was nonsignificantly lower in the right lateral position versus the left lateral position. There was 1 case of supine hypotensive syndrome associated with fetal heart rate decelerations when the mother shifted from the left lateral to the supine position. In all other cases, fetal heart rate was normal in all maternal positions.

Conclusions.—Fetal oxygen saturation is lower when the mother lies in the supine position, compared to the left lateral position, during labor. As suggested by previous studies using fetal heart rate monitoring, lying in the left lateral position improves fetal oxygenation. Studies of the clinical value of pulse oximetry for fetal monitoring are under way.

► The future role of fetal pulse oximetry during labor remains unclear. However, the present study provides further confirmation of the hazards of the supine position—with its attendant aortocaval compression—in laboring women.

D.H. Chestnut, M.D.

Intravenous Nitroglycerin: A Potent Uterine Relaxant for Emergency Obstetric Procedures. Review of Literature and Report of Three Cases

Riley ET, Flanagan B, Cohen SE, et al (Stanford Univ, Calif)

Int J Obstet Anesth 5:264–268, 1996 3–36

Background.—Obstetric emergencies such as retained placenta, uterine inversion, and breech extraction may require immediate uterine relaxation. The use of nitroglycerin for this purpose has been reported. Three case reports of IV nitroglycerin for emergency uterine relaxation were presented, along with a review of the literature on this topic.

Patients.—In 1 patient, incomplete uterine inversion with a tight cervical ring developed after vaginal delivery and oxytocin infusion. The cervical ring prevented manual uterine replacement. Intravenous nitroglycerin was administered in a single bolus of 100 µg. The uterus relaxed significantly within 60 to 90 seconds, permitting easy manual replacement of the uterus.

Another patient had cervical contraction with placental retention after spontaneous abortion of an 18-week fetus. The patient was sedated and given doses of IV nitroglycerin every 30 to 60 seconds. The doses escalated from 50 to 100, 200, and finally 500 µg. After a total dose of 1,850 µg, the uterus relaxed sufficiently for manual removal of the placenta. The third patient was undergoing elective cesarean section because of breech presentation. Delivery of the baby was complicated by increased uterine tonus and malpresentation. Within 30 seconds after a 100-µg IV bolus of nitroglycerin, the uterus relaxed sufficiently to permit delivery.

Discussion.—This and previous reports show that IV nitroglycerin is a safe and effective technique of achieving rapid uterine relaxation in obstetric emergencies (Table). Indications include retained placenta, uterine inversion, and certain complications of twin delivery. Intravenous nitroglycerin also may be useful in preterm labor and pregnancy-induced hypertension.

► This series of 3 cases provides further anecdotal evidence of the efficacy of IV nitroglycerin as a potent uterine relaxant in obstetric patients. Both anesthesiologists and obstetricians should be aware that IV administration of small bolus doses of nitroglycerin results in profound but *transient* uterine relaxation. Thus, in some cases, it may be necessary to administer additional doses to facilitate completion of the procedure. The fact that the uterine relaxation is transient increases the likelihood of achieving effective uterine tone and hemostasis at the completion of the procedure.

D.H. Chestnut, M.D.

TABLE.—Summary of the Literature on IV Nitroglycerin Use in Obstetric Emergencies

Indication	Number of cases	Dose used	Onset of action	Adverse effects
Retained placenta post partum	15	500 μg i.v.	75–95 s	Mild decrease in blood pressure
Retained placenta post partum	22	50–100 μg i.v.	30–40 s	None
Upper uterine segment head entrapment of double footling breech during cesarean delivery under epidural anesthesia	1	1000 μg i.v.	Rapid uterine relaxation	Hypotension, blood pressure 70/30 with rapid response to ephedrine
Uterine contraction during internal podalic version for breech extraction of second twin	1	Sublingual aerosol 2 doses of 400 μg	30 s	None
30 wk. twin pregnancy, intense uterine contraction and inability to deliver during cesarean section under spinal anesthesia	1	100 μg i.v.	60–90 s	Mild hypotension with rapid response to ephedrine
Uterine inversion at cesarean delivery under spinal anesthesia	1	200 μg i.v. bolus	60 s	None
Complete uterine inversion with attached placenta	1	50 μg i.v. 2 doses	90–120 s	Mild hypotension after second dose
External version for 2nd twin transverse lie	1	50 μg i.v.	90–120 s	None
Internal podalic version of 2nd twin	2	Sublingual aerosol	35–65 s except for 1 pt with 2 doses	None
Abnormal presentation at cesarean delivery	2	2 doses of 400 μg		
Retained placenta	3			
Post partum uterine inversion	1	100 μg i.v.	60–90 s	None
Breech extraction during cesarean delivery under spinal anesthesia	1	100 μg i.v.	30 s	None
2nd trimester retained placenta	1	1850 μg i.v. total	Increasing over 5 min	None

Note: For reference information, see the original article.

(Courtesy of Riley ET, Flanagan B, Cohen SE, et al: Intravenous nitroglycerin: A potent uterine relaxant for emergency obstetric procedures. Review of literature and report of three cases. *Int J Obstet Anesth* 5:264–268, 1996.)

Comparison of Thrombelastography With Common Coagulation Tests in Preeclamptic and Healthy Parturients

Wong CA, Liu S, Glassenberg R (Northwestern Univ, Chicago)

Reg Anesth 20:521–527, 1995 3–37

Background.—The epidural administration of analgesia/anesthesia often benefits patients with preeclampsia. However, coagulopathy contraindicates regional anesthesia. Patients are commonly assessed by a routine coagulation battery (RCB) to determine their coagulation status. The RCB consists of prothrombin time, partial thromboplastin time, platelet count, and bleeding time. Thrombelastography (TEG) permits assessment of overall coagulation activity. The ability of TEG to predict normal and abnormal coagulation as diagnosed by RCB in healthy and preeclamptic parturients was investigated prospectively.

Methods.—Forty-seven women were included in the study. Tests were performed in the first stage of labor. The RCB and TEG were performed in 21 healthy women (group 1); 19 patients with mild preeclampsia/eclampsia (group 2); and 8 with severe preeclampsia/eclampsia (group 3).

Findings.—Normal RCB findings but mildly abnormal TEG results were documented in 1 patient in group 1, 3 in group 2, and 1 in group 3. One group 2 patient and 4 group 3 patients had abnormal RCBs. In 3 of these 5 women, thrombocytopenia with normal bleeding times and TEGs were noted. Two women had thrombocytopenia, prolonged bleeding times, and abnormal TEG results.

Conclusions.—In these preeclamptic parturients, TEG did not effectively predict abnormal coagulation, as diagnosed by RCB and using currently defined normal TEG values for nonpregnant women. However, because an abnormal TEG maximum amplitude value was always associated with prolonged bleeding time, TEG may be of value in determining platelet function in the presence of thrombocytopenia.

▶ It remains to be seen whether TEG will prove useful in preeclamptic women. These and other investigators have expressed hope that further studies might enable them to make recommendations for using TEG to guide clinical decisions regarding the administration of epidural anesthesia. However, anesthesiologists should remember that the incidence of epidural hematoma in preeclamptic women is very low. Although TEG may provide an estimate of the risk of surgical bleeding, I question whether it will allow anesthesiologists to predict the risk of epidural hematoma.

D.H. Chestnut, M.D.

Bolus Metoclopramide Does Not Enhance Morphine Analgesia After Cesarean Section

Driver RP Jr, D'Angelo R, Eisenach JC (Wake Forest Univ, Winston-Salem, NC)

Anesth Analg 82:1033–1035, 1996 3–38

Background.—The analgesic effects of opioids are postoperatively potentiated by IV metoclopramide. The mechanism that underlies this effect may be increased spinal concentrations of acetylcholine from metoclopramide-induced acetylcholinesterase inhibition.

Methods.—Sixty women who underwent elective cesarean section with subarachnoid anesthesia were enrolled in a randomized, placebo-controlled study. Thirty to 60 minutes before subarachnoid injection, the patients received an IV of either 20 mg metoclopramide, or saline. Before local anesthetic was injected, 2 mL of cerebrospinal fluid (CSF) was aspirated for assessment of cholinesterase activity. Pain was evaluated on a visual analog scale (VAS) before drug administration, at the first request for analgesia, and at discharge from the postanesthesia care unit. In addition, total morphine use was documented in the recovery room and for 1 day after surgery.

Findings.—The groups did not differ significantly in VAS scores, morphine use, or cerebrospinal cholinesterase activity. The CSF cholinesterase activity was comparable to that previously reported in nonpregnant patients.

Conclusions.—The women in this study did not demonstrate enhanced analgesia after IV metoclopramide was given in doses previously found to be analgesic after minor operative procedures. Also, there was no evidence that 20 mg of metoclopramide inhibited CSF acetylcholinesterase activity 45 minutes after it was administered.

▶ Metoclopramide is my preferred antiemetic agent for prevention and treatment of nausea and vomiting during or after administration of anesthesia for cesarean section. In an earlier study,[1] we observed that metoclopramide reduced the incidence of nausea and vomiting during or after administration of epidural anesthesia for cesarean section. In this article, investigators observed that prophylactic administration of 20 mg of metoclopramide did not enhance analgesia provided by patient-controlled intravenous morphine after cesarean section.

D.H. Chestnut, M.D.

Reference

1. Chestnut DH, Vandewalker GE, Owen CL, et al: Administration of metoclopramide for prevention of nausea and vomiting during epidural anesthesia for elective cesarean section. *Anesthesiology* 66:563–566, 1987.

Adding Fentanyl 0.0002% to Epidural Bupivacaine 0.125% Does Not Delay Gastric Emptying in Laboring Parturients

Zimmermann DL, Breen TW, Fick G (Univ of Calgary, Alberta, Canada)
Anesth Analg 82:612–616, 1996 3–39

Background.—Gastric emptying is reportedly delayed by as much as 45 minutes when administering bolus doses of fentanyl (50 and 100 μg) with epidural bupivacaine to laboring women. The effects of small-dose infusions of fentanyl coupled with local anesthetic on gastric emptying were evaluated in a group of women in active labor.

Patients and Methods.—Twenty-eight laboring women who had requested epidural anesthesia were randomly assigned to receive 10 mL bupivacaine 0.125% followed by an infusion of 0.125% bupivacaine at 10 mL/hour or 10 mL bupivacaine 0.125% with 50 μg fentanyl followed by an infusion of 0.125% bupivacaine and 0.0002% fentanyl at 10 mL/hour. Each patient ingested 20 mg/kg acetaminophen in a suspension of 150 mL of water 2 hours after initiation of epidural analgesia. Venous blood samples were obtained at baseline, and repeat samples were collected every 15 minutes for 2.5 hours thereafter.

Results.—Age, weight, height, gestational age, cervical dilation, mode of onset of labor, and number of top-ups required were similar between treatment groups. All patients showed a clear peak in the acetaminophen

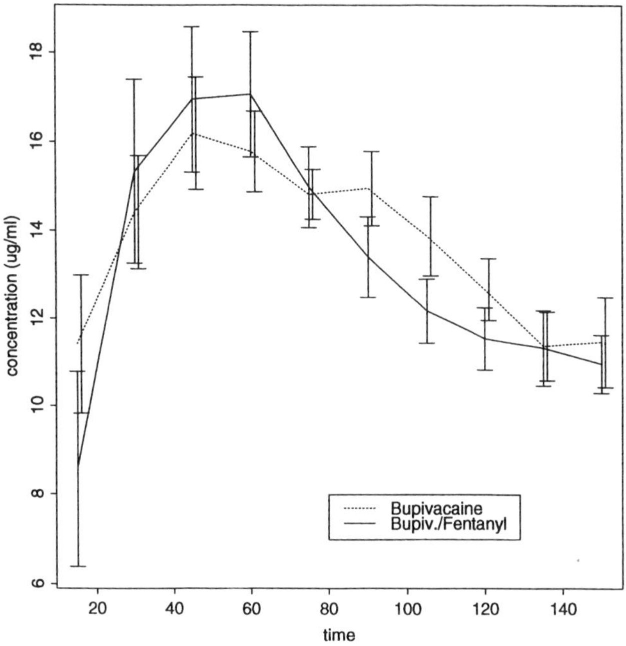

FIGURE 1.—The mean plasma acetaminophen concentration profiles over time for the 2 groups. (Courtesy of Zimmermann DL, Breen TW, Fick G: Adding fentanyl 0.0002% to epidural bupivacaine 0.125% does not delay gastric emptying in laboring parturient. *Anesth Analg* 82:612–616, 1996.)

concentration curve. There were no significant differences in peak plasma concentrations of acetaminophen noted between groups (Fig 1). Likewise, time to achieve peak plasma concentrations and areas under the curve at 45 and 90 minutes did not significantly differ between groups.

Conclusions.—Epidural infusions using 0.125% bupivacaine and 0.00025 fentanyl do not delay gastric emptying compared with infusion of bupivacaine 0.0125% in laboring patients. These findings suggest that concerns about delayed gastric emptying when adding small-dose fentanyl to local anesthetic continuous epidural infusions are unfounded. The risk of aspiration is, however, still present. Caution is therefore encouraged for pregnant laboring patients, since gastroesophageal reflux can occur in some pregnant women at term.

▶ Two decades ago, anesthesiologists told laboring women that one of the advantages of epidural analgesia was the fact that systemic opioid administration could be avoided during labor. Administration of epidural analgesia allowed physicians to avoid the effects of systemic opioids on the infant, as well as the adverse effects of systemic opioids on maternal gastric emptying. During the last decade, epidural administration of both a lipid-soluble opioid and a local anesthetic has become a common practice in laboring women. Initial studies suggested that epidural opioid administration during labor resulted in delayed gastric emptying. The present study suggests that any delay in gastric emptying as a result of epidural fentanyl administration is of short duration; gastric emptying times were normal 2 hours after epidural administration of a 50 μg bolus dose of fentanyl. Also, continuous epidural administration of 20 μg/hour of fentanyl did not delay gastric emptying.

D.H. Chestnut, M.D.

Neostigmine, Atropine, and Glycopyrrolate: Does Neostigmine Cross the Placenta?

Clark RB, Brown MA, Lattin DL (Univ of Arkansas, Little Rock)
Anesthesiology 84:450–452, 1996 3–40

Background.—Drugs given to pregnant women can cross the placenta and affect the fetus. In the following case report, neostigmine apparently crossed the placenta in a pregnant patient undergoing open reduction for an elbow fracture.

> *Case Report.*—Woman, 22, about 31 weeks' pregnant, fractured her elbow and required open reduction. Her history was remarkable for paranoid schizophrenia, which had been treated with haloperidol and lorazepam. The open reduction was performed under general endotracheal anesthesia. Isoflurane and nitrous oxide were the main anesthetics used. Thiopental was adminsitered to induce anesthesia, succinylcholine to facilitate intubation, and ve-

curonium to prevent movement. Neostigmine and glycopyrolate were given intravenously to reverse the muscle relaxant effect at the end of surgery. The fetal heart rate was observed to drop to 90 to 110 beats/min after neostigmine and glycopyrolate administration. Eventually, the heart rate returned to 120 beats/min. Although the open reduction was performed with no other complications, 4 days later the repair was judged unsatisfactory. The surgery was repeated as before, with left uterine displacement and careful monitoring of fetal heart rate and uterine contractions. This time, however, neostigmine and atropine were given to antagonize the muscle relaxant, and there was no change in fetal heart rate. A healthy infant was subsequently delivered at term.

Conclusions.—Significant placental crossing of neostigmine appeared to occur in this patient. The authors recommend the use of atropine with neostigmine rather than glycopyrrolate for reversing nondepolarizing muscle relaxants in pregnant women to ameliorate the marked bradycardia induced by the neostigmine.

▶ Several years ago, a colleague of mine made a similar observation during administration of anesthesia for a thyroidectomy in a pregnant patient. At the conclusion of the procedure, he observed fetal bradycardia after administration of neostigmine and glycopyrrolate to reverse the nondepolarizing muscle relaxant. He correctly concluded that the bradycardia resulted from the transplacental transfer of the neostigmine. The fetal heart rate gradually returned baseline, and the outcome was good for both mother and baby.

D.H. Chestnut, M.D.

Ilioinguinal Iliohypogastric Nerve Blocks: Before or After Cesarean Delivery Under Spinal Anesthesia?

Huffnagle HJ, Norris MC, Leighton BL, et al (Thomas Jefferson Univ, Philadelphia)

Anesth Analg 82:8–12, 1996 3–41

Background.—Surgical incisions and other perioperative events can trigger sustained changes in central neural function, leading to subsequent postoperative pain. Local anesthetic block of the involved somatosensory pathways before surgery may mitigate the postoperative pain response, thereby decreasing postoperative pain and analgesic use. The Pfannenstiel incision lies within the L1 dermatome; thus, bilateral ilioinguinal iliohypogastric nerve blocks (IINBs) should furnish analgesia after low transverse cesarean section. To test this hypotheses, the analgesic effects of IINBs placed pre- and postoperatively were evaluated in patients undergoing cesarean sections.

Patients and Methods.—Forty-six patients scheduled to undergo cesarean section deliveries were included in the study, with 22 randomly as-

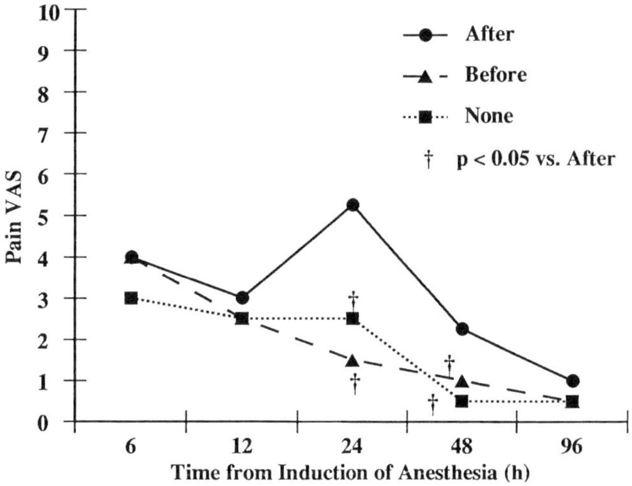

FIGURE 4.—Overall pain (median) at rest for 96 hours after induction of anesthesia. Women in the Before and After groups had bilateral ilioinguinal iliohypogastric nerve block placed before and after surgery, respectively; women in the None group had no block. Women in the After group had the most pain at 24 and 48 hours. *Abbreviation: VAS*, visual analogue scale. (Courtesy of Huffnagle HJ, Norris MC, Leighton BL, et al: Ilioinguinal iliohypogastric nerve blocks: Before or after cesarean delivery under spinal anesthesia? *Anesth Analg* 82:8–12, 1996.)

signed to before-surgery block, 12 to after-surgery block, and 12 to no-block treatment groups. Age, height, weight, and previous number of cesarean deliveries were similar between groups. No intraoperative medications, with the exception of antibiotics or ephedrine, were administered. Patients assigned to nerve block treatment had bilateral IINBs placed, and 10 mL of 0.5% bupivacaine was administered to each side. Additional postoperative morphine was provided as needed through a patient-controlled analgesia pump. Twenty-four hour use of morphine was evaluated by an observer blinded to treatment groups. Patient satisfaction and incisional-related and overall pain scores also were recorded during a 96–hour period.

Results.—Eleven of the patients assigned to before-surgery treatment had failed blocks at 6 hours and were eliminated from the analysis. No between-group differences in morphine use were noted. There also were no consistent between-group differences in pain scores. However, patients in the before-surgery treatment group had less incisional pain at rest, compared with the no-treatment group at 6 hours, and with the after-surgery treatment group at 24 hours. The greatest amount of incisional pain with movement was observed in women receiving after-surgery treatment at the 48-hour evaluation. The after-surgery treatment group also had the most overall pain at rest 24 and 48 hours after surgery (Fig 4). At the 96-hour assessment, patients in the after-surgery treatment group had the greatest amount of overall pain with movement. Similar satisfaction scores were noted across all 3 treatment groups throughout the study period.

Conclusions.—Patients receiving spinal anesthesia during elective cesarean delivery do not benefit from IINBs placed either before or after surgery. Surprisingly, postoperative blocks appear to increase postoperative pain. These findings suggest that there is currently no need to use IINBs in this particular patient population.

► I have no experience with the performance of IINBs in obstetric patients undergoing cesarean section. The negative results observed in the present study suggest that, for now, there is little reason for me to add this block to my armamentarium in obstetric anesthesia practice.

D.H. Chestnut, M.D.

Airway Management Issues

Some Important Details in the Technique of Percutaneous Dilatational Tracheostomy via the Modified Seldinger Technique

Marx WH, Ciaglia P, Graniero KD (State Univ of New York, Syracuse; St Elizabeth Hosp, Utica, NY)

Chest 110:762–766, 1996 3–42

Objective.—A tracheostomy performed to maintain an airway in patients needing ventilatory support is a safe and reliable procedure that is acceptable to patients. A prospective study of the results of percutaneous dilatational tracheostomy led to recommendations of changes in operative technique to improve the procedure.

Methods.—Percutaneous dilational tracheostomies were performed on 254 patients in a 10-year period.

> *Technique.*—After the endotracheal cuff is deflated and the tube is withdrawn, the catheter introducer needle is passed into the trachea through a 1- to 2-cm incision between the first and second tracheal rings. If end-tidal CO_2 increases or arterial oxygen saturation decreases, the endotracheal tube is advanced or the cuff is reinflated. The trachea is anesthetized and a J wire is inserted. Dilation is performed with the short 11 F dilator, which is then removed. An 8 F guiding catheter with a new ridge is inserted, and the trachea is serially dilated. Care should be exercised when removing the largest dilators so that the double guide is not also withdrawn. The tracheostomy tube flanges are secured with sutures, and the patient's neck is taped to secure the tube, which is attached to the ventilator with a double-swivel connector. A bronchoscope is used to confirm placement and positioning.

Results.—There were 4 major complications, including 1 death, 1 tension pneumothorax, 1 tube displacement, and 1 left main-stem intubation, and 18 minor complications, including 5 patients who could not be intubated. Seven late complications included 2 patients with tracheal stenosis,

1 patient with persistent stoma, 1 with cellulitis, 1 with left main-stem bronchial intubation, 1 with tube displacement, and 1 with partial obstruction as a result of tube twisting.

Conclusion.—Percutaneous dilational tracheostomy can be safely performed with the procedural modifications recommended in this study. Complications were similar to those from open tracheostomy. Complications rates were 1. 5% for major and 5.5% for minor complications. The mortality rate was 0.39%.

Comparison of Percutaneous and Surgical Tracheostomies

Friedman Y, Fildes J, Mizock B, et al (Cook County Hosp, Chicago; Finch Univ of Health Sciences/Chicago Med School, North Chicago, Ill, Univ of Illinois, Chicago)

Chest 110:480–485, 1996 3–43

Introduction.—Surgical tracheostomy is considered a simple and safe procedure; however, complication rates range up to 66%. A simpler procedure performed at bedside would eliminate the risks involved in transporting critically ill patients. The percutaneous tracheostomy is such a procedure and was modifed in 1985 as the percutaneous dilational tracheostomy. A randomized, prospective comparison of surgical tracheostomy and percutaneous dilational tracheostomy was performed to evaluate the potential logistic benefits and to confirm the relative safety of percutaneous dilational tracheostomy.

Methods.—Twenty-seven patients were randomized to surgical tracheostomy and 26 were randomized to percutaneous dilational tracheostomy. All were 18 years of age or older. Percutaneous dilational tracheostomies were done at the patient's bedside and surgical tracheostomies were performed in the operating room under general anesthesia. Patients having percutaneous dilational tracheostomies had 100% fraction of inspired oxygen, local anesthesia, and IV sedation to control pain and anxiety. The procedure involved repositioning the endotracheal tube above the site of the proposed tracheostomy. At the level of the first or second tracheal interspace, a guidewire was placed in the trachea. At the site of the skin puncture, a 1-cm incision was made. Over the guidewire, a series of dilators were introducted to enlarge the stoma and the tracheostomy tube was inserted.

Results.—The time was shorter from randomization into the study until tracheostomy for the percutaneous dilational tracheostomy (28.5±27.9 hours) than the surgical tracheostomy (100.4±95.0 hours) after randomization. Percutaneous dilational tracheostomy took significantly less time (8.2±4.9 minutes) to perform than surgical tracheostomy (33.9±14 minutes). Between the groups, there was no significant difference in intraprocedureal complications. For the percutaneous dilational tracheostomy group, postprocedure complication rate was 12%, and for the surgical

TABLE 3.—Postprocedure Complications

	Percutaneous $n=26$	Surgical $n=27$
Major		
Accidental decannulation	1 (4)	4 (15)
Moderate bleed (150–250 mL)	0	0
Severe bleed (>250 mL)	1 (4)	1 (4)
Minor		
Small bleed (25–100 mL)	1 (4)	3 (11)
Wound/stomal infection	0	4 (15)
Total	3 (12)	12 (41)*

Note: Numbers in parentheses denote percentage.
$^*P = 0.008$.
(Courtesy of Friedman Y, Fildes J, Mizock B, et al: Comparison of percutaneous and surgical tracheostomies. *Chest* 110:480–485, 1996.)

tracheostomy group, the postprocedure complication rate was 41% (Table 3).

Conclusion.—Logistically, percutaneous dilational tracheostomy is superior to surgical tracheostomy because it can be performed at bedside and eliminates the risks of patient transport. Percutaneous dilational tracheostomy can be performed earlier because operating room scheduling is not necessary. There are fewer postprocedure complications, less cost, and better cosmetic results with percutaneous dilational tracheostomy.

▶ These 2 articles describe percutaneous dilational tracheostomy, a technique that may prove to be useful in those institutions in which surgical tracheostomy is associated with logistic and/or medical complications. While procedurally this does not appear to be a difficult skill to achieve, it should not be attempted without experienced guidance.

D.M. Rothenberg, M.D.

Postextubation Laryngeal Edema in Adults: Risk Factor Evaluation and Prevention by Hydrocortisone

Ho LI, Harn HJ, Lien TC, et al (Veterans Gen Hosp Taipei, Taiwan, Republic of China)

Intensive Care Med 22:933–936, 1996 3–44

Background.—Endotracheal intubation has become standard, life-saving treatment for critically ill patients who need respiratory support. Although it is generally well tolerated, complications from injury to the hypopharynx, larynx, and trachea can occur during intubation and after extubation. Evidence of injury often includes mucosal ulceration and inflammation, and edema. Edema of the laryngeal structure can cause significant morbidity and death. Risk factors for postextubation stridor were identified and the ability of steroids to prevent this complication was determined.

Methods.—Intubation was performed in 77 patients via the orotracheal or nasotracheal route with a low-pressure, high-volume cuff tube. The tube cuffs were checked at least once every 8 hours, and cuff pressure was maintained at 25–30 cm H_2O. Possible risk factors, such as age, gender, diagnosis, internal diameter of the endotracheal tube, and route and duration of intubation were recorded. Patients were given 100 mg of hydrocortisone sodium succinate or placebo IV 1 hour before extubation. Patients were monitored every 6 hours for 24 hours.

Results.—Laryngeal edema was defined as clinical signs of upper airway obstruction, and stridor was defined as a crowing sound on inspiration. The overall incidence of postextubation stridor was 22%. Stridor occurred in 39% of females and 17% of males. The relative risk of stridor was 2.29 in female patients. Postextubation stridor occurred in 7 of 39 patients given hydrocortisone and 10 of 38 patients in the control group. Reintubation was required in only 1 patient, who was from the control group.

Discussion.—The major finding was that 100 mg of hydrocortisone administered IV 1 hour before extubation did not affect the risk of postextubation stridor. No correlation between postextubation stridor and duration of intubation was found. Female gender was the only significant risk factor for the development of stridor. The use of corticosteroids to prevent stridor is not supported. Darmon, et al. reported that the risk of postextubation laryngeal edema is higher in females and in patients who are intubated for more than 36 hours. It is believed that postextubation laryngeal edema or stridor results from trauma to the laryngeal mucosa. More research is needed to identify the actual risk factors of postextubation stridor.

▶ This simple study confirms previous data that also failed to support the use of corticosteroids to prevent postextubation stridor. Although this study assessed only the efficacy of single dose therapy, prior studies with multiple dose treatment showed no improvement either. Unfortunately, old myths die hard and clinicians continue to prescribe corticosteroids on an all too routine basis, often with little regard for the potential side effects.

D.M. Rothenberg, M.D.

Myasthenia Gravis and Upper Airway Obstruction

Putman MT, Wise RA (Johns Hopkins Hosp, Baltimore, Md)

Chest 109:400–404, 1996 3–45

Background.—Although most cases of respiratory impairment in myasthenia gravis are attributed to weakness of the diaphragm and other muscles, some are caused by upper airway obstruction. The latter cause is not often reported and may go unrecognized; however, it may be more common than the literature suggests. A retrospective study was prompted by a case of symptomatic upper airway obstruction in a patient with myasthenia gravis.

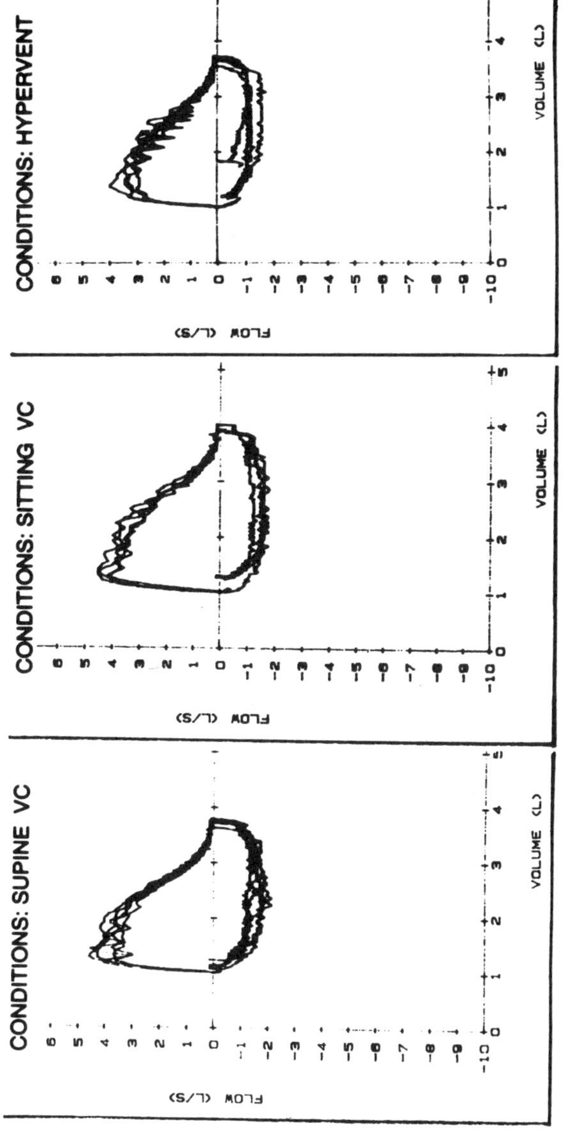

FIGURE 1.—Flow volume loops of the patient reported in the supine and sitting position and after hyperventilating for 1 min. *Abbreviation: VC,* vital capacity. (Courtesy of Putman MT, Wise RA: Myasthenia gravis and upper airway obstruction. *Chest* 109:400–404, 1996.)

Case Report.—Woman, 54, who had had myasthenia gravis for 5 years was referred for evaluation of acute shortness of breath. All of the episodes occurred at night, beginning with persistent coughing and followed by shortness of breath and wheezing. The patient's forced vital capacity and forced expiratory volume in 1 sec were normal in supine and sitting positions and after hyperventilation. However, under all 3 of these conditions, her maximal inspiratory pressure was reduced. Flow volume loops showed significant reductions in forced inspiratory flow, suggesting variable extrathoracic airway obstruction (Fig 1).

Study Findings.—In a review of 61 patients with myasthenia gravis tested in a pulmonary function laboratory, 12 were found to have flow volume loops. Seven of these 12 patients had a pattern consistent with extrathoracic upper airway obstruction, and 5 of the 7 had a forced vital capacity of 80% or more.

Conclusions.—Upper airway obstruction in myasthenia gravis may be more frequent than generally thought. Respiratory evaluation of patients with myasthenia gravis, especially those with bulbar muscle weakness or respiratory symptoms of unknown origin, should include the inspiratory and expiratory flow volume loop.

▶ Recognizing that postoperative respiratory failure may occur in patients with myasthenia gravis, anesthesiologists often request that a preoperative workup include baseline vital capacity or peak flow so that the degree, if any, of respiratory muscle dysfunction can be assessed. This study would suggest that a flow volume loop should also be performed to diagnose upper airway obstruction. Those who manifest changes consistent with extrathoracic obstruction may require additional anticholinesterase therapy, immunotherapy, or, possibly, plasmapheresis before an elective procedure.

D.M. Rothenberg, M.D.

Preoperative Fasting

Preoperative Fasting Time: Is the Traditional Policy Changing?: Results of a National Survey

Green CR, Pandit SK, Schork MA (Univ of Michigan, Ann Arbor)

Anesth Analg 83:123–128, 1996 3–46

Background.—The "nothing by mouth" (NPO) after midnight order is a routine preoperative order, although there are clear detrimental effects of prolonged fasting. Several recent studies have challenged this preoperative fasting practice, and a relaxation of the traditional NPO policy has been reported. To determine current policies and practices regarding the NPO order, anesthesiologists in the United States were surveyed.

Methods.—A questionnaire regarding NPO policy, practice guidelines, and adverse outcomes was mailed to randomly selected university anesthesiology programs and ambulatory surgery facilities.

Results.—The traditional NPO policy, with nothing allowed by mouth after midnight, was supported for adults by 59% of the respondents. However, either flexibility or the allowance of clear liquids up to 4 hours before elective surgery was reported by 41% with adult patients and 68% with pediatric patients. Among those allowing clear liquids, water was acceptable for adults in 100% and for children in 94%. Apple juice was allowed for both adults and children by more than 90% of the respondents. Only 19% reported using routine aspiration prophylaxis in elective surgery outpatients. No adverse outcomes associated with a change in the NPO policy were reported.

Conclusions.—A substantial number of anesthesiologists have changed or relaxed NPO guidelines for elective surgery in adults and especially in children.

▶ This is a national survey in which "none of the respondents reported any medical adverse event associated with the institution of flexible NPO policy." Do the authors really expect survey respondents to report adverse events? Only 64% of the anesthesiologists who were sent the questionnaire even responded at all! The response bias of this article is likely to render it completely invalid. I do not doubt that we are becoming more flexible in our NPO policy, but the numbers contained in this survey are subject to the problems contained in any kind of survey in which there could be medical or legally damaging events that would be unprotected or poorly protected from discovery. At least, the authors do tell us what "NPO" means, namely, in the Latin, *nulla per os.*

J.H. Tinker, M.D.

Postoperative Feeding

The Clear Liquid Diet Is No Longer a Necessity in the Routine Postoperative Management of Surgical Patients

Jeffery KM, Harkins B, Cresci GA, et al (Med College of Georgia, Augusta; Eisenhower Army Med Ctr, Augusta)

Am Surg 62:167–170, 1996 3–47

Introduction.—The return of bowel sounds is the accepted indicator for when to advance from a liquid diet after abdominal surgery. Little scientific evidence supports the need for restricting patients with abdominal surgery to a liquid diet in the presence of a postoperative ileus. Nor does evidence exist that beginning a regular diet in the immediate postoperative period is acceptable. The recent interest in challenging traditional views regarding the immediate postoperative diet has prompted this large, prospective randomized investigation to address this uncertainty.

Methods.—All patients from 3 large medical centers scheduled to undergo elective or emergent abdominal surgery were randomized to receive either a clear-liquid or regular diet in the immediate postoperative period. Patients in the clear-liquid diet group were advanced to a regular diet as tolerated. Patients were observed postoperatively for nausea, vomiting, abdominal distention, and other signs of dietary intolerance.

Results.—Of 241 patients, 106 were assigned to a regular diet and 135 to a clear-liquid diet for the first postoperative meal. The regular diet group received significantly more calories and protein than did patients in the clear-liquid diet group. The most common symptoms of dietary intolerance were nausea and vomiting. Eight (7.5%) patients in the regular diet group and 11 (8.1%) patients in the clear-liquid diet group developed intolerance. All patients in the clear liquid diet group and 6 patients in the regular diet group were switched to nothing-by-mouth status. The remaining 2 patients in the regular diet group were given a liquid diet until symptoms resolved. No significant differences occurred in dietary intolerance according to type of surgery performed. No significant between-group differences occurred in diet-associated morbidity.

Conclusion.—Findings suggest that no increased morbidity was associated with the use of a regular meal as the first postoperative meal. Patients should proceed cautiously and eat only food that is appealing when starting with a regular diet in the immediate postoperative period. It would be interesting to see if hospital stays are shorter because of the additional nutritional support received when a regular diet is served.

▶ This is an important study as it debunks one of the "old wives' tales" of medicine. The standard has always been to start with clear liquids when resuming oral intake in patients who have had intra-abdominal surgery and advance the patient's diet in a stepwise fashion. This study randomly allocated patients to the two groups and then started one of the groups with a regular diet. The authors don't show any benefit, other than for the intermediate variable of amount of intake of total calories, but then they also show that starting with a regular diet is not harmful.

Another caveat in this study is that esophageal surgery, surgery for obesity, Whipple procedures, prolonged intubation or ICU stay, or tube feedings begun immediately were important exclusion criteria. I encourage you to read this study as it appears to be both well done and important for our specialty.

M.F. Roizen, M.D.

Cardiovascular Anesthesia Issues

Nonlinear Measures of Heart Rate Variability After Fentanyl-based Induction of Anesthesia

Storella RJ, Kandell RB, Horrow JC, et al (Hahnemann Univ, Philadelphia; Drexel Univ, Philadelphia)

Anesth Analg 81:1292–1294, 1995 3–48

Introduction.—The new nonlinear methods of measuring heart rate variability (HRV) have yet to be applied in the operating room. To determine whether these methods would be of value in detecting changes in

HRV that occur during anesthetic management, 2 nonlinear methods were used to measure the effect of induction of anesthesia on HRV.

Methods.—The nonlinear methods evaluated were approximate entropy (ApEn) and point correlation dimension (PD2). The first method, ApEn, is calculated by identifying patterns within a time series and determining the effect of increasing pattern size, assuming that patterns repeat themselves. The second method, PD2, estimates the "dimension" at each point in a series, even if it changes during the measurement period. Calculation with PD2 is complex, and involves breaking a time series into vectors of many dimensions. The nonlinear methods were evaluated in a study of ECGs from 12 patients who were undergoing cardiac surgery.

Results.—Neither the mean R-R interval nor the standard deviation of the R-R intervals changed significantly after induction of anesthesia. Although the *r* value at which peak ApEn occurred was not altered with anesthesia induction, significant decreases in total power, ApEn, peak ApEn, and mean PD2 were observed. Mean percent decreases after anesthesia induction were 37% for ApEn and 32% for mean PD2, both greater than the mean decrease in peak ApEn (13%). Decreases in mean PD2 were seen in all 12 patients, and only 1 of the 2 patients with atrial fibrillation failed to show decreases in ApEn and peak ApEn.

Discussion.—Both the nonlinear methods of HRV measurement revealed changes after the induction of anesthesia. Peak ApEn changed less with induction than ApEn, but peak ApEn also varied less and can be calculated independently for each time series. Because the magnitude of periodic change does not affect ApEn, this method is preferable when changes in position and respiratory rate are confounding factors. In contrast, PD2 is appropriate for non-stationary data. Both nonlinear measures may supplement spectral analysis of HRV.

► This study stems from the use of HRV as a potentially valuable sign of both preoperative autonomic neuropathy and intraoperative depth of anesthesia. Some of the measures of HRV are interval variation, and this newer application described here is the approximate entropy of the HRV. This is the first report that I have seen using this and showing a 30% or greater reduction in HRV by this measure with induction of an opioid-based anesthetic. I encourage you to notice where this article comes from so that if this method gains popularity, you will be able to go back and trace its origins, problems, and promises.

M.F. Roizen, M.D.

Cardiopulmonary Resuscitation on Television: Miracles and Misinformation

Diem SJ, Lantos JD, Tulsky JA (Durham Veterans Affairs Med Ctr, NC; Duke Univ, Durham, NC; Univ of Chicago)

N Engl J Med 334:1578–1582, 1996 3–49

Background.—Patients must be educated about the risks and benefits of CPR before they can take part in decision making about its potential use. Because television is an important source of information, the portrayal of CPR on 3 popular medical shows was analyzed.

Methods.—All episodes of "ER" and "Chicago Hope" from the 1994–1995 television season and 50 consecutive episodes of "Rescue 911" broadcast during 3 months in 1995 were analyzed. All portrayals of CPR in each episode were documented, and the causes of cardiac arrest, identifiable demographic features of the characters who underwent CPR, underlying diseases, and outcomes were considered in the analysis.

Findings.—Sixty depictions of CPR were documented in the 97 television episodes. Thirty-one occurred in "ER," 11 in "Chicago Hope," and 18 in "Rescue 911." In most instances, trauma caused cardiac arrest. Only 28% resulted from primary cardiac causes. Sixty-five percent of the cardiac arrests depicted were in children, adolescents, or young adults. Seventy-five percent of the fictional patients survived the immediate arrest. Sixty-seven percent apparently survived to hospital discharge.

Conclusions.—In these television shows, the survival rates associated with cardiac arrest were significantly higher than the best survival rates reported in the medical literature. The portrayal of CPR on television may lead the public to have unrealistic expectations of the success of this procedure. When discussing the use of CPR with patients and their families, physicians should be aware of the misperceptions that television images of CPR may foster.

▶ After my initial reading, I asked myself a simple question: Do we really need an article in a prestigious medical journal to tell us that we shouldn't believe everything we see on television? Let alone on "Chicago Hope"? Upon further review, however, I became more concerned with the physicians who were forced to sit through 50 consecutive episodes of "Rescue 911"! After that ordeal I know that, irrespective of the success of resuscitation commonly portrayed, I'd have asked to have a do-not-resuscitate order placed in my *TV Guide*!

D.M. Rothenberg, M.D.

Systemic Inflammatory Response Syndrome After Cardiac Operations
Cremer J, Martin M, Redl H, et al (Hannover Med School, Germany)
Ann Thorac Surg 61:1714–1720, 1996 3–50

Background.—After open heart surgery, hyperdynamic circulatory instability and organ dysfunction may result from a systemic inflammatory response. The current study determined the extent to which mediator release is involved.

Methods.—Ten patients with postoperative hyperdynamic circulatory dysregulation requiring α-constrictors (group 1) and 10 undergoing routine cardiac procedures and stable postoperative hemodynamic indices (group 2) were studied. Mediator release and metabolic and hemodynamic changes until the third day after surgery were documented.

Findings.—Cardiac index was significantly increased and systemic vascular resistance decreased after bypass and at 3 hours in group 1. These patients also had significantly higher serum levels of interleukin-6. Though nonsignificant, increases in elastase, tumor necrosis factor, soluble tumor necrosis factor receptor, and interleukin-8 were also noted in group 1. In the early postoperative period, soluble E-selectin and soluble intercellular adhesion molecules were elevated (nonsignificantly) in group 1. Only 3 of 10 group 1 patients had continuously increased levels of endotoxin. Severe lactic acidosis was observed only in group 1 patients.

Conclusions.—Postoperative hyperdynamic instability is apparently associated with a certain pattern of mediator release after open heart surgery. Interleukin-6 seems to be involved in circulatory dysregulation and metabolic derangement.

▶ The literature is now replete with studies similar to this that show elevated cytokine levels during or shortly after cardiopulmonary bypass. (Previous experimental and clinical studies were cited in the 1995 Year Book.[1, 2]) Unfortunately these studies are not easily comparable as they fail to control for such factors as temperature, steroid use, or blood product administration. We have all witnessed the patient who develops a profoundly vasodilated state after cardiopulmonary bypass, and have speculated on complement or cytokine mediation, but there are little data out there to help us discern which of these patients are preoperatively at risk. Once this is defined, the task of prophylactic therapy will then need to be addressed.

D.M. Rothenberg, M.D.

References

1. Menasché P, Haydar S, Peyret J, et al: A potential mechanism of vasodilation after warm heart surgery: The temperature-dependent release of cytokines. *J Thorac Cardiovasc Surg* 107: 293–299, 1994. (1995 Yearbook of Anesthesiology and Pain Management, p 204.)
2. Kawamura T, Wakusawa R, Okada K, et al: Elevation of cytokines during open heart surgery with cardiopulmonary bypass: Participation of interleukin 8 and 6 in reperfusion injury. *Can J Anaesth* 40: 1016–1021, 1993. (1995 Yearbook of Anesthesiology and Pain Management, p 208.)

Mental Stress–induced Myocardial Ischemia and Cardiac Events
Jiang W, Babyak M, Krantz DS, et al (Duke Univ, Durham, NC; Uniformed Services Univ of the Health Sciences, Bethesda, Md)
JAMA 275:1651–1656, 1996 3–51

Objective.—Although mental stress has been shown to induce myocardial ischemia in patients with stable coronary artery disease (CAD), the prognostic significance is unknown. The association of mental stress-induced ischemia with clinical events in patients with documented CAD and positive exercise tests during a follow-up period was determined prospectively.

Methods.—Antianginal medications were withdrawn from 126 CAD patients (112 men, 14 women; mean age, 59 years) with exercise-induced ischemia 48 hours before they took 5 mental stress tests, including mental arithmetic, public speaking, mirror tracing, reading, and a taped interview to assess type-A behavior. After a 20-minute rest, radionuclide ventriculography (RNV) was performed at rest and after exercise testing on a bicycle ergometer to 90% of predicted maximal heart rate or until standard clinical endpoints were reached. Patients were followed for up to 5 years to assess medical status.

Results.—There were no clinical or demographic differences between patients who experienced a cardiac event and those who did not. There were 28 patients (22%) with at least 1 cardiac event, 2 of them fatal, and 2 noncardiac deaths. Patients with mental stress–induced ischemia were almost 3 times as likely to have a cardiac event. Regression analysis showed that reduction of left ventricular ejection fraction during mental stress was significantly related to a decrease in event-free survival. Every 1% reduction in left ventricular ejection fraction was associated with an 8% increase in risk of a cardiac event. The exercise ischemic threshold was not prognostic of cardiac events.

Conclusion.—Patients with mental stress–induced ischemia had significantly more fatal and nonfatal cardiac events than did patients with exercise-induced ischemia, possibly because they may have had more severe CAD. Patients with mental stress–induced ischemia may have heightened sympathetic discharge, increased neurohumoral responses to stress, and altered circulatory, coagulation, electrolyte, or platelet responses. Studies that examine the effect of stress management on the incidence of cardiac events may be helpful.

▶ Read this article but, please, not out loud or in a public domain. Analyze the data, but feel free to use a calculator and by all means take your time. And finally, have a couple of aspirins, some vitamin E, and a clove of garlic after your next unexpected, difficult intubation.

D.M. Rothenberg, M.D.

Normothermic Continuous Blood Cardioplegia Improves Electrophysiologic Recovery After Open Heart Surgery

Gozal Y, Glantz L, Luria MH, et al (Hadassah Univ, Jerusalem)

Anesthesiology 84:1298–1306, 1996 3–52

Purpose.—Oxygenated blood cardioplegia can protect the myocardium during open heart surgery. The optimal temperature of cardioplegia is still open to debate, however. Cold blood cardioplegia plus systemic hypothermia provides safe and reliable myocardial preservation. Retrograde warm blood cardioplegia is an attractive alternative that avoids the adverse impact of hypothermia on the heart while reducing ischemia and subsequent reperfusion injury. These 2 approaches were compared for their effect on the quality of myocardial protection and on functional recovery of the heart in a randomized, controlled trial.

Methods.—The study included 42 patients undergoing coronary artery bypass grafting. They were assigned to undergo either normothermic or hypothermic cardioplegia, at temperatures of 33.5° and 10.0°C, respectively. Anesthesia was induced and maintained with fentanyl and midazolam. The operations were performed under continuous ECG Holter monitoring, and a coronary sinus cannula was used to obtain blood samples during surgery.

Results.—Seventy-five percent of patients in the hypothermic bypass group had transition through ventricular fibrillation at the start of cardio-

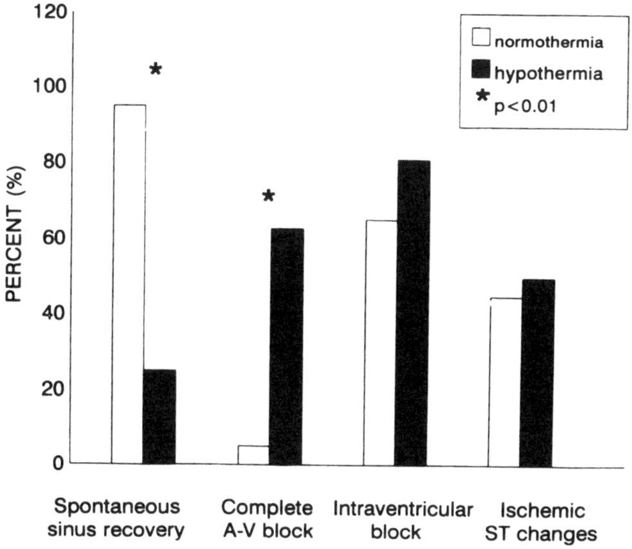

FIGURE 1.—ECG characteristics in the post–cardiopulmonary bypass period as obtained by continuous ECG (Holter) recordings. A comparison between myocardial protection by normothermic blood cardioplegia (n = 20) and hypothermic blood cardioplegia (n = 16). *Significant difference between the 2 groups (P < .01). (Courtesy of Gozal Y, Glantz L, Luria MH, et al: Normothermic continuous blood cardioplegia improves electrophysiologic recovery after open heart surgery. *Anesthesiology* 84: 1298–1306, 1996.)

pulmonary bypass, whereas 65% of those in the normothermic bypass group had atrial fibrillation. Reperfusion was followed by spontaneous resumption of sinus rhythm in 95% of patients in the normothermic group compared with 25% of patients in the hypothermic group. Ventricular fibrillation occurred in three fourths of patients in the latter group. Complete atrioventricular block sometimes followed, requiring temporary pacing for a mean of 168 minutes. There was no difference in the incidence of intraventricular block and ST segment changes, although patients in the hypothermic group had a significantly greater incidence of ventricular premature beats in the first 16 hours after bypass (Fig 1). In both groups, concentrations of lactate, creatinine phosphokinase, epinephrine, and norepinephrine increased gradually during the operation, with no differences between groups.

Conclusions.—Hypothermic blood cardioplegia appears to make patients more susceptible to ventricular fibrillation and dysrhythmia, and to delay recovery of the conduction system. These changes seem to stem from temperature-induced alterations in the cellular functions of the conduction tissue after ischemia. Myocardial protection is adequate with both techniques; however, the heart may recover more quickly after bypass with normothermic oxygenated blood cardioplegia.

▶ It is becoming clearer and clearer that, although moderate hypothermia may exert reasonable cerebral protection, normothermic cardioplegia may be better for the heart! I have little idea how to resolve this dilemma, but I would opine that we may have to find a reasonable compromise between the two.

J.H. Tinker, M.D.

Large-dose Intrathecal Morphine for Coronary Artery Bypass Grafting

Chaney MA, Smith KR, Barclay JC, et al (Loyola Univ, Maywood, Ill)

Anesth Analg 83:215–222, 1996 3–53

Background.—In cardiac surgical patients, aggressive pain control in the immediate postoperative period can reduce the incidence and severity of myocardial ischemia. In addition, by reducing blood catecholamine levels, aggressive pain control also may reduce morbidity and mortality. The intense and prolonged analgesia produced by intrathecal morphine may help to control postoperative pain and/or to reduce the stress response after cardiac surgery. The effects of large-dose intrathecal morphine in patients undergoing coronary artery bypass grafting (CABG) were assessed.

Methods.—The randomized trial included 60 patients undergoing primary, elective CABG. Intraoperative anesthesia consisted of fentanyl, midazolam, and vecuronium. In the postoperative period, the patients received either intrathecal morphine or saline placebo. Otherwise, the 2 groups received the same perioperative care, including patient-controlled analgesia with IV morphine. Catecholamine levels were compared by arterial blood sampling.

Results.—The postoperative IV morphine requirement from ICU arrival to the morning of the second postoperative day was significantly lower in the patients receiving intrathecal morphine. Patients receiving morphine tended to have lower perioperative norepinephrine and epinephrine levels than those in the saline group, but the difference was not significant. Disadvantages of intrathecal morphine included inability to extubate immediately after surgery and the possibility of postoperative urinary retention and somnolence.

Conclusions.—Large-dose intrathecal morphine provides reliable postoperative analgesia. However, it does not reliably reduce the stress response after CABG. It is unknown whether such aggressive control of postoperative pain affects patient outcomes, but the clinical disadvantages appear to outweigh the theoretical benefits.

▶ Whenever I see a paper like this, in which the authors have tried to demonstrate that a clinical effect occurs and have not been able to do so, I always wonder whether the study design had enough "power" to discriminate. This one, with 60 patients in it, probably did have such power, and it clearly shows that large-dose intrathecal morphine "does not reliably attenuate the stress response during and after cardiac surgery." Shades of "stress-free" anesthesia! Pain does not equal stress; it does not necessarily produce physiologic stress, contrary to popular belief; and stress does not equal pain in the sense of the physiologic trespass involved. I cannot for the life of me understand why we persist in such simplistic linkages. The authors here have lowered norepinephrine and epinephrine levels and provided adequate pain relief, yet did not attenuate other aspects of the stress response to any significant degree. Given the debacle of "stress-free" high-dose fentanyl anesthesia of a few years ago, I am not surprised.

J.H. Tinker, M.D.

Heparin-coated Circuits Reduce the Formation of TNFα During Cardiopulmonary Bypass

Yamada H, Kudoh I, Hirose Y, et al (Yokohama City Univ, Japan)

Acta Anaesthesiol Scand 40:311–317, 1996 3–54

Background.—Previous research has shown that the inflammatory response associated with cardiopulmonary bypass (CPB) can be reduced by heparin coating of the extracorporeal circuits, which decreases complement and granulocyte activation. The effects of heparin coating on the formation of tumor necrosis factor-α (TNFα), a major inflammatory mediator found in the circulation during and after CPB, were investigated.

Methods and Findings.—By random assignment, 18 patients scheduled for coronary artery bypass grafting underwent extracorporeal perfusion with either heparin-coated or uncoated circuits. Plasma levels of TNFα were found to increase only during CPB in patients with the uncoated circuits. Plasma levels of interleukin-8 (IL-8) increased during and after CPB in both groups. Heparin coating did not influence IL-8 levels. The neutrophil count increased after aortic cross-clamp release and remained increased for 3 days in both groups. However, in the group with coated circuits, the increase in neutrophil count was significantly lower than in the group with uncoated circuits. Both groups showed significant increases in plasma levels of neutrophil elastase during and after CPB. Elastase levels were significantly lower at certain time points in the patients with the coated circuits.

Conclusions.—Heparin-coated circuits significantly decrease TNFα formation, followed by a reduction in levels of neutrophil count and neutrophil elastase. Heparin coating of extracorporeal circuits appears to improve biocompatibility, which is beneficial to the patient.

▶ It is becoming understood that "neutrophil activation" is one of the culprits for activation of the stress response and the subsequent inflammatory damage done by CPB. We have long known that CPB is decidedly unphysiologic. Now, our colleagues are beginning to figure out why. It seems that a substance that originally was entitled TNFα is known now to be a major mediator of inflammation. It also is known now that this substance is responsible for at least some of the problems that are seen after CPB. This paper reports that heparin-coated circuits reduce the release of this substance and may improve outcomes in terms of inflammation and other problems after CPB. It is not obvious, but is possible, that some parts of the still-high incidence of cerebral dysfunction after CPB might be due to these kinds of mediators.

J.H. Tinker, M.D.

The Relationship Between Intelligence and Duration of Circulatory Arrest With Deep Hypothermia

Oates RK, Simpson JM, Turnbull JAB, et al (Univ of Sydney, Australia; Children's Hosp, Camperdown, Australia)

J Thorac Cardiovasc Surg 110:786–792, 1995 3–55

Background.—Studies that have examined whether cerebral anoxia with hypothermia is consistent with normal neurologic outcomes have yielded contradictory findings. The association between the duration of total circulatory arrest and various measures of cognitive function in a large group of children old enough for accurate psychological and neuropsychological testing was determined.

Methods.—One hundred fourteen children were included. Fifty-one had tetralogy of Fallot, 30 had transposition of the great arteries, and 33 had ventricular septal defect. Repair of these defects involved deep hypothermia and circulatory arrest in all patients. At a mean 9 to 10 years postoperatively, intellectual and neuropsychological function was assessed.

None of the subjects had preoperative intellectual deficits or postoperative neurologic complications. Fifty-four patients with atrial septal defects repaired with the use of cardiopulmonary bypass comprised a comparison group.

Findings.—The bypass group had reaction times 2 to 3 seconds shorter on average than the hypothermic circulatory arrest group. This was the only significant difference. Although intelligence quotient (IQ) did not differ between groups, IQ was found to be related to arrest time. In a regression analysis, IQ declined significantly with increased arrest time, with a decrease of 3 to 4 IQ points for each 10 minutes of arrest.

Conclusions.—Deep hypothermia with circulatory arrest apparently does not fully protect the brain in children who undergo cardiac surgery. Amount of impairment is linearly related to duration of circulatory arrest.

► These authors studied 114 children at about 10 years after they survived operations that involved deep hypothermia, and compared them with children who had atrial septal defects repaired with ordinary cardiopulmonary bypass. Despite this nearly absurd "apples vs. pomegranates" comparison, the authors concluded "It appears that deep hypothermia with circulatory arrest for cardiac operations in children does not fully protect the brain." An amazing leap of faith. The authors make an assumption that children with tetralogy of Fallot, transposition of the great arteries, and other major cardiac defects are in exactly the same category, from the beginning, as those with much more minor cardiac defects, such as atrial septal defect. Another interesting aspect of this paper is its title: "*The* (my italics) Relationship Between Intelligence and Duration of Circulatory Arrest With Deep Hypothermia." A rather arrogant title, wouldn't you think? These authors have shown that children seriously ill enough to have one of the most major physiologic trespasses we do in the operating room performed on them at a very early age may not always grow up with quite as great an intellectual capacity as children who had much more minor anomalies. I don't think the authors have proved their conclusion in any way at all.

J.H. Tinker, M.D.

Differential Age Effects of Mean Arterial Pressure and Rewarming on Cognitive Dysfunction After Cardiac Surgery

Newman MF, Kramer D, Croughwell ND, et al (Duke Heart Ctr, Durham, NC)

Anesth Analg 81:236–242, 1995 3–56

Background.—The outcomes of cardiac surgery have improved, but the trend toward operating on higher-risk patients has inevitably resulted in increased morbidity and mortality. The incidence of neurologic dysfunction is especially high. The causes of neurologic and neuropsychological dysfunction after cardiac surgery are controversial. The effects of mean arterial pressure (MAP) during cardiopulmonary bypass (CPB) and the

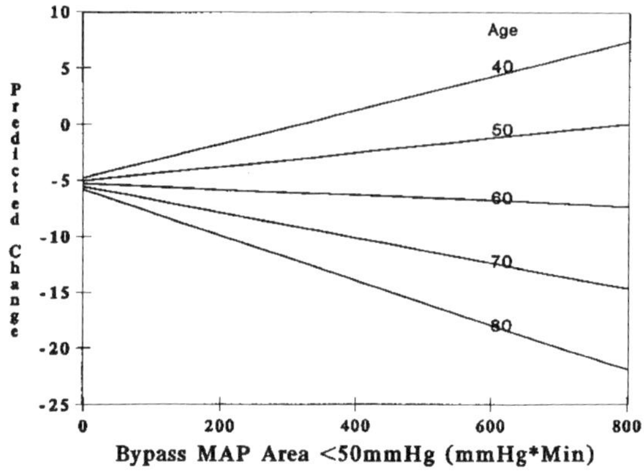

FIGURE 1.—Model-predicted change in Digit Symbol Subtest of Wechsler Adult Intelligence Scale-Revised score, preoperative to predischarge, with preoperative score as a constant in the model set to sample mean and varying age. Mean arterial pressure <50 mm Hg during cardiopulmonary bypass, and Age (the area >50 mm Hg at each minute during cardiopulmonary bypass) interaction. *Abbreviation: MAP* mean arterial pressure. (Courtesy of Newman MF, Kramer D, Croughwell ND, et al: Differential age effects of mean arterial pressure and rewarming on cognitive dysfunction after cardiac surgery. *Anesth Analg* 81:236–242, 1995.)

rate of rewarming on cognitive decline after cardiac surgery were investigated.

Methods.—Two hundred thirty-seven patients underwent neuropsychological tests before surgery and again before discharge. The MAP and temperature were recorded at 1-minute intervals. The MAP area of less than 50 mm Hg and maximal rewarming rate were determined.

Findings.—In a multivariate linear regression analysis, the rate of rewarming and MAP were unassociated with cognitive decline. However, there were significant interactions associated with cognitive decline between age and MAP area of less than 50 mm Hg on 1 measure and between age and rewarming rates on another, which indicates that elderly persons are susceptible to these factors. Although MAP and rewarming were not the main determinants of cognitive decline overall, hypotension and rapid rewarming significantly contributed to cognitive dysfunction in elderly patients (Fig. 1).

Conclusions.—The MAP during CPB and rewarming rate are apparently not the main predictors of cognitive decline after cardiac surgery. However, as the age of the patient population that requires cardiac surgery increases, MAP during CPB and the rewarming rate may play a role in more complex spatial and figural memory deficits. Greater caution for the maintenance of MAP and a slowing of the rewarming rate may be indicated in older patients.

▶ This is one of a series of studies that have attempted to understand the determinants of the well-known cognitive problems that occur, mostly temporarily, after CPB. The authors found that age had something to do with these problems after bypass. The authors also resurrected an old idea from the work of Stockard and Bickford, that the area under the mean blood pressure time curve, when that pressure was below 50 mm Hg might have something to do with cognitive decline. It is the first recent article to resurrect the old blood pressure correlate with cognitive decline after CPB.

J.H. Tinker, M.D.

Cerebral Oximetry in Patients Undergoing Carotid Endarterectomy Under Regional Anesthesia

Samra SK, Dorje P, Zelenock GB, et al (Univ of Michigan, Ann Arbor)
Stroke 27:49–55, 1996 3–57

Background.—Near-infrared spectroscopy may be useful to monitor changes in cerebral oxygenation. Currently, there is little clinical information on the value of this technology in its ability to relate neurologic outcome to cerebrovascular hemoglobin oxygen saturation (Sco_2). Changes in Sco_2 from carotid cross-clamping during carotid endarterectomy in awake patients were reported.

Methods.—Thirty-eight adults who underwent 41 carotid endarterectomies under regional anesthesia were monitored. Ipsilateral and contralateral hemispheres were monitored simultaneously during 36 operations. In the remaining 5, ipsilateral monitoring alone was performed.

Findings.—There were no significant differences between ipsilateral and contralateral Sco_2 during preclamp or postclamp periods. Carotid cross-clamping significantly reduced the ipsilateral Sco_2 from 71.8% to 65.8%. The contralateral Sco_2 remained stable at about 70.5%. Ipsilateral Sco_2 changes varied from +2.6% to −28.6% of the preclamp value. Ipsilateral and contralateral Sco_2 differed significantly during cross-clamping. The mean duration of cross-clamping was 39 minutes. The reduction in ipsilateral Sco_2 varied greatly from one patient to another and was unassociated with duration of cross-clamping.

Conclusions.—Carotid artery occlusion causes a significant but variable reduction in Sco_2 in most patients. A range of Sco_2 values unassociated with clinically detectable neurologic dysfunction was observed.

▶ It is now possible to do "near-infrared" cerebral oxygen saturation spectrometry in an apparently noninvasive way. My head is still reeling as to how this can penetrate scalp, skull bone, etc., but apparently it can. Virtually nothing seems sacred if "Big Brother" can penetrate our skulls. Seriously, this article also shows that cerebral oxygen saturation decreased during regional anesthesia. As I am not a big fan of regional anesthesia for carotid endarterectomy, this article goes along with my biases that oxygen is generally good (though maybe not in gross excess), definitely with some reserves as a margin for error.

J.H. Tinker, M.D.

Tranexamic Acid Reduces Transfusions and Mediastinal Drainage in Repeat Cardiac Surgery

Shore-Lesserson L, Reich DL, Vela-Cantos F, et al (Mount Sinai Med Ctr, New York)

Anesth Analg 83:18–26, 1996 3–58

Background.—Increasing concern about transfusion-related risks and complications has prompted increasing use of blood-sparing drugs during cardiac surgery. These may be particularly important during repeat cardiac operations, which are associated with longer cardiopulmonary bypass times, more tissue dissection, and increased bleeding and demand for transfusions. Therefore, the hematologic and blood-sparing effects of tranexamic acid (TA) during cardiac re-operations were evaluated in a prospective, controlled, double-blind clinical trial.

Methods.—Thirty-one patients were randomly assigned to receive either TA or saline after the induction of anesthesia with fentanyl/oxygen/muscle relaxant. Laboratory tests were done before and after surgery to measure prothrombin time, activated partial thromboplastin time, fibrinogen level, Hb, hematocrit reading, platelet count, fibrin degradation products, activated clotting time, D-dimer levels, and thromboelastography. Blood loss was rated by the surgeon. Mediastinal tube drainage was measured at 25, 48, and 72 hours postoperatively. Transfusion requirements were compared in the 2 groups. Patients were followed up for 72 hours, with monitoring for any thrombosis-related adverse events.

Results.—None of the coagulation variables varied significantly between the 2 groups at any time point. Allogeneic transfusions were required for 10 of 17 patients in the TA group and 12 of 13 patients in the placebo group. In comparison with the placebo group, the TA group had significantly reduced mediastinal tube drainage at all time points. The thrombosis-related adverse events included perioperative myocardial infarction in 1 patient in the TA group and 2 patients in the placebo group, perioperative transient cerebral ischemia in 2 patients in the TA group, and embolic stroke in 1 patient in the placebo group.

Conclusions.—Tranexamic acid reduces postoperative mediastinal tube drainage and the incidence of transfusion in patients requiring repeat cardiac surgery. It is likely that TA produces this effect by inhibiting fibrinolysis and plasmin-related deleterious effects on the coagulation system.

► Not that many years ago, epsilon amino caproic acid was touted to decrease postcardiac surgical mediastinal bleeding. Tranexamic acid is the latest of these antifibrinolytics. In between these 2 agents came aprotinin which, although not antifibrinolytic, if you believe the reports, cures everything from fungus to flat feet. Over the years, I have been impressed with how wonderful these kinds of drugs are *said* to work in the early enthusiastic studies but do not seem to be all that great in and around the operating rooms! Time will tell us whether TA is in that category, because you can rest assured that surgeons will use it, at least until something "even better" comes along.

J.H. Tinker, M.D.

The Effect of Posture on the Induction of Epidural Anesthesia for Peripheral Vascular Surgery

Whalley DG, D'Amico JA, Rybicki LA, et al (Cleveland Clinic Found, Ohio)

Reg Anesth 20:407–411, 1995 3–59

Background.—Epidural anesthesia has relatively benign effects on the cardiovascular and respiratory systems, and in patients having peripheral vascular surgery, it is associated with a lower rate of reoperation for graft occlusion. Factors that may affect the epidural spread of local anesthesia are volume of injectate, speed of injection, and age, body weight, height, and patient position at the time of injection. Studies on the effect of position on spread of anesthesia have reported inconsistent results. The effect of a seated or supine position on the quality and time to maximum anesthesia using lumbar epidural anesthesia before infrainguinal arterial reconstruction was determined.

Methods.—There were 40 patients scheduled for infrainguinal arterial reconstruction. Mean patient age was 68 years. An epidural catheter was inserted at the L3–L4 interspace. Patients were assigned to 1 of 2 groups. In group 1, a test dose of 3 mL of lidocaine 1.5% with 5 µg/mL of epinephrine was administered to seated patients, followed by 12 mL of bupivacaine 0.75%. The patients remained seated for 5 minutes and then were placed supine. In group 2, the epidural catheter was inserted while patients were seated, but the patients were then immediately placed supine. Lidocaine and bupivacaine were administered as in group 1. Onset of anesthesia was determined by a loss of sensation to pinprick and the Bromage scale. Maximum cephalad spread of anesthesia, maximum motor block, time to maximum cephalad spread of anesthesia, and time to maximum motor block in each group were compared and correlated to age, height, weight, and body surface area.

Results.—Maximum cephalad spread of anesthesia, motor block, and time to maximum motor block were similar in both groups. In group 1, the time to maximum cephalad spread of anesthesia was shorter than in group 2. In both groups, quality and time to maximum anesthesia were unaffected by age or weight. In group 1, a significant relation was noted between height and body surface area and time to maximum cephalad spread of anesthesia.

Discussion.—In these elderly patients, the time to maximum cephalad spread of anesthesia was shorter and directly related to patient height and body surface area when lumbar epidural anesthesia was administered with the patient in the sitting position. The final level of cephalad spread and degree of motor block were not affected by the position of the patient during induction of anesthesia. These findings are limited by the identification of the L3–L4 interspace by its relationship to the iliac crest and by the insertion of the catheter only 3 cm into the epidural space.

▶ Is this a bad effect—a more rapid onset with sitting? It clearly could be a bad effect if you have more rapid hemodynamic changes that aren't accounted for, and thus more hemodynamic instability and its consequences of ischemia to organs especially if those organs are the brain stem and the heart. It may be that this article says "yes" you can get the patient ready for the surgeon quicker by having them sitting up, and that is not an insignificant time difference of 13 minutes vs. 18 minutes, but that you also risk increased hemodynamic change by doing so. I wish that the American Society of Anesthesiologists closed claim study reported the position of the patient when the spinals and epidurals were done in those studies to see if similar problems also developed.

M.F. Roizen, M.D.

Intestinal Permeability, Gastric Intramucosal pH, and Systemic Endotoxemia in Patients Undergoing Cardiopulmonary Bypass

Riddington DW, Venkatesh B, Boivin CM, et al (Univ of Birmingham, England; Queen Elizabeth Hosp, Birmingham, England)

JAMA 275:1007–1012, 1996 3–60

Purpose.—Although progressive or sequential multiple organ system failure is regarded as the major cause of late mortality in critically ill patients, its pathogenesis remains unclear. It has been suggested that shock leads to endotoxemia through the gut, and thence to failure of remote organ systems. However, this sequence has never been documented in humans. The links between gastric intramucosal pH, intestinal permeability, endotoxemia, and oxygen delivery were evaluated in patients undergoing cardiopulmonary bypass (CBP).

Methods.—The prospective, observational study included 50 patients undergoing elective cardiac surgery and a reference group of 10 patients scheduled for elective cardiac operations. Intestinal permeability was assessed using chromium 51–labeled ethylenediaminetetraacetic acid (^{51}Cr-EDTA), and intramucosal pH (pHi) was measured by a nasogastric tonometer. Systemic oxygen delivery and consumption were assessed by pulmonary artery catheter, and arterial blood samples were obtained for detection of plasma endotoxin by the *Limulus* amebocyte assay. The study hypothesis was that gut ischemia would lead to increased intestinal permeability, with subsequent effects on endotoxemia, systemic oxygen supply and consumption, and clinical outcomes.

Results.—Over 24 hours, the median percentage of ^{51}Cr-EDTA recovered in urine was 11% in the patients undergoing CPB versus 1% in the reference patients. The findings indicated increased intestinal permeability during CPB. The median value for lowest pHi after CPB was 6.98, but no decline in pHi occurred until after the end of CPB, when the heart regained control of the circulation. Forty-two percent of the patients had endotoxin levels of greater than 0.2 U/mL during the study, and most of these patients had endotoxemia by the end of CPB. Episodes of endotoxemia tended to cluster after 1 hour of CPB, with an additional peak 2 to 6 hours after the end of CPB . However, intestinal permeability was apparently unrelated to endotoxemia, gut ischemia, or systemic oxygen supply and consumption.

Conclusions.—Patients undergoing CPB have increased gut permeability, which occurs before ischemia of the gut mucosa. However, a low pHi in this group of patients is not necessarily associated with negative clinical effects. Many patients undergoing CPB have detectable endotoxemia. Increased intestinal permeability and gastric mucosal acidosis are independent events, related in neither severity nor onset.

► I selected this article because it demonstrates the association between systemic endotoxemia and CPB. It is of interest that endotoxemia was observed before CPB, after the induction of anesthesia, and after 60 minutes of CPB. The fact that this effect occurred so early is surprising. However, the authors failed to find a causal relation for the occurrence of systemic endotoxemia in patients undergoing cardiac surgery.

M. Wood, M.D.

Orthopedic Anesthesia Issues

Evaluation of the Usefulness of Intrathecal Bupivacaine Infusion for Analgesia After Hip and Knee Arthroplasty
Niemi L, Pitkänen M, Dunkel P, et al (Helsinki Univ)
Br J Anaesth 77:544–545, 1996 3–61

Introduction.—Technical problems with microcatheters and opioid side effects with intrathecal administration occur too frequently. The use of continuous low-dose intrathecal bupivacaine infusion was evaluated in the treatment of postoperative pain in 47 patients in ASA I–III who were undergoing hip or knee arthroplasty.

Methods.—Spinal anesthesia was induced with 0.5% bupivacaine 2 mL using a 28-gauge spinal catheter inserted with a 22-gauge needle at the L3-4 interspace. Incremental doses of bupivacaine 0.5 mL were delivered for a maximum of four 2-mL doses with the goal of reaching T6. Patients were randomizly assigned to receive 0.5% bupivacaine 0.4 mL h^{-1}(2 mg h^{-1}) (12 patients), 0.5% bupivacaine 0.2 mL h^{-1} (1 mg h^{-1}) (12 patients), or saline 0.2 mL h^{-1} (11 patients). There were 12 exclusions, mostly because of technical problems. A dose of 0.1–0.14 mg oxycodone per $kilogram^{-1}$ was administered IM on request. Patients were interviewed at 3, 6, 12, and 24 hours after initiation of intrathecal infusion. A visual analogue scale was used to assess the intensity of pain at rest and on movement.

Results.—The 12 patients receiving bupivacaine 2 mg h^{-1} needed significantly less oxycodone, compared with the 12 patients receiving bupivacaine 1 mg h^{-1} and the 11 receiving saline (19, 36, and 52 doses, respectively). Five patients who received bupivacaine 2 mg h^{-1} experienced apparent sensory and motor block 12 hours after start of infusion, compared with 2 patients in the bupivacaine 1 mg h^{-1} group and no patients in the saline group. Three patients in the bupivacaine 2 mg h^{-1} group and 1 patient in the bupivacaine 1 mg h^{-1} group experienced an increase in the spinal block in their patient ward. These patients also had motor block. Transient hypotension associated with increased block occurred in 2 patients in the bupivacaine 2 mg h^{-1} group.

Conclusions.—Patients who underwent hip or knee arthroplasty with intrathecal infusion of bupivacaine 2 mg h^{-1} for 24 hours received satisfactory postoperative analgesia. This regimen cannot be recommended as a routine method for relief of postoperative pain because of technical problems, unpredictability of the spread of intrathecal bupivacaine with reappearance of spinal block in some patients, and occasional sudden hypotension.

► Although intrathecally administered bupivacaine alone appears to be less than optimal for postoperative intrathecal infusion, combinations of bupivacaine plus opioids may be quite satisfactory. If spinal microcatheters are re-introduced in the United States, optimal protocols for postoperative intrathecal infusions will need to be developed.

S.E. Abram, M.D.

Continuous Postoperative Infusion of a Regional Anesthetic After an Amputation of the Lower Extremity

Pinzur MS, Garla PGN, Pluth T, et al (Loyola Univ, Maywood, Ill)

J Bone Joint Surg (Am) 78A:1501–1505, 1996 3–62

Background.—The use of continuous perineural infusion of a long-acting local anesthetic to alleviate pain after lower extremity amputation is increasing in popularity. Whether continuous bupivacaine infusion reduces the need for narcotics for pain relief after amputation was determined in a prospective, randomized clinical trial.

Methods.—Twenty-one patients scheduled for lower extremity amputation because of ischemic necrosis caused by peripheral vascular disease were assigned to a treatment or a control group. After the amputation, a Teflon catheter was placed next to the transected end of the sciatic or posterior tibial nerve, and bupivacaine or normal saline solution was infused for 72 hours. Intravenous morphine delivered by a patient-controlled pump was allowed during infusion.

Findings.—Compared to patients in the control group, patients in the treatment group used less morphine on the first and second days after surgery. The groups did not differ in amount of morphine used on day 3. Overall, 11 of 14 patients completing a questionnaire reported reduced pain between the third- and sixth-month assessment.

Conclusions.—Continuous perineural infusion of bupivacaine appears to be safe and effective for relieving pain after amputation. However, it did not prevent residual or phantom pain in this patient population.

▶ It is not surprising that the technique described failed to prevent the development of chronic pain after amputation. There is evidence that aggressive treatment of pre-existing persistent pain with regional anesthetic techniques prior to initiation of surgery is a requirement for modification of the incidence of chronic postoperative pain. Although the technique described here may be a helpful adjunct, it does not eliminate the necessity for preemptive control of existing pain plus aggressive intraoperative management with regional anesthetic techniques.

S.E. Abram, M.D.

Analgesia for Acute Musculoskeletal Trauma: Low-dose Subcutaneous Infusion of Ketamine

Gurnani A, Sharma PK, Rautela RS, et al (Univ College of Med Sciences, Shahdara, Delhi, India; GTB Hosp, Shahdara, Delhi, India)

Anaesth Intensive Care 24:32–36, 1996 3–63

Background.—Analgesia is often underused in victims of acute musculoskeletal trauma. Subcutaneous infusion of an analgesic may be a good alternative to conventional intermittent intramuscular or intravenous injections (the effects of which tend to wear off between doses) or to con-

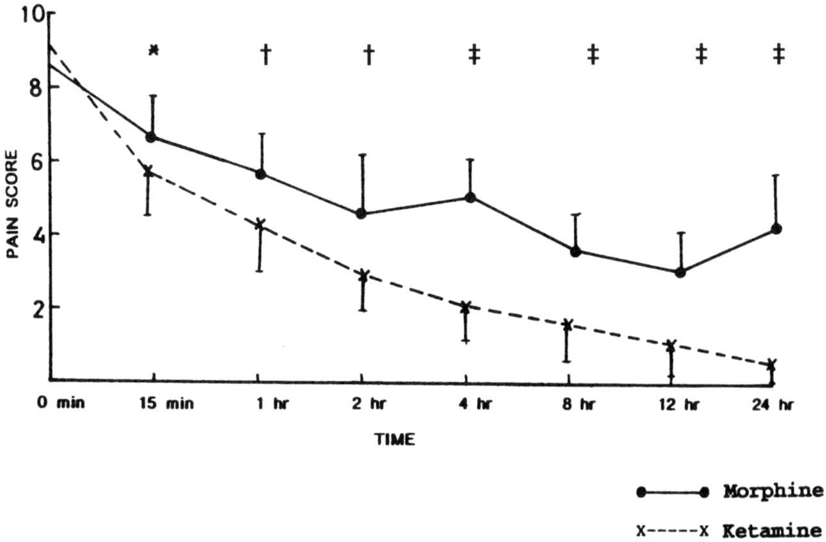

FIGURE 1.—Mean (SD) visual analogue pain scale scores in the 2 groups. *$P < 0.05$. †$P < 0.01$. ‡$P < 0.001$. (Courtesy of Gurnani A, Sharma PK, Rautela RS, et al: Analgesia for acute musculoskeletal trauma: Low-dose subcutaneous infusion of ketamine. *Anaesth Intensive Care* 24:32–36, 1996.)

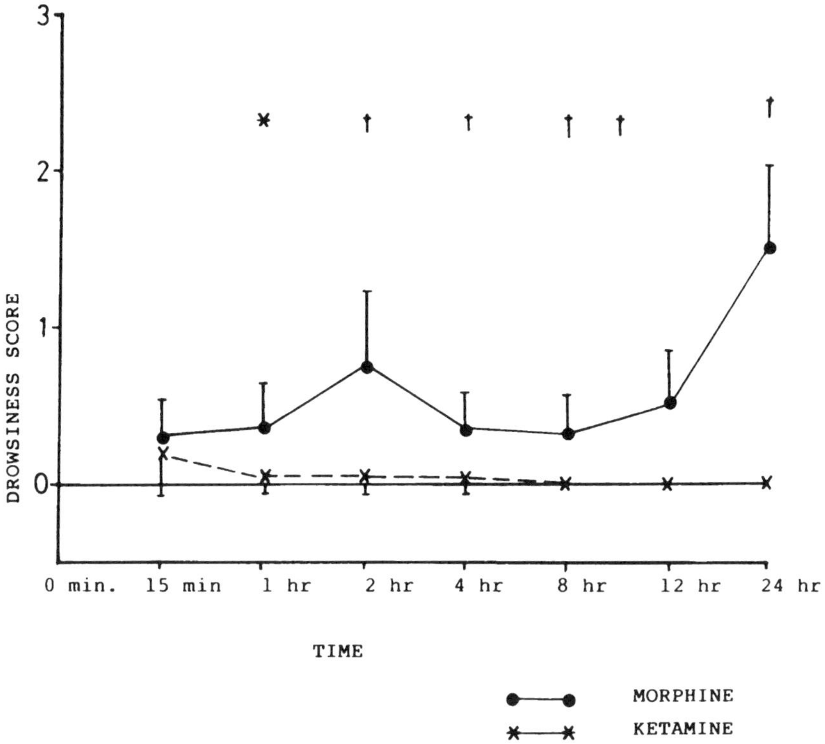

FIGURE 2.—Mean (SD) drowsiness score in the 2 groups. *$P < 0.05$. †$P < 0.001$. (Courtesy of Gurnani A, Sharma PK, Rautela RS, et al: Analgesia for acute musculoskeletal trauma: Low-dose subcutaneous infusion of ketamine. *Anaesth Intensive Care* 24:32–36, 1996.)

tinuous intravenous infusion (which carries risk of accidental overdosage). A pilot study of 8 patients revealed that subcutaneous infusion of ketamine causes minimal side effects and provides effective analgesia to patients with acute musculoskeletal trauma. The analgesic efficacy of this regimen is compared with that of intermittent intravenous morphine.

Methods.—Forty adults with acute musculoskeletal trauma not requiring immediate surgery received either low-dose ketamine by subcutaneous infusion (0.1 mg/kg/h) or intermittent morphine (0.1 mg/kg intravenously every 4 hours). In double-blind fashion, visual analogue scales were used to assess pain, and a 4-point rank drowsiness score was used to assess sedation. Cardiovascular and respiratory status were determined objectively; subjective patient acceptability was related to supplementary analgesia required and early mobilization.

Results.—The ketamine infusion provided better pain relief than did intermittent morphine (Fig 1). Ketamine infusion also resulted in the patients being more awake and alert (Fig 2) and in a significant improvement in peak expiratory flow rate. Patients receiving the ketamine infusion were more easily mobilized for traction or splintage and none required supplementary analgesia. Patients treated with morphine experienced a high incidence of nausea and vomiting.

Conclusions.—Continuous subcutaneous infusion of ketamine safely and effectively provides adequate pain relief for victims of acute musculoskeletal trauma. The regimen may be more effective than conventional opioid administration (provided that tissue perfusion is not compromised) and carries minimal risk of acute complications from accidental overdose.

► Whereas the results of this study are sufficient to arouse our interest, the study design is problematic because ketamine infusion was compared with intermittent IV injections of morphine given at 4-hour intervals. This morphine schedule is clearly suboptimal, and predisposes the patient to alternating periods of oversedation and inadequate analgesia.

S.E. Abram, M.D.

Postoperative Complaints After Spinal and Thiopentone-Isoflurane Anaesthesia in Patients Undergoing Orthopaedic Surgery: Spinal Versus General Anaesthesia

Standl T, Eckert S, Schulte am Esche J (Univ Hosp Eppendorf, Hamburg, Germany)

Acta Anaesthesiol Scand 40:222–226, 1996 3–64

Background.—Small-bore and blunt spinal needles have been associated with a reduction in the incidence of postdural puncture headache, but they can be difficult to use. Thus, general anesthesia is often preferred to spinal anesthesia in patients at greater risk for postdural puncture headache. The impact of a standardized technique of spinal and general anesthesia on the incidence and consequences of postanesthetic complaints, dependent on the age and sex of the patients, was studied.

Methods.—Four hundred thirty-three orthopedic patients who underwent lower limb surgery were assigned randomly to spinal or general anesthesia. In the spinal anesthesia group, 0.5% hyperbaric bupivacaine was delivered through a 26-gauge Quincke needle. In the general anesthesia group, thiopentone, fentanyl, and atracurium were injected, with 65% nitrous oxide and 1 to 1.5 Vol% isoflurane in oxygen for maintenance. Patients were interviewed 4 days after surgery.

Findings.—The patients who received general anesthesia had a higher overall incidence of nausea and/or vomiting and sore throat. The incidence of nausea and/or vomiting was also greater among patients 20 to 60 years of age in the general anesthesia group compared with the spinal anesthesia group. The incidence of urinary dysfunction was higher in men after spinal anesthesia, and that of nausea and/or vomiting was greater in women after general anesthesia. Patients who received general anesthesia had greater analgesic requirements, longer postoperative surveillance, and more frequent treatment of postoperative complaints.

Conclusions.—Compared with general anesthesia, spinal anesthesia was associated with a lower incidence of postoperative complaints and treatments as well as a shorter surveillance. The complications associated with spinal anesthesia did not depend on age or sex. This technique may be preferable even in younger patients and in women who undergo orthopedic surgery.

▶ This is another European comparison of regional vs. general anesthesia, of which there have been many designs in the past. As usual for these studies, the authors find that spinal anesthesia was associated with less postoperative problems. They found less nausea and vomiting, less sore throat, and a shorter time of postoperative surveillance. Obviously, this kind of a study cannot be double-blinded. Most likely, the authors' pre-study biases were in favor of regional anesthesia. It is interesting to me that so very few people whose biases are in favor of general anesthesia ever seem to bother to do such studies! Anyway, even though many studies, of which this is one, purport to show various positive effects for regional anesthesia vs. general anesthesia, this conclusion has not been clinically widely accepted. I included this article because there is the very distinct possibility that these folks might be right.

J.H. Tinker, M.D.

Effect of Preoperative Donation of Autologous Blood on Deep-vein Thrombosis Following Total Joint Arthroplasty of the Hip or Knee

Anders MJ, Lifeso RM, Landis M, et al (VA Med Ctr, Buffalo, NY)

J Bone Joint Surg Am 78A:574–580, 1996 3–65

Background.—Without prophylaxis, deep-vein thrombosis after elective total joint arthroplasty can occur in as many as 84% of patients. Many prophylactic strategies have been described in an attempt to reduce the prevalence of potentially fatal pulmonary embolism. Preoperative donation of autologous blood has been routine since the mid-1980s. The effect of preoperative autologous blood donation on postoperative deep-vein thrombosis was investigated.

Methods and Findings.—Two hundred thirty-seven men at high risk for deep-vein thrombosis undergoing elective total hip or knee arthroplasty for noninflammatory degenerative joint disease were included. In 54 patients, venography showed evidence of deep-vein thrombosis of the lower extremity. Most of these patients had asymptomatic clots distal to the knee. Deep-vein thrombosis occurred in 16% of 116 patients after total hip arthroplasty and in 29% of 121 patients after total knee arthroplasty. This complication developed in 17% of the 161 patients who had donated blood before surgery and in 34% of the 76 patients who had not. Logistic regression analysis indicated that autologous blood donation significantly reduced the development of postoperative deep-vein thrombosis for patients undergoing total knee arthroplasty but not for those having total hip arthroplasty. In an additional neural network analysis, autologous blood donation was the most important prognostic factor in predicting the absence of postoperative deep-vein thrombosis.

Conclusions.—Although autologous blood donation alone is not sufficient for prophylaxis against deep-vein thrombosis after total joint arthroplasty, it appeared to protect against this complication after total knee arthroplasty in this high-risk population. This is an added benefit of preoperative donation of autologous blood, which also reduces the need for homologous blood transfusion.

▶ Advocates of preoperative blood donation before major surgery have taken some blows in recent years because it is not all that obvious that predonation is in fact cost-effective. This paper is interesting because it takes a new tack, namely it provides some evidence that perhaps preoperative donation of autologous blood can protect to some degree against postoperative deep-vein thrombosis, at least after total knee surgery. The authors believe that this is the first study to specifically report the above effect. The mechanism by which this occurs is unclear, but may involve the simple fact that reasonably large quantities of predonated blood result in a patient for surgery who is somewhat hemodiluted! In other words, we are drawing the autologous blood from the patient preoperatively to be able to give it back perioperatively, but in fact if we give back as little as possible, we may be able to prevent deep-vein thrombosis! I find the above to be fascinating.

J.H. Tinker, M.D.

Mild Hypothermia Increases Blood Loss and Transfusion Requirements During Total Hip Arthroplasty

Schmied H, Kurz A, Sessler DI, et al (Hosp of Amstetten, Austria; Univ of California, San Francisco; Univ of Vienna)

Lancet 347:289–292, 1996 3–66

Introduction.—There is in vitro evidence that hypothermia adversely affects platelet function and the coagulation cascade. However, it is unknown whether mild perioperative hypothermia in surgical patients has any impact on bleeding during surgery. The effects of mild hypothermia on blood loss and transfusion requirements were studied in patients undergoing hip arthroplasty.

Methods.—The study included 60 patients who were undergoing primary, unilateral total hip arthroplasty. This operation was selected because it is a relatively standardized procedure that carries substantial microvascular blood loss. The patients were randomly assigned to normothermic and mild hypothermic groups. In the normothermic group, core temperature was maintained around 36.5°C with active skin and fluid warming; in the hypothermic group, core temperature was allowed to decrease to about 35°C. Strict criteria were applied for the administration of crystalloid, colloid, scavenged red cells, and allogeneic blood. The study hypothesis was that patients in the normothermic group would have less blood loss and less need for allogeneic blood transfusion.

Results.—Both groups had normal and similar bleeding parameters before surgery. Cumulative blood loss was nearly 2.2 (0.5) L in the hypothermic group, compared with 1.7 (0.3) L in the normothermic group (Table 2). Seven patients in the hypothermic group received a total of 8 U of allogeneic blood, whereas 1 patient in the normothermic group required 1 U of blood. On the day after surgery, the hemoglobin concentration was lower, although not significantly so, in the hypothermic patients.

Conclusions.—Maintaining normal body temperature during hip replacement surgery reduces blood loss and the need for blood transfusion. A typical perioperative decline in core temperature during hip arthroplasty increases blood loss by about 500 mL. For this, as well as for patient comfort and other reasons, it seems best to maintain normal body tem-

TABLE 2.—Hemoglobin, Blood Loss, Administered Fluid, and Allogeneic Transfusion Requirements

	Normothermic	Hypothermic	*P*
Hemoglobin (mg/dL)			
Pre-operative	12.7 (1.3)	12.2 (1.2)	NS
After hemodilution	10.9 (1.1)	10.8 (1.4)	NS
End of surgery	10.6 (1.3)	10.4 (1.2)	NS
Next morning	10.6 (1.5)	10.2 (1.3)	NS
Cumulative blood loss (mL)			
End of surgery	690 (230)	920 (400)	0.008
3 hr postoperatively	1310 (330)	1700 (510)	<0.001
12 hr postoperatively	1500 (310)	1970 (560)	<0.001
Next morning	1670 (320)	2160 (550)	<0.001
Intraoperative fluid administration (mL)			
Colloid (hemodilution)	880 (260)	870 (290)	NS
Crystalloid	2500 (500)	2900 (600)	0.007
Colloid (additional)	80 (173)	217 (303)	0.036
Blood (hemodilution)	450 (320)	470 (340)	NS
Postoperative fluid administration (mL)			
Crystalloid	960 (390)	1150 (290)	0.04
Colloid	12 (19)	40 (12)	<0.001
Blood (hemodilution)	320 (330)	320 (340)	NS
Cell scavenger	400 (240)	520 (260)	0.07
Allogeneic blood			
Patients (no/total)	1/30	7/30	0.06
3 hr postoperaively (mL/patient)	10 (55)	60 (120)	0.04
Within 24 hr (mL/patient)	10 (55)	80 (154)	0.02

Note: Total blood loss was significantly greater in the hypothermic patients at each measured time (2-tailed, unpaired *t*-tests). The hypothermic patients required more intraoperative crystalloid and hetastarch. Seven of the 30 hypothermic patients required the transfusion of 8 U of allogeneic blood within 24 hours of surgery, whereas only 1 of the 30 normothermic patients required 1 U of allogeneic blood. The section labeled "postoperative fluid resuscitation" refers to the first 3 hours after surgery. Results are presented here as means (SD). *NS* indicates $P \geq 0.05$. *P* values for the volume of intraoperative colloid administration and allogeneic blood requirement were virtually identical when calculated using a nonparametric (Wilcoxon) statistic.

(Courtesy of Schmied H, Kurz A, Sessler DI, et al: Mild hypothermia increases blood loss and transfusion requirements during total hip arthroplasty. *Lancet* 347:289–292, 1996. Copyright by The Lancet Ltd., 1996.)

perature during surgery, unless hypothermia is indicated for some specific reason.

▶ Although anesthesiologists like to prevent intraoperative hypothermia, until recently, objective evidence of adverse outcome resulting from mild hypothermia simply did not exist. This well-performed study shows the value of maintaining intraoperative normothermia. Although the patient group studied was undergoing unilateral total hip arthroplasty, it would be of enormous interest and importance if the data could be extrapolated to other patient groups.

M. Wood, M.D

Transplant Anesthesia Issues

Desensitization of Myocardial β-Adrenergic Receptors and Deterioration of Left Ventricular Function After Brain Death

D'Amico TA, Meyers CH, Koutlas TC, et al (Duke Univ, Durham, NC)

J Thorac Cardiovasc Surg 110:746–751, 1995 3–67

Background.—Brain death can lead to a series of hemodynamic changes in potential organ donors before transplantation. Although the deterioration of myocardial performance after brain death has been documented, the pathophysiologic process of the myocardial dysfunction occurring after brain death has not been well defined. The function of the myocardial β-adrenergic receptor and the development of left ventricular dysfunction were studied in a porcine model of brain death.

Methods.—Experimental brain death was induced in 6 animals. For comparison, another group of 6 animals not subjected to brain death was studied. To analyze the β-receptor, receptor density and adenylate cyclase activity were determined after stimulation independently at the receptor protein, the G protein, and the adenylate cyclase moiety.

Findings.—Myocardial β-receptor density was unaffected by brain death induction. Stimulated adenylate cyclase activity was reduced within the first hour after brain death at the level of the β-receptor, G protein, and adenylate cyclase moiety, suggesting rapid desensitization of β-receptor function. Myocardial performance also deteriorated significantly in the first hour after brain death, as evidenced by a reduction in preload-recruitable stroke work compared with the baseline value.

Conclusions.—In this porcine model, significant dysfunction occurred within 1 hour after brain death and was unrelated to β-receptor number. β-Receptor desensitization may be involved in the pathophysiologic process of cardiac dysfunction after brain death. The deterioration of myocardial performance is temporally associated with a defect in β-receptor/G protein/adenylate cyclase coupling. Apparently, this defect is localized to the adenylate cyclase moiety itself.

▶ This is an incredibly important study, on which our colleague, Debra Schwinn, served as the senior investigator (Debbie, you continue to do great work!). In any case, this study shows that there is an impairment in cardiovascular β-receptor function after brain death, and that this impairment increases with time after brain death, appearing to reach an (at least) intermediate phase 1 to 2 hours after brain death, as also evidenced by a decrease in myocardial contractile performance, and paralleled by a decline in β-adrenergic receptor function localized to the adenylate cyclase moiety.

M.F. Roizen, M.D.

Perioperative Mucosal pH and Splanchnic Endotoxin Concentration in Orthotopic Liver Transplantation

Welte M, Pichler B, Groh J, et al (Ludwig-Maximilians-Univ, Munich)

Br J Anaesth 76:90–98, 1996 3–68

Background.—Impairment of splanchnic perfusion can induce mucosal hypoxia and endotoxemia during orthotopic liver transplantation (OLT). However, the changes in mucosal oxygenation during and after OLT are unknown. The effects of liver surgery on mucosal pH (pH_i) and the response of pH_i to acute changes in portal flow were studied.

Methods and Findings.—Gastric pH_i was measured during 6 liver resections using tonometry. After hepatoduodenal ligament clamping in 2 patients, pH_i declined within 30 minutes, recovering promptly after reperfusion. Gastric and sigmoid pH_i then were assessed during the perioperative phase in 18 patients undergoing OLT. Median pH_i values were low preoperatively. Mucosal pH was decreased during the anhepatic phase, despite the constancy of global oxygen delivery and hemodynamic variables, and portal flow maintenance by veno-venous bypass (VVB). After graft reperfusion, pH_i recovered. By the end of OLT, it did not differ from baseline values. Gastric pH_i increased further postoperatively, peaking 30 hours after ICU admission. No significant endotoxemia occurred intraoperatively in portal or systemic blood. The maximum decrease in pH_i was unassociated with VVB duration, OLT, or number of red cell units transfused. After reperfusion, pH_i was uncorrelated with graft viability or dysfunction of the lung or kidney.

Conclusions.—Measures of pH_i indicate mucosal ischemia during OLT, not necessarily associated with endotoxemia. Intraoperative pH_i monitoring is apparently not a good predictor of postoperative graft failure and organ dysfunction.

▶ Is this an appropriate model to answer the question that the authors have posed? I do not know the answer to that, but it is clear that these surgeons and this technique were not of benefit. Like all good studies, this one appears to bring up more questions than it answers.

M.F. Roizen, M.D.

Pulmonary Allograft Ischemic Time: An Important Predictor of Survival After Lung Transplantation

Snell GI, Rabinov M, Griffiths A, et al (Alfred Hosp, Prahran, Australia)

J Heart Lung Transplant 15:160–168, 1996 3–69

Background.—The number of human lungs available for transplantation has been limited by the requirement to keep graft ischemic time to less than 6 hours. In Australia, where the population is widely spread, such organs often are obtained after 6 hours. The clinical consequences of a prolonged allograft ischemic time were analyzed.

Methods.—One hundred six lung or heart-lung transplantations performed between 1990 and 1994 were reviewed. Mean graft ischemic time was 323 minutes. Lungs were preserved with an infusion of 40 to 80 ng/kg/min of prostacyclin for 10 minutes and cold modified Euro-Collins solution flush. Organs were stored and transported on ice at temperatures of 6° to 10°C.

Findings.—Survival and graft ischemic times for heart-lung, single-lung, and double-lung transplantation did not differ significantly. Graft ischemic time independently predicted survival. In a subgroup analysis, the effect of graft ischemic time was most pronounced past 5 hours.

Conclusions.—Although survival is reduced, the outcomes of pulmonary allograft ischemic times beyond 5 hours are acceptable. Graft ischemic times should be kept to a minimum, with careful coordination of transport and personnel.

▶ This is an important article because it strongly looks at outcome, it looks at an established program, and it comes to the conclusion that there is a time of allograft ischemia beyond which mortality increases substantially, and that time appears to be 5 hours.

M.F. Roizen, M.D.

Regional Anesthesia Issues

Hemodynamic Responses to Intravascular Injection of Epinephrine-containing Epidural Test Doses in Adults During General Anesthesia

Liu SS, Carpenter RL (Virginia Mason Med Ctr, Seattle; Wake Forest Univ, Winston-Salem, NC)

Anesthesiology 84:81–87, 1996 3–70

Introduction.—Sometimes, a patient under general anesthesia will undergo initiation of epidural anesthesia and analgesia. Test doses containing local anesthetic and epinephrine commonly are given, to identify subarachnoid injection and prevent unintentional intravascular injection. However, little is known about the efficacy of these test doses. The hemodynamic criteria for a positive response to intravascular injection of test doses during general anesthesia were assessed.

Methods.—Thirty-six patients undergoing elective surgery were randomly assigned to receive either 0.5 minimum alveolar concentration (MAC) of isoflurane, 1 MAC of isoflurane, or 0.5 MAC each of isoflurane and nitrous oxide. After they were given IV saline, the patients received 3 tests doses consisting of 45 mg of lidocaine with 7.5, 15, and 30 µg of epinephrine. After each injection, the heart rate and systolic, diastolic, and mean blood pressures were measured. Peak hemodynamic increases during saline administration were used to determine the positive hemodynamic criteria associated with intravascular injection. Linear regression was performed to determine the minimum epinephrine dose required to produce peak positive hemodynamic increases.

Results.—The positive hemodynamic criteria identifying intravascular injection were increases equal to or greater than 8 beats/min for heart rate, 13 mm Hg for systolic blood pressure, 7 mm Hg for diastolic blood pressure, and 9 mm Hg for mean blood pressure. There were significant dose-effect relations between epinephrine and peak increases in hemodynamics, with correlation coefficients ranging from 0.61 to 0.91. Depending on the hemodynamic measurement under consideration and the anesthetic the patient received, the minimum dose of epinephrine required to produce peak positive hemodynamic increases ranged from 6 to 19 µg.

Conclusions.—In patients receiving intravascular test doses during general anesthesia, the hemodynamic response is affected by the dose of epinephrine and the depth and type of general anesthesia. For patients under anesthesia with 0.5 MAC of isoflurane, with or without 0.5 MAC of nitrous oxide, a standard test dose containing 15 µg of epinephrine should produce multiple positive hemodynamic responses. For patients under anesthesia with 1 MAC of isoflurane, a larger dose of epinephrine may be needed or systolic blood pressure should be monitored.

► The use of epinephrine in a local anesthetic solution to detect intravascular injection after epidural administration is common; the typical adult epidural "test dose" is 15 µg of epinephrine and is based on studies of the cardiovascular effects of epinephrine, 15 µg, given IV to healthy, awake individuals. If an intravascular injection occurs, the anesthesiologist may observe a sudden increase in heart rate and systolic blood pressure, unless the patient is concurrently receiving medication such as β-adrenergic blocking agents.

Epidural anesthesia frequently is administered during general inhalational anesthesia, and this study shows that it is important for the anesthesiologist to recognize that a standard test dose may not produce the expected effect.

M. Wood, M.D.

The Effects of Epidural Anesthesia on Ventilatory Response to Hypercapnia and Hypoxia in Elderly Patients

Sakura S, Saito Y, Kosaka Y (Shimane Med Univ, Izumo, Japan)

Anesth Analg 82:306–311, 1996 3–71

Purpose.—Epidural anesthesia commonly is used for surgery in elderly patients. However, this form of anesthesia could decrease ventilation through various mechanisms. The effects of epidural anesthesia on resting ventilation, arterial blood gas tension, ventilatory response to hypercapnia, and progressive isocapnic hypoxia were studied in elderly patients.

Methods.—Sixteen unpremedicated elderly patients were studied, 8 of whom received lumbar epidural blocks for lower abdominal surgery and 8 of whom received thoracic epidural blocks for upper abdominal surgery. The mean ages in these groups were 70 and 71 years, respectively. The patients were studied before and 20 minutes after the instillation of 10 mL

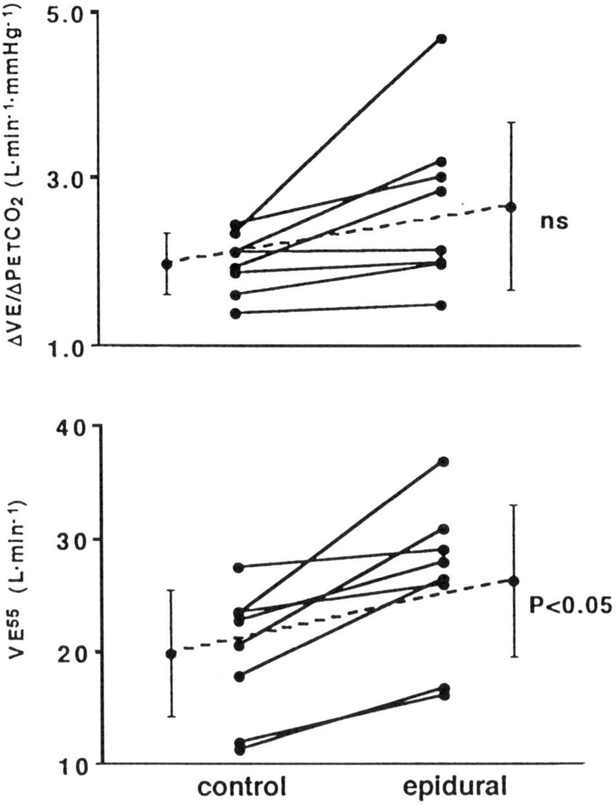

FIGURE 1.—Slope of the hypercapnic response curve ($\Delta V_E/\Delta P_{ETCO_2}$) and minute ventilation at a P_{ETCO_2} of 55 mm Hg (V_E^{55}), before and after lumbar epidural block in each of the patients. The *dotted lines* connect mean values. *Error bars* represent ± 1 SD. (Courtesy of Sakura S, Saito Y, Kosaka Y: The effects of epidural anesthesia on ventilatory response to hypercapnia and hypoxia in elderly patients. *Anesth Analg* 82:306–311, 1996.)

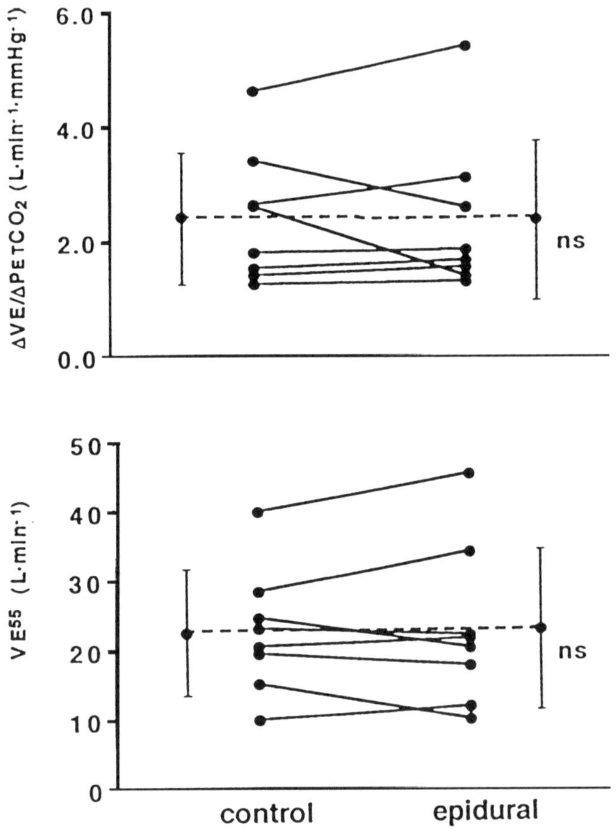

FIGURE 2.—Slope of the hypercapnic response curve ($\Delta V_E/\Delta P_{ETCO_2}$) and minute ventilation at a P_{ETCO_2} of 55 mm Hg (V_E^{55}), before and after thoracic epidural block in each of the patients. The *dotted lines* connect the mean values. *Error bars* represent ±1 SD. (Courtesy of Sakura S, Saito Y, Kosaka Y: The effects of epidural anesthesia on ventilatory response to hypercapnia and hypoxia in elderly patients. *Anesth Analg* 82:306–311, 1996.)

of 2% lidocaine into the lumbar or thoracic epidural space. A hypercapnic stimulation test and a progressive isocapnic hypoxic stimulation test were performed to test the hypothesis that thoracic epidural anesthesia would adversely affect the response to hypercapnia and hypoxia, compared with lumbar epidural anesthesia.

Results.—Resting ventilation was unaffected by lumbar epidural anesthesia. In contrast, patients who received thoracic epidural anesthesia had a 13% decrease in minute ventilation along with a 14% decrease in tidal volume. Lumbar epidural anesthesia led to a significant increase in the ventilatory response to hypercapnia (Fig 1) , whereas no change occurred after thoracic epidural anesthesia (Fig 2). Neither type of epidural anesthesia altered the slope of the hypoxic response curve. However, lumbar epidural anesthesia was associated with a significant increase in minute ventilation at an SpO_2 of 90%.

Conclusions.—Thoracic epidural anesthesia can cause a slight decline in resting ventilatory function in elderly patients. However, neither lumbar nor thoracic epidural anesthesia appears to reduce the ventilatory response to hypercapnia and hypoxia. Lumbar and thoracic epidural anesthesia appear to be safe for use in elderly patients with normal cardiopulmonary function.

▶ Two groups of elderly patients aged 70 ± 5 and 71 ± 6 years were studied. I would have liked to have known the effect of regional anesthesia on the ventilatory response to hypercapnia and hypoxia in even older patients, because age limits for major surgery are nonexistent today. As the authors themselves point out, no control comparison was made between elderly and younger patients. In addition, the same experiment performed in a postoperative setting, when impaired responses might be more likely to result in adverse outcome, would be of interest. Nevertheless, the authors present physiologic data of clinical importance.

M. Wood, M.D.

Pediatric Anesthesia Issues

Effect of Anaesthesia on Lung Function in Children With Asthma

May HA, Smyth RL, Romer HC, et al (Royal Liverpool Children's NHS Trust, England)

Br J Anaesth 77:200–202, 1996 3–72

Objective.—Although childhood asthma has a prevalence of greater than 14% according to 1 Scottish study, and many children require general anesthesia for surgical or therapeutic procedures, the effect of inhalation agents on respiratory function has not been studied. The effect of balanced general anesthesia on respiratory function and patterns of postoperative overnight pulse oximetry were compared in children with and without asthma.

Methods.—Twenty children with asthma, aged 5 to 16 years, and an age- and sex-matched control group without asthma underwent elective surgery requiring general anesthesia. Those undergoing cardiothoracic or major abdominal surgery were not included. Regular medication was administered after operation. Spirometry measurements were obtained before and after operation. Pulse oximetry was recorded continuously and satisfactorily for 8 hours on the first night after surgery in 11 pairs of children. Statistical lung function changes were compared using the student's *t* test.

Results.—Spirometry measurements decreased after operation, and the decrease was significant for peak expiratory flow rate (PEFR) in the last postoperative period (Table 2). Early and late postoperative differences between groups in PEFR and forced expiratory volume in 1 second (FEV_1) were not significant. Differences in percentage oxygen saturation and time spent with oxygen saturations of less than 90% were not significant between groups.

TABLE 2.—Percentage Decreases in PEFR and FEV_1 From Baseline (Mean [95% Confidence Intervals])

	Asthmatics	*P*	Controls	*P*
"Early" PEFR	19.9 (10.8–29.0)	0.001	19.3 (10.7–27.8)	0.04
"Early" FEV_1	16.0 (9.3–22.8)	0.0007	11.0 (2.9–19.2)	0.001
"Late" PEFR	18.6 (11.2–25.9)	0.0007	14.9 (7.9–22.0)	0.03
"Late" FEV_1	8.2 (0.8–1.56)	0.007	6.8 (−0.8 to 14.4)	0.12

Note: P values relate to significance of decreases from baseline.
Abbreviations: PEFR, peak inspiratory flow rate; *FEV_1*, forced expiratory volume in 1 second.
(Courtesy of May HA, Smyth RL, Romer HC, et al: Effect of anaesthesia on lung function in children with asthma. *Br J Anaesth* 77:200–202, 1996.)

Conclusion.—Measurements of FEV_1 and PEFR decline similarly in children with and without asthma after procedures requiring general anesthesia.

▶ I selected this article because there is evidence that the prevalence of asthma may have increased recently. The decline in FEV_1 and PEFR appeared to be most important in the early postoperative period; do these changes that have been demonstrated in only a small group of children have implications for the time of discharge of ambulatory pediatric patients?

M. Wood, M.D.

Prevention of Vomiting After Paediatric Strabismus Surgery: A Systematic Review Using the Numbers-needed-to-treat Method

Tramèr M, Moore A, McQuay H (Churchill Hosp, Oxford, England)

Br J Anaesth 75:556–561, 1995 3–73

Background.—Although nausea and vomiting are common, unpleasant complications of the postoperative period, the best approach to treatment has not been defined. The effectiveness of various pharmacologic interventions to prevent vomiting after pediatric strabismus surgery were compared in a systematic literature review using odds ratio and numbers-needed-to-treat methods.

Methods.—Only published, randomized, controlled trials that examined the pharmacologic prevention of vomiting after pediatric strabismus surgery were reviewed. Medline was searched by the keyword method and additional papers were identified from reference lists and review articles.

Results.—Thirty-three publications were identified, but 6 were excluded because of inadequate randomization or the use of a historical control group, or because the data combined adult and pediatric procedures. Of the 27 studies included, 23 were in English, 3 were in German, and 1 was in French. These studies included 2,033 children and 38 treatment arms.

The combined rate of early vomiting in placebo and no-treatment control groups was 54%. The combined rate of late vomiting in placebo and no-treatment control groups was 59%. The best documented treatments,

TABLE 1.—Numbers Needed-to-treat (NNT) to Prevent Early and Late Vomiting With Various Drugs

Drug	Dose	Absence of early vomiting				Absence of late vomiting			
		Active	Control	Odds ratio (95% CI)	NNT (95% CI)	Active	Control	Odds ratio (95% CI)	NNT (95% CI)
Droperidol	10 μg kg^{-1}	23/26	23/28	1.6 (0.4, 7.2)	15.8 (4, ∞)				
	20 μg kg^{-1}	22/34	16/33	1.9 (0.7, 5)	6.2 (2.5, ∞)				
	50 μg kg^{-1}	30/57	24/57	1.5 (0.7, 3.2)	9.5 (3.5, ∞)	16/32	14/32	1.3 (0.5, 3.4)	16.0 (3.3, ∞)
	75 μg kg^{-1}	204/269	131/277	3.3 (2.4, 4.7)	3.5 (2.8, 4.8)	149/228	98/231	2.5 (1.7, 3.6)	4.4 (3.1, 7.1)
Metoclopramide	0.10 mg kg^{-1}	24/25	23/28	3.9 (0.7, 20.9)	7.2 (3.3, ∞)				
	0.15 mg kg^{-1}	69/120	40/124	2.8 (1.7, 4.6)	4.0 (2.7, 7.6)	9/33	1/34	6.6 (1.7, 25.1)	4.1 (2.5, 12.3)
	0.25 mg kg^{-1}	42/58	18/56	5.0 (2.4, 10.3)	2.5 (1.8, 4.3)	14/30	10/30	1.7 (0.6, 4.8)	7.5 (2.6, ∞)
Dixyrazine	0.25 mg kg^{-1}	17/20	9/20	5.6 (1.5, 20)	2.5 (1.5, 7.6)	64/78	33/78	5.4 (2.8, 10.2)	2.5 (1.9, 3.9)
Ondansetron	0.15 mg kg^{-1}	27/30	15/30	6.5 (2.2, 19.5)	2.5 (1.6, 5.2)	21/30	10/30	4.2 (1.6, 11.6)	2.7 (1.7, 7.6)
Lignocaine	2 mg kg^{-1}					20/25	12/25	3.9 (1.2, 12.2)	3.1 (1.8, 14.5)
Scopolamine TTS (hyoscine)	0.375–0.75 mg					21/25	13/25	4.2 (1.3, 13.7)	3.1 (1.8, 13)
Atropine	10 μg kg^{-1}	20/25	19/25	1.3 (0.3, 4.7)	25.0 (3.7, ∞)	7/25	13/25	0.4 (0.1, 1.2)	∞
Lorazepam	10 μ kg^{-1}	34/43	31/43	1.5 (0.6, 3.9)	14.3 (4, ∞)	27/39	24/42	1.7 (0.7, 4.1)	8.3 (3, ∞)

Note: The drugs evaluated included droperidol, metoclopramide, dixyrazine, ondansetron, lignocaine, hyoscine, atropine, and lorazepam. For reference information, refer to the original article.
(Courtesy of Tramèr M, Moore A, McQuay H: Prevention of vomiting after pediatric strabismus surgery: A systematic review using the numbers-needed-to-treat method. *Br J Anaesth* 75:556–561, 1995.)

with more than 100 patients each, were droperidol, metoclopramide, and propofol. In the regimen with the best documentation, droperidol 75 µg/kg, 4 children had to be given the drug to prevent 1 from vomiting, 2 would not have vomited anyway, and the remaining child may have vomited after receiving the drug (Table 1). Fewer than 1 child in 100 may have an extrapyramidal reaction to this drug, whereas 16 may experience minor adverse effects. Metoclopramide was significantly better than placebo only for the control of early vomiting. Propofol had a high incidence of oculocardiac reflex, without a significant anti-emetic effect. Propofol should not be used as an anti-emetic.

Conclusions.—Although preventing vomiting in children undergoing strabismus surgery would be desirable, the benefits of any prophylactic anti-emetic therapy remain unproven. Because only 50% of these children vomit without any treatment and the best-studied regimen has a 75% no-vomit rate, the real rate of prevention by this regimen is only 25%. It may be better to see who vomits and then treat that specific patient.

► I chose this article to highlight the importance of determining the number of patients needed to treat, and the number of patients that need to be treated to prevent 1 specific outcome when assessing the effectiveness of a particular therapy. Studies of postoperative nausea and vomiting are very difficult to conduct; the authors question whether it is better to treat prophylactically or wait and see who vomits and then treat. We do not know the answer.

M. Wood, M.D.

Other Perioperative Anesthesia Management Issues

Magnetic Resonance Imaging of the Upper Airway: Effects of Propofol Anesthesia and Nasal Continuous Positive Airway Pressure in Humans

Mathru M, Esch O, Lang J, et al (Univ of Texas, Galveston)

Anesthesiology 84:273–279, 1996 3–74

Background.—Anesthetic agents depress ventilation by inhibiting the upper airway respiratory muscles more than the diaphragm. This leads to the potential for narrowing or closure of the pharyngeal airway during anesthesia. This airway obstruction has been attributed to reduced genioglossus activity and the resulting posterior displacement of the tongue. Because the underlying mechanisms of airway obstruction in sleep apnea are similar to those in apnea associated with anesthesia, and because sleep apnea can be treated by nasal continuous positive airway pressure (CPAP), the effects of CPAP on anesthesia-induced pharyngeal narrowing were examined.

Methods.—Anesthesia was induced in 10 healthy male and female volunteers aged 25 to 34 years by IV administration of propofol in 50-mg increments increased every 30 seconds until the eyelash reflex disappeared, to a maximum dose of 300 mg. Magnetic resonance imaging of the upper airway was conducted when volunteers were awake, during anesthesia, and during anesthesia plus 10 cm of nasal CPAP.

Results.—The minimum anteroposterior diameter of the pharynx at the level of the soft palate decreased significantly during propofol anesthesia and increased significantly after nasal CPAP. The anteroposterior diameter of the pharynx at the level of the dorsum of the tongue increased during anesthesia and increased further during CPAP. The administration of nasal CPAP significantly increased pharyngeal volume during propofol anesthesia.

Conclusions.—The administration of nasal CPAP counteracted propofol anesthesia–induced pharyngeal narrowing. The results of MRI studies during anesthesia suggest that airway obstruction is not caused by relaxation of the tongue, but occurs at the level of the soft palate. Further studies are necessary to determine whether these results apply to other anesthetic agents.

▶ I selected this article because of the current interest in the use of nasal CPAP. It also illustrates the novel use of MRI of the upper airway to define the factors involved in airway patency.

M. Wood, M.D.

Laparoscopic Cholecystectomy as a Day Surgery Procedure

Singleton RJ, Rudkin GE, Osborne GA, et al (Royal Adelaide Hosp, South Australia)

Anaesth Intensive Care 24:231–236, 1996 3–75

Background.—Laparoscopic cholecystectomy has become an accepted alternative to the open procedure. In Australia, there is skepticism as to whether laparoscopic cholecystectomy is appropriate as day surgery. An experience with laparoscopic cholecystectomy in a day surgery unit was reviewed.

Patients.—The experience included 40 consecutive patients undergoing elective laparoscopic cholecystectomy in the day surgery unit of a public teaching hospital. There were 27 women and 13 men, with a mean age of 43 years. All but 1 patient were American Society of Anesthesiologists grade 1 or 2.

Outcomes.—All but 2 procedures were completed laparoscopically. The mean duration of these procedures was 98 minutes, and the mean intraoperative fentanyl dose was 2.7 $\mu g/kg^{-1}$. Seven patients were admitted to the hospital, for an unanticipated hospital admission rate of 17.5%. Five admissions resulted from surgery-related considerations and 2 from nausea and vomiting (Table 1). The subsequent hospital stay was uneventful in all 7 patients.

The average time in the recovery room before discharge was 272 minutes, and each patient received an average of 3 home visits by a community nurse. Eighty-five percent of patients resumed their normal activities of

TABLE 1.—Details of Unanticipated Admissions on the Day of Surgery

Case No.	Age	Sex	ASA Status	Reason for admission
1*	40	F	1	Open cholecystectomy (further biliary tree exploration required)
5†	42	F	1	PONV
10†	36	F	1	PONV/Pain (bile spillage/drainage)
12*	69	M	2	Oozing from gall bladder bed/drainage
13*	28	F	2	Oozing from gall bladder bed/drainage
36†	47	F	2	Oozing from gall bladder bed/drainage
40*	56	M	2	Open cholecystectomy (difficult access)

*The decision to admit these patients was made intraoperatively.
†The decision to admit these patients was made in second-stage recovery.
Abbreviation: PONV, postoperative nausea and vomiting.
(Courtesy of Singleton RJ, Rudkin GE, Osborne GA, et al: Laparoscopic cholecystectomy as a day surgery procedure. *Anaesth Intensive Care* 24:231–236, 1996.)

daily living within 2 weeks. Although 76% of patients reported that they were happy spending the first night after surgery at home, 21% would have preferred to stay in the hospital.

Conclusions.—Laparoscopic cholecystectomy can be performed on a day surgery basis. However, operating and recovery room times and hospital admission rates may be greater than for other day surgery procedures. These factors must be taken into account when assessing the cost implications of outpatient laparoscopic cholecystectomy.

▶ This is a very small series in which only 40 patients were evaluated. Laparoscopic cholecystectomy is being performed in an outpatient setting, but I thought that the unanticipated high admission rate was of interest, especially because 12.5% (5 patients) was a result of surgical causes. In a much larger study of 758 patients,[1] 4.7% of operations were converted to open cholecystectomy and the mean hospital stay was 1.2 days (range 6 hours to 30 days). Thus, some patients essentially did have outpatient surgery, although this was not clearly reported. Clearly, larger studies reporting outcome after laparoscopic cholecystectomy in an outpatient setting are required.

M. Wood, M.D.

Reference

1. The Southern Surgeons Club: A prospective analysis of 1518 laparoscopic cholecystectomies. *N Engl J Med* 324:1073–1078, 1995.

Treatment of Hereditary Angioedema With a Vapor-heated C1 Inhibitor Concentrate

Waytes AT, Rosen FS, Frank MM (NIH, Bethesda, Md; Children's Hosp, Boston; Harvard Med School, Boston)

N Engl J Med 334:1630–1634, 1996 3–76

Background.—Hereditary angioedema is characterized by profoundly reduced levels of C1 inhibitor activity. The lack of inhibition of C1 results in low levels of the early-acting complement components C4 and C2. The periodic attacks of angioedema can affect various areas and may be life-threatening if they affect the trachea. These attacks can be treated or prevented by androgen or antifibrinolytic therapy. However, these therapies are not effective in all patients. The efficacy of infusions of C1

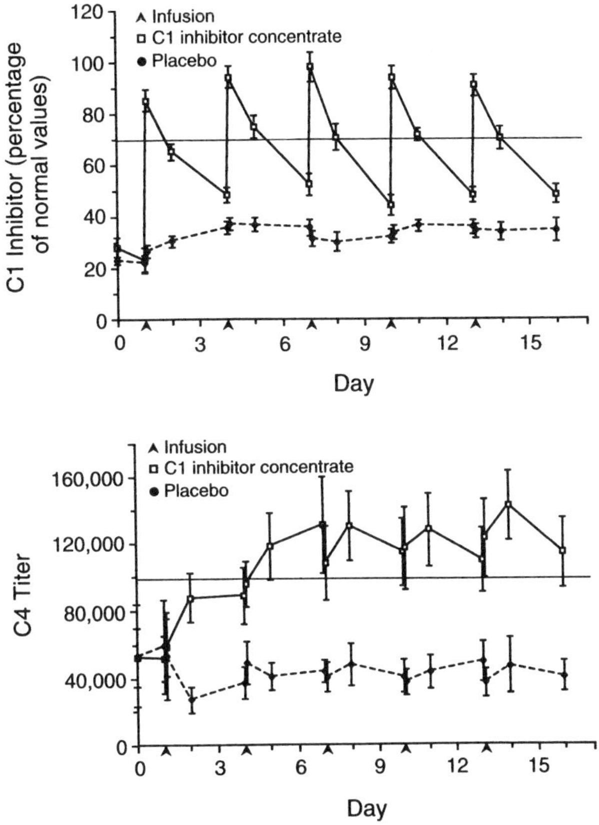

FIGURE 1.—Mean functional C1 inhibitor levels and C4 levels in patients with hereditary angioedema after infusions of C1 inhibitor concentrate or placebo. Each *point* represents the mean plasma level of 6 recipients. The *bars* show the range. The lower limits of normal are represented by the *solid horizontal lines*. (Courtesy of Waytes AT, Rosen FS, Frank MM: treatment of hereditary angioedema with a vapor-heated C1 inhibitor concentrate. *N Engl J Med* 334:1630–1634, 1996, Massachusetts Medical Society.)

inhibitor concentrate in the prevention and treatment of hereditary angioedema attacks was investigated in a randomized, placebo-controlled, double-blind study.

Methods.—Prophylactic infusions of either purified C1 inhibitor concentrate or placebo were given to 6 patients with hereditary angioedema every 3 days for 17 days. After a 3-week washout period, the patients were given infusions of the alternate preparation on the same schedule for 17 days. Each attack of angioedema was rated for severity overall and for abdominal, extremity, laryngeal, and genitourinary edema. Plasma levels of complement were measured at 2, 24, and 72 hours after the infusion.

In the treatment study, the patients reported within 5 hours after an attack began to receive an infusion of either placebo or viral-inactivated C1 inhibitor. The time until the symptoms abated was recorded.

Results.—With C1 inhibitor concentrate, but not placebo, plasma levels of C1 inhibitor decreased immediately after infusion and were almost normal by 24 hours, whereas levels of C4 increased significantly at a slower pace but reached normal levels by 24 hours (Fig 1). There was at least a 60% decrease in the mean daily symptomatic scores for edema of the extremities, larynx, abdomen, and genitourinary tract during treatment with C1 inhibitor concentrate, compared with treatment with placebo.

Eleven patients received C1 inhibitor concentrate to treat 55 attacks, and 11 patients received placebo to treat 49 attacks. Symptoms began to abate at a mean of 55 minutes after infusion of C1 inhibitor and 563 minutes after infusion of placebo. Within 30 minutes after the start of the infusion, 69% of the attacks treated with C1 inhibitor and 2% of the attacks treated with placebo had responded.

Conclusions.—Infusion of viral-inactivated C1 inhibitor concentrate is safe and effective for the treatment and prophylaxis of hereditary angioedema.

▶ Angioedema (formerly known as angioneurotic edema) is a relatively uncommon disease, but investigators predict a rise in its incidence as the number of spontaneous gene mutations increases. It is imperative, therefore, that anesthesiologists familiarize themselves with the etiology, precipitating factors, and treatment modalities of C1 inhibitor deficiency to appropriately manage these patients perioperatively. It is of critical importance to recognize the ineffectiveness of antihistamines, corticosteroids, and epinephrine in the treatment of acute laryngeal edema. The apparent safety profile and efficacy of vapor-heated C1 inhibitor concentrate will likely make this the primary therapy of both prophylaxis and treatment in the perioperative setting.

D.M. Rothenberg, M.D.

The Acute and Residual Effects of Subanesthetic Concentrations of Isoflurane/Nitrous Oxide Combinations on Cognitive and Psychomotor Performance in Healthy Volunteers

Zacny JP, Yajnik S, Lichtor JL, et al (Univ of Chicago)

Anesth Analg 82:153–157, 1996 3–77

Background.—Research has shown that 25% to 30% nitrous oxide premixed with oxygen along with low concentrations of isoflurane is an effective analgesic combination for painful procedures. This drug combination at subanesthetic concentrations may be useful for patients who undergo ambulatory surgery. The acute and residual effects of subanesthetic concentrations of combined nitrous oxide and isoflurane on psychomotor and cognitive performance were investigated.

Methods.—Ten healthy volunteers were included in the blind, randomized, cross-over trial. The volunteers inhaled 100% oxygen-placebo, 30% nitrous oxide in oxygen, and 0.2% and 0.4% isoflurane in oxygen alone and combined with 30% nitrous oxide in different sessions.

Findings.—The combination of inhaled anesthetics resulted in profound impairment. Isoflurane appeared to produce more impairment than did nitrous oxide. Recovery was very rapid. Control-level function returned 5 minutes after cessation of drug inhalation (Fig 1).

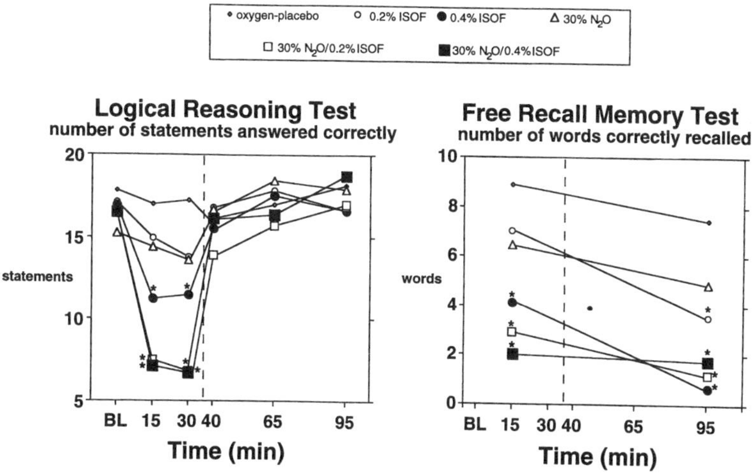

FIGURE 1.—*Left frame*, mean number of statements answered correctly on the Logical Reasoning Test as a function of drug condition and time. Baseline represents the time point when volunteers (n = 10) were inhaling oxygen prior to the onset of the 35-minute inhalation period. Measures were also taken 15 and 30 minutes after initiation of the inhalation period, and 5, 30, and 60 minutes after termination of the period. *Right frame*, mean number of words correctly recalled 15 minutes during and 60 minutes after the cessation of drug inhalation. *Vertical dashed line* separates the inhalation period from the 60-minute recovery period. *The given time point that the drug or drug combination is associated with significantly greater impairment than is the oxygen-placebo condition, as determined by Tukey post-hoc comparison testing. Symbols that represent a given drug condition are shown above the graph. *Abbreviations: BL*, baseline; *ISOF*, isoflurane. (Courtesy of Zacny JP, Yajnik S, Lichtor JL, et al: The acute and residual effects of subanesthetic concentrations of isoflurane/nitrous oxide combinations on cognitive and psychomotor performance in healthy volunteers. *Anesth Analg* 82:153–157, 1996.)

Conclusions.—The combination of isoflurane and nitrous oxide appears to have promise for conscious sedation procedures. More systematic study of its analgesic and mood-altering effects is now needed.

▶ I included this article because it utilizes sophisticated and relatively new methodology for the study of psychomotor performance. Although I don't think the results are particularly surprising (namely that nitrous oxide plus low dose isoflurane in combination seems to be a reasonable candidate for conscious sedation), nonetheless, the reader may be interested in the sophisticated methods by which these authors studied their subjects. Clear headedness after general anesthesia or conscious sedation in today's world of outpatient procedures has become quite important.

J.H. Tinker, M.D.

Large-dose Propofol Alone in Adult Epileptic Patients: Electrocorticographic Results

Cheng MA, Tempelhoff R, Silbergeld DL, et al (Washington Univ, St Louis, Mo)

Anesth Analg 83:169–174, 1996 3–78

Background.—Propofol is useful for "awake" craniotomy, in which the patient must be awake and responsive for intraoperative mapping of eloquent brain areas. However, propofol reportedly has both proconvulsant and anticonvulsant properties, which is potentially hazardous in patients with epilepsy. Previous studies of seizure activity during electrocorticography (ECoG) have not considered the effects of the large doses of propofol required during general anesthesia for craniotomy. The electrophysiologic effects of large-dose propofol, used as the sole anesthetic, in patients with epilepsy were examined.

Methods.—The study included 9 adult patients with medically intractable complex partial epilepsy. All were undergoing a 3-stage approach to surgical management of their seizure disorder: stage I, placement of the intracranial electrode array; stage II, extraoperative localization of the seizure focus; and stage 3, electrode removal and resection of the seizure focus. For stage III, the patients were given induction anesthesia with propofol infusion, 0.5 $mg/kg^{-1}/—^{-1}$. The patients received no premedication. The propofol infusion continued until electrical seizure activity or burst suppression occurred, or up to a total dose of 10 mg/kg. Continuous ECoG recordings were made throughout.

Results.—Two patients were slow to wake after stage I and were excluded from the analysis. In both these patients, propofol had been given in combination with other anesthetics. None of the remaining 7 patients showed any ECoG evidence of seizure activity. Six patients showed burst suppression at a mean propofol dose of 5.7 mg/kg.

Conclusions.—No electrical seizure activity was observed during anesthesia with large-dose propofol alone in patients undergoing surgery for intractable epilepsy. However, other studies have suggested that seizure activity can occur when propofol is given in combination with other anesthetics. Other anesthetics may block propofol's anticonvulsant effects, or potentiate its proconvulsant effects.

► Commenting on this article is E.J. Heyer, M.D., Ph.D., Assistant Professor of Anesthesiology and Neurology, Columbia University College of Physicians and Surgeons, New York:

► The article by Cheng and associates deals with the effect of large doses of propofol on electroencephalographic (EEG) recordings. The investigators used 3 end points to evaluate this effect: EEG evidence of seizure activity, burst suppression, and a total dose of 10 mg/kg. No patients had evidence of seizure activity. All but 1 had burst suppression; that patient required a large dose of propofol to become adequately anesthetized. The authors' conclusion was that when propofol is used alone, without agents such as fentanyl (which may augment seizure activity), it produces burst suppression.

This paper addresses the question of whether propofol increases seizures in patients with epilepsy. However, it does not address another critical issue, whether propofol alters the EEG so as to make it difficult to assess "true" interictal spike activity from an epileptogenic focus. This problem was addressed in part in a paper by Drummond and colleagues[1]. They described a situation in which propofol produced high frequency, large-amplitude EEG activity throughout the cerebral cortex. This activity was seen after a propofol infusion was stopped that did not produce unresponsiveness, and made localization of the seizure focus impossible.

E.J. Heyer, M.D., Ph.D.

Reference

1. Drummond JC, Iraqui-Madoz VJ, Alksne JF, et al: Masking of epileptiform activity by propofol during seizure surgery. *Anesthesiology* 76:652–654, 1992.

Effect of Pneumoperitoneum and Trendelenburg Position on Gastro-oesophageal Reflux and Lower Oesophageal Sphincter Pressure

Tournadre JP, Chassard D, Berrada KR, et al (Hôpital de l'Hôtel Dieu, Lyon, France)

Br J Anaesth 76:130–132, 1996 3–79

Background.—Esophageal barrier pressure (BrP) (the difference between lower esophageal sphincter pressure [LESP] and gastric pressure) is usually increased by factors that increase LESP. The effects of pneumoperitoneum, the Trendelenburg position, and anesthesia on LESP and gastroesophageal reflux were studied.

Methods.—In 11 anesthetized pigs, the effect on LESP and BrP of pneumoperitoneum and the Trendelenburg position were measured; a pH electrode was used to measure incidence of gastroesophageal reflux. Anesthesia was induced with propofol, sufentanil, and pancuronium.

Results.—No effect was seen on LESP or BrP in response to anesthesia. Lower esophageal sphincter pressure and BrP increased significantly with adoption of the Trendelenburg position along with a pneumoperitoneum of 15 mm Hg (LESP also could be increased by either alone). Regurgitation did occur, however, in 2 pigs with low pre-induction BrP. When all the pigs were placed supine, gastric pressure decreased to levels similar to those measured during pneumoperitoneum.

Conclusions.—According to these data, on an individual patient basis, predicting that the adaptive response of the lower esophageal sphincter will protect against regurgitation during laparoscopy is not possible. In general, however, LESP does increase significantly in response to increased intra-abdominal pressure.

▶ Although this study gives some hope that in fact, increasing the Trendelenburg position and pneumoperitoneum do not promote gastric reflux, it is clear that because 2 of the pigs did regurgitate, this extra pressure barrier is not uniformly effective.

M.F. Roizen, M.D.

Preoperative Marijuana Inhalation: An Airway Concern

Mallat A, Roberson J, Brock-Utne JG (Stanford Univ, Calif; California Ear Inst, Palo Alto)

Can J Anaesth 43:691–693, 1996 3–80

Introduction.—*Cannabis sativa* (marijuana) can cause respiratory disorders, including asthma, bronchitis, oropharyngitis, and uvular edema. The case of a healthy patient in whom severe uvular edema developed after preoperative marijuana smoking and general anesthesia was reported.

> *Case Report.*—Boy, 17 years, with chronic otitis media was scheduled for tympanomastoidectomy. The patient had a history of marijuana use. Because the patient exhibited very little response to placement of the IV catheter and appeared unusually calm, marijuana use was suspected. An unsymptomatic, reddened, class I airway with enlarged tonsils and uvula was observed. In the recovery room, the patient complained of feeling that something was lodged in his throat. Examination revealed an even larger, swollen, elongated uvula. The uvula was estimated to be 10 to 12 cm. Dexamethasone, 10 mg, was administered IV and the patient was discharged the next day. He admitted to marijuana use 4 to 6 hours before hospital admission.

Discussion.—Uvular edema caused by marijuana inhalation is a potentially serious postoperative problem. The edema is easily diagnosed and treated. Elective surgical procedures should be canceled for patients with an acute history of marijuana use because prophylactic treatment may not be sufficient.

▶ This case report represents a warning that marijuana use can lead to uvular edema and airway obstruction, a finding hitherto unreported in the literature.

M. Wood, M.D.

Peri-operative Management of Diabetic Patients: Any Changes for the Better Since 1985?

Eldridge AJ, Sear JW (John Radcliffe Hosp, Oxford, England)

Anaesthesia 51:45–51, 1996 3–81

Introduction.—The perioperative management of patients with diabetes is controversial. In 1985, the anesthetists in the Oxford region of England were surveyed regarding their practices for the perioperative management of this patient population, with particular attention to the perioperative blood glucose maintenance level and methods of controlling the blood glucose level during anesthesia. The survey was repeated in the Oxford region to investigate changes in clinical practice.

Methods.—All practicing anesthetists at 7 hospitals were sent a questionnaire addressing the perioperative management of both non–insulin-dependent diabetic (NIDDM) patients and IDDM patients undergoing minor, intermediate, or major surgery. The respondents indicated their choice of 6 ranges of blood glucose concentrations they maintain during the perioperative and postoperative periods and of 6 methods of controlling the blood glucose level. They were asked to report changes in their practices since 1985.

Results.—Of the 172 respondents, 62% indicated that 7–10 mmol/L was the ideal blood glucose level for perioperative maintenance, although 16% chose 4–7 mmol/L and 22% chose a concentration greater than 10 mmol/L. However, the normoglycemic range of 4–7 mmol/L was preferred during the immediate postoperative period by 30%, and only 9% maintained a blood glucose concentration greater than 10 mmol/L postoperatively. These patterns indicate a tighter control of perioperative and particularly postoperative blood glucose concentration, compared with the responses in 1985.

The anesthetists were more likely to adopt a minimally interventional approach of omitting both hypoglycemic agents and extraneous glucose with NIDDM patients, particularly those undergoing minor surgery, although 17% would take this initial approach even with NIDDM patients undergoing major surgery. Active management was advocated with IDDM patients by all anesthetists. Compared with the anesthetists involved in the 1985 survey, current practice has moved away from the use of a combined intravenous glucose, insulin, and potassium infusion and of subcutaneous insulin administration. Anesthetists are currently most likely to use separate infusions of insulin and either glucose or sodium chloride 0.9% to maintain glucose concentrations.

The anesthetists reported little change in their practices since 1985. The reported changes were mainly related to the development of reliable infusion pumps and bedside measurement of blood glucose concentration. The hospital's standardized protocols changed the management practices of 2 respondents.

Conclusions.—There is a trend toward more frequent perioperative maintenance of normoglycemia among anesthetists managing patients with diabetes. This change may reflect a greater recognition of the benefits of the normoglycemic state and the greater ability to perform frequent measurements of blood glucose concentrations with bedside glucosimetry, allowing more confidence in the ability to avoid hypoglycemia.

▶ This report looks at the change in practice patterns of 172 British anesthetists in 1995, as compared with 1985. Although there is a trend toward glucose and insulin infusions and in tighter control of blood sugar in 1995 than in 1985, these changes appear to be minor adjustments in the management of diabetic patients. Perhaps no major ones were needed.

M.F. Roizen, M.D.

Perioperative Normothermia to Reduce the Incidence of Surgical-Wound Infection and Shorten Hospitalization

Kurz A, for the Study of Wound Infection and Temperature Group (Univ of California, San Francisco; Univ of Vienna)

N Engl J Med 334:1209–1215, 1996 3–82

Background.—Perioperative hypothermia in which the core body temperature is about 2°C less than normal commonly occurs in patients undergoing colonic surgery. Vasoconstriction and impaired immunity can result, increasing a patient's susceptibility to perioperative wound infections. Hypothermia may increase susceptibility to surgical-wound infection and length of hospital stay.

Methods.—Two hundred patients undergoing colorectal surgery were studied. Half were randomly assigned to receive routine intraoperative thermal care, and half were assigned to receive additional warming. All patients were given cefamandole and metronidazole, and their anesthetic care was standardized.

Findings.—More transfusions of allogeneic blood were needed in the patients assigned to hypothermia. Mean final intraoperative core temperatures were 34.7°C in the hypothermia group and 36.6°C in the normothermia groups (Fig 1). Nineteen percent of patients assigned to hypothermia and 6% assigned to normothermia had surgical-wound infections (Table 2). Patients in the hypothermia group had sutures removed 1 day later than patients in the normothermia group. Hospital stays were prolonged by 2.6 days (about 20%) in patients assigned to hypothermia.

Conclusions.—Forced-air warming combined with fluid warming maintained normothermia. Unwarmed patients had core temperatures of about

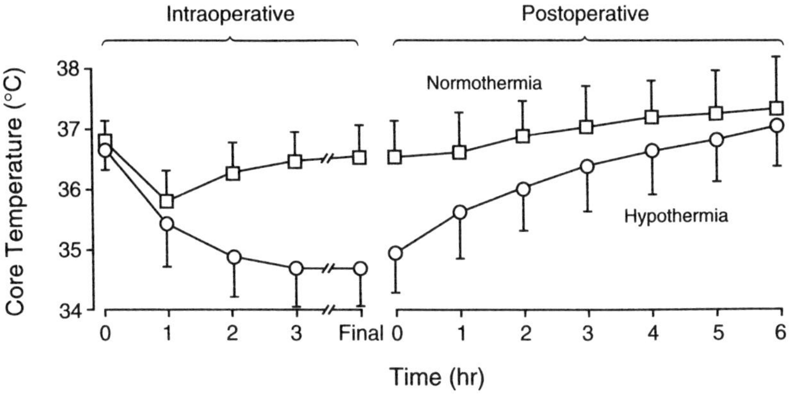

FIGURE 1.—Core temperatures during and after colorectal surgery in the study patients. The mean (±SD) final intraoperative core temperature was 34.7 ± 0.6 ° C in the 96 patients assigned to the hyperthermia group, who received routine thermal care, and 36.6 ± 0.5 ° C in the 104 patients assigned to the normothermia group, who were given extra warming. The core temperatures in the 2 groups differed significantly at each measurement, except before the induction of anesthesia (first measurement) and after 6 hours of recovery. (Courtesy of Kurz A, for the Study of Wound Infection and Temperature Group: Perioperative normothermia to reduce the incidence of surgical-wound infection and shorten hospitalization. *N Engl J Med* 334:1209–1215, 1996. Reprinted by permission of *The New England Journal of Medicine*. Copyright 1996, Massachusetts Medical Society.)

2°C less than normal. Perioperative hypothermia lasted for more than 4 hours and included the period decisive for establishment of an infection.

▶ This well-designed study brings into question the popular misconception that a cold operating room imparts protection against infection. Indeed, with the exception of offering neurologic protection during intracranial or cardiopulmonary bypass procedures, intraoperative hypothermia appears to lead to

TABLE 2.—Postoperative Findings in the 2 Study Groups*

Variable	Normothermia (*n* = 104)	Hypothermia (*n* = 96)	*P* Value
All patients			
Infection—no. of patients (%)	6 (6)	18 (19)	0.009
ASEPSIS score	7 ± 10	13 ± 16	0.002
Collagen deposition—µg/cm	328 ± 135	254 ± 114	0.04
Days to first solid food	5.6 ± 2.5	6.5 ± 2.0	0.006
Days to suture removal	9.8 ± 2.9	10.9 ± 1.9	0.002
Days of hospitalization	12.1 ± 4.4	14.7 ± 6.5	0.001
Uninfected patients			
No. of patients	98	78	
Days to first solid food	5.2 ± 1.6	6.1 ± 1.6	<0.001
Days to suture removal	9.6 ± 2.6	10.6 ± 1.6	0.003
Days of hospitalization	11.8 ± 4.1	13.5 ± 4.5	0.01

*Plus-minus values are means ± SD.

(Courtesy of Kurz A, for the Study of Wound Infection and Temperature Group: Perioperative normothermia to reduce the incidence of surgical-wound infection and shorten hospitalization. *N Engl J Med* 334:1209–1215, 1996. Reprinted by permission of *The New England Journal of Medicine*. Copyright 1996, Massachusetts Medical Society.)

a number of deleterious consequences. In addition to the increased rates of surgical wound infection and prolonged hospitalization found in the study, the hypothermic group had an increased incidence of blood transfusion. This corroborates prior data suggesting that hypothermia induces coagulopathy. In an era in which discharge time is critical for controlling cost, it would seem imperative that anesthesiologists and surgeons practice the simple measures stated in this article so that patients' temperatures are maintained in a normal range during the perioperative period.

D.M. Rothenberg, M.D.

Exacerbation or Unmasking of Focal Neurologic Deficits by Sedatives

Thal GD, Szabo MD, Lopez-Bresnahan M, et al (Harvard Med School, Boston; Massachusetts Gen Hosp, Boston)

Anesthesiology 85:21–25, 1996 3–83

Background.—Patients with carotid disease or brain tumors may awaken from general anesthesia with a focal neurologic deficit that resolves quickly. This may have a pharmacologic etiology. This phenomenon, recently called "differential awakening," has not been fully charac-

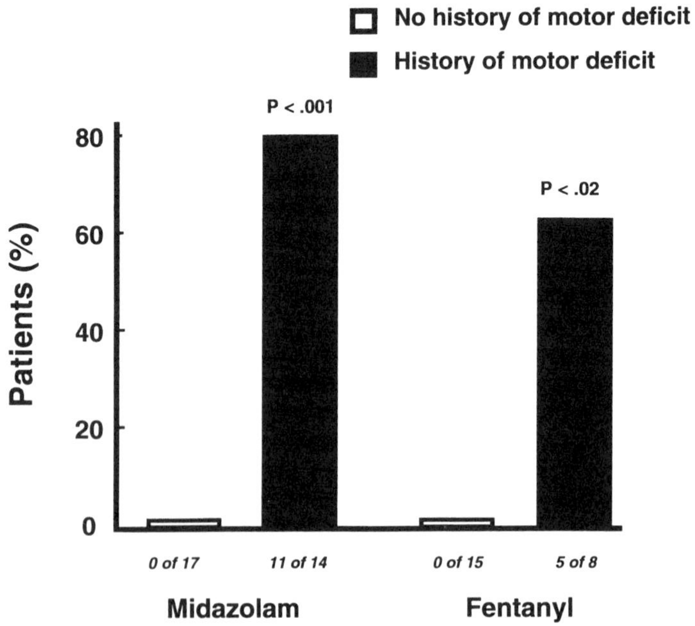

FIGURE 1.—The percentage of patients with sedative-induced neurologic dysfunction. None of the 32 patients without a history of prior focal motor deficit had motor changes after the administration of midazolam or fentanyl (*open bars*). Of the 22 patients with prior motor dysfunction, 79% of those given midazolam and 63% of those given fentanyl experienced worsening of motor function with sedation (*shaded bars*). (Courtesy of Thal GD, Szabo MD, Lopez-Bresnahan M, et al: Exacerbation or unmasking of focal neurologic deficits by sedatives. *Anesthesiology* 85:21–25, 1996.)

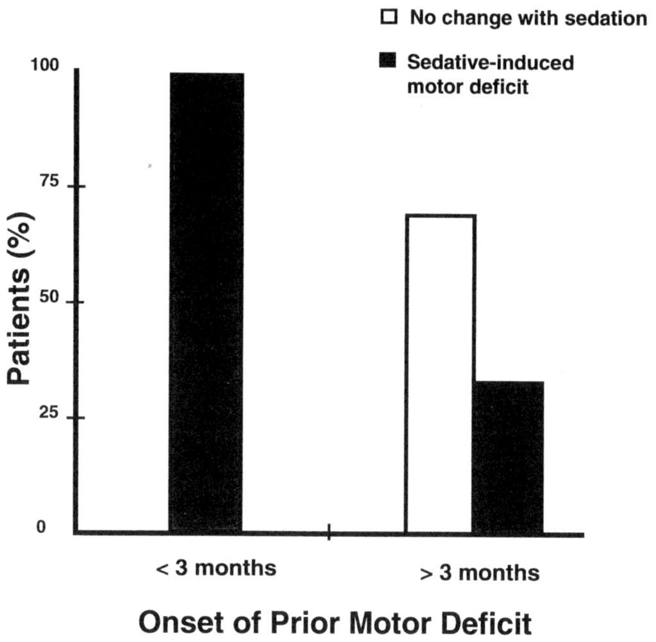

FIGURE 2.—The percentage of patients with sedative-induced neurologic dysfunction as a function of time of onset of a pre-existing motor deficit (less than 3 months vs. more than 3 months). All patients with a history of a new motor deficit within the 3 months before surgery exhibited sedative-induced changes in the neurologic examination. In contrast, in patients with long-standing prior motor deficits (onset more than 3 months previously, *shaded bars*), exacerbation with sedation developed in only 33%. (Courtesy of Thal GD, Szabo MD, Lopez-Bresnahan M, et al: Exacerbation or unmasking of focal neurologic deficits by sedatives. *Anesthesiology* 85:21–25, 1996.)

terized. Patients with underlying neurologic dysfunction were studied to determine whether sedatives can worsen or unmask focal neurologic deficits in this population.

Methods.—Intravenous midazolam, 2.8 mg, or fentanyl, 170 µg, was administered before surgery to 54 adult patients with carotid disease or brain tumors. A motor examination and a mental status examination were performed before and after sedation.

Results.—The patients were fully cooperative, although mildly sedated. In 30% of the patients, focal motor deterioration occurred after sedation (Fig 1). This incidence was similar in patients given midazolam or fentanyl. In 73% of the patients with a focal motor abnormality at baseline or a resolved prior motor deficit, exacerbation or unmasking of these signs occurred after sedation (Fig 2). No sedative-induced change occurred in the patients without a prior history of motor dysfunction. The changes in neurologic function ranged from unilateral mild weakness to complete plegia. These changes appeared to be transient.

Conclusions.—Midazolam or fentanyl can exacerbate or unmask focal motor deterioration in patients with prior motor dysfunction, especially those with acute or subacute focal motor neurologic dysfunction. These patients were examined perioperatively only, but transient focal neurologic deficits early after surgery also may be drug related. A pharmacologic effect should be added to the differential diagnosis of seemingly new postoperative focal motor deficits.

▶ This interesting study highlights the observation that patients recovering from general anesthesia who have carotid disease or brain tumor lesions may exhibit a focal neurologic deficit that rapidly improves. It is well recognized that elderly patients who receive long-acting hypnotics (often benzodiazepines) have an increased incidence of hip fractures, and this has been attributed to an impairment of balance or lack of attention. However, this study suggests that drugs may worsen neurologic deficits in patients with subacute neurologic dysfunction, and has much wider implications than the perioperative period.

M. Wood, M.D.

4 Anesthesia-related Pharmacology and Toxicology

Sevoflurane Issues

Clinical Characteristics

Induction, Recovery, and Safety Characteristics of Sevoflurane in Children Undergoing Ambulatory Surgery: A Comparison With Halothane
Lerman J, Davis PJ, Welborn LG, et al (Univ of Toronto; Hosp for Sick Children, Toronto; Children's Hosp of Pittsburgh, Pa; et al)
Anesthesiology 84:1332–1340, 1996 4–1

Background.—Sevoflurane is a polyfluorinated methyl, isopropyl ether anesthetic that may be a good alternative to halothane for ambulatory surgery in infants and children. The induction, recovery, and safety characteristics of sevoflurane were compared with those of halothane in an open-label, multicenter, randomized, controlled, phase III study of children undergoing ambulatory surgery.

Methods.—Three hundred seventy-five children with American Society of Anesthesiologists physical status 1 or 2 were assigned in a 2:1 ratio to receive sevoflurane or halothane. Both agents were given in 60% N_2O and 40% O_2. Anesthesia was induced using a mask with an Ayre's t piece or Bain circuit or a mask with a circle circuit. During induction, maximum inspired concentrations were 7% for sevoflurane and 4.3% for halothane. Tracheal intubation was not used. End-tidal concentrations of both agents were adjusted to 1 minimum anesthetic concentration (MAC) for at least 10 minutes before surgery was finished.

Findings.—Time to loss of eyelash reflex during induction was 0.3 minute faster with sevoflurane than with halothane. The incidence of airway reflex responses was infrequent and similar between groups. Total MAC-per-hour exposure to sevoflurane was 11% less than exposure to halothane. However, the end-tidal MAC multiple during the final 10 minutes of anesthesia was similar for both groups. Early recovery after sevoflurane was 33% faster than after halothane, although time to hospital discharge was similar in the 2 groups (Fig 1). One hour after sevoflu-

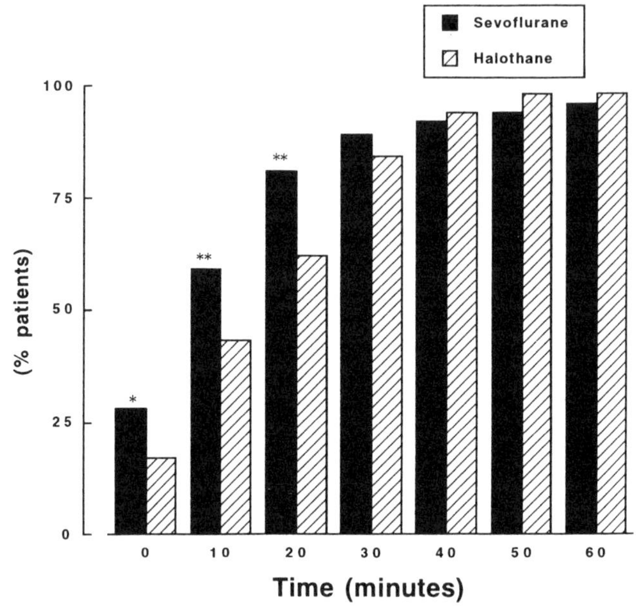

FIGURE 1.—Proportion of children who achieved a modified Aldrete recovery score of 8 or greater (appendix A) during the first 60 minutes of recovery after sevoflurane or halothane anesthesia. The proportion of children in the sevoflurane group who achieved a score of 8 or greater at 0, 10, and 20 minutes after arrival in recovery was significantly greater than that in the halothane group. $*P < .03$ between treatments. $**P < .003$ between treatments. (Courtesy of Lerman J, Davis PJ, Welborn LG, et al: Induction, recovery, and safety characteristics of sevoflurane in children undergoing ambulatory surgery: A comparison with halothane. *Anesthesiology* 84:1332–1340, 1996.)

TABLE 3.—Complications During Induction and Emergence

	Sevoflurane	Halothane
Induction		
Coughing	7 (3%)	9 (7%)
Laryngospasm	0	0
Breathholding	6 (2%)	4 (3%)
Bronchospasm	0	0
Secretions	3 (1%)	3 (2%)
Excitement	17 (7%)	4 (3%)
Vomiting	0	0
Emergence		
Coughing	18 (7%)	7 (6%)
Laryngospasm	1 (<1%)	0
Breathholding	1 (<1%)	0
Bronchospasm	0	0
Secretions	1 (<1%)	1 (1%)
Excitement	19 (8%)*	2 (2%)
Vomiting	1 (<1%)	2 (2%)

Note: More than 1 complication may have been experienced by a patient during the same study interval.

$*P < .017$ vs. halothane.

(Courtesy of Lerman J, Davis PJ, Welborn LG, et al: Induction, recovery, and safety characteristics of sevoflurane in children undergoing ambulatory surgery: A comparison with halothane. *Anesthesiology* 84:1332–1340, 1996.)

TABLE 4.—Incidence of Study Drug–Related Adverse Experiences

	Sevoflurane	Halothane	*P*
Respiratory	47 (19%)	20 (16%)	0.57
Cardiovascular	37 (15%)	33 (26%)	0.007
Bradycardia*	0	3 (2%)	0.036
Digestive*	62 (25%)	46 (37%)	0.021
Vomiting	54 (22%)	44 (35%)	0.006
Nervous system*	75 (30%)	26 (21%)	0.064
Agitation	45 (18%)	9 (7%)	0.004
Overall	160 (64%)	90 (72%)	0.131

Note: Data are the number of patients (percentage of the total patients in each group). The adverse events here summarize the incidence over a 24-hour period. Cardiovascular events included arrhythmias, hypotension, and hypertension.

*Bradycardia was defined as a heart rate greater than 100 bpm. Digestive events included dyspepsia, flatulence, nausea, and vomiting. Nervous system events included dizziness, somnolence, agitation, myoclonus, and insomnia.

(Courtesy of Lerman J, Davis PJ, Welborn LG, et al: Induction, recovery, and safety characteristics of sevoflurane in children undergoing ambulatory surgery: A comparison with halothane. *Anesthesiology* 84:1332–1340, 1996.)

rane discontinuation, mean plasma concentration of inorganic fluoride was 10.3 µM. The incidences of adverse effects were comparable in the 2 groups, with the exception of agitation, which was 3-fold greater with sevoflurane than with halothane (Tables 3 and 4).

Conclusions.—Early recovery was predictably faster after sevoflurane than after halothane, although hospital discharge was not sooner. Clinically, the 2 agents are comparable in induction, recovery, and safety characteristics. Thus, sevoflurane is an acceptable alternative to halothane for children undergoing minor ambulatory surgery.

► Despite theoretical objections to sevoflurane, namely excessive fluoride release with possible kidney and/or liver problems and breakdown in soda lime with possible toxicity from compound A, it is gaining wide clinical acceptance in very rapid fashion with clinical anesthesiologists. It does not seem to be associated with those problems mentioned above. Also important, sevoflurane is proving to be quite "user friendly." Clearly, there is a "learning curve" with this and any other new drug. Equally obvious, the rapid awakening that one sees with sevoflurane must be modulated by proper clinical practices. Nonetheless, this drug is clearly "taking off." This paper contains information that will be useful to those who anesthetize children and who are thinking about trying sevoflurane, if they have not already done so.

J.H. Tinker, M.D.

A Comparison of the Induction Characteristics of Sevoflurane and Halothane in Children

Black A, Sury MRJ, Hemington L, et al (Great Ormond Street Hosp for Children NHS Trust, London; Inst of Child Health, London)
Anaesthesia 51:539–542, 1996 4–2

Background.—Sevoflurane is a rapid-acting, nonirritating, pleasant-smelling inhalational induction agent that may be ideal for use in children. The induction characteristics of sevoflurane and halothane in children were compared as part of a multicenter international phase 3 trial.

Methods and Findings.—Eighty-one children, aged 6 months to 6 years, were included in the analysis. The children were undergoing general surgical, urologic, plastic, or orthopedic procedures. Those given sevoflurane had a significantly shorter mean time to loss of eyelash reflex than those given halothane (1 minute, 41 seconds versus 2 minutes, 17 seconds, respectively). Mean time to achieve steady spontaneous ventilation and small pupils with central gaze also was briefer in children receiving sevoflurane, (3 minutes, 58 seconds) compared with halothane (4 minutes, 50 seconds). The 2 agents had similar effects on heart rate, blood pressure, and oxygen saturation during induction. No major complications occurred in either patient group (Fig 1).

Conclusions.—Mean time to loss of eyelash reflex and to complete induction is significantly shorter in children given sevoflurane than in those given halothane. Neither agent results in major adverse effects.

▶ These authors studied and compared the induction characteristics of sevoflurane with those of halothane in children. Those of sevoflurane were clearly shorter, as would be expected by its blood gas solubility coefficient. This has now been validated by the growing experience that pediatric anesthetists are gaining with it. They saw no arrhythmias or other major compli-

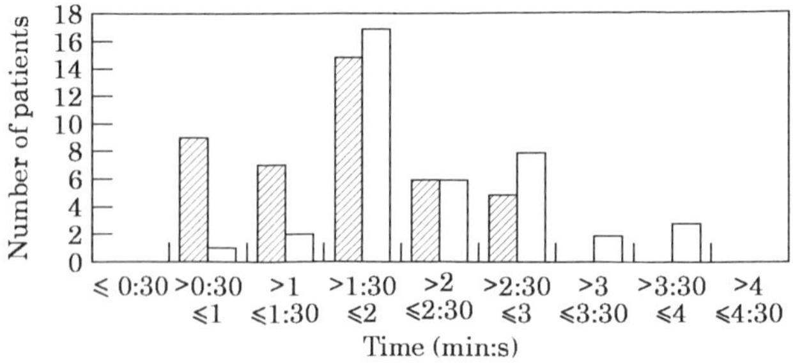

FIGURE 1.—Distribution of the time taken to cause loss of consciousness (loss of eyelash reflex) in children induced with either sevoflurane or halothane ($t = 4.11$, $P = < .01$). *Hatched column*, sevoflurane, mean time = 1 minute, 41 seconds (SD 35 seconds); *open column*, halothane, mean time = 2 minutes, 17 seconds (SD 43 seconds). (Courtesy of Black A. Sury MRJ, Hemington L, et al: A comparison of the induction characteristics of sevoflurane and halothane in children. *Anaesthesia* 51:539–542, 1996.)

cations. The authors did not see evidence of the "malignant" laryngospasm that seems to be possible with desflurane during inhalation induction.

J.H. Tinker, M.D.

A Comparison of the Recovery Characteristics of Sevoflurane and Halothane in Children

Sury MRJ, Black A, Hemington L, et al (Great Ormond Street Hosp for Children NHS Trust, London; Inst of Child Health, London)

Anaesthesia 51:543–546, 1996 4–3

Background.—Sevoflurane, approved by the FDA in 1995, has many features of an ideal inhalational agent for children. Anesthesia induction is rapid, and recovery may be faster than after halothane. The recovery characteristics of sevoflurane and halothane in children were compared as part of a multicenter international phase 3 trial.

Methods and Findings.—Forty children, aged 6 months to 6 years, were enrolled in the study. All were undergoing outpatient procedures. Mean time to opening eyes after surgery was 7 minutes, 52 seconds after sevoflurane, compared with 15 minutes, 50 seconds after halothane. This difference was significant. Mean time to discharge from the recovery unit to the ward also was significantly shorter after sevoflurane than after halothane (12 minutes, 46 seconds versus 19 minutes, 13 seconds, respectively). However, after sevoflurane, more children were in pain and given analgesia. In addition, the mean time to meeting criteria for discharge home was comparable in the 2 groups. No major complications occurred in either group.

Conclusions.—Children receiving sevoflurane awaken more quickly than those given halothane. However, children given sevoflurane have more discomfort, require more effective analgesia, and are not ready to go home earlier than children receiving halothane. Thus, adequate analgesia before recovery is needed.

► This paper illustrates the "learning curve" that experienced pediatric anesthesiologists are going through as we add sevoflurane to our armamentarium. The authors found no difference between times required to discharge the patients home. I would argue that this could well have been due to the fact that recovery personnel have certain times in mind that must be adhered to after "general anesthesia." Over time, I will bet that discharge times may come down somewhat with shorter-acting agents. The notion that these shorter-acting drugs, introduced into clinical practice, would rapidly lead to shorter discharge times has proved to be particularly resilient to change, probably in part because of various recovery "protocols," both formal and informal.

J.H. Tinker, M.D

Comparison of Sevoflurane and Halothane Anesthesia in Children Undergoing Outpatient Ear, Nose, and Throat Surgery

Greenspun JCF, Hannallah RS, Welborn LG, et al (Children's Natl Med Ctr, Washington, DC; George Washington Univ, Washington, DC)

J Clin Anesth 7:398–402, 1995 4–4

Background.—The rapid uptake and elimination of sevoflurane should permit more rapid emergence and recovery from anesthesia than with halothane. These 2 anesthetics were compared for use during short ear, nose, and throat surgical procedures in children.

Methods.—Thirty-nine children, 1 to 12 years of age, who underwent adenoidectomy with or without myringotomy participated in the randomized, open trial. Anesthesia was induced and maintained with either sevoflurane or halothane in 60% nitrous oxide. Oral midazolam, 0.5 mg/kg, was given as premedication and IV fentanyl, 1 μg/kg, was given immediately after induction. Mivacurium 0.2 mg/kg IV was given for tracheal intubation. The end-tidal concentration of anesthesia corresponded to 1 minimum alveolar concentration of the assigned drug. Outcome measures included emergence, recovery, and discharge times.

Results.—Children who received sevoflurane were quicker to emerge from anesthesia than those who received halothane (7 vs. 10 minutes). Recovery time was quicker with sevoflurane as well (20 vs. 31 minutes). Discharge time was similar, however: 184 minutes in the sevoflurane group, 189 minutes in the halothane group. For patients who received sevoflurane, heart rate was easily maintained at or greater than baseline. Patients who received halothane had significantly greater depression of blood pressure after fentanyl administration. The incidence of postoperative vomiting was similar with both anesthetics.

Conclusions.—In pediatric ear, nose, and throat procedures, sevoflurane anesthesia is associated with quicker emergence and recovery than halothane anesthesia. However, this does not translate into a quicker home discharge. Rapid emergence may not have a significant impact on current discharge criteria, or the discharge criteria may need to be modified to gain the benefits of sevoflurane.

▶ The authors concluded that, although there was a faster anesthetic emergence in recovery than with halothane in these children, the sevoflurane group did not go home earlier. I wonder whether this does not simply represent the edge of a "learning curve." Clearly, more rapid emergence in children with sevoflurane also produces excitement and, who knows, perhaps prejudice on the part of the postanesthesia care unit nurses? If the latter is true, what are the biases at play when criteria for readiness for discharge are met? This is a very subjective, difficult problem, as I am sure the reader can see. I suspect that, as we learn how to use sevoflurane, we will be able to discharge patients earlier.

J.H. Tinker, M.D.

The Comparative Effects of Sevoflurane Versus Propofol in the Induction and Maintenance of Anesthesia in Adult Patients

Jellish WS, Lien CA, Fontenot HJ, et al (Loyola Univ, Maywood, Ill; Cornell Med Ctr, New York; Univ Hosp of Arkansas, Little Rock; et al)

Anesth Analg 82:479–485, 1996 4–5

Objective.—Previous comparisons of the IV anesthetic propofol with inhaled anesthetics have generally found that propofol promotes better recovery with fewer negative postoperative outcomes. The new inhaled anesthetic sevoflurane permits rapid induction and recovery and is agreeable to most patients. Propofol and sevoflurane were compared for use in anesthesia during elective surgical procedures.

Methods.—The randomized study included 186 patients undergoing elective surgical procedures expected to last for up to 3 hours. The patients were randomly assigned to receive either sevoflurane- or propofol-based anesthesia. In the sevoflurane group, anesthesia was induced by mask with sevoflurane starting at 0.5% and gradually increased to 3.5% to 4.0% inhaled concentration with 67% nitrous oxide in oxygen. In the propofol group, anesthesia was induced with propofol, 1.5–2.0 mg/kg IV. In both groups, anesthesia was maintained with the primary anesthetic and 67% nitrous oxide in oxygen. The 2 anesthetic regimens were compared for induction, maintenance, emergence, and safety characteristics.

Results.—Induction time was 2.2 minutes with propofol vs. 3.1 minutes with sevoflurane. Tracheal intubation time was 5.1 vs. 7.2 minutes, respectively. However, emergence time was 13 minutes with propofol vs. 9 minutes with sevoflurane. Patients in both groups were equally likely to remain free of complications during the induction, maintenance, and emergence phases. However, airway excitement was more common during induction with sevoflurane. After surgery, the patients became oriented and required analgesia much earlier in the sevoflurane group. Hemodynamic variables remained stable throughout the study in both groups, and postoperative nausea, vomiting, and pain-discomfort scores were similar. Patients anesthetized with sevoflurane had decreased urine specific gravity.

TABLE 6.—Analysis of Changes from Baseline to Postanesthesia Determinations of Renal Function

Variable	Treatment group	Baseline	Postanesthesia
Creatinine (mmol/L)	Sevoflurane	83.22 ± 1.98	85.79 ± 3.73
	Propofol	78.12 ± 1.78	78.83 ± 2.03
Urine pH	Sevoflurane	6.05 ± 0.11	6.25 ± 0.11
	Propofol	5.94 ± 0.10	6.13 ± 0.13
Specific gravity	Sevoflurane	1.018 ± 0.001	1.015 ± 0.001*
	Propofol	1.017 ± 0.001	1.016 ± 0.001

Note: Values are mean ± SEM. No significant differences were found between groups.
* $P < 0.05$ vs. baseline.
(Courtesy of Jellish WS, Lien CA, Fontenot HJ, et al: The comparative effects of sevoflurane versus propofol in the induction and maintenance of anesthesia in adult patients. *Anesth Analg* 82:479–485, 1996.)

Neither group had any significant changes in serum creatinine levels or urinary pH from baseline (Table 6).

Conclusions.—Sevoflurane is a useful alternative to propofol for anesthesia for elective surgical procedures lasting 1–2 hours. The 2 anesthetics are similar in terms of ease of induction and emergence from anesthesia, and in the incidence of nausea and vomiting. Although immediate emergence is quicker with sevoflurane, there is no significant difference in time to discharge or ambulation.

▶ The authors compared sevoflurane/nitrous oxide vs. propofol also with nitrous oxide. Perhaps not surprisingly, there was little difference between the 2 groups with respect to nausea and vomiting, despite the highly touted antinauseant and antiemetic properties of propofol. I wonder why? Could it have been the presence of that old bugaboo, namely nitrous oxide? Many observers, including me, have long believed that our problems with nausea and vomiting after anesthesia will be linked even closer to the presence of nitrous oxide.

J.H. Tinker, M.D.

Sevoflurane Versus Isoflurane: Induction and Recovery Characteristics With Single-Breath Inhaled Inductions of Anesthesia

Sloan MH, Conard PF, Karsunky PK (Univ of Connecticut, Farmington)

Anesth Analg 82:528–532, 1996 4–6

Introduction.—Single-breath inhalation of volatile anesthetics provides rapid induction of anesthesia without IV drugs. The anesthetic sevoflurane has properties that make it well-suited for this purpose: it has little odor, does not irritate the airways, and has a low blood-gas solubility coefficient. Sevoflurane and isoflurane were compared for use in single-breath inhaled induction of anesthesia.

Methods.—The single-blind, randomized, prospective trial included 50 adult patients undergoing ambulatory surgery. Anesthesia was induced with a single breath of either 5.0% sevoflurane or 5.0% isoflurane in a 1:1 N_2O/O_2 mixture. Maintenance anesthesia was obtained by administering the assigned anesthetic in 70% N_2O until the end of surgery. Induction time was assessed by the loss of the eyelash reflex. Recovery characteristics and the awakening concentration were evaluated as well.

Results.—Mean induction times were similar—75 seconds with sevoflurane and 67 seconds with isoflurane. Complications were less likely to occur during sevoflurane induction—patients receiving isoflurane were more likely to cough. Although both anesthetics caused the heart rate to increase, the increase was greater with isoflurane. Time to eye opening was not significantly different. However, eye opening occurred at an end-tidal minimum alveolar anesthetic concentration fraction of 0.12 with sevoflurane vs. 0.15 with isoflurane. Patients in the sevoflurane group reported less clumsiness and less confusion during recovery, but higher pain scores than those in the isoflurane group.

Conclusions.—Sevoflurane is preferable to isoflurane for single-breath induction of anesthesia. Induction is smoother and complications are less frequent with sevoflurane, and patient acceptance is better as well. Single-breath sevoflurane induction could be a useful alternative to IV induction in adult patients undergoing outpatient surgery.

► In the old-time movies, the villain would pour some mysterious liquid on a handkerchief and hold it for 1 or 2 seconds over the face of the heroine. She would fall to the ground in a swoon, almost instantaneously. Until sevoflurane, absent cyclopropane (thankfully), this was not really possible. Single-breath inductions *are* possible with sevoflurane, as this article indicates. Precisely how useful this is, because these were ambulatory adults, I don't know. Will people be tempted to do short ambulatory anesthetics without establishing an IV line?

J.H. Tinker, M.D.

The Effects of Sevoflurane, Isoflurane, Halothane, and Enflurane on Hemodynamic Responses During an Inhaled Induction of Anesthesia via a Mask in Humans

Tanaka S, Tsuchida H, Nakabayashi K, et al (Sapporo Med Univ, Japan)
Anesth Analg 82:821–826, 1996 4–7

Background.—A rapid increase in isoflurane or desflurane concentration is known to induce tachycardia and hypertension and to increase plasma catecholamine levels. It has not been established that sevoflurane, halothane, and enflurane induce comparable responses during anesthesia induction by mask.

Methods.—Fifty patients, 20 to 40 years of age with American Society of Anesthesiologists physical status I, were included in the study. All were scheduled for elective minor surgery. Sevoflurane, isoflurane, halothane, or enflurane were delivered. After anesthesia induction with thiamylal, patients inhaled 0.9 minimum alveolar anesthetic concentration (MAC) of the anesthetic in 100% oxygen by mask. Inspired anesthetic concentration was increased every 5 minutes by 0.9 MAC to a maximum of 2.7 MAC. Heart rate and systolic blood pressure were measured before and every minute for 15 minutes during anesthetic inhalation.

Findings.—Increases in inspired isoflurane concentration to 1.8 MAC and 2.7 MAC resulted in sustained increments in heart rate. Transient increases in systolic blood pressure were also observed after the inspired concentration of isoflurane was increased to 2.7 MAC. By contrast, hyperdynamic responses did not result from changes in sevoflurane and halothane concentrations. In the isoflurane group, plasma norepinephrine levels were significantly greater than that in the sevoflurane group during 2.7 MAC (Fig 1).

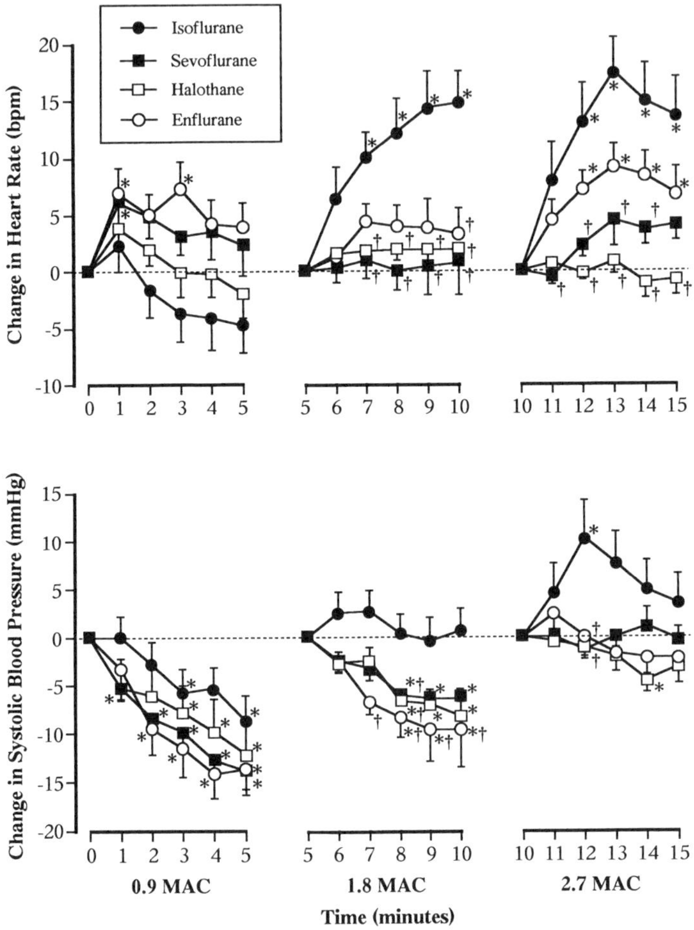

FIGURE 1.—Changes in heart rate (upper panel) and systolic blood pressure (lower panel) from the respective baseline (the time the inspired anesthetic concentration was increased) in the 4 groups. Data are expressed as mean ± SEM. *$P < 0.05$ compared with baseline within the group; †$P < 0.05$ compared with the isoflurane group. *Abbreviation: MAC,* minimum alveolar anesthetic concentration. (Courtesy of Tanaka S, Tsuchida H, Nakabayashi K, et al: The effects of sevoflurane, isoflurane, halothane, and enflurane on hemodynamic responses during an inhaled induction of anesthesia via a mask in humans. *Anesth Analg* 82:821–826, 1996.)

Conclusions.—Tachycardia and hypertension are induced by a large, abrupt, stepwise increase in isoflurane and enflurane concentration given by mask. Sevoflurane and halothane do not induce hyperdynamic responses after increases in anesthetic concentration by 0.9 to 2.7 MAC. Airway irritation appears to be a factor in the observed hypertension and tachycardia.

▶ I included this article with some reluctance because it basically tells us what we already knew, namely that sevoflurane is very smooth compared to drugs like isoflurane and enflurane for mask induction. This detailed scientific study does put numbers on that belief for those who are interested.

J.H. Tinker, M.D.

Cardiovascular Effects of Sevoflurane Compared With Those of Isoflurane in Volunteers

Malan TP Jr, DiNardo JA, Isner RJ, et al (Univ of Arizona, Tucson)

Anesthesiology 83:918–928, 1995 4–8

Background.—Sevoflurane, a new inhalational anesthetic, has the desirable properties of a low blood-gas partition coefficient and nonpungent character. The hemodynamic effects of sevoflurane in healthy volunteers who did not have surgery were investigated.

Methods.—Twenty-one volunteers were randomly assigned to receive sevoflurane, isoflurane, or sevoflurane, 60% N_2O. The subjects inhaled the designated anesthetic for induction and maintenance. Hemodynamic measures were obtained before anesthesia, during controlled ventilation, during spontaneous ventilation, and again during controlled ventilation after 5.5 hours of anesthesia.

Findings.—At high concentrations of anesthetic, a few subjects became excessively hypotensive, which prevented data collection. Heart rate was unaffected by sevoflurane. However, mean arterial pressure (MAP) and mean pulmonary artery pressure were reduced. Cardiac index declined at 1 and 1.5 minimum alveolar concentration (MAC). In subjects with MAP of 50 mm Hg or greater, it returned to baseline values at 2.0 MAC when systemic vascular resistance dropped. Sevoflurane did not change echocardiographic indices of ventricular function, but reduced an index of afterload. Compared with isoflurane, sevoflurane resulted in a greater reduction in mean pulmonary artery pressure, but the cardiovascular effects of these 2 agents were otherwise similar. Sevoflurane with 60% N_2O, by

TABLE 3.—Differences Noted With Prolonged Sevoflurane Administration

Variable	MAC	Preanesthetic Value	Early Value	Late Value
HR (beats/min)	1.0	72 ± 4	67 ± 2	83 ± 3
CI ($L \cdot min^{-1} \cdot m^{-2}$)	1.0	3.8 ± 0.2	2.7 ± 0.2	3.8 ± 0.3
SVR ($dyne \cdot s \cdot cm^{-5}$)	1.0	974 ± 65	948 ± 41	712 ± 76
	2.0	974 ± 65	712 ± 53	373 ± 0
SVI (ml/m^2)	1.0	57 ± 4	41 ± 2	47 ± 3
Svo_2 (%)	1.0	78.0 ± 1.8	86.3 ± 1.1	90.2 ± 0.6

Note: Data are mean ± SEM. Variables included in this table are those for which there was a difference ($P<0.05$) between the early and late values. Early value is that obtained during first 150 minutes of anesthesia. Late value is that obtained after 320 to 400 minutes of anesthesia. Data could not be collected for some subjects at 2.0 minimum aveolar concentration (MAC) due to intolerable hypotension (mean arterial pressure <50 mmHg); n = 7 at 1.0 MAC, n = 5 at 2.0 MAC in the early period, and n = 4 at 2.0 MAC in the later period.

Abbreviations: MAC, minimum aveolar concentration; *HR,* heart rate; *CI,* cardiac index; *SVR,* systemic vascular resistance; *SVI,* stroke volume index; *SVO_2,* mixed venous oxyhemoglobin saturation.

(Courtesy of Malan TP Jr, DiNardo JA, Isner RJ, et al: Cardiovascular effects of sevoflurane compared with those of isoflurane in volunteers. *Anesthesiology* 83:918–928, 1995.)

prolonged administration or spontaneous ventilation, resulted in reduced cardiovascular depression (Table 3).

Conclusions.—These healthy volunteers tolerated sevoflurane well at 1.0 and 1.5 MAC. No adverse cardiovascular properties occurred at 2.0 MAC in subjects with MAP of 50 mm Hg or greater. The cardiovascular effects of sevoflurane were similar to those of isoflurane, which has been in use since 1981.

▶ This is 1 in a series of articles from Arizona that used volunteers to understand various effects of sevoflurane in detail. It puts into numbers the general impression many people have that sevoflurane is quite "user friendly" with respect to cardiovascular changes and other problems. The sponsorship of this study by the pharmaceutical company that makes sevoflurane is noted up front and prominently in the article, and I commend that. This is the kind of article that isn't novel or exciting, but it does provide the kind of solid documentary evidence that we need as we launch a new anesthetic.

J.H. Tinker, M.D.

Fluoride and Renal Issues with Sevoflurane

Sevoflurane Versus Isoflurane for Maintenance of Anesthesia: Are Serum Inorganic Fluoride Ion Concentrations of Concern?

Goldberg ME, Cantillo J, Larijani GE, et al (Univ of Medicine and Dentistry of New Jersey/Robert Wood Johnson Med School, Camden, NJ; Jefferson Med College, Philadelphia)
Anesth Analg 82:1268–1272, 1996 4–9

Background.—The administration of sevoflurane may increase inorganic fluoride ion levels in serum, which may result in the inhibition of renal concentrating ability. Serum fluoride levels, renal function, and re-

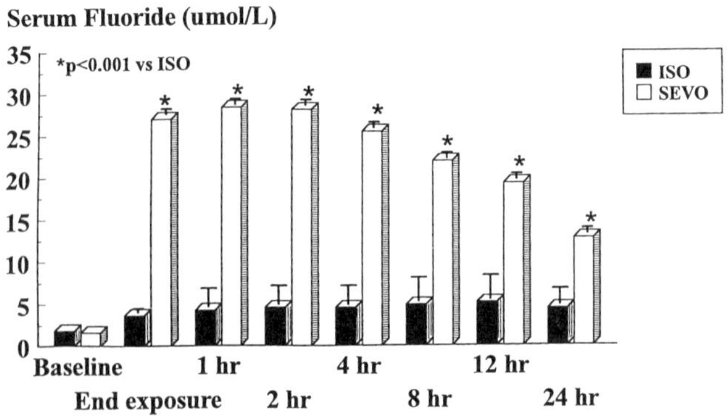

FIGURE 1.—Mean ± SEM serum inorganic fluoride ion levels for up to 24 hours after exposure in sevoflurane (*SEVO*) and isoflurane (*ISO*) groups. (Courtesy of Goldberg ME, Cantillo J, Larijani GE, et al: Sevoflurane versus isoflurane for maintenance of anesthesia: Are serum inorganic fluoride ion concentrations of concern? *Anesth Analg* 82:1268–1272, 1996.)

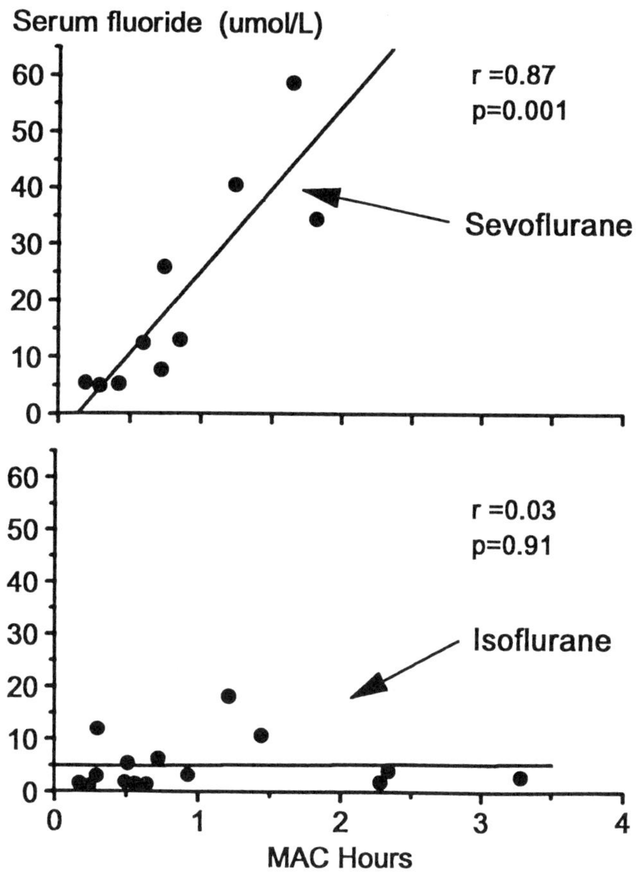

FIGURE 2.—Correlation between minimum alveolar anesthetic concentration (*MAC*) hours and serum fluoride ion concentration at 12 hours after administration of sevoflurane and isoflurane. (Courtesy of Goldberg ME, Cantillo J, Larijani GE, et al: Sevoflurane versus isoflurane for maintenance of anesthesia: Are serum inorganic fluoride ion concentrations of concern? *Anesth Analg* 82:1268–1272, 1996.)

covery variables as a function of time were measured in patients given sevoflurane or isoflurane for general anesthesia for at least 1 hour.

Methods and Findings.—Fifty patients with American Society of Anesthesiologists grade I to III physical status were given sevoflurane at a maximum of 2.4% inspired concentration or isoflurane at a maximum of 1.9% inspired concentration. Mean serum fluoride levels were significantly increased in the patients given sevoflurane compared with those given isoflurane at all time points (Fig 1). Mean peak serum levels were 28.2 μmol/L at 1 hour and 5.08 μmol/L at 12 hours, respectively. Increases in serum fluoride levels in the sevoflurane group peaked at 1 hour and generally declined rapidly after anesthesia was discontinued. Three of the 24 patients given sevoflurane had 1 or more fluoride levels exceeding 50 μmol/L. One had a serum inorganic fluoride ion level of more than 50 μmol/L at 12 hours after sevoflurane administration, and another had

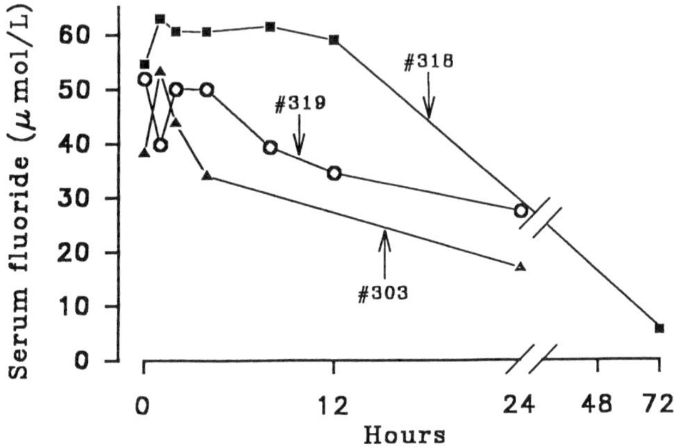

FIGURE 3.—Serum inorganic fluoride ion concentrations for patients 303, 318, and 319, the 3 patients exposed to sevoflurane with fluoride levels greater than 50 µmol/L. (Courtesy of Goldberg ME, Cantillo J, Larijani GE, et al: Sevoflurane versus isoflurane for maintenance of anesthesia: Are serum inorganic fluoride ion concentrations of concern? *Anesth Analg* 82:1268–1272, 1996.)

fluoride levels of more than 33 µmol/L for up to 24 hours after sevoflurane discontinuation. Both these patients also had increased serum blood urea nitrogen and creatinine levels at 24 hours after sevoflurane administration compared with baseline. Serum fluoride ion had an elimination half-life of 21.6 hours (Figs 2 and 3).

Conclusions.—Compared with isoflurane, sevoflurane resulted in significantly increased serum fluoride levels, which peaked early and rapidly declined. Some patients with increased fluoride levels had changes in blood urea nitrogen and creatinine levels, possibly because of sevoflurane exposure. Thus, sevoflurane may result in renal toxicity.

▶ This controversial paper did indeed find 2 patients in whom there was an increase in blood urea nitrogen and creatinine levels at 24 hours after sevoflurane administration. The authors found, as have many, that there are characteristically elevated fluoride concentrations after sevoflurane use. To my knowledge, this is 1 of the only recent studies that purports to link the fluoride release to renal problems, however temporary. Medicine is experiential and experimental. Accumulating experience will probably tell the story about this situation one way or the other.

J.H. Tinker, M.D.

The Hemodynamic and Renal Effects of Sevoflurane and Isoflurane in Patients With Coronary Artery Disease and Chronic Hypertension

Rooke GA, and the Sevoflurane Ischemia Study Group (Univ of Washington, Seattle; Med College of Wisconsin, Milwaukee; Veterans Affairs Med Ctrs, Seattle)

Anesth Analg 82:1159–1165, 1996 4–10

Background.—The hemodynamic effects of sevoflurane and isoflurane are similar in patients without significant cardiovascular disease. However, the hemodynamic effects of sevoflurane in patients with hypertension and ischemic disease are not known. The effects of sevoflurane were compared with those of isoflurane in this high-risk population.

Methods.—Two hundred fourteen patients with evidence of ischemic heart disease or multiple risk factors for ischemic heart disease undergoing elective surgery were studied. By random assignment, 106 patients received sevoflurane and 108 received isoflurane for anesthetic maintenance in conjunction with fentanyl and nitrous oxide in oxygen.

Findings.—Heart rate and arterial blood pressure responses to sevoflurane and isoflurane did not differ between patients with and without chronic hypertension. Therapy needed for hemodynamic deviation also was comparable between patients given sevoflurane and those given isoflurane. Postoperatively, creatinine and blood urea nitrogen declined in both the sevoflurane and isoflurane groups to a similar degree. The incidence of postoperative proteinuria also was comparable in the 2 groups.

Conclusions.—In these patients with ischemic heart disease and hypertension, the hemodynamic response to sevoflurane was very similar to that of isoflurane. Renal function also seemed to be preserved equally well with both agents.

► This is part of a continuing effort to expand, if possible, the useful indications for sevoflurane anesthesia. Expanding the use of sevoflurane to patients with cardiovascular instability and coronary artery disease seems to be occurring nationwide today, and with reasonable results. One thing that seems to be clear by now is that there is no hint of coronary steal with sevoflurane, a finding that makes sense based on the fact that blood pressure control seems quite easy with the drug. This paper is also a careful study of renal function and really finds no disruption of renal function postoperatively, compared to the isoflurane group.

J.H. Tinker, M.D.

Plasma Inorganic Fluoride Concentrations After Sevoflurane Anesthesia in Children

Levine MF, Sarner J, Lerman J, et al (Univ of Toronto; Hosp for Sick Children, Toronto; Children's Hosp of Pittsburgh, Pa; et al)
Anesthesiology 84:348–353, 1996 4–11

Purpose.—In adult surgical patients, sevoflurane degradation in vivo can lead to increased plasma concentrations of inorganic fluoride [F^-]. In some cases, the fluoride level can come close to the theoretical level for nephrotoxicity, which is 50 μM. The plasma [F^-] level in children who underwent sevoflurane anesthesia was investigated in a randomized study.

Methods.—One hundred twenty children who underwent elective surgery were randomized into 3 treatment groups before induction of anesthesia: sevoflurane in air/oxygen 30% (group 1); sevoflurane in 70% N_2O/30% O_2 (group 2); and halothane in 70% N_2O/30% O_2 (group 3). Inhalation anesthesia was induced through the use of a Mapleson D or F circuit with fresh gas flows between 3 and 61 per minute, and maintained with 1.0 to 1.3 minimum alveolar concentration (MAC) sevoflurane or halothane. Plasma [F^-] was measured in whole blood collected at induction and termination of anesthesia and postoperatively at intervals for 1 to 24 hours. Induction and postoperative measurements of plasma urea and creatinine were obtained as well.

Results.—Sevoflurane anesthesia lasted a mean of 2.7 hours and halothane anesthesia 2.5 hours. In most of the children who received sevoflurane, [F^-] concentration peaked at a mean level of 16 μM 1 hour after termination of anesthesia. This level dropped to less than 6 μM by 24 hours. As the MAC·hr of sevoflurane increased, so did the peak [F^-] concentration and the area under the plasma concentration of inorganic fluoride-time curve. The peak [F^-] concentration after halothane was only 2.0 μM and was unrelated to the duration of anesthesia. In both groups, plasma urea concentrations decreased for 24 hours after surgery and plasma creatinine concentrations were unchanged.

Conclusions.—Children who received sevoflurane anesthesia, 2.7 MAC·hr, showed low peak [F^-] concentrations, similar to those seen after enflurane. Inorganic fluoride is eliminated rapidly from children, which suggests a low risk of nephrotoxicity.

▶ One of the "targeted" groups of patients for sevoflurane anesthesia is obviously the pediatric age group because of the relative nonpungency and likelihood that mask induction is more rapid than with halothane (with fewer arrhythmias?). Therefore, the metabolism of sevoflurane into fluoride is of a special interest in this age group. This elegant study from 2 excellent pediatric anesthesia groups from Pittsburgh and Toronto indicates, as one would expect, that elimination of sevoflurane from children is sufficiently fast and/or metabolism sufficiently lower so that the peaks of fluoride are relatively small and unlikely to be important with respect to nephrotoxicity.

J.H. Tinker, M.D.

Prolonged Sevoflurane Inhalation Was Not Nephrotoxic in Two Patients With Refractory Status Asthmaticus

Mori N, Nagata H, Ohta S, et al (Akita Univ, Japan)

Anesth Analg 83:189–191, 1996 4–12

Background.—Inhalation of volatile anesthetics has a potent ventilatory benefit in patients with refractory status asthmaticus, but it could have nephrotoxic effects. Two patients with refractory status asthmaticus were treated with prolonged sevoflurane therapy without experiencing renal dysfunction.

Case 1.—Man, 55, was admitted to the ICU postoperatively. Endotracheal suction had induced an asthmatic attack that did not respond to treatment with theophylline and dexamethasone. Inhalation of sevoflurane at concentrations of 1% to 3% was initiated, which resulted in prompt ventilatory improvement. After 30 hours of sevoflurane administration, it was gradually reduced and discontinued, with weaning from the ventilator occurring on day 5. The inorganic fluoride level increased during sevoflurane inhalation, but there were no changes in serum creatinine level, urinary output, urine specific gravity, or serum electrolytes either during or after sevoflurane inhalation.

Case 2.—Man, 29, with refractory status asthmaticus, was admitted to the ICU with respiratory acidosis. Symptoms did not improve with dexamethasone and epinephrine treatment. Inhalation therapy with sevoflurane was started at a concentration of 2% and increased to 4%. Ventilation improved dramatically. The sevoflurane was gradually reduced and discontinued at 104 hours. The patient was weaned from the ventilator on day 7, 2 days after discontinuation of sevoflurane. Throughout treatment, the patient maintained normal urinary output, blood urea nitrogen, creatinine, serum electrolytes, and urine specific gravity.

Conclusions.—Administration of inhaled sevoflurane causes dramatic ventilatory improvement in patients with refractory bronchial asthma. This treatment can be administered for a prolonged period without causing renal dysfunction.

▶ Two patients were given sevoflurane—1 for 30 hours and 1 for 104 hours, in high concentrations. In case 1, which involved an exposure of 34.5 minimum alveolar anesthetic concentration hours, they had fluoride levels over 50 mmol for many hours. In case 2 the patient received 152.5 minimum alveolar anesthetic concentration hours but fluorides were not measured (no guts?). They also did not test renal tubular function. They "hauled out all the usual suspects," such as blood urea nitrogen and creatinine, etc., but did not really do exhaustive and definitive tests of renal tubular function. I present this article because it is possible to administer sevoflurane for long periods of time, and whether or not it works in status asthmaticus, it did not seem to hurt the kidneys, although the authors were not sophisticated in their testing for renal dysfunction.

J.H. Tinker, M.D.

The Effects of Sevoflurane and Isoflurane Anesthesia on Renal Tubular Function in Patients With Moderately Impaired Renal Function

Tsukamoto N, Hirabayashi Y, Shimizu R, et al (Jichi Med School, Tochigi, Japan)

Anesth Analg 82:909–913, 1996 4–13

Background.—Sevoflurane anesthesia causes an increased concentration of inorganic fluoride, which may induce nephrotoxicity. However, there is increasing evidence that sevoflurane anesthesia does not result in renal functional impairment in healthy patients. The effect of sevoflurane anesthesia on renal tubular function was evaluated in patients with pre-existing renal dysfunction.

Methods.—Fourteen patients with moderately impaired renal function and creatinine clearance between 10 and 55 mL/min were randomly assigned to anesthesia with either sevoflurane or isoflurane. The types of surgery were similar and anesthetic management was identical in the 2 groups. Plasma inorganic fluoride concentrations were measured in blood samples obtained hourly during anesthesia and daily for the first postoperative week and on day 14. Urine samples were collected daily for the first postoperative week and on day 14 and were analyzed to determine concentrations of *N*-acetyl-β-D-glucosaminidase (NAG), γ-glutamyltranspeptidase (γ-GTP), and β_2-microglobulin (β_2MG).

Results.—There were no differences between the 2 groups in plasma creatinine or urea nitrogen concentrations before and after anesthesia. The plasma inorganic fluoride concentration was significantly greater in the sevoflurane group than in the isoflurane group. The urine NAG, γ-GTP, and β_2MG excretions were similar in the 2 groups both before and after anesthesia, with no significant increases after anesthesia in NAG and γ-GTP and increasing urine β_2MG excretions in both groups after anesthesia.

Conclusions.—Sevoflurane had no significant effect on the renal tubules of patients with moderately impaired renal function. No evidence of any potentially serious kidney injury was found in these patients.

▶ The authors studied patients with moderately impaired renal function and found, as usual, relatively high inorganic fluoride concentrations in plasma and high fluoride "areas under the curve" than isoflurane, but no difference in resultant renal function, even though these patients started out with moderately impaired renal function. I think this is consistent with the experience that is occurring around the United States today. On the other hand, although the authors did use soda lime and a semi-closed circle absorber system, they used fairly high flows (some would consider these very high flows), namely, 6 L/min. Therefore, they probably had relatively little release of Compound A, a fact that might have made a difference in these patients with renal impairment.

J.H. Tinker, M.D.

Fluoride Ion Toxicity in Human Kidney Collecting Duct Cells

Cittanova M-L, Lelongt B, Verpont M-C, et al (Hôpital Pittié-Salpêtriére, Paris; Hôpital Tenon, Paris; Hôpital Bichat, Paris; et al)

Anesthesiology 84:428–435, 1996 4–14

Purpose.—Dose-related renal dysfunction can occur with several of the halogenated anesthetics, including methoxyflurane, enflurane, and possibly sevoflurane. This defect is associated with polyuria caused by impaired urine-concentrating ability. Fluoride ion toxicity in the collecting duct cells may play a role. The effects of fluoride ion in the human collecting duct were evaluated, focusing on the Na-K-ATPase activity and morphologic changes occurring after fluoride exposure.

Methods and Results.—Experiments were performed in a new simian-virus-40 immortalized human collecting duct cell line. Initial studies established the toxicity threshold of fluoride ion at 5 mmol/L. After 24 hours of exposure at this level, cell numbers were reduced by 23%, total protein content by 30%, and ^{3}H-leucine incorporation by 43%. Lactate dehydrogenase release increased by 236%. At the same concentration, Na-K-ATPase activity was reduced by 58%. The lowest concentration studied, 1 mmol/L, produced crystal formation and other major morphologic changes of the mitochondria.

Subsequent time-effect studies revealed significant signs of toxicity after only 6 hours of exposure at 5 mmol/L. At this time, cell number was decreased by 13%, ^{3}H-leucine by 48%, and Na-K-ATPase activity by 20%, while lactate dehydrogenase release was increased by 145%. As in the toxicity threshold experiments, mitochondrial crystal deposits were a sensitive marker of cell injury; these crystals appeared within 2 hours of exposure to fluoride ion.

Conclusions.—Fluoride ion has toxic effects on the human collecting duct cells. Exposure can cause morphologic alterations of mitochondria, characterized by crystal formation. The mitochondrion thus appears to be the target for fluoride toxicity in these cells, and the subsequent lack of high-energy phosphates may play a role in the urinary concentrating defect observed after anesthetic inhalation in patients.

► I was attracted to this paper by the authors' use of the term "immortalized human collecting duct cells ..."; I love the hype, but it seems a bit strong to me! Anyway, the authors did study fluoride as a toxin for these cells. Sure enough, fluoride *is* a toxin for these cells by inhibiting the Na-K-ATPase pump. I think the levels here are clinically relevant. The fanciful notion that extracellular concentrations of fluoride, related to serum concentrations of fluoride down all the usual gradients, arriving at the kidney from sevoflurane metabolism in the liver, somehow are not related to nephrotoxicity is spoken strongly against by this study. Clearly the fluoride in this study came from extracellular sources. It is clear (to me) that if there is to be nephrotoxicity from fluoride, then serum fluoride concentration must play a role.

J.H. Tinker, M.D.

Factors Affecting Production of Compound A From the Interaction of Sevoflurane With Baralyme® and Soda Lime

Fang ZX, Kandel L, Laster MJ, et al (Univ of California, San Francisco)

Anesth Analg 82:775–781, 1996 4–15

Background.—Various alkali convert sevoflurane to Compound A, a vinyl ether associated with a toxicity that raises concerns about the safe administration of sevoflurane through rebreathing circuits. Sevoflurane degradation and output of Compound A caused by standard Baralyme brand absorbent and standard soda lime, as well as Baralyme and soda lime with various water content, were investigated.

Methods and Findings.—A flow-through system was used, and a gas flow rate relative to absorbent volume that roughly equaled the rate/volume found in clinical practice was applied. The 2 absorbents produced roughly equal concentrations of Compound A at similar water contents, temperatures, and sevoflurane concentrations. Compared with standard absorbents, dry and nearly dry absorbents produced less Compound A early in exposure to sevoflurane, with more produced later. The output of Compound A was increased by elevations in temperature and sevoflurane concentration. The 2 absorbents also destroyed Compound A, especially when dry. The concentration that exited from absorbent resulted from a complex sum of production and destruction.

Conclusions.—The variability of concentrations of Compound A observed in clinical practice may be largely explained by the inflow rate used, sevoflurane concentration, and the temperature and dryness of the absorbent. The effect of dryness is complex. Fresh dry absorbent destroys Compound A as it is produced, and dry absorbent exposed to sevoflurane for some period yields a Compound A output that is sometimes unusually high.

▶ I trust our readers are familiar with the concept of "academic straw man," with apologies for the apparent sexist sound of the term. Academicians need to have timely and apparently portentious phenomena to study. There is no question that Compound A emerges from soda lime and Baralyme. The reaction goes considerably faster if the temperature is high (47°C to 50°C). This article indicates that there are numerous other complex nuances with respect to the release of Compound A from soda lime/Baralyme. What does it all mean? Is Compound A really as dangerous as Dr. Eger and his colleagues would have us believe? Or is it an academic straw man (person)?

J.H. Tinker, M.D.

Desflurane Issues

Hepatotoxicity After Desflurane Anesthesia

Martin JL, Plevak DJ, Flannery KD, et al (Johns Hopkins Med Insts, Baltimore, Md; Mayo Clinic and Mayo Found, Rochester, Minn; Luther Hosp, Eau Claire, Wis; et al)

Anesthesiology 83:1125–1129, 1995 4–16

Background.—Several fluorinated inhalation anesthetics have been associated with hepatotoxicity, but desflurane has never been reported to cause liver damage in humans. The development of hepatitis after a desflurane anesthetic in a patient who may have been sensitized by previous halothane exposure was described.

Case Report.—Woman, 65, with a history of hypertension underwent a left hemithyroidectomy for a thyroid adenoma. She had been exposed to halothane anesthetics during previous operations. In the current procedure, general anesthesia was induced with 100 mg propofol, 100 μg fentanyl citrate, 40 mg atracurium, and 130 mg lidocaine, given intravenously before tracheal intubation, and maintained with 37% to 39% O_2 in nitrous oxide with 3% to 7% desflurane and IV fentanyl. The day after surgery, the patient was discharged in good condition. Eleven days later, however, pruritus, malaise, nausea, and polyarthralgias developed. A macular erythematous rash appeared over the buttocks and thighs, and the patient's urine was unusually dark. By 16 days after surgery, dermal jaundice and epigastric abdominal pain had developed, and the patient was readmitted. Examination revealed a rash, jaundice, and substantial increases in liver transaminases. On postoperative day 22, the patient was transferred to a hepatology unit for further assessment and possible liver transplantation. Diffuse hepatic parenchymal heterogeneity was observed on ultrasound, with normal bile ducts and normal Doppler examination of the hepatic, portal, and splenic vessels. By postoperative day 27, the patient's liver function and symptoms were improved, and she was discharged. By postoperative day 97, the patient was free of symptoms, with nearly normal liver function. Her medications were spironolactone and furosemide for ascites.

Conclusions.—The patient had several features commonly seen in hepatotoxicity after fluorinated anesthetic administration. Her negative serologic findings and medical history, and the presence of serum antibodies that reacted with trifluoroacetylated-liver microsomal proteins, support the diagnosis of desflurane-induced hepatitis. Previous halothane exposure may have sensitized this patient, and subsequent reexposure to desflurane or possibly other fluorinated anesthetics may have precipitated hepatotoxicity.

▶ The authors contend that they have reported the first case of desflurane-associated hepatotoxicity. The case report is clearly associative and no more definitive than that. I must point out that the first author, Dr. Jackie Martin, is a charismatic speaker who is often sponsored by Ohmeda, the manufacturer of desflurane. If anything, there is "reverse bias" in the publication of a punitive hepatotoxicity case that involves desflurane! Does that improve the credibility of this case report?

J.H. Tinker, M.D.

Desflurane Slightly Increases the Sweating Threshold But Produces Marked, Nonlinear Decreases in the Vasoconstriction and Shivering Thresholds

Annadata R, Sessler DI, Tayefeh F, et al (Univ of California, San Francisco)
Anesthesiology 83:1205–1211, 1995 4–17

Background.—Because shivering is rare during general anesthesia, it may be profoundly impaired by anesthetic agents. The effects of surgical doses of volatile anesthetics on control of shivering have not yet been assessed. The effects of desflurane on sweating and thermoregulatory vasoconstriction are also unknown. The concentration-dependent effects of desflurane on sweating, vasoconstriction, and shivering were investigated.

Methods.—Nine volunteers were included in the study. On separate, randomly ordered days, the subjects were given no anesthesia, a target end-tidal desflurane concentration of 0.5 minimum alveolar concentration (MAC, 3.5%), and a target concentration of 0.8 MAC (5.6%). On each day, the volunteers were warmed until they began to sweat, then cooled until peripheral vasoconstriction and shivering occurred. Changes in skin temperature were compensated arithmetically with the established linear cutaneous contributions to control each response. The concentration-response relationship was determined from the calculated thresholds.

Findings.—Desflurane significantly and linearly increased the sweating threshold. The mean values were 37.1° C on the control day, 37.6° C at 0.5 MAC, and 38.1° C at 0.8 MAC. Vasoconstriction and shivering thresholds were significantly but nonlinearly decreased by desflurane. Thus, the sweating-to-vasoconstriction range increased from 0.5° C to 2.3° C at 0.5 MAC and further to 4.6° C at 0.8 MAC. The range of vasoconstriction to shivering remained between 1.1° C and 1.5° C on the 3 study days (Fig 1).

Conclusions.—The statistically significant and linear, but slight, increase in the sweating threshold is similar to that produced by most general

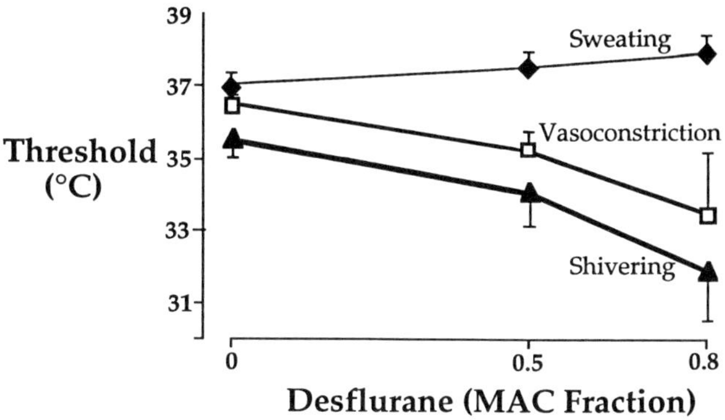

FIGURE 1.—The sweating threshold increased linearly, but slightly, during desflurane anesthesia. Desflurane markedly, although nonlinearly, reduced the vasoconstriction threshold. Consequently, the interthreshold range (temperatures not triggering autonomic thermoregulatory defenses) increased enormously during desflurane administration. In contrast, the vasoconstriction-to-shivering range remained essentially unchanged. All thresholds differed significantly from control and from each other. *Abbreviation: MAC,* minimum alveolar concentration. (Courtesy of Annadata R, Sessler DI, Tayefeh F, et al: Desflurane slightly increases the sweating threshold but produces marked, nonlinear decreases in the vasoconstriction and shivering thresholds. *Anesthesiology* 83:1205–1211, 1995.)

anesthetics. The approximate 3° C decrease in the vasoconstriction threshold by 0.8 MAC desflurane is comparable to that seen previously in isoflurane and propofol anesthesia. At 0.5 MAC, however, the threshold declined less than expected, which suggests that the dose-response relationships for vasoconstriction may be nonlinear. Shivering during general anesthesia is probably rare because thermoregulatory vasoconstriction usually prevents the body temperature from a decline of 1° to 1.5° C.

► This is another in the long series of articles from Dr. Sessler and his colleagues. I included it because it is an elegant human physiologic study in which the authors are able to determine the so-called "inter threshold," i.e., the range from sweating to vasoconstriction in response to increased and decreased body core temperatures. During general anesthesia with isoflurane at 0.8 MAC, this threshold went from about a half degree centigrade to about 4.6°C. This is quite a major physiologic change and has all sorts of implications for our patients and their protection.

J.H. Tinker, M.D.

Halothane Hepatotoxicity

Identification of the Enzyme Responsible for Oxidative Halothane Metabolism: Implications for Prevention of Halothane Hepatitis

Kharasch ED, Hankins D, Mautz D, et al (Univ of Washington, Seattle)
Lancet 347:1367–1371, 1996 4–18

Introduction.—Severe hepatic necrosis can occur after halothane anesthesia. This "halothane hepatitis" is an immunologic complication mediated by sensitization to trifluoroacetylated liver protein neoantigens formed by oxidative halothane metabolism. However, the enzyme that causes oxidative halothane metabolism and trifluoroacetylated neoantigen formation is unknown. Cytochrome P450 2E1 was investigated for its possible role in human halothane metabolism in vivo.

Methods.—Twenty patients scheduled for elective surgical procedures were investigated. The night before their operation, 10 patients received disulfiram, 500 mg orally, and 10 received no treatment. Because disulfiram is converted in vivo to an effective inhibitor of P450 2E1, it served as a metabolic probe for it. All operations were performed with standard halothane anesthesia, with a 10% end-tidal concentration maintained for 3 hours. The levels of halothane in the patients' blood and the levels of trifluoroacetic acid, bromide, and fluoride in their urine were monitored for up to 96 hours after surgery.

Results.—The 2 groups received a similar total halothane dose, as measured by cumulative end-tidal and blood halothane concentrations. However, the patients treated with disulfiram had significantly reduced oxidative and total halothane metabolism, as evidenced by decreased plasma concentrations and urinary excretion of trifluoroacetic acid and bromide. By 96 hours after surgery, cumulative trifluoroacetic acid excretion was 12,900 μmol in the control group vs. 2,010 μmol in the disulfiram group. Figures for bromide excretion were 1,720 μmol and 160 μmol, respectively.

Conclusions.—Treatment with disulfiram before halothane anesthesia results in significantly reduced trifluoroacetic acid production. Thus P450 2E1 appears to play a major role in human oxidative halothane metabolism. Giving oral disulfiram before surgery inhibits P450 2E1, thereby reducing production of the halothane metabolite that leads to formation of the neoantigen that causes halothane hepatitis. Thus preoperative disulfiram administration may prevent halothane hepatitis.

▶ It is amazing, isn't it, how many studies and how much incredible talent is still being expended on trying to understand halothane hepatotoxicity. I seldom include these studies any more in the YEAR BOOK, but this one caught my eye. These authors have solidly identified a particular isozyme of cytochrome P450 (namely 2E1) as the predominant enzyme responsible for human oxidative metabolism of halothane (not necessarily sevoflurane). They next tested a single preoperative dose of the old drug disulfiram, a known P450 2E1 inhibitor, as a possible way to dramatically decrease halothane metabolism. It seems to have worked. The next question is whether something like this could also be done as an adjunct to sevoflurane anesthesia, not because sevoflurane has necessarily been shown to be toxic, but because it is relatively highly metabolized. The idea that perhaps we could "metabolically condition" patients with a few days' pretreatment before anesthesia has many possible applications.

J.H. Tinker, M.D.

Isoflurane vs. Enflurane on Splanchnic Oxygenation

Effects of Enflurane and Isoflurane on Splanchnic Oxygenation in Humans

Berendes E, Lippert G, Loick HM, et al (Univ of Munster, Germany)

J Clin Anesth 8:456–461, 1996 4–19

Objective.—Twenty patients scheduled for elective thoracic and/or abdominal surgery were prospectively studied to determine the effects of enflurane on human hepatic oxygenation. The influences of enflurane on splanchnic oxygen (O_2) extraction and O_2 content difference, hepatic venous oxygen saturation ($ShvO_2$), and hepatic venous lactate concentration were compared with the alterations associated with isoflurane. No previous study has examined the influence of enflurane on human hepatic oxygenation.

Methods.—Seven patients had implantation of an aortobifemoral bypass, 7 underwent abdomino-thoracic esophagogastrectomy, and 6 had a duodenohemipancreatectomy. Ten were randomly assigned to receive enflurane and 10 to receive isoflurane. The 2 groups were similar in mean age, weight, and height, and in gender distribution. One hour after operation, after placement of catheters in the pulmonary artery, radial artery, and peripheral and right hepatic vein, either enflurane or isoflurane was administered. Each anesthetic drug was applied to achieve end-expiratory concentrations of 0.5, 1.0, and 1.5 minimum alveolar concentration (MAC) in a randomized order. Study parameters were determined before and 10 minutes after the administration of each desired end-expiratory anesthetic concentration.

Results.—Cardiac output and mean arterial pressure decreased in both groups at all MAC levels in a dose-dependent manner. Arterial and mixed venous oxygen saturations and systemic O_2 extraction remained unchanged with each anesthesia, but enflurane led to decreases in $ShvO_2$ with increasing inhalational concentrations. In contrast to isoflurane, the decrease in $ShvO_2$ with enflurane reflected an increase in splanchnic O_2 extraction (Fig 1).

Discussion.—Enflurane anesthesia was associated with a dose-dependent decrease in mean arterial pressure and cardiac output that was paralleled by a reduction in $ShvO_2$. Isoflurane anesthesia, despite reductions in CO, preserves the splanchnic and hepatic O_2 supply/demand ratio.

► Years ago, radiologists knew that if they needed to perform hepatic angiograms, they should not do them during halothane anesthesia because it virtually made the hepatic artery do a disappearing act. Indeed, this was so dramatic that inhibition of splanchnic perfusion was implicated at that time as a possible contributor to the mechanism of halothane hepatotoxicity. Readers will recall the concern about the reductive metabolic pathway for halothane, which turned out to be a bit of a straw man (i.e., true but not likely relevant). Nonetheless, the reduction of splanchnic flow by halothane is well

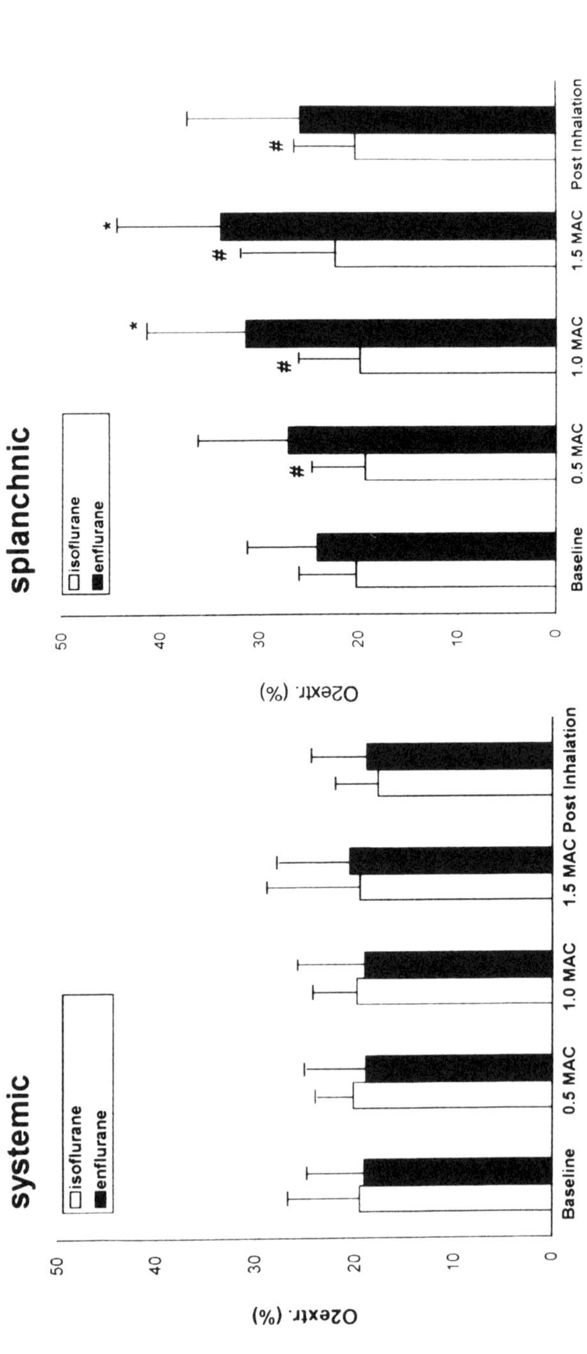

FIGURE 1.—Systemic and splanchnic oxygen extraction (O_2 *extr.*), isoflurane compared with enflurane. Splanchnic oxygen extraction increases during enflurane compared with isoflurane anesthesia. Means ± SD; n = 10/group; **P* <.05 *vs.* baseline; #*P* <.05 isoflurane *vs.* enflurane. (Reprinted by permission of the publisher from Berendes E, Lippert G, Loick HM, et al: Effects of enflurane and isoflurane on splanchnic oxygenation in humans. *J Clin Anesth* 8:456–461. Copyright 1996 by Elsevier Science Inc.)

known. This paper indicates that the same or similar effects are true with enflurane but not so much with isoflurane. This makes sense because halothane and enflurane are similar, with a predominance of myocardial depression and a relative dearth of peripheral vasodilation. Isoflurane has more of the latter and less of the former.

J.H. Tinker, M.D.

Expired Ethanol During Isoflurane Anesthesia

Analysis of Ethanol in Expired Air During Low-Flow Isoflurane Anaesthesia

Olsson J, Hahn RG (Sundsvall Central Hosp, Sweden; Stockholm Söder Hosp)

Br J Anaesth 76:85–89, 1996 4–20

Background.—Ethanol concentration in expired air is monitored to assess fluid absorption during transurethral prostatic surgery and endometrial resection. However, the validity of this method in low-flow ventilation systems has not been studied.

Methods.—Ten healthy women, 24 to 62 years of age, who had been admitted for elective ear, nose, and throat surgery were included in the current study. The concentration-time profiles of ethanol in expired gas and venous blood during an IV infusion of 0.4 g kg^{-1} ethanol over 30 minutes during isoflurane anesthesia and in the awake state were compared.

Findings.—Anesthesia increased the ethanol concentration by 13% in expired gas and by 34% in venous blood. The expired gas-blood difference during infusion was eliminated. The central volume of distribution for ethanol was decreased on average from 20.9 to 8.6 L.

Conclusions.—Breath sampling during low-flow isoflurane anesthesia is a good indicator of alcohol load. However, a change in ethanol disposition slightly increases the values compared with the awake state.

▶ This complex article further evaluates the idea that we may not be able to use low concentrations of ethanol in the irrigating solution during transurethral resections of the prostate, measure it in exhaled air, and generate an indication as to whether there was excessive water absorption. It seemed like a great idea at first, but these authors have concluded that the measurements of ethanol are also effected by utilization of a low flow anesthesia system. Although I warmly embraced the idea at first, these authors have added a note of caution. It may be that the single best "monitor" with respect to water absorption during transurethral resection of the prostate is still the length of surgery.

J.H. Tinker, M.D.

Propofol Issues

Performance of Computer-controlled Infusion of Propofol: An Evaluation of Five Pharmacokinetic Parameter Sets

Vuyk J, Engbers FHM, Burm AGL, et al (Leiden Univ Hosp, The Netherlands)

Anesth Analg 81:1275–1282, 1995 4–21

Background.—The use of computer-controlled propofol infusion for inducing and maintaining anesthesia is becoming more popular. The performance of such devices relies on the match between the implemented pharmacokinetic parameter set and the pharmacokinetics of the patient. The performance of a computer-controlled infusion device with 5 different pharmacokinetic parameter sets of propofol was investigated.

Methods.—Infusion rate-time data on 19 women who had received propofol by computer-controlled infusion, using the pharmacokinetic parameter set from Gepts and colleagues, were stored on a disk. These data then were entered into a computer simulation program to re-calculate predicted propofol levels that would have been obtained with 4 other pharmacokinetic parameter sets of propofol (as described by Shafer, Kirkpatrick, Cockshott, and Tackley and their colleagues).

Findings.—The initial pharmacokinetic parameter set resulted in a median performance error of 24% and a median absolute performance error of 26%. Computer simulations demonstrated that 1 of the other pharmacokinetic parameter sets (of Kirkpatrick and colleagues) had a significantly worse performance. The remaining 3 sets did not differ significantly. For

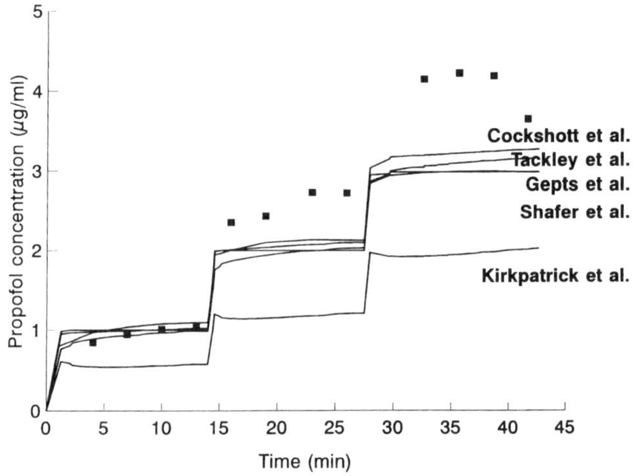

FIGURE 1.—Measured and predicted propofol concentrations versus time of a representative patient from group A. The *squares* represent the measured blood propofol concentrations and the *lines* represent the propofol concentrations as predicted by the computer when provided with the 5 studied pharmacokinetic parameter sets of propofol. (Courtesy of Vuyk J, Engbers FHM, Burm AGL, et al: Performance of computer-controlled infusion of propofol: An evaluation of five pharmacokinetic parameter sets. *Anesth Analg* 81:1275–1282, 1995.)

all 5 sets, the divergence in median and range in patients receiving a stepwise increasing target propofol concentration was significantly greater than that in patients receiving a single constant target propofol concentration. Thus, the performance error increased with target propofol concentration rather than with time (Fig 1).

Conclusions.—In the patients described, the pharmacokinetic parameter sets of propofol of Gepts, Shafer, Cockshott, and Tackley and their colleagues permit a clinically acceptable (although less than optimal) computer-controlled propofol infusion performance. The underprediction of the measured concentration increases as the target concentration increases with all the sets examined.

▶ Underprediction of the measured concentration increases with increasing target concentration over time. The most important point to recognize is that pharmacokinetic parameters provide a starting point for infusion schemes, and after that, one must titrate to clinical effect. For prolonged surgery, turn off the infusion pump earlier than one might predict, because measured propofol concentrations exceeded predicted concentrations.

M. Wood, M.D

Remifentanil Clinical Studies

Remifentanil: A Novel, Short-Acting, μ-Opioid

Bürkle H, Dunbar S, Van Aken H (Westfälische Wilhelms-Universität, Münster, Germany; Tufts Univ, Medford, Mass)

Anesth Analg 83:646–651, 1996 4–22

Objective.—Remifentanil is a novel, potent, μ-opioid receptor agonist with a half-life of 8 to 10 minutes. The anesthetic, analgesic, and sedative properties of remifentanil were reviewed.

Basic Pharmacology and Metabolism.—Remifentanil is a rapidly metabolized anilidopiperidine whose renally excreted major metabolite is much less potent. The easily hydrolyzed N-acyl side chain of remifentanil is responsible for its short-acting effect. The opioid is lipophilic and highly selective for the μ-opioid receptor.

Spinal Administration.—Spinal or epidural administration is not recommended because of motor dysfunction problems caused by the glycine vehicle.

Clinical Pharmacology.—The clearance rate is 2.9 L/min, the systemic half-life is 9 to 11 minutes, and the "context-sensitive" half-life is about 4 minutes. Abruptly discontinuing administration of this drug could result in sudden onset of pain. The 50% effective dose for all surgical stimuli was found to be 0.52 μg/kg/min, and the 50% effective dose for loss of consciousness was shown to be 4.25 μg/kg/min.

Organ-Specific Pharmacology.—The CNS effects of remifentanil in dogs were similar to those of alfentanil. The hemodynamic responses were similar to those of other anilidopiperidines. Remifentanil produces respiratory depression in a dose-dependent fashion. Liver clearance is similar in patients with and without liver disease. Remifentanil does not cause the release of histamine. The drug is not suitable as a general anesthetic.

Conclusion.—Remifentanil is a potent, systemic, fast-acting μ-opioid that has a short analgesic effect. The drug does not accumulate, even after long infusions. However, new anesthetic techniques may be required to prevent immediate postoperative pain.

▶ I have chosen this article as an important review because remifentanil is now available for clinical use. Although remifentanil will dramatically change how we administer opioid anesthesia, its correct use will require education. The pharmacology of remifentanil predicates rapid onset and offset, but these characteristics also bring dangers. Abrupt discontinuation of the drug may lead to extreme pain and other adverse effects, whereas its administration to provide postoperative analgesia will require careful monitoring. Opioid side effects such as respiratory depression, muscle rigidity, hypotension, and bradycardia may occur in the postoperative recovery room and require immediate attention.

M. Wood, M.D.

Remifentanil vs. Alfentanil in the Rat

Continuous Intrathecal Administration of Short-Lasting μ Opioids Remifentanil and Alfentanil in the Rat

Buerkle H, Yaksh TL (Univ of California, San Diego)

Anesthesiology 84:926–935,1996 4–23

Background.—Intrathecal lipid-soluble μ opioids produce a potent, dose-dependent analgesic response. Because these opioids are cleared rapidly, the response is brief. Continuous infusion of lipid-soluble μ opioids can result in systemic accumulation and significant extraspinally mediated adverse effects. The effects of intrathecal infusion of remifentanil, an esterase metabolized agent with an inactive metabolite, and alfentanil were studied.

Methods.—Remifentanil or alfentanil was infused intrathecally in flow rates of 1 μL/min and 0.1 μL/min in rats with chronic lumbar intrathecal catheters. The rats were then tested for hind paw thermal withdrawal latency, supraspinal side effects, and motor impairment. Remifentanil delivered either in a glycine formulation (R_g) or in a saline vehicle (R_s) was studied separately.

Findings.—At an infusion rate of 0.1 μL/min, the 2 agents produced naloxone-reversible, dose-dependent analgesia and supraspinal side effects. The intrathecal median effective dose (ED_{50}) for analgesia was 1.5 μg/min for R_s, 1.2 μg/min for R_g, and 1.5 μg/min for alfentanil. For supraspinal effects, it was 1.7 μg/min for R_s, 1.9 μg/min for R_g, and 1.5 μg/min for alfentanil. Potency or time to onset for analgesia did not differ at either delivery rate. For supraspinal effects, the infusion rate of 1.0 μL/min resulted in a faster R_g onset. After equianalgesic doses, recovery of normal thresholds was faster in R_s than alfentanil, and for the supraspinal index faster in the R_s and R_g groups. At a flow rate of 0.1 µl/min, only R_g produced a dose-dependent motor impairment after 90 minutes of infusion. Glycine in R_g and glycine alone had parallel time courses for motor impairment and similar intrathecal ED_{50} for this nonnaloxone reversible effect. No significant motor effects were associated with intrathecal bolus administration of the same total dose of glycine.

Conclusions.—Like alfentanil, remifentanil has a rapid onset. However, recovery of action is faster after intrathecal infusion. Although it has a rapid clearance, remifentanil induces supraspinal side effects at analgesic effective doses. Furthermore, a reversible motor impairment can occur after intrathecal delivery with glycine.

▶ Spinal and epidural administration of highly lipid-soluble opioids result in very transient spinal effects and, with continuous administration, systemic accumulation and supraspinal effects. Remifentanil is unique among these drugs because of its rapid clearance from plasma. It was hoped, therefore, that continuous neuraxial infusion might produce a more selective spinal effect than fentanyl or sufentanil. The data from this study suggest that may not be the case. In addition, the commercial preparation contains glycine, which produces motor blockade at analgesic doses in the rat.

S.E. Abram, M.D.

Opioid-induced Priorities

Transnasal Butorphanol for the Treatment of Opioid-induced Pruritus Unresponsive to Antihistamines

Dunteman E, Karanikolas M, Filos KS (Washington Univ, St Louis, Mo; Univ of Patras, Greece)

J Pain Symptom Manage 12:255–260, 1996 4–24

Introduction.—Pruritus is somewhat common during neuraxial opioid administration and rare with oral dosing. Pruritus ranges from being a minor nuisance (8% for epidural opioids to 46% for intrathecal opioids) to so severe for some patients that opioid therapy must be modified or discontinued (1%). Antihistamines, opioid antagonists, and propofol are not universally effective in treating pruritus. Only a small number of trials have tested the effectiveness of butorphanol in the prevention of opioid-induced side effects. The effects of intranasal butorphanol administration on pruritus, pain, and sedation were evaluated in patients with severe opioid-induced pruritus after opioid administration unresponsive to diphenhydramine.

Methods.—Six patients receiving opioids by IV, subcutaneous, or epidural routes for postoperative pain experienced severe pruritus unresponsive to diphenhydramine 50 mg IV. Patients reported pruritus, pain, and sedation on separate visual analogue scales (VAS). They received 2 mg intranasal butorphanol every 4 to 6 hours. The VAS scores were collected at 15, 30, and 60 minutes after butorphanol administration.

TABLE 2.—Visual Analogue Scale Scores for Pruritus, Pain, and Sedation after Butorphanol Administration

Variable	VAS score baseline	VAS score baseline + 15 min	VAS score baseline + 30 min	VAS score baseline + 60 min
Pruritus (N = 6)	62.3 ± 12.5	41 ± 21.8	15.3 ± 25.3*	8.2 ± 16.3**
Pain (N = 4)	41.5 ± 39.2	42.7 ± 32.6	34 ± 32.5	25 ± 36.4
Sedation (N = 4)	36.5 ± 41.4	66.8 ± 36.1	57 ± 30.2	50.5 ± 34.4

Note: N, number of patients for which data are available; VAS scores reported as mean ± standard deviation.
*$P < 0.01$, **$P < 0.001$ for comparisons to baseline (1-way analysis of variance, post hoc test).
Abbreviation: VAS, visual analogue scale.
(Reprinted by permission of Elsevier Science, Inc. from Transnasal butorphanol for the treatment of opioid-induced pruritus unresponsive to antihistamines, by Dunteman E, Karanikolas M, Filos KS. *Journal of Pain and Symptom Management*, Vol. 12 No. 4, pp. 255–260. Copyright 1996 by the U.S. Cancer Pain Relief Committee.)

Results.—All patients reported significant relief at 30 minutes and 60 minutes after intranasal butorphanol administration (Table 2). Five patients reported an improvement within 15 minutes. There were no significant differences in pain or sedation VAS scores at any time point, compared with baseline VAS scores.

Conclusions.—Intranasal butorphanol had a significant effect on opioid-induced pruritus that was unresponsive to antihistamines. Controlled studies are now needed to confirm these findings.

▶ This appears to be an effective method of controlling pruritus associated with neuraxial opioids without affecting analgesia. A particular advantage is the minimal increase in manpower cost. The principal downside is sedation, which could be a problem, because this symptom is ordinarily followed closely as an indicator of impending respiratory depression.

S.E. Abram, M.D.

Morphine on Gastroduodenal Motility

Systemic and Central Effects of Morphine on Gastroduodenal Motility
Thörn S-E, Wattwil M, Lindberg G, et al (Örebro Med Ctr Hosp, Sweden; Huddinge Univ, Sweden)
Acta Anaesthesiol Scand 40:177–186, 1996 4–25

Introduction.—The gastrointestinal side effects of opioids continue to be a problem for patients who require both short- and long-term use of these agents for pain control. The extent to which the systemic effects of morphine after epidural administration contribute to the action on gastrointestinal motility was evaluated in a study of healthy volunteers.

Methods.—Study participants were 20 young men without a history of gastrointestinal disease or abdominal surgery. After an overnight fast, participants had a catheter inserted for continuous registration of pressure activity in the duodenum over an 11- to 12-hour period. Ten patients received single doses of both intrathecal (0.4 mg) and IM (4 mg) morphine (IT-IM group). The second group of 10 volunteers was given intrathecal morphine (0.4 mg) and IM saline (IT group). Gastroduodenal activity was evaluated by gastric emptying, manometry, and electrogastrography. Plasma and urine samples were obtained for determination of morphine concentrations.

Results.—Both groups of volunteers demonstrated the characteristic 3-phase pattern of gastrointestinal activity during the fasted state. After intrathecal administration of morphine, the intense activity of phase III occurred significantly earlier in the IT-IM group (median 31 minutes) than in the IT group (median 82 minutes). During the first 4 hours after the administration of morphine, the number of phase IIIs was higher in the IT-IM group. No differences were observed between the IT-IM and IT groups after 6 hours. Both groups exhibited a significant and similar decrease in the propagation velocity of phase III and in tachygastria. The area under the concentration curve in the acetaminophen absorption test was significantly smaller in the IT-IM group compared to the IT group. The latter group showed no measurable plasma concentrations of morphine or the glucuronidated metabolites M3G and M6G.

Conclusion.—Intrathecal morphine influenced gastroduodenal motility and IM morphine had additional effects, providing indirect evidence that the gastroduodenal effects of epidural morphine are the result of both central and systemic actions.

► An important issue in the management of cancer pain is the relative effect of systemic vs. epidural intrathecal opioids. Patients often become tolerant to all the opioid side effects except constipation as the dosage is escalated. This study suggests that there is a decrease in gastrointestinal motility associated with neuraxial opioid administration that is independent of systemic effects. It is not clear, therefore, whether changing from systemic to epidural or intrathecal administration will improve gastric motility in any given patient. It would be helpful to study gastrointestinal motility in patients receiving long-term opioids who are changed from systemic morphine to equi-analgesic epidural or intrathecal doses.

S.E. Abram, M.D.

Flumazenil/Midazolam

Effect of Flumazenil on Ventilatory Drive During Sedation With Midazolam and Alfentanil

Gross JB, Blouin RT, Zandsberg S, et al (Univ of Connecticut, Farmington)

Anesthesiology 85:713–720, 1996 4–26

Introduction.—Flumazenil is a benzodiazepine antagonist that has been shown to effectively reverse benzodiazepine-induced depression of the ventilatory responses to carbon dioxide and hypoxemia. Some reports indicate that it causes a further decrease in ventilatory drive in patients who have previously received both a benzodiazepine and an opioid. The effect of flumazenil on the ventilatory responses to carbon dioxide and hypoxemia was investigated in 12 volunteers sedated with a combination of a benzodiazepine and an opioid in a randomized, placebo-controlled, double-blind, crossover trial.

Methods.—Four treatment phases were undertaken to determine ventilatory responses to carbon dioxide and isocapnic hypoxia: (1) baseline, (2) alfentanil infusion, (3) combined midazolam and alfentanil infusions, and (4) combined alfentanil, midazolam, and "study drug" (consisting of either flumazenil or flumazenil vehicle) infusions. Volunteers received the alternate study drug 2 to 6 weeks later.

Results.—With the administration of alfentanil, the slope of the carbon dioxide response curve was decreased from 2.14 to 1.43 $L/min^{-1}/mm\ Hg^{-1}$ and decreased the minute ventilation at $P_{ET}CO_2$ = 50 mm Hg from 19.7 to 14.8. These variables were reduced further with midazolam: 0.87 $L/min^{-1}/mm\ Hg^{-1}$ and 11.7 L/min^{-1}, respectively. Slope and $\dot{V}_E$ 50 increased to 1.47 $L/min^{-1}/mm\ Hg^{-1}$ and 16.4 L/min with the addition of flumazenil. After placebo, the respective values of 1.02 $L/min^{-1}/mm\ Hg^{-1}$ and 12.5 L/min^{-1} did not change significantly from their values during the combined administration of alfentanil and midazolam. The effect of flumazenil was significantly different from that of placebo. The slope and the displacement of the hypoxic ventilatory response ($P_{ET}CO_2$ = 46 ± 1 mm Hg) were similarly affected, with flumazenil demonstrating a significant improvement, compared to placebo.

Conclusion.—Flumazenil effectively reverses the benzodiazepine component of ventilatory depression during conscious sedation in the presence of concomitant opioid-induced depression of ventilatory drive.

▶ We know that flumazenil (a benzodiazepine antagonist) reverses the effect of benzodiazepine-induced depression of the ventilatory responses to both carbon dioxide and hypoxemia. However, in an ambulatory anesthetic setting, we often administer a benzodiazepine and an opioid together to provide sedation. Flumazenil does not reverse alfentanil-induced respiratory depression, but does reverse the benzodiazepine component of ventilatory depression. The volunteers in this study were all young and healthy, so I would advise caution in extrapolating these results to elderly patients.

M. Wood, M.D.

Midazolam Sedation

Effect of Epidural Bupivacaine Block on Midazolam Hypnotic Requirements

Tverskoy M, Shifrin V, Finger J, et al (Rebecca Sieff Hosp, Safed, Israel; Harvard Med School, Boston)

Reg Anesth 21:209–213, 1996 4–27

Purpose.—Systemic local anesthetics may decrease the need for hypnotic drugs. This raises the possibility that epidural block might have equal or greater potential to decrease hypnotic drug requirements. The effects of epidural bupivacaine block on midazolam requirements were studied.

Methods.—The randomized, double-blind, placebo-controlled trial included 60 unpremedicated male patients. All patients, aged 45 to 65 years and with American Society of Anesthesiologists physical status I or II, were undergoing elective surgical procedures in the lower abdomen, pelvis, or lower limb. Before they were given midazolam, the patients received either an IM injection of saline, 15 mL (M); an IM injection of 0.5% bupivacaine, 15 mL (MIB); or an epidural injection of 0.5% bupivacaine, 15 mL (MEB), at the L3–L4 level. Thirty minutes after these injections, IV midazolam was given in predetermined doses (5 patients per dose). The effects were assessed in terms of loss of response to verbal commands, and the dose-response curves were determined by probit analysis.

Results.—The median effective doses to achieve a hypnotic effect with midazolam were 0.20 mg/kg (95% confidence limit 0.10 to 0.27 mg/kg) in the M group, 0.01 mg/kg (0.05 to 0.22 mg/kg) in the MIB group, and 0.04 mg/kg (0.03 to 0.07 mg/kg) in the MEB group. The differences between all groups were highly significant (Fig 1).

Conclusions.—Epidural bupivacaine in surgical patients can reduce the median effective dose of midazolam by 80%. A 50% decrease also can be

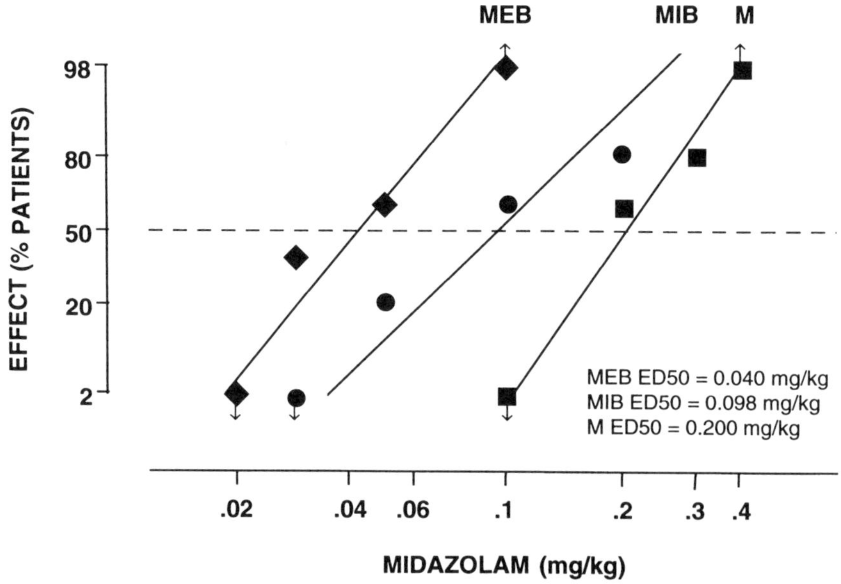

FIGURE 1.—The effect of epidural bupivacaine block (at the L3–L4 level) on the hypnotic dose-response curve for midazolam. The *vertical axis* shows the percentage of patients (on a probit scale) who did not open their eyes in response to the command. The *horizontal axis* represents the doses of midazolam (on a logarithmic scale). *Abbreviations: M*, midazolam dose-response curve without bupivacaine; *MIB*, midazolam dose-response curve with IM bupivacaine (0.5%, 15 mL); *MEB*, midazolam dose-response curve with epidural bupivacaine (0.5%, 15 mL). Each symbol represents a subgroup of 5 patients at the indicated dosage (*dots* for MIB). *Arrows* superimposed on symbols indicate that their actual locations are higher or lower (restriction due to probit scale of the figure). The midazolam ED_{50} values are presented in the right bottom corner. The levels of significance for the differences were $P < 0.00001$ for MEB versus M, $P < 0.002$ for MEB vs. MIB, and $P < 0.01$ for MIB vs. M. (Courtesy of Tverskoy M, Shifrin V, Finger J, et al: Effect of epidural bupivacaine block on midazolam hypnotic requirements. *Reg Anesth* 21:209–213, 1996.)

achieved by IM injection of bupivacaine. The reduced hypnotic requirements after central neural block with bupivacaine probably result from decreased brain afferent input.

▶ This interesting clinical study showed that midazolam hypnotic requirements are reduced in the presence of epidural bupivacaine blockade. The authors attribute this effect to a reduction in afferent input secondary to regional anesthesia, but another explanation for this interaction may be the effect of even very low concentrations of local anesthetic on the CNS. Obstetric anesthesiologists for many years have observed that when higher concentrations of bupivacaine are used, patients often fall asleep after having received epidural analgesia for their labor pain.

M. Wood, M.D.

Midazolam: Periodic Ventilation

Periodic Cardiovascular and Ventilatory Activity During Midazolam Sedation

Galletly DC, Williams TB, Robinson BJ (Wellington School of Medicine, New Zealand)

Br J Anaesth 76:503–507, 1996 4–28

Objective.—Heart rate variability (HRV) analysis provides a useful, noninvasive indicator of cardiac autonomic tone. Various techniques of HRV analysis have been used to study the cardiovascular effects of IV, volatile, and inhalation anesthetics. Midazolam has clinically significant cardiovascular effects, including the ability to obtund sympathetic and baroreflex function. The effects of midazolam sedation on HRV, systolic arterial pressure (SAP), and photoplethysmograph amplitude (PLA) were studied.

Methods.—Eight healthy male volunteers were studied during sedation with midazolam, 0.1 mg/kg^{-1}. Cardiovascular and ventilatory activity were studied in terms of beat-to-beat heart rate (HR), HRV, SAP, finger PLA, and impedance pneumography. The effects of reversing sedation with flumazenil, 0.5 mg, also were evaluated.

Results.—At the start of sedation, there was a small but nonsignificant decrease in SAP and an increase in HR. On spectral analysis of HR over time, the proportion of power in the high-frequency "ventilatory" band (greater than 0.15 Hz) decreased, suggesting the presence of midazolam-induced vagolysis. Low-frequency (less than 0.05 Hz) oscillations of PLA, HR, SAP, and ventilation were observed during sedation, probably the result of activity of coupled cardiorespiratory neurones within the brain stem. The ventilatory periodic effect was comparable to that observed in the early stages of sleep. Flumazenil reversal of sedation also reversed the midazolam-induced diminished high-frequency and increased low-frequency oscillations.

Conclusions.—Midazolam sedation causes alterations in HR and HRV that are suggestive of vagolysis. In some healthy individuals, midazolam may induce periodic oscillations in HR, PLA, and systolic blood pressure, sometimes coupled to periodic ventilatory activity. Even when a drug has little effect on standard hemodynamic measures, significant cardiorespiratory effects may be apparent on detailed time series analysis.

▶ Even though standard hemodynamic parameters such as blood pressure and HR are little changed by midazolam sedation, this study demonstrates that HRV is affected. Heart rate variability has been used to assess vagal and sympathetic cardiac autonomic tone in different clinical settings, and has become recognized as a new tool in cardiovascular physiologic methodology. It is of interest that flumazenil reversed these effects. The clinical significance of drug-induced effects on cardiorespiratory control is not clear from this study.

M. Wood, M.D.

Intranasal Midazolam vs. Sufentanil Premedication

Comparison of Intranasal Midazolam and Sufentanil Premedication in Pediatric Outpatients

Zedie N, Amory DW, Wagner BKJ, et al (UMDNJ-Robert Wood Johnson Med School, New Brunswick, NJ; Rutgers Univ, Piscataway, NJ)

Clin Pharmacol Ther 59:341–348, 1996 4–29

Introduction.—The growing use of outpatient surgery in children has led to the need for rapid, reliable, and short-acting premedications. Intranasal premedication avoids needles and provides direct and rapid drug absorption, reducing the necessary dose. Intranasally administered midazolam and sufentanil were studied for their safety and efficacy as premedications for children undergoing outpatient surgery.

Methods.—The randomized study included 60 children, 6 months to 6 years old, who were undergoing elective surgical procedures lasting 2 hours or less. Thirty minutes before surgery, the children received either midazolam, 0.2 mg/kg, or sufentanil, 2 μg/kg, intranasally in double-blind fashion. Anesthesia was induced with halothane in 50% nitrous oxide/oxygen. The children's preoperative emotional state was assessed, along with their response to premedication, induction, and emergence from anesthesia and side effects.

Results.—Of those children who had not cried before intranasal administration, 71% cried when midazolam was given compared to 20% when sufentanil was given. Nasal irritation occurred in about two thirds of the children who received midazolam. By 20 minutes after intranasal administration, most children in both groups could be separated from their parents without undue distress. During induction, the patients who received sufentanil were better sedated and more cooperative. Neither premedication was associated with significant changes in vital signs or oxygen saturation before or after surgery. Two patients in the sufentanil group did have a moderate reduction in ventilatory compliance after the induction of anesthesia. Nausea and vomiting occurred in 34% of the sufentanil

TABLE 3.—Incidence of Side Effects

	Midazolam (*n* = *31*)		*Sufentanil* (*n* = *29*)	
	No.	%	No.	%
PACU				
Apnea	0	0	2	7
Nausea/vomiting	2	6	10	34*
Pruritus	0	0	1	3
Recovery at home				
Nausea/vomiting	9	29	8	28
Sleepiness	2	5	2	7

*Significant difference ($P = 0.0169$) by χ^2 test.
Abbreviation: PACU, postanesthesia care unit.
(Courtesy of Zedie N, Amory DW, Wagner BKJ, et al: Comparison of intranasal midazolam and sufentanil premedication in pediatric outpatients. *Clin Pharmacol Ther* 59:341–348, 1996.)

group versus 6% of the midazolam group (Table 3). Children who received midazolam were discharged about 40 minutes earlier.

Conclusions.—In children undergoing outpatient surgery, premedication with intranasal midazolam and sufentanil produces rapid, safe, and effective sedation. Sufentanil is somewhat more effective at induction and emergence, but it causes more postoperative nausea and vomiting. Midazolam causes more nasal irritation, but it permits timely separation from the parents with less sedation and fewer side effects.

▶ Oral midazolam has become a popular premedication in pediatric patients, but the dose is difficult to predict accurately because of first-pass metabolism by the liver. The intranasal route more accurately approximates systemic administration; however, the administration of intranasal midazolam produces a burning sensation that children do not like. A new commercial preparation formulated for intranasal use might be of benefit.

M. Wood, M.D.

Clonidine as Shivering Prophylaxis

The Effect of Prophylactic Clonidine on Postoperative Shivering

Vanderstappen I, Vandermeersch E, Vanacker B, et al (Westfälische Wilhelms Universität, Münster, Germany)

Anaesthesia 51:351–355, 1996 4–30

Introduction.—Involuntary muscle activity frequently accompanies recovery from anesthesia and surgery. In patients with coronary heart disease or heart failure, postoperative pain can be exacerbated by shivering, which has been attributed to uninhibited spinal reflexes, decreased sympathetic activity, pain, thermoregulatory shivering in response to intraoperative hypothermia, and adrenal suppression. In treating shivering, meperidine 25 mg has been found to be more effective than other opioids. Other useful treatments for postoperative shivering are clonidine and doxapram. The influence of clonidine administered at induction on postoperative shivering after elective peripheral surgery was evaluated.

Methods.—The double-blind study included 280 males who had elective peripheral surgery with the use of general anesthesia with an anticipated duration of 10–180 minutes and limited blood loss. Warmed infusions, a warmed blanket, a heat and moisture exchanger, and a warming device in the inspiratory breathing system were used to minimize body cooling. The patients were divided into 2 groups, with 1 group receiving clonidine 2 $\mu g/kg^{-1}$ and another group receiving placebo. An esophageal thermometer was used to measure body temperature after intubation and at the end of anesthesia. Every 5 minutes and for 30 minutes after the end of anesthesia, postoperative shivering was measured using a scale of none, if no tension of muscles was observed, to severe, when there was uncontrolled shivering of the whole body.

Results.—The group taking clonidine had less shivering that the placebo group. In the clonidine group, 61% had at least 1 episode of postoperative shivering compared to 74% in the placebo group. Postoperative sedation was not increased and overall consciousness was not diminished by clonidine. Moderate/severe shivering occurred in 21% of the clonidine group compared to 35% of the placebo group.

Conclusion.—Preventive IV administration of clonidine 2 $\mu g/kg^{-1}$ during peripheral surgery slightly, but significantly, reduces visible postoperative shivering.

▶ A number of pharmacologic modalities have been employed to treat postoperative shivering, a disorder that in addition to patient discomfort, can increase myocardial oxygen consumption and lead to postoperative ischemia. These agents include meperidine, chlorpromazine, and clonidine. In severe instances nondepolarizing muscle relaxants may be necessary in those patients who are still sedated and receiving mechanical ventilation. In addition to maintaining body temperature by actively warming both the patient and IV fluids intraoperatively, this study suggests that prophylactic management with clonidine may also help to minimize postoperative shivering. Clonidine administered in this fashion may also add to postoperative analgesia and lower the amount of general anesthetic required for surgery (variables not assessed in this study). The effect of clonidine in preventing shivering secondary to epidural anesthesia would be interesting to assess in future studies.

D.M. Rothenberg, M.D.

Clonidine Enhances Ephedrine Response

Enhancement of Pressor Response to Ephedrine Following Clonidine Medication

Tanaka M, Nishikawa T (Tsuchiura Kyodo Gen Hosp, Japan; Univ of Tsukuba, Japan)

Anaesthesia 51:123–127, 1996 4–31

Objective.—Premedication with clonidine can enhance the pressor response to IV ephedrine, perhaps by increasing peripheral catecholamine storage. The enhanced response could involve peripheral accumulation and increased release of catecholamine by IV ephedrine, or an exaggerated cardiovascular response to ephedrine and/or to catecholamine release by ephedrine. Pressor responses and changes in plasma catecholamine concentrations after ephedrine administration with and without clonidine premedication were studied.

Methods.—The study included 20 patients undergoing various major surgical procedures using general anesthesia with enflurane and nitrous oxide. The patients were studied after receiving 2 consecutive 0.1-mg/kg^{-1} doses of ephedrine, with or without premedication with clonidine, 5 μg/kg^{-1}. The arterial blood pressure and heart rate responses to each dose were measured each minute for 10 minutes. Plasma catecholamine levels were measured before and 3 minutes after each dose of ephedrine.

Results.—The change in mean blood pressure from baseline was greater for the patients who received clonidine from 3 to 8 minutes after the first dose of ephedrine and from 4 to 9 minutes after the second dose. There were no significant changes in heart rate for the patients who received clonidine pretreatment. Plasma noradrenaline and adrenaline concentrations showed no significant changes from baseline in either group. Throughout the study, the clonidine-treated patients had somewhat lower plasma catecholamine concentrations.

Conclusions.—In anesthetized surgical patients, premedication with clonidine enhances the pressor response to ephedrine injections with no significant increase in plasma catecholamine levels. Thus, the recognized augmentation of the pressor effect to ephedrine by clonidine most likely results from increased cardiovascular reactivity to ephedrine and/or to catecholamines released by ephedrine.

▶ The idea that clonidine premedication augments the pressor response to ephedrine is fascinating. Plasma catecholamine levels did not increase after ephedrine administration, and the authors infer that exaggerated catecholamine release is not the mechanism for this phenomenon, but rather an enhanced cardiovascular response. Plasma catecholamine levels during surgery can be very difficult to interpret, and more work is required to define the mechanism. We know that β-blockers in the presence of catecholamine excess can aggravate hypertension because unopposed β-adrenergic vasoconstriction occurs—classically seen in the message that propranolol should not be given to a patient with pheochromocytoma until adequate β-blockade is established. We also know that clonidine suppresses the catecholamine secretion-clonidine suppression test. Thus, in a setting of clonidine-induced suppression of catecholamine secretion, there is an enhanced response to ephedrine. As α_2-adrenergic agonists are used more frequently during anesthesia as "adjuncts" to anesthesia, their side effects may require careful monitoring.

M. Wood, M.D.

Clonidine Interaction with Neostigmine

Interaction Between Intrathecal Neostigmine and Epidural Clonidine in Human Volunteers

Hood DD, Mallak KA, Eisenach JC, et al (Wake Forest Univ, Winston-Salem, NC)

Anesthesiology 85:315–325, 1996 4–32

Background.—The analgesic effects of α_2-adrenergic agonists may be related to their activation of spinal acetylcholine release. Animal studies have demonstrated a synergistic interaction between opioids and α_2-adrenergic agonists administered intraspinally. The interaction between intrathecal neostigmine and epidural clonidine was studied in humans, with examination of both analgesia and side effects. The hypothesized involvement of acetylcholine release and nitric oxide synthase stimulation in the action of these agents also was investigated.

Methods.—Healthy adult volunteers were positioned either sitting (32 subjects) or lateral (26 subjects). An epidural needle was inserted at the L3-4 or L4-5 interspace and either vehicle or neostigmine (at doses of 50, 100, or 200 μg) was injected intrathecally. Seventy minutes later, either normal saline or clonidine was injected through an epidural catheter to targeted CSF concentrations of 50, 100, 200, or 400 ng/mL. The epidural infusion was repeated for a second hour. Drug assignments were made with an isobolographic design to obtain dose responses for each drug alone and for the combination. Analgesia was assessed after a 60-second immersion of the hand and foot in ice water before intrathecal injection, 60 to 65 minutes after intrathecal injection, and 60 to 65 minutes after each epidural infusion. Cerebrospinal fluid was sampled just before and after drug administration to determine changes in the concentrations of acetylcholine, norepinephrine, and cyclic guanosine monophosphate (cGMP). Side effects were recorded.

Results.—Analgesia with intrathecal neostigmine was dependent on subject position; it was effective in the lateral position, but not in the sitting position. Analgesia with each drug alone and with the combination was dose-dependent in the foot and was minimal, although statistically significant, in the hand. The 2 agents had an additive analgesic interaction. Epidural clonidine alone caused a dose-related increase in CSF acetylcholine, which was increased further with intrathecal neostigmine only when the subject was in the lateral position. There were no drug-related effects on CSF cGMP concentrations. Epidural clonidine alone was associated with hypotension and reduced plasma norepinephrine, whereas intrathecal neostigmine alone was associated with increased plasma norepinephrine with the subject in the lateral, but not seated, position, and had no effect on blood pressure. The combination did not influence blood pressure if administered in the lateral position, but reduced blood pressure if administered in the sitting position. Neostigmine antagonized the clonidine effect on plasma norepinephrine when administered in the lateral, but not the sitting, position. When neostigmine was administered in the lateral position, it caused nausea, weakness, and mild sedation. Clonidine caused intense sedation. None of the adverse effects were magnified by combined treatment with both agents.

Conclusions.—Intrathecal neostigmine and epidural clonidine produce analgesia individually and additively when combined. Lumbar administration of both drugs produces greater analgesia in the foot than in the hand. Neostigmine analgesia is greater when the patient is in the lumbar position than in the sitting position. Neostigmine partially counteracts the adverse effects of clonidine on blood pressure and plasma norepinephrine. There are no other alterations or enhancements in the side effect profile of either drug when administered in combination. Therefore, this combination has clinical promise, deserving further study.

▶ The additive analgesic effect of these 2 intrathecal agents may allow enough dose reduction of each drug to significantly reduce side effects. The introduction of new, non-neurotoxic classes of neuraxial analgesics should expand our ability to provide improved analgesia with fewer side effects for patients with acute and chronic pain who have difficult management problems.

S.E. Abram, M.D.

Nitric Oxide Pharmacology

Nitric Oxide: Physiology and Pharmacology

Schroeder RA, Kuo PC (Univ of California, San Francisco; Stanford Univ, Calif)

Anesth Analg 81:1052–1059, 1995 4–33

Objective.—Nitric oxide (NO) is now recognized as a chemical messenger for various biological systems, with homeostatic activity in the maintenance of cardiovascular tone, platelet regulation, and CNS signaling. It is also involved in gastrointestinal smooth muscle relaxation and immune regulation and may be an effector molecule for the volatile anesthetics. The biochemistry of NO activity was reviewed, including the current clinical applications.

Synthesis, Transport, and Regulators.—Nitric oxide is produced by oxidation of the guanidino nitrogen of L-arginine in the presence of oxygen, a reaction catalyzed by NO synthase (NOS). Molecular NO is a free radical that can be oxidized, reduced, or complexed with other molecules, dependent on the microenvironment. Nitric oxide synthesis occurs through cell-specific isoforms of NOS, which is broadly classified into constitutive and inducible subtypes. It is unknown how NO is transported to its molecular targets. There are many different pharmacologic regulators of NO synthesis, such as nitroglycerin and sodium nitroprusside as promoters, and flavoprotein and calmodulin as inhibitors.

Pulmonary System.—In the pulmonary system, NO appears to play a role in the neural regulation of bronchial and pulmonary vascular smooth muscle. When NO synthesis is inhibited, the vasoconstrictor response is inhibited. Nitric oxide deficit appears to cause chronic pulmonary hypertension, which suggests that inhaled NO could be used clinically as a selective pulmonary vasodilator. Its main clinical indication is persistent pulmonary hypertension in the newborn. Its applications in adults are less clear—it is unknown whether NO can improve outcomes for patients with adult respiratory distress syndrome. The toxicity and administration of inhaled NO continue to pose difficult challenges.

Cardiovascular System.—In the cardiovascular system, NO from platelets and other sources may modulate platelet adhesion and aggregation, among other functions. Deranged NO production has been identified in various disease states, and some protective effects of NO have been evaluated as well. The role of NO in the fibrinolytic and thrombolytic consequences of endothelial injury may point the way to a new method of pharmacologic "anticoagulation" in patients with arterial injury. The role of NO in the regulation of platelet activity is of interest. There is also evidence that it may be a myocardial depressant factor in sepsis and may be involved in the development of hypotension in septic shock. Recent reports have described NO inhibition in patients with pressor-resistant shock or multisystem organ failure. Studies of the role of NO in vascular homeostasis suggest that its protective or toxic effects may be concentration dependent.

Anesthetic Interactions.—Many reports have described interactions between NO and anesthetics. Halogenated drugs disrupt the arginine-NO-cyclic guanosine monophosphate pathway and thus suppress vasodilation, although the mechanism of this effect is uncertain. Halogenated drugs may reduce the significant pressor responses to NOS inhibition. There is also evidence that NO may be involved in the cerebral hyperemia that occurs with halogenated anesthetics. Other studies have suggested that NO may affect anesthetic effects on awareness; studies of its role in pain perception have yielded contradictory results.

Discussion.—The role of NO as a chemical messenger in various physiologic systems is not completely understood. Inhaled NO may be a useful treatment for pulmonary disorders that involve derangements of vascular function or oxygenation, and manipulation of the NO pathway could be useful in selected cardiovascular disorders and cancer immunotherapy. Much more experimental and clinical research into the potential applications of NO must be performed before it can be used as a systemic treatment for specific conditions.

▶ When I first heard that a major American pharmaceutical company would devote a considerable amount of its time and energies to the development and commercialization of NO, I couldn't for the life of me see a large enough "market" to justify the effort. I still don't, although the possible uses for NO will undoubtedly grow. At the moment, there is no question that NO improves neonatal survival in severe instances of respiratory distress syndrome as it allows continued life while lungs continue to mature (I think). In adult respiratory distress syndrome, whether NO therapy allows more than simply improvement of numbers (i.e., actually allows increased survival) is much more debatable. I am not sure we will ever come to the answer, because as NO becomes more commonly used, the argument will inevitably arise as to whether given patients would have survived without, vs. with, NO. This article will bring our readers up to date on numerous aspects of this fascinating poison.

J.H. Tinker, M.D.

Nitrous Oxide Kinetics in Labor

Gas Kinetics During Nitrous Oxide Analgesia for Labour
Einarsson S, Stenqvist O, Bengtsson A, et al (Sahlgrenska Univ Hosp, Göteborg, Sweden)
Anaesthesia 51:449–452, 1996 4–34

Background.—Hyperventilation with nitrous oxide during labor may result in hypoxemia. Whether use of nitrous oxide for analgesia during labor in a clinical setting is associated with risk of diffusion hypoxia was examined.

Methods.—Participants included 24 women undergoing vaginal delivery who were randomly assigned to receive either 50% or 70% nitrous oxide in oxygen. The nitrous oxide/oxygen mixture was available to patients at all times; the women were not trained to control their respiratory rates or tidal volumes and were given no restrictions in use of the analgesic.

Results.—Median nitrous oxide inhalation time per contraction measured 58 seconds for those breathing 50% nitrous oxide and 33 seconds for those breathing 70% nitrous oxide. Minute ventilation and end-tidal carbon dioxide remained unchanged. End-tidal oxygen concentration reached a low after 120 seconds and dipped to 15.4% in both groups. No difference between groups was noted in terms of oxygen saturation. Desaturation occurred in 2 women. The desaturation episodes could not be attributed to diffusion hypoxia, however, because both women had low end-tidal nitrous oxide concentrations as well as low end-tidal oxygen concentrations.

Conclusions.—Diffusion hypoxia appeared to be of minor importance in desaturation among women using nitrous oxide for labor analgesia. No indications were found that 70% nitrous oxide imparts a greater risk of desaturation than does 50% nitrous oxide. The degree of desaturation reached during apnea is affected by oxygen consumption and oxygen reserve in the functional residual capacity; parturient women are more likely than are nonpregnant women to have hypoxemia develop when hypoventilating.

► The reader of this study should not be distracted from the following fact: maternal and fetal hypoxemia may occur after hyperventilation with nitrous oxide during labor. In this study, 2 of the 24 women had hypoxemia (i.e., an arterial oxygen saturation of 80% and 84%, respectively). Further, nitrous oxide does not consistently provide satisfactory analgesia during labor.

D.H. Chestnut, M.D.

Neuromuscular Blocking Drugs

A Two-center Comparison of the Cardiovascular Effects of Cisatracurium (Nimbex) and Vecuronium in Patients With Coronary Artery Disease

Konstadt SN, Reich DL, Stanley TE III, et al (Mt Sinai Med Ctr, New York; Duke Heart Ctr, Durham, NC; Burroughs Wellcome Co, Research Triangle Park, NC)

Anesth Analg 81:1010–1014, 1995 4–35

Background.—Cisatracurium, a stereoisomer of atracurium and intermediate-acting benzylisoquinolinium neuromuscular blocker, produces no clinically significant cardiovascular effects or histamine release when given to healthy patients in doses up to 8 × ED_{95}. The effects of a 2 × ED_{95} dose of cisatracurium injected over 30 or 60 seconds on hemodynamics in patients undergoing coronary artery bypass graft surgery (CABG) during oxygen-fentanyl-midazolam anesthesia were examined in a pilot study. In addition, the effects of a 2 × ED_{95} dose of cisatracurium or vecuronium in a rapid 5- to 10-second bolus were investigated in a randomized, controlled trial.

Methods.—Ten patients participated in the pilot study and 60 participated in the controlled trial. All were undergoing elective myocardial revascularization. Anesthesia consisted of 100% oxygen, fentanyl, and midazolam. Succinylcholine was administered to facilitate tracheal intubation. Baseline hemodynamic measures were obtained at least 5 minutes after tracheal intubation and again 2, 5, and 10 minutes after cisatracurium or vecuronium injection. In the pilot study, the patients received 0.10 mg/kg of cisatracurium or 0.10 mg/kg of vecuronium, with cisatracurium delivered over 60 seconds (group A) or 30 seconds (group B). In the controlled study, cisatracurium was delivered over 5 to 10 seconds (group C), and vecuronium was delivered over 5 to 10 seconds (group D).

Findings.—No episodes of cutaneous flushing occurred. Fifteen patients were excluded from the final analysis for various reasons. Multiple significant hemodynamic changes occurred between pre-injection and post-injection. However, findings in groups C and D were comparable. None of the patients given cisatracurium had a mean arterial pressure decrease of 20% or more.

Conclusions.—The hemodynamic changes in patients given cisatracurium were minor, comparable to those observed in patients receiving vecuronium. A rapid bolus dose of cisatracurium produces minimal hemodynamic side effects in patients with coronary artery disease.

▶ Cisatracurium (Nimbex) is one of the stereoisomers of atracurium, and constitutes about 15% of the mixture. It is said to be devoid of histamine-releasing effects when given in large doses (i.e., 2 × ED_{95}), and thus preferable to atracurium. It will be interesting to see what happens to this new muscle relaxant in a health care cost-conscious market in which anesthesia pharmacy budgets are being scrutinized closely.

M. Wood, M.D.

Pharmacokinetics of Cisatracurium in Patients Receiving Nitrous Oxide/Opioid/Barbiturate Anesthesia

Lien CA, Schmith VD, Belmont MR, et al (New York Hosp-Cornell Med Ctr; Glaxo Wellcome Inc. Research Triangle Park, NC)

Anesthesiology 84:300–308, 1996 4–36

Introduction.—The non-depolarizing muscle relaxant cisatracurium is 1 of the 10 stereoisomers of atracurium. It has an intermediate duration of action and is more potent than atracurium, although less likely to lead to histamine release. Because it is an isomer of atracurium, cisatracurium is presumed to be subject to Hofmann elimination. The pharmacokinetics of cisatracurium and its metabolites were studied, including dose proportionality after a cisatracurium dose of 2 or 4 times the ED_{95}.

Methods.—The study sample comprised 20 patients with American Society of Anesthesiologists physical status 1 or 2 who were undergoing elective surgery with nitrous oxide/opioid/barbiturate anesthesia. Each patient was given a rapid IV bolus dose of 0.1 or 0.2 mg/kg^{-1} of cisatracurium, which corresponded to 2 or 4 times the ED_{95} of 0.05 mg/kg^{-1}. The patients' recovery from cisatracurium-induced neuromuscular block then was monitored to a train-of-4 ratio of 0.70 or greater. Plasma samples were obtained and prepared for analysis of cisatracurium and its metabolites.

Results.—The mean cisatracurium clearance was 5.28 mL/min^{-1}/kg^{-1} with the 0.1-mg/kg^{-1} dose and 4.66 mL/min^{-1}/kg^{-1} with the 0.2-mg/kg^{-1} dose; the difference was not significant. Terminal elimination half-lives also were similar, being 22.4 and 25.5 minutes, respectively (Table 2). For the metabolite laudanosine, the average maximum concentration value was 38 ng/mL^{-1} for patients receiving the 0.1-mg/kg^{-1} dose vs. 103 ng/mL^{-1} for patients receiving the 0.2-mg/kg^{-1} dose. For monoquaternary alcohol, the values were 101 vs. 51 ng/mL^{-1}, respectively. None of the plasma samples showed detectable monoquaternary acid.

Conclusions.—In patients receiving the atracurium isomer cisatracurium, laudanosine is formed by the process of Hofmann elimination. After

TABLE 2.—Pharmacokinetics of Cisatracurium

	Noncompartmental (elimination from central compartment only)		Compartmental (elimination from both compartments)	
	2× ED_{95} (0.1 mg·kg^{-1})	4× ED_{95} (0.2 mg·kg^{-1})	2× ED_{95} (0.1 mg·kg^{-1})	4× ED_{95} (0.2 mg·kg^{-1})
Clearance (ml±min^{-1}·kg^{-1})	5.28 ± 1.23	4.66 ± 0.67	5.09 ± 0.84	4.58 ± 0.64
$t_{1/2}\beta$ (min)	22.4 ± 2.7	25.5 ± 4.1	24.8 ± 2.1	25.0 ± 3.8
V_{ss} (ml·kg^{-1})	144 ± 34	121 ± 22	175 ± 48	155 ± 36

Note: Values are mean ± SD.
*V_{ss} determined using noncompartment methods is underestimated.
Abbreviations: V_{ss}, volume of distribution at steady state; $t_{1/2}\beta$, elimination half-life.
(Courtesy of Lien CA, Schmith VD, Belmont MR, et al: Pharmacokinetics of cisatracurium in patients receiving nitrous oxide/opioid/barbiturate anesthesia. *Anesthesiology* 84:300–308, 1996.)

doses equivalent to 2 or 4 times the ED_{95}, the pharmacokinetics of cisatracurium are dose-independent. The pharmacodynamics of cisatracurium are consistent with the dose-proportional pharmacokinetic findings.

▶ Atracurium has become an extremely popular muscle relaxant, but it has 2 disadvantages: (1) it produces histamine release at 2 to 3 times the ED_{95}, so the dose must be limited for use during rapid tracheal intubation; and (2) its metabolite, laudanosine, may accumulate during prolonged infusion of atracurium in the ICU. Cisatracurium is a single isomer of atracurium and is said to be about 3 times more potent than atracurium and less likely to release histamine. Thus, the pharmacokinetics of cisatracurium and its metabolites are of direct clinical relevance. This investigation suggests that like atracurium, cisatracurium undergoes Hofmann elimination, but in contrast, it does not undergo ester hydrolysis to any appreciable extent. In addition, plasma levels of laudanosine are lower than those seen after atracurium administration.

M. Wood, M.D.

Mivacurium When Preceded by Pancuronium Becomes a Long-acting Muscle Relaxant

Erkola O, Rautoma P, Meretoja OA (Helsinki City Hosp; Univ of Helsinki)

Anesthesiology 84:562–565, 1996 4–37

Objective.—When a long-acting muscle relaxant is used for deep neuromuscular block, it may seem appropriate to follow it with a short-acting muscle relaxant to facilitate recovery. The effects of giving mivacurium during recovery from pancuronium neuromuscular block were studied.

Methods.—The study included 41 adult patients undergoing general anesthesia with propofol, alfentanil, nitrous oxide, and oxygen. All underwent electromyographic (EMG) monitoring of neuromuscular function. Once the EMG calibration response stabilized, the patients received cumulative doses of pancuronium to produce 95% neuromuscular block. Control patients received mivacurium, instead of pancuronium, in an ED_{95} dose of 100 µg/kg. After the EMG calibration response returned to 25% of baseline, the patients received 1 IV bolus dose of mivacurium, 10 or 70 µg/kg. They were monitored thereafter for spontaneous recovery of neuromuscular function.

Results.—The patients were similar in their baseline characteristics. The mean time to 25% EMG recovery was 38 minutes after pancuronium. For patients in the pancuronium group, the mean time to 25% recovery was 28 minutes after 10 µg/kg of mivacurium and 54 minutes after 70 µg/kg of mivacurium. For those in the mivacurium group, these times were 3 and 10 minutes, respectively (Fig 1 and Table 2). The mean time to 95% recovery in the pancuronium group was 77 minutes after 10 µg/kg of mivacurium and 97 minutes after 70 µg/kg of mivacurium. In the mivacurium group, these times were 11 and 20 minutes, respectively. The mean recovery index

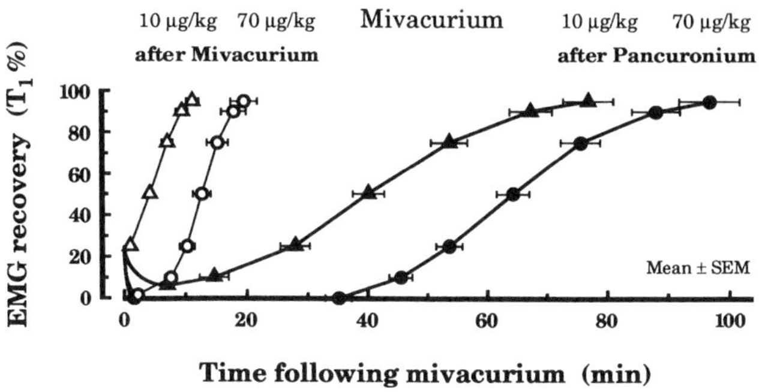

FIGURE 1.—Spontaneous EMG recovery of neuromuscular block after 10 (*triangles*) or 70 (*circles*) μg/kg of mivacurium given at T_1 25% during recovery from pancuronium (*closed symbols*) or mivacurium (*open symbols*) block. Groups differed ($P < 0.05$) from each other at every EMG recovery level besides mivacurium groups at 90% and 95% T_1 recovery levels. (Courtesy of Erkola O, Rautoma P, Meretoja OA: Mivacurium when preceded by pancuronium becomes a long-acting muscle relaxant. *Anesthesiology* 84:562–565, 1996.)

in the pancuronium group was 26 minutes after 10 μg/kg of mivacurium and 22 minutes after 70 μg/kg of mivacurium, compared with 7 and 5 minutes, respectively, in the mivacurium group. Finally, the mean time to reach a train-of-4 ratio of 0.7 in the pancuronium group was 94 minutes after 10 μg/kg of mivacurium and 111 minutes after 70 μg/kg of mivacurium, compared with 12 and 22 minutes, respectively, in the mivacurium group.

Conclusions.—Giving even a small dose of mivacurium during recovery from pancuronium-induced neuromuscular block prolongs recovery time. Thus, mivacurium given after pancuronium does not behave as a short-

TABLE 2.—Spontaneous Recovery Times After 10 or 70 μg/kg of Mivacurium at T_1 25% During Recovery From Pancuronium or Mivacurium Block

T_1 %	PcMIV 10	MivMiv 10	PcMiv 70	MivMiv 70	P*
T_1 10%	15 ± 8	—	46 ± 6	8 ± 3	< 0.0001
T_1 25%	28 ± 8	—	54 ± 7	10 ± 4	< 0.0001
T_1 50%	40 ± 9	4 ± 2	64 ± 9	13 ± 5	< 0.0001
T_1 75%	54 ± 10	7 ± 3	76 ± 10	15 ± 5	< 0.0001
T_1 90%	67 ± 12	9 ± 3	88 ± 13	18 ± 7	< 0.001
T_1 95%	77 ± 14	11 ± 3	97 ± 16	20 ± 7	< 0.0001
T_1 25–75%	26 ± 4	—	22 ± 6	5 ± 2	< 0.0001
TR 0.7	94 ± 16	12 ± 4	111 ± 14	22 ± 8	< 0.0001

Note: Values are given in minutes (mean ± SD). Data are missing in the MivMiv 10 group because 10 μg/kg of mivacurium did not increase twitch depression enough.

*Between-groups comparison (ANOVA).

Abbreviations: PcMiv 10 or 70, pancuronium followed by mivacurium 10 or 70 μg/kg; *MivMiv 10 or 70*, mivacurium followed by mivacurium 10 or 70 μg/kg; *TR 0.7*, time from the administration of mivacurium until train-of-4 ratio 0.7.

(Courtesy of Erkola O, Rautoma P, Meretoja OA: Mivacurium when preceded by pancuronium becomes a long-acting muscle relaxant. *Anesthesiology* 84:562–565, 1996.)

acting neuromuscular blocker. The pharmacodynamic or pharmacokinetic nature of this interaction remains to be determined.

▶ Many regimens combining expensive and inexpensive muscle relaxants have been advocated to reduce costs. Thus, to ensure rapid recovery of neuromuscular block, a short-acting muscle relaxant might be administered after an inexpensive, long-acting one. Do not do it! In the absence of careful studies, combinations of muscle relaxants should not be used.

M. Wood, M.D.

Comparison of Duration of Neuromuscular Blocking Effect of Atracurium and Vecuronium in Young and Elderly Patients

Slavov V, Khalil M, Merle JC, et al (Univ of Paris)

Br J Anaesth 74:709–711, 1995 4–38

Background.—Atracurium and vecuronium, non-depolarizing neuromuscular blocking agents of intermediate duration of action, are thought to be noncumulative. However, vecuronium may have a prolonged, cumulative effect in elderly patients. The clinical durations of action of atracurium and vecuronium were investigated in elderly and younger adults.

Methods.—Eighty patients undergoing routine abdominal surgery were enrolled in the controlled, randomized study. Forty were older than 65 years, and 40 were aged 18 to 50 years. Normal plasma creatinine levels were documented in all patients. After anesthesia was induced, patients were randomly assigned to receive either atracurium, 0.5 mg/kg^{-1}, or vecuronium, 0.1 mg/kg^{-1}, to facilitate tracheal intubation. The evoked response of the adductor pollicis muscle to supramaximal single twitch ulnar nerve stimulation was assessed every 10 seconds with a strain gauge. When adductor pollicis responses recovered to 25% of the control twitch height, repeated doses of atracurium at 0.1 mg/kg^{-1}, or vecuronium, 0.02 mg/kg^{-1}, were administered.

Findings.—The initial atracurium dose had a similar duration of action in the elderly and younger adults. The duration of action did not vary after repeated doses. However, the initial vecuronium dose significantly prolonged clinical block in the elderly patients compared with the younger ones. Repeated doses' duration of action also was longer in the elderly patients.

Conclusions.—The administration of vecuronium to elderly patients is associated with a risk of prolonged duration of action. Neuromuscular function monitoring is recommended in such patients. By contrast, atracurium had the same effect in elderly and younger adults, even after prolonged, repeated administration. Thus, this is the preferred agent for prolonged surgery.

▶ Atracurium is the drug of choice in patients with renal insufficiency; these investigators suggest that atracurium should be preferred in another subgroup, elderly patients. I firmly believe that the intermediate-acting muscle relaxants, atracurium and vecuronium, exhibit less variability and less risk of prolonged effect, and therefore are much more "forgiving" than the long-acting muscle relaxants such as pancuronium in elderly patients. I also would argue that just because studies have failed to show a statistically significant difference in outcome for different neuromuscular blocking agents (because of inadequate sample size) does not mean that there is not a difference. Absence of evidence is not evidence of absence.[1]

M. Wood, M.D.

Reference

1. Altman DG, Bland JM: Absence of evidence is not evidence of absence. *BMJ* 311:485, 1995.

Atracurium Versus Vecuronium in Asthmatic Patients: A Blinded, Randomized Comparison of Adverse Events

Caldwell JE, Lau M, Fisher DM (Univ of California, San Francisco)

Anesthesiology 83:986–991, 1995 4–39

Objective.—Because initial trials of atracurium produced adverse effects that were linked to histamine release, patients with asthma were excluded from further clinical trials. Since then, studies have suggested that atracurium has a lower incidence of adverse effects than vecuronium or other muscle relaxants. In addition, these nonrandomized studies did not look specifically at adverse effects occurring in patients with known asthma. Atracurium and vecuronium were compared for adverse effects in patients with asthma.

Methods.—The prospective, blinded, randomized study included 61 patients with known asthma who were undergoing anesthesia with midazolam, fentanyl, nitrous oxide, and isoflurane. All patients had a history of bronchospasm for which they were receiving long-term bronchodilator therapy. Tracheal intubation was performed without paralysis. Once the patients were under stable anesthesia and mechanical ventilation, they received either 0.5 mg/kg of atracurium or 0.1 mg/kg of vecuronium given over 5 to 10 seconds. For 6 minutes thereafter, any cardiovascular, pulmonary, or cutaneous evidence of adverse reactions was recorded. Cardiovascular effects were defined as a decrease in blood pressure or a change in heart rate. Noncardiovascular adverse effects included an increase in peak airway pressure of greater than 5 cm H_2O, a tidal volume decrease of greater than 10%, rashes, and wheezing.

Results.—Small decreases in arterial pressure and heart rate occurred after atracurium administration, whereas vecuronium administration was followed by small declines in systolic pressure and heart rate. About 60% of patients in both groups had cardiovascular effects of greater than 10% (Table 3). Thirty-seven percent of patients had cardiovascular effects of greater than 20% with atracurium, compared to 13% of patients with vecuronium. Noncardiovascular adverse events occurred in 17% of the

TABLE 3.—Percentage of Patients Who Experienced Adverse Effects After 0.5 mg/kg of Atracurium or 0.1 mg/kg of Vecuronium

	Atracurium (n = 30)	Vecuronium (n = 30)
Heart rate changes		
>10%	17	33
>20%	3	3
>40%	0	0
Blood pressure (systolic, diastolic, or mean) decreases		
>10%	57	37
>20%*	37	10
>40%	10	3
Cardiovascular changes (heart rate or blood pressure)		
>10%	60	57
>20%*	37	13
>40%	10	3
Noncardiovascular changes		
Peak airway pressure increase >5 cm H_2O	0	3
Tidal volume decrease >10%	0	3
Rashes (erythema only)	10	0
Wheezing (expiratory only)	10	7
Decrease in Sp_{O2} >5%	0	0
Any of these noncardiovascular changes	17	7

*$P < 0.05$ by chi-square with the Yates continuity correction or Fisher's exact test.

(Courtesy of Caldwell JE, Lau M, Fisher DM: Atracurium versus vecuronium in asthmatic patients: A blinded, randomized comparison of adverse events. *Anesthesiology* 83:986–991, 1995.)

patients who received atracurium and 7% of those who received vecuronium—the difference was not significant. With 1 exception (a patient in the vecuronium group), none of the patients had more than a 10% increase in tidal volume. There were no instances of wheezing, marked decreases in arterial oxygen saturation, or marked increases in end-tidal carbon dioxide tension.

Conclusions.—Patients with asthma are more likely to experience adverse cardiovascular effects with atracurium than with vecuronium. There is no difference between the 2 muscle relaxants in the incidence of mild cardiovascular effects, or in the incidence of noncardiovascular effects. With midazolam, fentanyl, nitrous oxide; and isoflurane anesthesia, few adverse effects occur with either atracurium or vecuronium in patients with asthma.

▶ Atracurium is known to produce histamine release in some patients, and many anesthesiologists preferentially choose an alternative muscle relaxant when anesthetizing patients with asthma. This outcome study in patients with known asthma demonstrated that adverse cardiovascular events were more common with atracurium than with vecuronium. However, the incidence of noncardiovascular adverse events did not differ between the 2 groups, and no patient experienced an important increase in airway pressure or decrease in arterial oxygen saturation. It is of note that of the severe adverse reactions that occurred, a severe histaminoid reaction occurred with vecuronium!

M. Wood, M.D.

Thiopental: High Dose in Open Hearts

High-Dose Thiopentone for Open-Chamber Cardiac Surgery: A Retrospective Review

Pascoe EA, Hudson RJ, Anderson BA, et al (Univ of Manitoba, Canada)

Can J Anaesth 43:575–579, 1996 4–40

Introduction.—High-dose thiopentone anesthesia has been reported to decrease the incidence of neurologic complications during open-chamber cardiac procedures, but it has important side effects. To determine the safety of high-dose thiopentone, the records of investigators reviewed their experience for the 34-month period all patients who underwent elective, open-chamber surgery at one institution between March 1987 and December 1989 were reviewed.

Methods.—Of the 236 patients who were operated on during the review period, 9 were excluded from analysis because they had emergency procedures, were transferred from an ICU, or underwent deep hypothermic arrest. Eighty of the remaining patients received high-dose (>15 mg/kg^{-1}) thiopentone (group T) and 147 were given high-dose opioid anesthesia (group O). The choice of anesthesia was at the discretion of the attending anesthetist. The thiopentone infusion was titrated to achieve electroencephalographic burst-suppression, with isoelectric periods lasting about 60 seconds.

Results.—The mean thiopentone dose in group T was 38.1 mg/kg^{-1}. Seventeen group O patients received thiopentone (mean dose 5.7 mg/kg^{-1}), primarily at induction. The 2 anesthesia groups were similar in demographics, type of operation, and management of cardiopulmonary bypass. The overall mortality rate was 6.6%; group T had a lower mortality rate (1.2%) than group O (9.5%). There were 4 strokes in group O and none in group T, a difference that was not significant. The stroke rate was computed after excluding from analysis 5 intraoperative deaths, all in group O. The mean time to extubation was prolonged in group T (39 hours) vs. group O (27 hours), as was the duration of ICU stay (66 hours vs. 51 hours, respectively). Thiopentone anesthesia did not increase the need for inotropic or mechanical support after bypass.

Discussion.—High-dose thiopentone did not increase mortality or the frequency with which inotropic agents or intra-aortic balloon counterpulsation were used after cardiopulmonary bypass. The incidence of stroke, however, was not significantly reduced, and extubation was delayed in these patients undergoing open-chamber procedures. The risk-benefit ratio of high-dose thiopentone anesthesia has yet to be defined.

► In this study, the authors attempted to repeat the controversial "Nussmeier" study from the Texas Heart Institute in which extraordinarily high doses of thiopentone (about 39.5 mg/kg) were used in an attempt to protect patients from neurologic injury after cardiopulmonary bypass. The Nussmeier study reported a statistically significant decrease in adverse neurologic outcomes, both temporary and probably permanent. The present study did not find such an effect. On the other hand, in the Nussmeier study, the patients were nearly normothermic and no arterial inflow line filtration devices were in use during bypass. In this study, the authors used moderate hypothermia and arterial inflow line filtration. There were no strokes in the thiopentone group and 4 in the group not given thiopentone. Although this was not statistically significant, it is of interest, because there were also zero neurologic complications in the Nussmeier thiopentone group. The authors clearly observed the same thing that Nussmeier and colleagues did, namely that prolonged extubation time is a concern in today's "fast-track" environment. I have never believed that this high-dose pentothal technique would catch on, and it has not. On the other hand, this is the second paper in which there were zero neurologic complications in the treatment group, even though the statistical significance is not quite there. In other words, I wonder if thiopentone really does work, despite all its problems!

J.H. Tinker, M.D.

Thiopental: Taste

The Taste of Intravenous Thiopentone

Nor NBM, Fox MA, Metcalfe IR, et al (Royal Adelaide Hosp, South Australia)

Anaesth Intensive Care 24:483–485, 1996 4–41

Objective.—Although a significant number of patients report an onion or garlic taste shortly before induction of anesthesia with thiopental, not all patients have this experience. The results of a survey to ascertain the incidence and pattern of the taste of thiopental and the factors that might change it are presented.

Methods.—Patients (N = 116, (50 females) aged 6 to 85 being anesthetized with 2.5% thiopental at an initial dose of 1 mg/kg were asked shortly before they lost consciousness whether they had a taste in their mouths and, if so, whether the taste was onion or garlic. The answers were analyzed statistically.

Results.—Ten patients said that they tasted onions and 39 said that they tasted garlic for a positive response rate of 43%. Thirty-one of 63 males (49%) and 18 of 50 females (36%) noticed a taste. When the patients were divided into 3 groups by age, 39 (51%) patients were younger than 17, 53 (45%) patients were 17–59, and 21 (24%) patients were 60 or older. The reduction in proportion of tasters as age increases is significant. Significantly fewer premedicated than nonpremedicated patients noticed a taste. However, 60% of the patients 60 years or older were premedicated.

Conclusion.—The taste sensation was probably the result of stimulation in the tongue. The lower incidence of reported taste in patients receiving premedication is probably related to the fact that more older people, whose sense of taste is impaired by age, received premedication. The thiopental taste may also be genetic.

▶ I selected this article to show that it really is true! Patients do experience an onion or garlic taste following thiopental administration—42% noticed this taste.

M. Wood, M.D.

Methohexital vs. Thiopental in Infants

Faster Recovery After Anesthesia in Infants After Intravenous Induction With Methohexital Instead of Thiopental
Beskow A, Werner O, Westrin P (Univ Hosp, Lund, Sweden)
Anesthesiology 83:976–979, 1995 4–42

Background.—With the availability of EMLA topical anesthetic cream, IV anesthesia induction has become a viable option in children. One disadvantage is the potential for residual effects of the IV anesthetic during the recovery phase. Thiopental may cause such problems, especially in young infants. Recovery after anesthesia was compared for infants undergoing induction with IV methohexital vs. thiopental.

Methods.—Forty-one infants, aged 1 to 12 months, were studied during scheduled hernia repair or circumcision. The infants were randomly assigned to receive equipotent doses of methohexital or thiopental, 3 and 7.3 mg/kg, respectively. The infants then were intubated and given maintenance anesthesia with isoflurane in nitrous oxide/oxygen, as well as 0.75 mL/kg of caudal bupivacaine. Maintenance isoflurane was stopped as soon as skin closure began, and nitrous oxide was stopped after the last suture was placed. In the recovery room, postanesthetic recovery scores were evaluated in blinded fashion at intervals ranging from 5 to 120 minutes.

Results.—The 2 groups were comparable in age, weight, duration of surgery, and time from termination of nitrous oxide to extubation. Patients in the methohexital group spontaneously opened their eyes a mean of 23 minutes after induction, compared with 55 minutes in the thiopental group. From arrival in the recovery room to 45 minutes afterward, postanesthetic recovery scores were significantly more rapid in the infants who received methohexital (Fig 1). Nearly all the infants in both groups were awake by 120 minutes. There were no differences in pain between groups.

Conclusions.—For infants undergoing brief surgical procedures, IV induction anesthesia with methohexital permits quicker recovery than thiopental. The slower recovery from thiopental suggests that small plasma concentrations of this drug can produce substantial sedation in infants. A dose equivalent to 115% of the ED_{50} was used when giving IV induction anesthesia in children; the resulting anesthesia was deep enough to permit a brief period of mask ventilation.

▶ The use of EMLA has revolutionized the induction of anesthesia in children, and IV anesthesia has become much more common over the last 5 years.[1] As expected from the well-recognized pharmacokinetic parameters of thiopental and methohexital (thiopental clearance 3.4 to 3.6 mL/kg/min, and methohexital clearance 10.9 to 12.1 mL/kg/min), there is a faster recovery after methohexital than after thiopental.

M. Wood, M.D.

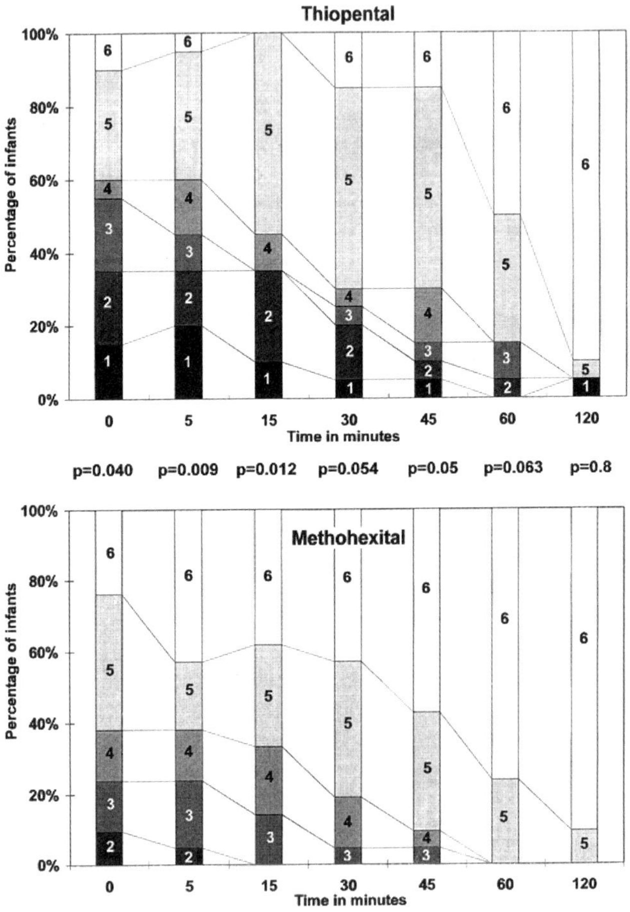

FIGURE 1.—Percentage of infants with each recovery score at different times after arrival in the recovery room. Recovery scores 1 to 6 are indicated. There were 21 infants in the methohexital group. The groups were compared with the Mann-Whitney U test. Obtained *P* values are indicated. (Courtesy of Beskow A, Werner O, Westrin P: Faster recovery after anesthesia in infants after intravenous induction with methohexital instead of thiopental. *Anesthesiology* 83:976–979, 1995.)

Reference

1. Wood U: Intravenous anesthetic agents, in Wood M, Wood AJJ (eds): *Drugs and Anesthesia,* Pharmacology for Anesthesiologists, ed 2. Baltimore, Williams & Wilkins, 1990.

Ketorolac: Postoperative Pain and Bleeding in Children

Effect of Ketorolac on Bleeding Time and Postoperative Pain in Children: A Double-Blind, Placebo-Controlled Comparison With Meperidine
Bean-Lijewski JD, Hunt RD (Scott & White Clinic and Mem Hosp, Temple, Tex; Texas A&M Univ, Temple)
J Clin Anesth 8:25–30, 1996 4–43

Background.—Nonsteroidal anti-inflammatory drugs (NSAIDs) are an attractive alternative to opioids for children undergoing outpatient surgery, because NSAIDs are not correlated with cardiorespiratory or CNS depression and may produce less postoperative vomiting. However, concerns have been raised about possible postoperative bleeding from NSAID-induced platelet dysfunction and the limits of analgesic efficacy. Whether ketorolac, 0.75 mg/kg provides analgesia comparable to that of meperidine, 1 mg/kg, was determined in children undergoing operations resulting in mild-to-moderate pain.

Methods.—Ninety healthy children with ASA status I and II were enrolled in the randomized, prospective, placebo-controlled, double-blinded trial. The children were scheduled for elective general, orthopedic, or genitourinary procedures. Ketorolac, 0.75 mg/kg, meperidine, 1 mg/kg, or normal saline was given IM at the beginning of surgery. Bleeding times were measured before and 180 minutes after these agents were delivered.

Findings.—Children given placebo required earlier rescue and twice the rescue dose compared with children given ketorolac or meperidine. Time to first rescue, cumulative proportion needing rescue, and number of rescue doses needed were comparable in the ketorolac and meperidine groups. A single IM ketorolac dose prolonged bleeding time by a mean of 53 seconds.

Conclusions.—The analgesia provided by ketorolac is comparable to that of meperidine. Ketorolac also significantly decreased opioid requirements. However, ketorolac administration did not reduce postoperative vomiting or length of stay. Because of this and the uncertain risk of bleeding associated with it, ketorolac offers no advantage over meperidine in the management of mild-to-moderate postoperative pain in children.

▶ Although the prolongation in bleeding time after ketorolac was statistically significant, it did not appear to be clinically significant, and no excessive bleeding was encountered. Ketorolac may be the better choice for patients with known problems with opioid side effects and may be particularly helpful as an adjunctive analgesic in opioid-tolerant patients.

S.E. Abram, M.D.

Non-anesthetic Adjuvants

A Pilot Study of the Effects of a Perflubron Emulsion, AF 0104, on Mixed Venous Oxygen Tension in Anesthetized Surgical Patients

Wahr JA, Trouwborst A, Spence RK, et al (Univ of Michigan, Ann Arbor; Univ of Amsterdam, The Netherlands; Univ of Medicine and Dentistry of New Jersey, Camden; et al)

Anesth Analg 82:103–107, 1996 4–44

Background.—AF 0104 is a concentrated, stable perfluorocarbon (PFC) emulsion that contains perflubron 90% wt/vol, 45% by volume. This synthetic oxygen-carrying solution has an intravascular half-life of less than 24 hours and so is most likely to be useful in situations requiring a temporary increase in oxygen transport. One possible application is during intraoperative acute normovolemic hemodilution (ANH). The effects of AF 0104 on hemodynamics and oxygen transport were studied in patients undergoing ANH.

Methods.—The pilot study included 7 surgical patients who were undergoing perioperative ANH and pulmonary artery catheter placement. After ANH was carried out and it was time to transfuse the first unit of blood, an IV dose of perflubron emulsion, 0.9 PFC/kg, was given instead over about 10 minutes. Hemodynamic and oxygen transport variables were assessed before and after ANH, immediately after AF 0104 infusion, and throughout the surgical procedure.

Results.—The administration of PFC emulsion brought no significant changes in hemodynamic variables. Mixed venous oxygen tension ($P\bar{v}O_2$) increased significantly, but there was no change in cardiac output or oxygen consumption. Hemoglobin declined with blood loss during the operation, but $P\bar{v}O_2$ stayed at or near pre-PFC levels. Perflubron blood levels peaked at 0.8 g/dL immediately after AF 0104 administration, declining to 0.3 g/dL at 1 hour.

Conclusions.—The administration of the perflubron emulsion AF 0104 produces significant changes in $P\bar{v}O_2$, with no change in oxygen consumption and cardiac output, in patients undergoing intraoperative ANH. If perflubron emulsion could be used as a supplemental oxygen-carrying solution during ANH, it might reduce the need for allogeneic blood while improving patient outcomes. Such clinical parameters will have to be evaluated in a controlled clinical trial.

▶ An oxygen-carrying solution to replace hemoglobin in situations where a blood transfusion otherwise would be required has been a vague, shadowy dream for a long time. Perfluoro chemicals are inert substances that have a high solubility for oxygen and carbon dioxide; the emulsion has a linear dissociation curve (like plasma), in contrast to the classic dissociation curve for hemoglobin. This study was an efficacy trial involving only 7 patients. The next step is to await the results of controlled, randomized trials.

M. Wood, M.D.

Cytokines in Stored Red Blood Cell Concentrates: Promoters of Systemic Inflammation and Simulators of Acute Transfusion Reactions?
Kristiansson M, Soop M, Saraste L, et al (Huddinge Hosp, Sweden; Umeå Hosp, Sweden)
Acta Anaesthesiol Scand 40:496–501, 1996 4–45

Background.—Cytokines exogenously given to trauma victims and patients with infection may affect their systemic inflammatory and metabolic response. The cytokine content of stored red blood cells (RBCs) were characterized, and the possible influence of storage time was assessed.

Methods.—Sixteen units of RBCs stored at +4°C for 40 days were analyzed for tumor necrosis factor (TNF)-α, interleukin-1 β (IL-1), interleukin-6 (IL-6), and interleukin-8 (IL-8). The RBC samples were obtained every tenth day. Healthy volunteers were studied for comparison.

Findings.—Compared with controls, IL-1 and IL-8 in RBCs were increased. On days 1 and 40, TNF-α was increased. The TNF-α was highest during storage on day 1. Concentrations of IL-1 increased during storage from 5 pg/mL to 174 pg/mL. Levels of IL-6 were 6 pg/mL on day 1 and did not change during storage. Concentrations of IL-8 were greatest on day 40.

Conclusion.—Tumor necrosis factor-α, IL-1, IL-6, and IL-8 are present in stored RBCs. Concentrations vary greatly during storage and among RBC units. In some RBC samples, the content of cytokines reached levels that may contribute to systemic inflammation and the symptomatology of acute transfusion reactions.

► This article may explain the etiology of febrile transfusion reactions and may stimulate future research into the area of cytokine detection and elimination in stored blood.

D.M. Rothenberg, M.D.

Evaluation of Recombinant Human Erythropoietin to Facilitate Autologous Blood Donation Before Surgery in Anaemic Patients With Cancer of the Gastrointestinal Tract
Braga M, Gianotti L, Vignali A, et al (Univ of Milan, Italy)
Br J Surg 82:1637–1640 1995 4–46

Background.—Using autologous blood for transfusion during surgery may reduce the incidence of transfusion-related complications, which are more common with homologous blood transfusions. However, patients with anemia may be unable to predonate blood. This contraindication is common among patients undergoing elective gastrointestinal cancer surgery. These patients may have reduced endogenous erythropoietin production in addition to iron deficiency. Therefore, the effect of treatment with recombinant human erythropoietin (rHuEPO) on the ability to predonate autologous blood was examined in anemic patients scheduled for surgery for the treatment of gastric or colorectal cancer.

Methods.—Twenty-two patients with cancer of the stomach or colorectum were randomly assigned to treatment with either iron saccharate 200 mg/day by intravenous slow infusion for 12 consecutive days or subcutaneous injection of rHuEPO 300 units/kg in addition to the iron saccharate infusion given on days 1, 4, 8, and 12. Hematologic parameters were evaluated at baseline and on days 4, 8, and 12. If the hematocrit exceeded 34%, the patients donated 1 unit of autologous blood, with a maximum of 2 units collected.

Results.—The patients in the 2 groups had similar baseline hematologic parameters. In the iron group, the serum iron level increased significantly after 12 days of treatment, but there were no significant changes in the reticulocyte count or hematocrit. None of the patients in the iron group donated autologous blood. In the rHuEPO group, there were significant increases in both the reticulocyte count and the hematocrit, although the serum iron level did not normalize. All of the patients in the rHuEPO group donated blood, with 8 patients donating 2 units and 3 patients donating 1 unit. During surgery, homologous blood transfusions were required by 4 patients in the iron group and no patients in the rHuEPO group.

Conclusions.—Treatment with rHuEPO enabled autologous blood transfusion in anemic patients with cancer, whereas iron supplementation alone did not facilite preoperative blood donation. The administration of rHuEPO stimulated erythropoiesis in these patients. This treatment approach requires validation in larger clinical trials.

▶ This is an important study in which patients with gastric or colorectal cancer were randomized to receive either iron or iron plus erythropoietin preoperatively and to determine if erythropoietin could stimulate perioperative autologous donation and decrease the incidence of required homologous blood transfusion. The reason to avoid homologous blood transfusion or cancer surgery is to avoid the risk of disease transmission and, more importantly, to decrease the loss of immunity that homologous transfusion causes with the anecdotally reported increased incidence of metastatic cancer. This regimen of 300 units/kg followed 4, 8 and 12 days later with 100 units/kg of erythropoietin allowed these previously anemic patients to be able to donate autologous blood in every case. Treatment with iron alone failed to do so.

M.F. Roizen, M.D.

Heparin-Protamine Complexes Cause Pulmonary Hypertension in Goats

Horiguchi T, Enzan K, Mitsuhata H, et al (Akita Kumiai Hosp, Japan; Akita Univ, Japan; Jichi Med School, Minamikawachi, Japan; et al)

Anesthesiology 83:786–791, 1995 4–47

Background.—Experimental research on sheep and pigs has found that protamine reversal of heparin-induced anticoagulation results in thromboxane release and pulmonary vasoconstriction. The possibility that heparin-protamine (H-P) complexes cause thromboxane release followed by pulmonary hypertension associated with protamine reversal of heparin was investigated in goats.

Methods.—Heparin-protamine and non–H-P complexes were separated from heparinized defibrinated human plasma neutralized with protamine by chromatography. Changes in hemodynamics, airway pressure, and thromboxane B_2 concentration were studied after H-P or non–H-P com-

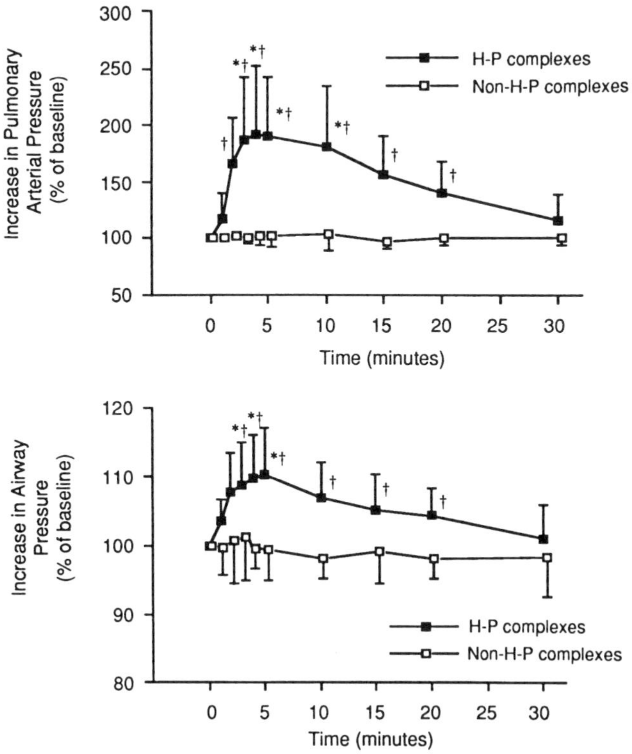

FIGURE 2.—The time course of pulmonary arterial pressure and airway pressure changes after the injection of heparin-protamine (*H-P*) or non–heparin-protamine (*non–H-P*) complexes in goats. Pulmonary arterial pressure and airway pressure increased significantly in the H-P complexes group, but no changes were observed in the non–H-P complexes group. Values represent percentage of baseline (before) and are given as mean ±SD. $^*P < 0.05$ vs. before injection; $†P < 0.05$ vs. non–H-P complexes group. (Courtesy of Horiguchi T, Enzan K, Mitsuhata H, et al: Heparin-protamine complexes cause pulmonary hypertension in goats. *Anesthesiology* 83:786–791, 1995.)

plexes were injected into 7 goats. Five goats pretreated with cyclo-oxygenase inhibitor and 5 pretreated with thromboxane synthetase inhibitor were studied to determine whether these pulmonary responses were blocked.

Findings.—Pulmonary arterial and peak airway pressures were increased by a very small dose of H-P complexes. This was followed by thromboxane B_2 release. No significant changes occurred in goats who received non–H-P complexes. The increases in pulmonary arterial pressure and thromboxane B_2 concentration were totally blocked by indomethacin and partially blocked by OKY-046 (Fig 2).

Conclusions.—Heparin-protamine complexes play an important role in pulmonary hypertension after heparin-induced protamine reversal. Thromboxane A_2 was a primary mediator of the pulmonary hypertensive response to H-P complexes in this animal model.

► Adverse reactions to protamine are potentially life-threatening, and include pulmonary vasoconstriction and bronchospasm. The mechanisms by which acute protamine reactions occur are not completely understood, but H-P complexes might lead to pulmonary artery hypertension through thromboxane release; thromboxane is a well-recognized pulmonary vasoconstrictor. This study confirms that H-P complexes are causative agents of pulmonary hypertension after protamine administration in a goat model. The adverse severe pulmonary hemodynamic response during protamine reversal of heparin is so rare in humans that whether cyclo-oxygenase inhibition with a drug such as indomethacin (which reduces thromboxane concentration) is warranted is not clear.

M. Wood, M.D.

Prevention of Bleeding After Cardiopulmonary Bypass With High-Dose Tranexamic Acid: Double-Blind, Randomized Clinical Trial

Karski JM, Teasdale SJ, Norman P, et al (Univ of Toronto)

J Thorac Cardiovasc Surg 110:835–842, 1995 4–48

Background.—Excessive bleeding occurs in 20% of patients undergoing cardiac surgery with cardiopulmonary bypass (CPB). The effects of high-dose tranexamic acid given before CPB were investigated.

Methods.—One hundred fifty patients were enrolled in the prospective, double-blind, randomized trial. Group 1 received 10 g of tranexamic acid IV for 20 minutes before sternotomy and placebo infusion for 5 hours; group 2, 10 g of tranexamic acid for 20 minutes and another 10 g infused IV during 5 hours; and group 3, a placebo bolus and placebo infusion for 5 hours.

Findings.—Eighteen percent of patients in group 3 lost more than 750 mL of blood in 6 hours, compared with 2% of patients in groups 1 and 2. Intravenous tranexamic acid, 10 g, infused before CPB decreased blood loss by 50% over 6 hours and by 35% over 24 hours. Continued tranexamic acid infusion did not further reduce bleeding. The coagulation profiles before surgery did not differ significantly between patients with and without excessive bleeding. Postoperatively, however, coagulation testing indicated ongoing fibrinolysis and platelet dysfunction in patients bleeding excessively.

Conclusions.—A single 10-g dose of IV tranexamic acid before sternotomy decreases the percentage of patients who bleed excessively after CPB. This dose also reduces blood loss postoperatively. Overall, the red blood cell transfusion requirement did not differ between groups.

▶ This study was done in patients who were not undergoing repeated operations, but of course these patients were from Canada, so they may have had a longer wait and more ongoing myocardial ischemia than those in the United States. Use of this antifibrinolytic prebypass seems to be all that was needed to decrease blood loss in a consistent and repeatable fashion. One wishes there were data on the patients who had the greatest benefit to determine if, in fact, all the benefit occurred in those patients who were undergoing not straightforward bypass, but a combination of valve and bypass or valve operations alone, or who were receiving aspirin beforehand.

Surprisingly, the abstract of the paper does not seem to correspond to the data. In fact, the difference in red blood cell transfusions between the treatment and control groups was not significantly different. I wonder why that did not make it into the abstract of the paper? Nonetheless, there is a difference in blood loss, but not in transfusion requirements.

M.F. Roizen, M.D.

Hydroxyethylstarch Compared With Modified Gelatin as Volume Preload Before Spinal Anaesthesia for Caesarean Section

Vercauteren MP, Hoffmann V, Coppejans HC, et al (Univ Hosp Antwerp, Belgium)

Br J Anaesth 76:731–733, 1996 4–49

Background.—The risks and benefits of hydrating obstetric patients before spinal anesthesia are being still debated. Smaller volumes are required of colloids as opposed to crystalloids, which might make them advantageous for such an application. However, the different properties of the available colloids have not been thoroughly explored. Gelatin and hydroxyethylstarch colloids were compared in a study of 90 patients undergoing elective cesarean section.

Methods.—Patients were randomly assigned to receive 1 of 3 regimens: (1) 1,000 mL lactated Ringer's solution with up to 1,000 mL of modified gelatin, (2) 1,000 mL of lactated Ringer's solution with up to 1,000 mL of 6% hydroxyethylstarch, or (3) up to 1,000 mL of 6% hydroxyethylstarch. After infusion of 500 mL of the colloid, lumbar puncture was performed.

Results.—The 3 groups were equivalent in terms of mean age, weight, and duration of pregnancy, and no patient required extradural supplementation before delivery. Patients in group 2 had a lower rate of severe hypotension (1 in 10 patients) than did patients in groups 1 or 3 (at least 1 of every 3 patients). Only 11 patients in group 2 required ephedrine, as opposed to 22 patients in group 1 and 20 patients in group 3. The mean dose requirement for ephedrine was also lower for patients in group 2. No patient showed respiratory or cardiac evidence of fluid overload, although packed cell volume decreased more than 20% in patients in groups 1 and 2. Patients in group 3 had a 14% reduction in packed cell volume.

Conclusions.—Volume preloading appears worthwhile, provided that a correct regimen is selected. Hydration should not be abandoned routinely without justification from further studies. The most optimal hemodynamic stability was accomplished with use of the crystalloid-hydroxyethylstarch combination (group 2). Cardiovascular instability, however, may not be prevented by high volumes, even if gelatins are used. A decrease in packed cell volume may be a concern for patients with mild pre-existent anemia.

▶ In this study, women who received both 1,000 mL of Ringer's lactate and approximately 1,000 mL of hydroxyethylstarch were less likely to have severe hypotension during spinal anesthesia for elective cesarean section than women in the other 2 groups. However, even this aggressive regimen did not eliminate hypotension altogether. Severe hypotension (i.e., systolic blood pressure of less than 90 mm Hg) occurred in 3 of the 30 women in the Ringer's lactate–hydroxyethylstarch group. It seem clear that no regimen of hydration will eliminate the risk of hypotension altogether. I continue to favor modest volume expansion (approximately 1,500 mL of Ringer's lactate) with prophylactic ephedrine to reduce the likelihood of hypotension during the administration of spinal anesthesia for cesarean section.

D.H. Chestnut, M.D.

Effects of Selenium Supplementation for Cancer Prevention in Patients With Carcinoma of the Skin: A Randomized Controlled Trial

Clark LC, for the Nutritional Prevention of Cancer Study Group (Univ of Arizona, Tucson; Cornell Univ, Ithaca, NY; Georgia Dermatology and Skin Cancer Clinic, Macon; et al)

JAMA 276:1957–1963, 1996 4–50

Introduction.—The trace element selenium plays a role in normal metabolism and may have cancer prevention properties when administered at levels greater than those associated with nutritional needs. Areas of the United States with high selenium levels have lower mortality rates for certain cancers than areas with reduced levels of the element. The hypothesis that increased selenium intake can reduce the risk of basal cell carcinoma (BCC) and squamous cell carcinoma (SCC) of the skin was tested in a multicenter trial.

Methods.—The double-blind, randomized trial enrolled 1,312 patients from 7 dermatology clinics in the eastern United States. All had a history of BCC or SCC skin cancers, with 1 of the carcinomas occurring in the previous year. Excluded were individuals with an internal malignancy treated within the previous 5 years or with a history of significant liver or kidney disease. Randomization took place from 1983 through 1991, with 653 patients allocated to selenium (200 μg daily) and 659 to placebo. Treatment continued for a mean of 4.5 years; mean total follow-up was 6.4 years. Patients were assessed every 6 months for new dermatologic problems and toxicity. Secondary end points, identified in 1990, included total mortality, cancer mortality, and the incidence of lung, colorectal, and prostate cancer.

Results.—Compliance was good in both selenium and placebo groups, and the 2 groups did not differ significantly in number of years receiving treatment or length of follow-up. The mean plasma selenium concentration was in the lower normal range at baseline. With selenium treatment, levels increased by about 67% within 6 to 9 months in that group of patients. The placebo and selenium groups showed no statistically significant differences in the incidence of skin cancers. There were 377 new cases of BCC and 218 of SCC in the selenium group versus 350 of BCC and 190 of SCC in the control group. Compared with control subjects, however, patients receiving selenium had significant reductions in total cancer incidence (77 versus 119 cancers), total cancer mortality (29 versus 57 deaths), and the incidence of lung, colorectal, and prostate cancer. All-cause mortality was lower in the selenium group than in the placebo group (108 versus 129 deaths), but this difference was not significant. There were no cases of selenium toxicity.

Discussion.—Although selenium treatment did not prevent the development of BCC or SCC of the skin, it was associated with reductions in total cancer incidence, total cancer mortality, and the incidence of and mortality from carcinomas of several sites. The lack of an effect on BCC and SCC may be attributed to the fact that ultraviolet radiation increases the risk of these lesions at both the initiation and promotion-progression stages of carcinogenesis.

Selenium and Cancer Prevention: Promising Results Indicate Further Trials Required

Colditz GA (Harvard Med School, Boston)

JAMA 276:1984–1985, 1996 4–51

Introduction.—Although previous studies examining a potential role for dietary supplements in the prevention of cancer have reported mixed results, there is still considerable public interest in the question. The interpretation of prevention studies was discussed and a study of selenium supplementation and skin cancer was reported.

Primary and Secondary End Points.—The primary outcome of the study was selenium's effect on the risk of developing new basal cell and squamous cell skin cancers in patients with a history of these lesions. Selenium supplementation did not reduce the incidence of these skin cancers, but a reduction in total carcinomas was observed. Specifically, selenium had an apparent rapid and large preventive effect for cancers of the lung, prostate, colon, and rectum, but not for those of the breast or bladder. Preventive inference, however, should not be based solely on randomized trials, and the effects of selenium must be confirmed by several studies with consistent findings.

Study Design.—The study cited the effectiveness of selenium in animal tumor models, but such trials included breast cancer cell lines, and there are no reports of a relation between selenium and the risk of breast cancer. Furthermore, the dose of selenium used in the study did not produce blood levels higher than those found in residents of high-selenium areas. And with men making up about 75% of trial participants, more research is needed before the results can be generalized safely to women.

Preventive Strategies.—If selenium proves to be of value in preventing cancer, strategies to provide supplementation to the U.S. population need to be considered. A population-wide approach, as has been used to increase folate intake, is 1 possibility. The dose-dependent adverse effects of selenium must be evaluated, however, before such a strategy is implemented. At the current time, any changes in public health recommendations or moves toward marketing of selenium supplements is premature.

▶ This article is interesting for several reasons that pertain to anesthesia very importantly, although one might not think so from the title or even from what is presented in the summary or abstract. Nevertheless, it is important from a couple of perspectives. The first is that it found something greatly different than it sought to find. Why is that important to anesthesia? Because it is the basis of the scientific process, that is, the prepared mind may well discover many more things about a patient, about a technique, or about science than the unprepared mind.

The second important point is what it tells us about cancer therapy, and the movement of health care in general. I truly believe that we have lived in the disease treatment era and that will continue even as gene therapy gets better and better. I believe more emphasis will be placed on disease prevention, from a standpoint of early disease detection, as with mammography and perhaps prostate-specific antigen levels, but even more on how we can influence the rate at which diseases develop.

This article looks at selenium treatment, a nutritional supplement of an essential trace element that may have other beneficial effects. Both the focus of the article on this nutritional supplement and the mechanism by which cancer may be prevented are important to anesthesiologists and pain management specialists for many reasons. First, it is our basic desire to understand science. Second, it it our desire to understand what our patients are going to be asking us about. Third, and most important, it is thought that selenium operates by a mechanism that may cause cancer cells to commit suicide.

This process relates to a basic change in the way we view things. In the future, we may use more therapies that cause healthy cells to live longer and diseased cells to commit suicide. No place, of course, is this more important to understand than in brain and nervous system function and vascular biology. Equally interesting is this concept for cancer cells and cells that are proliferating. Although this is a desirable cause-and-effect story, the editorial that accompanies the article points out some disturbing things with this study. For example, the authors emphasize the effectiveness of selenium in animal tumor moderated studies, perhaps because of the large effects observed. These studies suggest a specificity of the molecular mechanism that is perplexing. Laboratory studies cited to justify these mechanisms include breast cancer cell lines. Yet, this trial by Clark and colleagues, and numerous epidemiolgic studies, have found no relation between selenium and the risk of breast cancer. Further, if this possible magic bullet acts through the mechanism suggested by Clark and colleagues, it is not clear why it should be specific only to some cancers. Moreover, human populations have behaved differently from animals, and the laboratory findings are not consistent with human data. Both the article and the editorial reach similar conclusions:

> The promising set of results based on secondary endpoints from a skin cancer prevention trial require confirmation and further randomized studies. Given the results of this study and the expected effect to be large, the time frame will be short and such trials should be feasible. For now it is premature to change individual behavior to market specific selenium supplements or to modify public health recommendation on the results of one trial. Meanwhile, as we await the results of these trials, known lifestyle changes that can reduce cancer risk such as smoking cessation, consuming adequate amounts of fruits and vegetables each day, reducing intake of animal fat, and increasing physical activity should be implemented.

For the anesthesiologist, these are good recommendations to follow ourselves and to encourage in our patients; for now, I expect that we will find an increasing number of patients taking a variety of supplements, including selenium, and will learn whether selenium interacts with any of our current drugs. Selenium toxicity is well described, with the most common effect at low levels being pathologic nail changes, brittle hair, and garlic breath, and at high levels, severe liver injury and encephalopathy. None of the patients in this study had significant adverse effects, and the amount of supplement, 200 μg/day, is the amount that often is ingested by eating food grown in selenium-rich states such as North and South Dakota.

M.F. Roizen, M.D.

Dietary Flavonoids, Antioxidant Vitamins, and Incidence of Stroke: The Zutphen Study

Keli SO, Hertog MGL, Feskens EJM, et al (Natl Inst of Public Health and Environmental Protection, Bilthoven, The Netherlands)

Arch Intern Med 154:637–642, 1996 4–52

Background.—Epidemiologic studies have suggested an association between increasing consumption of fruit and vegetables and a declining trend in stroke mortality. It was hypothesized that dietary antioxidants, including flavonoids, provide a protective effect against stroke. Data from repeated dietary surveys of a cohort of middle-aged men were used to investigate this possible protective effect.

Methods.—A cohort of 552 men between the ages of 40 and 59 years in 1960 participated in a medical examination and repeated dietary surveys. Food intake was surveyed in 1960, 1965, and 1970, with reports of patterns of food consumption during the preceding 6–12 months and interviews with the man and his wife. The men underwent annual medical examinations between 1960 and 1973, and in 1977, 1978, and 1985. Information on risk factors, including blood pressure, cigarette smoking, and serum cholesterol levels, was obtained. Morbidity and mortality data were collected for the cohort between 1960 and 1985. Multivariate Cox models were used to determine the predictive significance of variables for stroke risk.

Results.—During the 15-year follow-up, 42 of the 552 men had a first fatal or nonfatal stroke. There was a significantly lower risk of stroke among the men in the highest quartile of β-carotene intake, compared with the men in the lowest quartile. There was no independent effect of vitamin C or E on stroke risk. Stroke risk was associated inversely with mean flavonoid intake in a dose-dependent fashion. Compared with the men in the lowest quartile of flavonoid intake, the relative risk of the men in the highest quartile was 0.27. Tea and solid fruit were the main sources of flavonoids, with tea providing 70% of the flavonoid intake. Compared with men who consumed less than 2.6 cups of tea per day, men who consumed an average of at least 4.7 cups of tea per day had a relative risk for stroke of 0.31. The risk of stroke was also significantly reduced in men who consumed the most solid fruit, compared with those who consumed the least solid fruit.

Conclusions.—Long-term flavonoid intake from black tea may reduce the risk of stroke. Solid fruit consumption and dietary β-carotene may also have a preventive effect. The protective role of these dietary factors requires further investigation.

▶ This is a fascinating study in that it examined men who were between the ages of 40 and 60 in 1960, surveyed 3 times during the decade of the 60s, and then followed up with them for disease and survival. It appears that important changes in survival were related to classic factors such as blood pressure and smoking, cholesterol, and energy used in physical activity.

Also, it appears the risk of stroke was reduced by 70% if one consumed 4.7 or more cups of tea a day. Of note, very few of the individuals took vitamin supplements and the level of vitamin E in their total diet was less than 1/25th of that recommended to prevent stroke and coronary artery disease; the level of vitamin C was 1/10 of that recommended to prevent myocardial infarction and stroke in the American studies. Thus, I am not sure that these results would pertain to people who consumed appropriate amounts of those vitamins. Nevertheless, these are important data on the ability of flavonoids such as may be found in black tea to be related to serious, morbid outcomes.

This is what would be called a prospective cohort study, and one tends not to believe cohort epidemiologic outcome studies unless the relative risk is threefold or more. That is what the relative risk in this study was found to be, and perhaps we will see that we can reduce our stroke risk and our risk of arterial aging by taking more flavonoids. This study follows earlier reports from the same group that flavonoids caused a similar, substantial reduction in coronary artery disease risk; one hopes that one can find confirmation in other populations. But, until that time, maybe I should switch from caffeine beverages without flavonoids, such as coffee, to flavonoid-rich black tea. Why do flavonoids do this? It is unclear. I recommend that you read this article to judge for yourself whether we should start drinking tea and teach our patients to do so as well.

M.F. Roizen, M.D.

Magnesium in Head Trauma

Effect of Magnesium Given 1 Hour After Head Trauma on Brain Edema and Neurological Outcome

Feldman Z, Gurevitch B, Artru AA, et al (Soroka Med Ctr, Beer-Sheva, Israel; Ben-Gurion Univ, Beer-Sheva, Israel; Univ of Washington, Seattle; et al)

J Neurosurg 85:131–137, 1996 4–53

Background.—Blood-brain barrier breakdown and extravasation of protein, as well as cytotoxic edema, are believed to produce posttraumatic brain edema. The reduction of brain edema associated with noncompetitive *N*-methyl-D-asparate receptor antagonist MK-801 treatment is mostly attributed to a reduction in the cytotoxic portion of the posttraumatic edema. In addition, the *N*-methyl-D-asparate receptor antagonist magnesium has been reported to reduce regional brain tissue water content and decrease memory impairment after fluid-percussion injury in rats. The effect of postinjury treatment with Mg^{++} on brain edema and neurologic outcomes after brain trauma was investigated.

Methods and Findings.—Sixty-nine rats that survived halothane anesthesia and closed head trauma (CHT) were assigned randomly to sham, CHT, or CHT with Mg^{++} administration 1 hour after injury. Mortality was comparable in the groups that received and did not receive Mg^{++}. Compared with baseline levels, brain tissue Mg^{++} levels were significantly increased at 48 hours. In addition, brain tissue-specific gravity in the contused hemisphere of rats given Mg^{++} was significantly greater than that in the contused hemisphere of untreated rats, which indicates attenuation of brain edema formation by Mg^{++}. At 18 and 48 hours, the neurologic severity scores of rats given Mg^{++} were significantly improved compared with values obtained 1 hour after CHT, but before Mg^{++} administration. Untreated rats showed no neurologic improvement.

Conclusion.—Treatment with Mg^{++} at 1 hour after CHT increased Mg^{++} concentrations in brain tissue at 48 hours. Brain tissue-specific gravity was also increased at 48 hours, and the neurologic severity score was improved at 18 and 48 hours.

► I couldn't possibly complete my yearly review of the critical care literature without an article that describes the wondrous effects of my most favorite divalent cation, magnesium. I have commonly used magnesium salts as replacement therapy in patients who received mannitol or furosemide intraoperatively as well as for potential neurologic protectant and antiarrhythmic effects during intracranial surgery.

D.M. Rothenberg, M.D.

Atenolol: Mortality After Noncardiac Surgery

Effect of Atenolol on Mortality and Cardiovascular Morbidity After Noncardiac Surgery

Mangano DT, for the Multicenter Study of Perioperative Ischemia Research Group (Univ of California, San Francisco; Ischemia Research and Education Found, San Francisco)

N Engl J Med 335:1713–1720, 1996 4–54

Introduction.—Many patients undergoing noncardiac surgery have or are at risk for coronary artery disease. In this group, myocardial ischemia and nonfatal myocardial infarction occurring in the week after surgery greatly increases the risk of mortality and cardiovascular morbidity. Preoperative or intraoperative beta-blockers have yielded encouraging effects on hemodynamics and measures of myocardial ischemia; however, the effects of giving this treatment throughout the postoperative period have not been investigated. The effects of intensive beta-blocker therapy before and after noncardiac surgery in patients with or at risk for coronary artery disease were studied over a 2-year follow-up period.

Methods.—The study included 200 patients undergoing elective noncardiac surgery who either had or were at risk for coronary artery disease. They were assigned to receive either atenolol or placebo before the induction of anesthesia, immediately after surgery, and then through up to 7 days of hospitalization. Before and immediately after surgery, the study medications were given IV. Each day thereafter, if the heart rate was greater than 55 bpm and the systolic blood pressure was at least 100 mm Hg, the patients received 2 tablets of atenolol (100 mg) or placebo. Just 1 tablet was given if the heart rate was 55 to 65 bpm or the systolic blood pressure was 100 mm Hg or greater. If the heart rate or blood pressure fell below these values, no treatment was given. Anesthetic and surgical management were not restricted by the study protocol. One hundred ninety-four patients survived to discharge, and outcome data were available for 192. The main outcome variable was all-cause mortality after 2 years; cardiovascular morbidity during the same period was a secondary outcome.

Results.—The overall mortality rate during 2 years of follow-up was 15.6%, with 21 of 30 deaths occurring in the placebo group. The overall mortality rate was 55% lower and the cardiac mortality rate was 65% lower with atenolol. In the atenolol group, there was 1 noncardiac death in the first 6 to 8 postoperative months; during the same time, there were 10 deaths in the placebo group, including 7 cardiac deaths. The early survival advantage with atenolol was preserved at 1 and 2 years.

The rate of cardiac events was lower with atenolol, with the main effect again occurring within 6 to 8 months. The time to the first adverse event was 6 days in the placebo group versus 158 days in the atenolol group. On multivariate analysis, factors associated with survival at 2 years were diabetes mellitus and atenolol therapy (Table 2). The risk of death was not increased for diabetic patients treated with atenolol, compared to a 4-fold increase in diabetic patients who received placebo. There was no difference between groups in the use of cardiovascular medications during follow-up. Atenolol had no serious adverse effects, such as hypotension or bradycardia.

Conclusions.—Giving atenolol throughout the hospitalization period can significantly reduce the risk of mortality and cardiovascular events after noncardiac surgery in patients with or at risk for coronary artery disease. The main effect of this treatment is apparent within the first 6 to 8 months after surgery. Beta-blockade is a safe and well-tolerated therapy.

TABLE 2.—Predictors of Death Among Patients Undergoing Noncardiac Surgery*

Predictor	Hazard Ratio (95% CI)	P Value
Univariable models		
Atenolol	0.4 (0.2–0.9)	0.03
Diabetes mellitus	3.1 (1.4–6.8)	0.01
Oral hypoglycemic treatment	2.6 (1.1–6.2)	0.03
Insulin treatment	2.6 (1.0–6.9)	0.05
Ischemia on Holter monitoring on postoperative days 0–2	2.3 (1.0–5.3)	0.04
Multivariable models		
Diabetes mellitus	2.8 (1.4–6.2)	0.01
Atenolol	0.5 (0.2–1.1)	0.06

*The patients included in these models were the 192 of the original randomized group of 200 who survived to hospital discharge and were followed up for 2 years after discharge; 30 of these 192 patients (15.6%) died during the 2 years of follow-up.

Abbreviation: CI, confidence interval.

(Courtesy of Mangano DT, for the Multicenter Study of Perioperative Ischemia Research Group: Effect of atenolol on mortality and cardiovascular morbidity after noncardiac surgery. *N Engl J Med* 335:1713–1720, copyright 1996, Massachusetts Medical Society. Reprinted by permission of *The New England Journal of Medicine*.)

Conservative cost estimates suggest that the overall cost per life-year saved with this therapy is $2,500.

▶ Intraoperative heart rate control long has been considered a mainstay of therapy in preventing myocardial ischemia, infarction, and death. Yet, as the authors are quick to surmise, postoperative heart rate control with beta-adrenergic antagonists often is avoided for fear of precipitating heart failure, bronchospasm, or heart block. This study also fails to address the consequences of treating tachycardia per se rather than its cause. What are the consequences of masking the tachycardic response to postoperative hemorrhage, infection, hypercarbia, or hypoxemia? I believe that, despite these compelling results, it is imperative to recognize that postoperative tachycardia often has cause that warrants investigation, and that cause-specific therapy may prove to be more beneficial to patient outcome. With this caveat in mind, it would seem prudent, based on the results of the study, to consider the perioperative use of beta-adrenergic antagonists for patients at risk (previous myocardial infarction, diabetes, angina pectoris, congestive heart failure) for cardiac morbidity and mortality.

D.M. Rothenberg, M.D.

Thyroid Hormone After Cardiopulmonary Bypass

Thyroid Hormone Treatment After Coronary-artery Bypass Surgery

Klemperer JD, Klein I, Gomez M, et al (Cornell Univ, New York; North Shore Univ Hosp, Manhassett, NY)

N Engl J Med 333:1522–1527, 1995 4–55

Objective.—Serum triiodothyronine concentrations fall during and immediately after cardiopulmonary bypass procedures, causing cardiac dysfunction. Studies suggest that IV administration of large doses of triiodothyronine might improve cardiac function in patients with postoperative cardiovascular problems. Triiodothyronine was administered to high-risk patients undergoing coronary artery bypass surgery.

Methods.—Immediately before surgery, 142 patients with ejection fractions of 40% or less during cardiac catheterization were given either placebo infusions of 5% dextrose or an IV bolus of 0.8 µg/kg of triiodothyronine followed by an IV infusion of 0.113 µg/kg/hr for 6 hours, then a tapered dose that was decreased by 50% every hour and finally stopped. Triiodothyronine concentrations were determined from arterial blood sampled at baseline, 30 minutes after the start of bypass, 6 hours after the start of infusion, and 15 hours after the end of infusion. Clinical and hemodynamic parameters were recorded.

Results.—Both the placebo and treatment groups required similar inotropic and vasodilator support, and similar numbers of patients in both groups received therapy for arrhythmias. Triiodothyronine concentrations in both groups decreased significantly by 40% 30 minutes after the start of cardiopulmonary bypass (Fig 1). Concentrations remained low in the placebo group but significantly increased to above normal in the treated

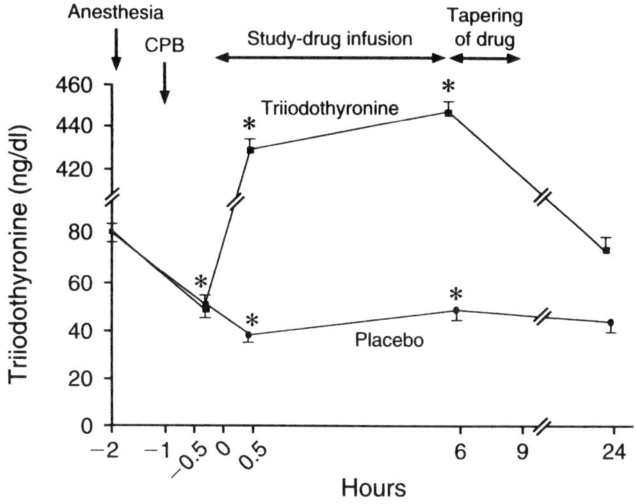

FIGURE 1.—Mean (±SE) serum triiodothyronine concentrations in patients who received triiodothyronine or placebo during coronary artery bypass surgery. Baseline serum samples were drawn in the operating room after the induction of anesthesia. Zero denotes the time when the aortic cross-clamp was removed and infusion of the study drug was begun. At 24 hours, serum triiodothyronine levels were measured in 11 patients in each study group. To convert values for triiodothyronine to nanomoles per liter, multiply by 0.015. Asterisks indicate $P < 0.001$ for the comparison with the baseline value. *Abbreviations: CPB,* cardiopulmonary bypass. (Courtesy of Klemperer JD, Klein I, Gomez M, et al: Thyroid hormone treatment after coronary-artery bypass surgery. *N Engl J Med* 333:1522–1527, 1995. Reprinted by permission of *The New England Journal of Medicine.* Copyright 1995, Massachusetts Medical Society.)

group and remained there throughout the infusion, then returned to normal for both groups at 24 hours. The cardiac index for the treated group was significantly higher and the systemic vascular resistance was lower than for the placebo group 2 hours after cross-clamp removal, and remained higher 4 and 6 hours thereafter (Fig 2). Incidences of perioperative mortality and major complications were similar in both groups.

Conclusions.—The administration of triiodothyronine was safe and effective in reducing cardiac dysfunction in patients after cardiopulmonary bypass. Because treatment did not lessen the need for inotropic support, the use of triiodothyronine is not a substitute for standard therapy.

▶ This study shows that triiodothyronine administration immediately after bypass increases cardiac output and lowers systemic vascular resistance, but has absolutely no effect on outcome or the need for inotropes or vasodilators. Anesthesiologists recognize that triiodothyronine concentrations are decreased in this clinical setting, but should we intervene? Probably not. Similarly, magnesium concentrations are decreased after cardiopulmonary bypass, but do all patients routinely require intervention with magnesium therapy?

M. Wood, M.D.

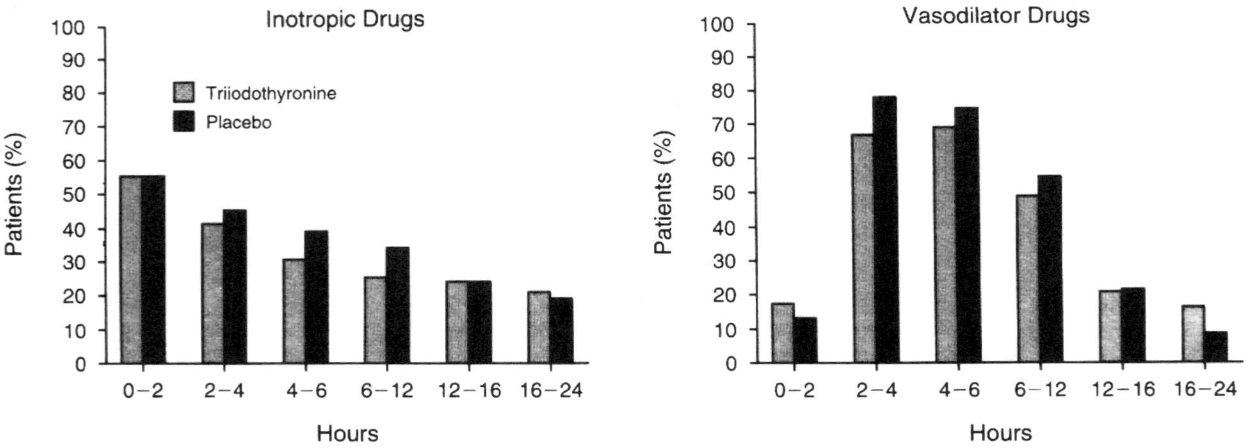

FIGURE 2.—Patients in the triiodothyronine and placebo groups who required inotropic or vasodilator drugs after coronary artery bypass surgery. Zero denotes the time when the aortic cross-clamp was removed and infusion of the study drug was begun. No statistically significant differences between groups were detected. (Courtesy of Klemperer JD, Klein I, Gomez M, et al: Thyroid hormone treatment after coronary-artery bypass surgery. *N Engl J Med* 333:1522–1527, 1995. Reprinted by permission of *The New England Journal of Medicine*. Copyright 1995, Massachusetts Medical Society.)

Prostacyclin: Pulmonary Vasodilation

Inhaled Aerosolized Prostacyclin as a Selective Pulmonary Vasodilator for the Treatment of Severe Hypoxaemia

van Heerden PV, Webb SAR, Hee G, et al (Sir Charles Gairdner Hosp, Perth, Western Australia)

Anaesth Intensive Care 24:87–90, 1996 4–56

Objective.—Given intravenously, prostacyclin is a powerful systemic and pulmonary vasodilator, although systemic hypotension and increased right-to-left shunting in the lung may limit this route of administration. Inhaled aerosolized prostacyclin (IAP) may be a useful selective pulmonary vasodilator; when given by inhalation, the drug is locally deposited in the lungs, with highest concentrations in the lung regions of highest

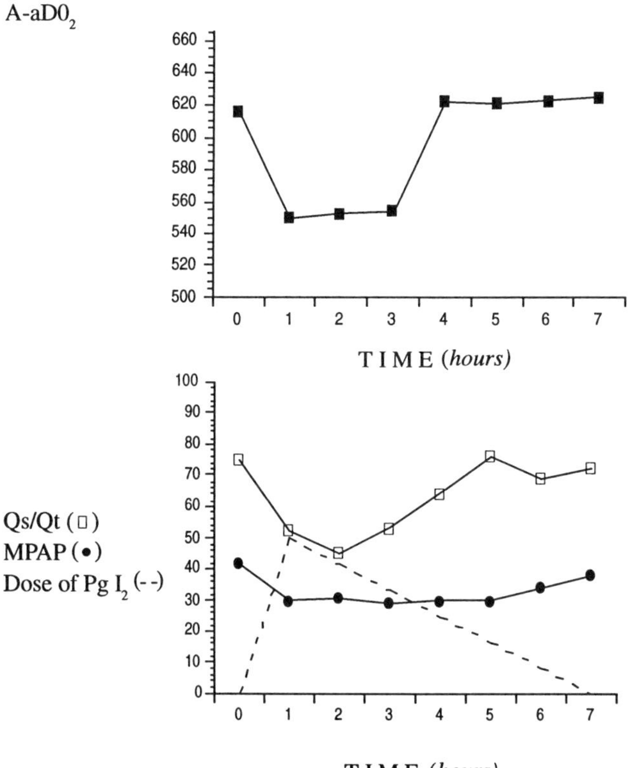

FIGURE 3.—Dose-response curves to inhaled aerosolized prostacyclin. *Abbreviations: A-aDO$_2$*, alveolar-arterial oxygen partial pressure gradient in millimeters of mercury (mm Hg); *Qs/Qt*, shunt fraction; *MPAP*, mean pulmonary artery pressure in mm Hg; *Time*, time in hours; *Dose of PgI$_2$*, dose of inhaled aerosolized prostacyclin in nanograms per kilogram per minute. (Courtesy of van Heerden PV, Webb SAR, Hee G, et al: Inhaled aerosolized prostacyclin as a selective pulmonary vasodilator for the treatment of severe hypoxaemia. *Anaesth Intensive Care* 24:87–90, 1996.)

ventilation. The effective use of IAP as a selective pulmonary vasodilator was described in 2 case reports.

Case 1.—Woman, 39, was transferred to the ICU with severe hypoxemia caused by amniotic fluid embolism. She received IAP through the ventilator in a dose of up to 50 ng/kg/min. This produced a striking improvement in PaO_2 within 2 hours, from 76 to 108 mm Hg. A maintenance IAP dose of 20 ng/kg/min was given, and the patient was gradually weaned off IAP over 48 hours. There were no signs of systemic hypotension or increased vasopressor requirements.

Case 2.—Young woman with acute-on-chronic liver failure and intra-abdominal sepsis was admitted to the ICU with hypoxemia related to acute respiratory distress syndrome. Oxygenation improved rapidly with administration of IAP in the same dose used in the first case. The 50-ng/kg/min dose was reduced in stepwise fashion in an attempt to identify the optimal IAP dose. At doses of 30 to 40 ng/kg/min, IAP maintained oxygenation at levels similar to those observed with the 50-ng/kg/min dose. When the IAP dose fell below 30 ng/kg/min, oxygenation deteriorated again (Fig 3).

Discussion.—Inhaled aerosolized prostacyclin appears to be a valuable selective pulmonary vasodilator that produces little or no systemic hypotension. It should be useful in patients with severe hypoxemia or pulmonary hypertension who might otherwise have been considered for inhaled nitric oxide therapy. Further studies are needed to establish the safety, optimal dosing, and long-term benefits of IAP.

► Selective pulmonary vasodilation is very difficult to achieve in clinical practice because most vasodilators are effective in both the systemic and pulmonary circulations. Systemic hypotension occurs, so that shunting and hypoxemia may worsen. Inhalation of nitric oxide does produce pulmonary vasodilation without systemic hypotension and so has great promise for the future, but of course is complicated to use and requires monitoring. Inhaled aerosolized prostacyclin has been used to treat adult respiratory distress syndrome[1]; this case report further extends the experience in 2 patients with severe hypoxemia.

M. Wood, M.D.

Reference

1. Walmrath D, Schneider T, Pilch J, et al: Aerosolised prostacyclin in adult respiratory syndrome. *Lancet* 342:961–962, 1993.

Tropisetron: Nausea Prevention

Tropisetron for the Prevention of Postoperative Nausea and Vomiting in Women Undergoing Gynecologic Surgery

Alon E, Kocian R, Nett PC, et al (Zurich Univ, Switzerland; Sandoz Wander Pharma Ltd, Berne, Switzerland)

Anesth Analg 82:338–341, 1996 4–57

Background.—As women recover from general anesthesia after gynecologic surgery, they commonly experience nausea, retching, and vomiting. None of the prophylactic antiemetic regimens currently used is completely successful, so new antiemetics such as serotonin antagonists have received much attention. The efficacy of tropisetron, a selective 5-hydroxytryptamine type 3 receptor antagonist, was investigated.

Methods.—Ten minutes before general anesthesia was induced, 80 patients were given a single IV injection of either 5 mg tropisetron or matching placebo in a double-blind manner. Thiopental was used to induce anesthesia, and nitrous oxide and enflurane in oxygen was used to maintain it.

Findings.—Within 24 hours of surgery, vomiting occurred in 17.5% of the patients given tropisetron and in 40% given placebo. Nausea occurred in 30% and 52%, respectively. Sixty-five percent in the tropisetron group and 40% in the placebo group had a total effective antiemetic response.

Conclusions.—Intravenous tropisetron administered before the induction of general anesthesia in patients who undergo gynecologic procedures significantly decreases postoperative nausea and vomiting compared with placebo. This drug causes no adverse effects.

► The authors tackled one of the most difficult problems in current outpatient medicine, namely postoperative nausea and vomiting in women who undergo gynecologic surgery. Tropisetron is a newer serotonin antagonist and is, perhaps, an improvement over ondansetron. This was a study against placebo and not a direct comparison against ondansetron. We now need a major assault on the issue of postoperative nausea and vomiting (which are possibly 2 separate problems).

J.H. Tinker, M.D.

Moving?

I'd like to receive my ***Year Book of Anesthesiology & Pain Management*** without interruption. Please note the following change of address, effective:

Name: ______________________________

New Address: ______________________________

____

City: ______________________ State: ________ Zip: ________

Old Address: ______________________________

____

City: ______________________ State: ________ Zip: ________

Reservation Card

Yes, I would like my own copy of ***Year Book of Anesthesiology & Pain Management***. Please begin my subscription with the current edition according to the terms described below.* I understand that I will have 30 days to examine each annual edition. If satisfied, I will pay just $75.95 plus sales tax, postage and handling (price subject to change without notice).

Name: ______________________________

Address: ______________________________

City: ______________________ State: ________ Zip: ________

Method of Payment

❍ Visa ❍ Mastercard ❍ AmEx ❍ Bill me ❍ Check (in US dollars, payable to Mosby, Inc.)

Card number: ______________________ Exp date: ________

Signature: ______________________________

LS-0909

*Your *Year Book* Service Guarantee:

When you subscribe to the *Year Book*, we'll send you an advance notice of future volumes about two months before they publish. This automatic notice system is designed to take up as little of your time as possible. If you do not want the *Year Book*, the advance notice makes it quick and easy for you to let us know your decision, and you will always have at least 20 days to decide. If we don't hear from you, we'll send you the new volume as soon as it's available. And, of course, the *Year Book* is yours to examine free of charge for 30 days (postage, handling and applicable sales tax are added to each shipment.).

NO POSTAGE
NECESSARY
IF MAILED
IN THE
UNITED STATES

BUSINESS REPLY MAIL
FIRST CLASS MAIL PERMIT No. 762 CHICAGO, IL

POSTAGE WILL BE PAID BY ADDRESSEE

Chris Hughes
Mosby-Year Book, Inc.
161 N. Clark Street
Suite 1900
Chicago, IL 60601-9981

NO POSTAGE
NECESSARY
IF MAILED
IN THE
UNITED STATES

BUSINESS REPLY MAIL
FIRST CLASS MAIL PERMIT No. 762 CHICAGO, IL

POSTAGE WILL BE PAID BY ADDRESSEE

Chris Hughes
Mosby-Year Book, Inc.
161 N. Clark Street
Suite 1900
Chicago, IL 60601-9981

5 Anesthesia Techniques and Monitoring

Monitoring Issues

Electroencephalogram Bispectral Analysis Predicts the Depth of Midazolam-induced Sedation
Liu J, Singh H, White PF (Univ of Texas, Dallas)
Anesthesiology 84:64–69, 1996 5–1

Purpose.—Patients receiving benzodiazepines during local and regional anesthesia need careful monitoring of sedation to prevent serious complications. Some reliable, noninvasive method of monitoring sedation would be useful in this situation. Electroencephalographic (EEG) studies of the effects of anesthetic and analgesic drugs have been reported previously. The use of EEG bispectral analysis to assess midazolam-induced sedation during regional anesthesia was evaluated in a retrospective study.

Methods.—The study included 26 men undergoing elective surgical procedures under regional anesthesia. All received IV midazolam in a dose of 4.5 to 20 mg, given in boluses of 0.5 to 1 mg until they stopped responding to mild tactile stimulation. Continuous EEG recordings were made from a bifrontal montage (FP_1-Cz and FP_2-Cz). These recordings were used to obtain the bispectral index (BI); 95% spectral edge frequency (SEF); median frequency (MF); and δ, θ, α, and β power bands. The Observer's Assessment of Alertness/Sedation (OAA/S) was used for clinical assessment of sedation, and the scores were correlated with the EEG parameters. Changes in EEG parameters reflecting the start and stop of midazolam-induced sedation also were analyzed.

Results.—The EEG parameter best correlated with the OAA/S scores was the BI, with Spearman's Rho statistics of 0.815 and 0.596 during the onset and recovery phases, respectively. As sedation increased, BI decreased, from 95 at an OAA/S score of 5 (wide awake) to 69 at an OAA/S score of 1 (unconscious). A similar pattern was observed in the relation between 95% SEF and the OAA/S score. As the patient recovered from midazolam-induced sedation, EEG-BI increased. None of the other EEG parameters were consistently related to level of sedation. At OAA/S scores of 3 to 2 and 2 to 1 during the onset and recovery phases, mean EEG_{50}

values were 79 for response to verbal command and 71 for response to shaking of the head for EEG-BI. For both these EEG_{50} values, EEG-BI had the smallest coefficients of variation.

Conclusions.—Midazolam-induced sedation during regional anesthesia can be assessed effectively using the EEG-BI. The information provided by EEG-BI monitoring can predict how likely it is that the patient will be able to respond to verbal commands or to shaking of the head while under midazolam sedation. An EEG-BI value of greater than 80 is associated with an OAA/S score of 3 or higher. More study is needed to determine the relation between OAA/S scores and EEG parameters in patients receiving other sedative and analgesic drugs in the operating room and ICU settings.

▶ Although this study demonstrated that bispectral analysis of the EEG (EEG-BI) predicts the depth of midazolam-induced sedation as assessed by an alertness/sedation score, this finding conversely also implies that the alertness/sedation score correlates with the EEG and is itself a good means of assessing sedation in a clinical setting. The really important question to be answered is: What is the clinical utility of EEG-BI in the operating room? Is EEG-BI a reliable noninvasive monitor that will permit better assessment of patient response during regional procedures? I remain unconvinced.

M. Wood, M.D.

Middle Latency Auditory Evoked Potentials During Repeated Transitions From Consciousness to Unconsciousness

Davies FW, Mantzaridis H, Kenny GNC, et al (Glasgow Univ, Scotland; Univ of Strathclyde, Glasgow, Scotland)

Anaesthesia 51:107–113, 1996 5–2

Background.—It would be useful to be able to measure anesthetic depth objectively and to produce a reliable indicator of awareness during anesthesia. The spontaneous electroencephalogram, the cerebral function monitor and analyzing monitor, fast Fourier transformation, and aperiodic waveform analysis have all been used in the past to measure anesthetic depth. More recent attempts have involved the change in lower esophageal contractility and have shown a relation to the end-tidal concentration of volatile anesthetics. However, it does not adequately discriminate at the transition between consciousness and unconsciousness and has been shown to be unrelated to blood concentration of anesthetics. It appears that the auditory-evoked potential shows changes in early cortical components related to anesthetic depth. Such changes are independent of the anesthetic agent and partially reversed by surgical stimulation. The changes in auditory-evoked potential parameters associated with alternating periods of consciousness and unconsciousness were examined.

Methods.—Twelve patients were scheduled for total knee replacement with the use of spinal anesthesia. The electroencephalogram produced middle latency auditory-evoked potential signals. After onset of anesthesia, the electrodes and earphone were placed and auditory-evoked potential signals were obtained. A propofol infusion was administered to induce alternating periods of consciousness and unconsciousness. Patient response to a verbal command and presence of an eyelash reflex were recorded.

Results.—Of the 12 patients, 11 finished the study. The mean patient age was 67 years. Of the 11 patients, 2 recalled events after onset of anesthesia. Heart rate and systolic arterial pressure were similar during conscious and unconscious periods. During the first transition from consciousness to unconsciousness, peak latencies increased significantly, and mean starting latency values increased from 20.0 msec to 22.5 msec for Na, from 31.7 ms to 39.3 msec for Pa, and from 42.8 ms to 57.8 msec for Nb. During successive transitions, awake latencies were somewhat higher than baseline awake latencies, and latencies during anesthesia were similar to latencies during the first period of unconsciousness.

Discussion.—Computer processing of the auditory-evoked potential may indicate the transition from anesthesia to awareness and awareness to anesthesia. The auditory-evoked potential latencies showed consistent change from consciousness to unconsciousness and vice versa. These findings suggest that the auditory-evoked potential may be a reliable monitor of awareness during anesthesia.

▶ This study represents a further continuation of efforts to find an acceptable measure of depth of anesthesia that is on line and will guarantee lack of awareness. The study appears promising in that there was a consistency of evoked potential readings during unconsciousness.

M.F. Roizen, M.D.

Processing Familiar and Unfamiliar Auditory Stimuli During General Anesthesia

Donker AG, Phaf RH, Porcelijn T, et al (Univ of Amsterdam; Hosp Prinsengracht, Amsterdam; Erasmus Univ, Rotterdam, The Netherlands)

Anesth Analg 82:452–455, 1996 5–3

Background.—During nonconscious states, only low-level information processing (such as activation learning) is considered possible. Whether information processing during general anesthesia is restricted to activation learning was investigated.

Methods.—Participating in the study were 58 patients undergoing day-case arthroscopic surgery with general propofol-sufentanil anesthesia. Memory priming was tested for auditory stimuli presented while the patients were unconscious. Common facts (group A) or familiar and unfamiliar full names of fictitious people (group B) were presented to the anesthetized patients via headphones. When tested postoperatively, patients in group A were expected to give more correct answers to questions about the common facts than were patients in group B. Patients in group

B were expected to attribute more fame to presented names than were patients in group A. Because general anesthesia may impair the process for learning new or unfamiliar information, more memory priming was expected for the familiar, as opposed to the unfamiliar, material.

Results.—Performance on tests of either type (common facts or fame attributed to names) did not differ significantly between patients in groups A and B. Priming was larger for familiar names than for unfamiliar names, but the degree of difference was not significant. Memory priming was correlated with preoperative anxiety on the Hospital Anxiety and Depression Scale but not on the State-Trait Anxiety Inventory.

Conclusions.—Although all differences were in the predicted direction, no significant memory-priming effects were shown. These data cannot answer the question of whether memory priming (in the Jelicic study) was based on elaboration of new or unfamiliar associations.

▶ I continue to remain skeptical about the amount of information processing and learning described during general anesthesia. These authors have only increased my skepticism because no difference was found between complex memory tasks and simple memory tasks.

M.F. Roizen, M.D.

End-tidal Carbon Dioxide for Monitoring Primary Closure of Gastroschisis

Puffinbarger NK, Taylor DV, Tuggle DW, et al (Univ of Oklahoma, Oklahoma City)

J Pediatr Surg 31:280–282, 1996 5–4

Objective.—In newborns with gastroschisis, primary closure can improve survival and minimize complications. However, the resulting increase in intra-abdominal pressure can cause compromised ventilation and other complications. Various intraoperative measurements have been used in an attempt to ensure the safety of closure, including intraoperative respiratory rate, cardiac indices, degree of visceroabdominal disproportion, size of defect, and lower extremity turgor. Since the availability of end-tidal carbon dioxide ($ETCO_2$) monitoring, primary reduction of gastroschisis has been performed in babies who could maintain an $ETCO_2$ of 50 mm Hg or less. One experience with $ETCO_2$ monitoring during primary closure of gastroschisis was reviewed.

Methods.—The study included 129 newborns who were treated for gastroschisis from 1976 through 1993. From 1976 through 1984, 64 patients underwent primary closure on clinical grounds. In 1985, intraoperative monitoring of $ETCO_2$ became available. The results of the 2 groups were compared in terms of primary closures, staged closures, and postoperative conversion to staged closure. Data on the effects of abdominal closure on $ETCO_2$ were analyzed to see whether there was any $ETCO_2$ level at which closure was not feasible.

TABLE 3.—End-tidal Carbon Dioxide Levels

No. of Patients	Closure	$ETCO_2$ Available	Highest $ETCO_2$	Average Birth Weight (g)
54	1°	40	44	2,585 ± 474
8	Silo	8	51	
2	Silo	2	20	2,427 ± 612
1	Silo	Not recorded	Not recorded	

(Courtesy of Puffinbarger NK, Taylor DV, Tuggle DW, et al: End-tidal carbon dioxide for monitoring primary closure of gastroschisis. *J Pediatr Surg* 31:280–282, 1996.)

Results.—The patients who were and were not monitored by $ETCO_2$ were similar in terms of overall mortality, birth weight, and postoperative ventilation requirements. The primary closure rate was higher after the introduction of $ETCO_2$ monitoring, with 38% of patients requiring staged closure from 1976 through 1984 versus 17% from 1985 through 1993. In the latter group, none of the patients who had primary closure subsequently required conversion to staged closure. Attempted closure produced an $ETCO_2$ level of more than 50 mm Hg for 73% of patients undergoing staged closure, compared with none of those having primary closure (Table 3).

Conclusions.—For patients with gastroschisis, $ETCO_2$ monitoring appears to be a useful and noninvasive adjunct in assessing the potential for primary closure. Primary closure may be unsafe for infants with $ETCO_2$ levels of 50 mm Hg or greater. Monitoring $ETCO_2$ during attempted closure may prevent the need for intragastric pressure monitoring or other invasive techniques.

► I thought this was an interesting report, but it was retrospective in nature. Undoubtedly, $ETCO_2$ monitoring is extremely useful for monitoring primary closure of gastroschisis, but it would have been interesting if other criteria for tolerance of a primary closure of gastroschisis also had been included, and related to $ETCO_2$ concentration.

M. Wood, M.D.

Fetal Pulse Oximetry: A Methodological Study

Maesel A, Mårtensson L, Gudmundsson S, et al (Univ of Lund, Sweden)

Acta Obstet Gynecol Scand 75:144–148, 1996 5–5

Background.—Pulse oximetry provides continuous information on arterial oxygen saturation levels in high-risk newborns. Fetal pulse oximetry is being developed as a potential complement to fetal heart rate monitoring during labor. The use of one type of sensor—an oxisensor—was reported.

Methods.—Data were collected on 96 singleton pregnancies. Obstetricians and midwives placed the sensors. Mean fetal arterial oxygen saturation levels were measured when the cervix was dilated 4 to 7 cm and 8 to 10 cm and in the second stage of labor.

Findings.—Ninety-five percent of the oxisensor placements were successful. One woman experienced pain, which disappeared after the sensor was removed. Two newborns had a mark caused by the sensor, but these marks completely resolved within 1 day. No cases of infection or increased bleeding developed. Recording lasted a mean of 134 minutes. Fetal arterial oxygen saturation values could be obtained during 69% of the recording time. A significant decline in mean fetal arterial oxygen saturation was seen between the first and second stages of labor.

Conclusions.—Fetal pulse oximetry monitored during labor with an oxisensor provides fetal arterial oxygen saturation values during two thirds of the recording period. This method appears to be safe for mothers and infants. Further research is needed to establish the possible clinical value of this method.

▶ Electronic fetal heart rate monitoring represents an indirect method of fetal assessment. Most randomized studies have failed to document a benefit associated with the use of electronic fetal heart rate monitoring during labor. We continue to await the availability of a direct method of measuring fetal oxygenation during labor. The present study suggests that much work needs to be done before fetal pulse oximetry is introduced into clinical obstetric practice. Investigators must overcome problems with the technology (in the present study, an acceptable signal was obtained in only 69% of patients), and further research must be done to determine whether this technique augments the information provided by fetal heart rate monitoring.

D.H. Chestnut, M.D.

Systemic Vascular Resistance Index Determined by Thoracic Electrical Bioimpedance Predicts the Risk for Maternal Hypotension During Regional Anesthesia for Cesarean Delivery

Ouzounian JG, Masaki DI, Abboud TK, et al (Univ of Southern California, Los Angeles; University of California, Los Angeles)

Am J Obstet Gynecol 174:1019–1025, 1996 5–6

Background.—Regional anesthesia delivered by epidural catheter or spinal blockade is most commonly used for cesarean delivery. Thirty to 60 percent of the patients experience hypotension, which reduces placental perfusion and can lead to fetal hypoxia and acidosis. The predictive value of a noninvasively derived baseline systemic vascular resistance index (SVRI) for maternal hypotension during regional anesthesia for cesarean delivery was investigated prospectively.

Methods.—Forty-two women received a standardized spinal or epidural anesthetic for nonurgent cesarean delivery. The NCCOM-3 cardiac output monitor (Biomed Medical Manufacturing, Irvine, Calif) was used to estimate stroke volume and cardiac output by thoracic electrical bioimpedance. Measures were indexed to body surface area. The SVRIs were

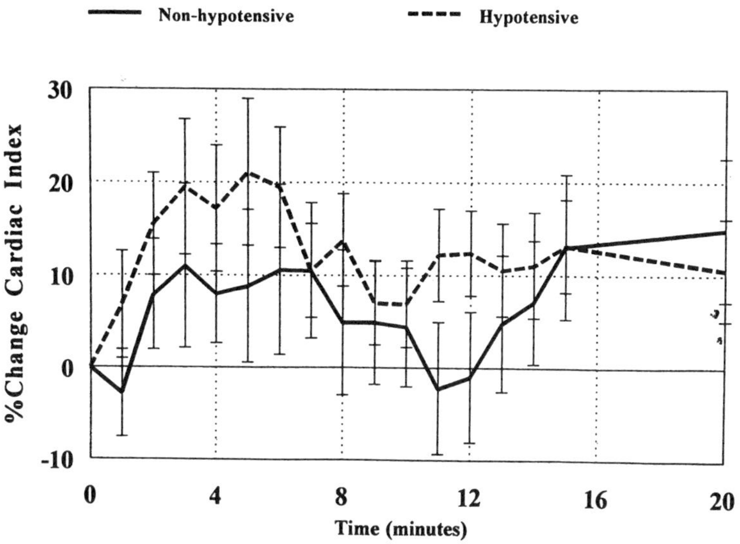

FIGURE 1.—Mean (SEM) of percent change in cardiac index from baseline values during regional anesthesia. There was no statistically significant difference in mean percent change in cardiac index between patients who had hypotension and those who did not. (Courtesy of Ouzounian JG, Masaki DI, Abboud TK, et al: Systemic vascular resistance index determined by thoracic electrical bioimpedance predicts the risk for maternal hypotension during regional anesthesia for cesarean delivery. *Am J Obstet Gynecol* 174:1019–1025, 1996.)

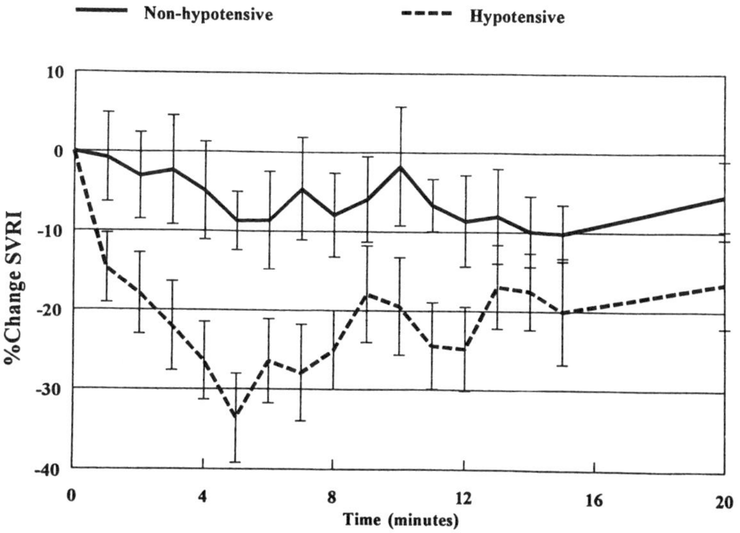

FIGURE 2.—Mean (SEM) of percent change in SVRI from baseline values during regional anesthesia. There was significantly larger decrease in mean percent change SVRI in patients who had hypotension compared with those who did not. (Courtesy of Ouzounian JG, Masaki DI, Abboud TK, et al: Systemic vascular resistance index determined by thoracic electrical bioimpedance predicts the risk for maternal hypotension during regional anesthesia for cesarean delivery. *Am J Obstet Gynecol* 174:1019–1025, 1996).

determined from mean arterial pressure and thoracic electrical bioimpedance-derived cardiac index.

Findings.—Fifty-seven percent of the women experienced hypotension. Hypotension incidence did not differ significantly between spinal and epidural anesthesthic delivery. The onset of hypotension occurred at a mean 12.2 minutes after anesthesia induction. Hypotensive women were found to have greater mean baseline systolic blood pressures than nonhypotensive women. Hypotensive women also had a higher mean baseline SVRI. With receiver-operator characteristic curves, the sensitivity, specificity, and positive and negative predictive values of a baseline SVRI of 500 were 83%, 78%, 83%, and 78%, respectively. The sensitivity and specificity of a baseline systolic blood pressure of 140 torr were 42% and 72%, respectively (Figs 1 and 2).

Conclusions.—Among women who underwent cesarean delivery with regional anesthesia, risk of maternal hypotension may be predicted by a baseline SVRI obtained by noninvasive output monitoring with thoracic electrical bioimpedance and systolic blood pressure. This risk is increased among patients with increased baseline SVRI or systolic blood pressure.

▶ It is interesting—but not surprising—that the mean baseline SVRI was higher in women who experienced hypotension than in those who did not. However, I disagree with the authors' suggestion that preanesthetic assessment with thoracic electrical bioimpedance is a useful tool for assessing the risk for maternal hypotension during administration of regional anesthesia for cesarean section. For example, the authors suggested that additional intravenous fluids might be administered to patients with increased baseline systemic vascular resistance, despite that aggressive hydration does not consistently reduce the incidence of hypotension during administration of spinal anesthesia for cesarean section.

D.H. Chestnut, M.D.

Transesophageal Echocardiography in Myocardial Revascularization: I. Accuracy of Intraoperative Real-Time Interpretation

Bergquist BD, Leung JM, Bellows WH (Univ of California, San Francisco; Kaiser Permanente Med Ctr, San Francisco)

Anesth Analg 82;1132–1138, 1996 5–7

Background.—The use of transesophageal echocardiography (TEE) to monitor ventricular function and volume during surgery is increasing. To determine whether data from TEE monitoring can be accurately interpreted on-line in real time, the performance of 5 community-based, full-time cardiac anesthesiologists during 75 operations was studied.

Methods.—Biplane TEE monitoring was used in all the procedures. Every 10 minutes during surgery, the anesthesiologists evaluated the video cine loop display of echocardiographic images, providing a real-time visual estimate of left ventricular ejection fraction area (EFA) and left ventricular filling at the level of the short axis and transgastric longitudinal views. A predefined scoring system was used. Two blinded investigators analyzed the same video images quantitatively off-line.

Findings.—Intraoperative real-time EFA estimates were moderately associated with off-line quantification. Fifty-five percent of the 662 cine loops analyzed by both off-line and real-time techniques were within ± 5% of one another, 75% were within ± 10%, 85% were within ± 15%, and 93% were within ± 20%. Real-time echocardiographic ischemia detection was 76% sensitive and specific, although individual variation occurred among the anesthesiologists. Recognition of normal and severe regional wall-motion abnormalities, such as akinesis, was more concordant with real-time and off-line analysis than was recognition of mild regional wall-motion abnormalities.

Conclusions.—Anesthesiologists can estimate ejection fraction and left ventricular filling fairly accurately in real time during surgery by visually inspecting 2-dimensional TEE images. When adjacent cine loops are compared with successive cardiac cycles, EFA can be estimated in real time to within ± 10% of off-line measurements in 75% of patients.

▶ This paper convinces me that ischemia detection in real time by echocardiography is, to quote the authors, "fairly" accurate. What they do not tell us, unfortunately, is the fact that ischemia detection by ECG is better. Transesophageal echocardiography in the anesthetic care of cardiac surgical patients still is a very fancy machine looking for neat things to do with the technology.

J.H. Tinker, M.D.

The Development of Hypercoagulability State, as Measured by Thromboelastography, Associated With Intraoperative Surgical Blood Loss
Ng KFJ, Lo JWR (Queen Mary Hosp, Hong Kong)
Anaesth Intensive Care 24:20–25, 1996 5–8

Introduction.—The practice of tolerating a lower "normal" hemoglobin level to reduce the need for blood transfusions is considered safe in most patients. The changes in blood coagulation associated with intraoperative blood loss and subsequent hemodilution have rarely been investigated. Thromboelastography (TEG) was used to analyze whether surgical blood loss with hemodilution is related to hypercoagulability.

Methods.—Twenty-one Chinese patients undergoing an elective or emergent surgical procedure for which a significant blood loss (up to 20% of total blood volume) was anticipated had blood samples drawn for measurement of coagulation and hemoglobin level: after induction of anesthesia, before surgical skin incision (control sample), at the termination of red blood cell transfusion (if required), at hourly intervals after the first sample until conclusion of surgery, and when estimated blood loss was 5%, 10%, and 15% of total blood volume. The estimated blood loss was replaced with intravenous normal saline. The time from sample placement in the TEG cuvette until TEG tracing amplitude reaches 2 mm was designated as R. The distance from R to the point where the amplitude of the tracing reaches 20 mm was designated as K. The angle formed by the slope of the TEG tracing from the R to the K value was designated α.

Results.—Significant shortening of R and K and widening of α was observed when patients' hemoglobin levels dropped to about 90% of the preoperative level. These patterns were also observed with further hemodilution when hemoglobin levels dropped to 85% of preoperative level. A comparison of TEG parameters taken at 60 minutes after induction showed that patients with blood loss and hemodilution had significant shortening of R and K and widening of α, compared to those without blood loss and hemodilution.

Conclusion.—Chinese patients with mild to moderate blood loss during surgery and volume replacement with normal saline experienced a hypercoagulable state that was not considered to be a result of the stress of surgery, anesthesia, or tissue trauma. These hypercoagulation changes associated with blood loss occur in a similar fashion in caucasian patients. These findings are significant, particularly for patients at high risk of thromboembolic complications and those undergoing intentional intraoperative hemodilution.

▶ The genesis of this study is interesting—the authors worried that hemodilution would promote a hypocoagulable state and thus, increase blood loss. It is logical that the body would respond to surgical blood loss by increasing its activated coagulation factors, increasing the receptor activation of platelets, and, in fact, showing an increased tendency to coagulate. That may be why we see it in the postoperative period. The authors did disprove their hypothesis showing that coagulation tendency increases with blood loss. Thus, this is an important study because it reaffirms the need to consider agents that decrease the tendency of coagulation in the immediate perioperative period.

M.F. Roizen, M.D.

The Clinical Usefulness of the Preoperative Bleeding Time

Gewirtz AS, Miller ML, Keys TF (Cleveland Clinic Found, Ohio)

Arch Pathol Lab Med 120:353–356, 1996 5–9

Background.—The bleeding time (BT) test is commonly performed as part of the preoperative evaluation. The implication that superficial skin bleeding predicts the risk for perioperative bleeding has been questioned by numerous investigators. The clinical usefulness of the BT test as a predictor of perioperative bleeding was examined retrospectively.

Methods.—The records of patients who had Simplate BT testing during a 6-month period were reviewed. Of 332 patients identified, 167 had BT testing as part of a preoperative evaluation. These 167 patients were divided into 2 groups: those with a normal and those with an abnormal BT. The groups were compared for the presence of indicators of bleeding risk and for excessive perioperative bleeding. The patients were also divided into groups defined by the presence or absence of clinically significant perioperative bleeding and compared for BT, indicators of bleeding risk, and blood product usage.

Results.—Of the 167 patients, 147 had normal and 20 had abnormal BTs. Nine patients had clinically significant perioperative bleeding, including 8 with normal BTs and 1 with an abnormal BT. The patient with both an abnormal BT and perioperative bleeding had no bleeding history and a normal prothrombin time, activated partial thromboplastin time, platelet count, and creatinine level, but was taking medications that interfere with platelet function. Preoperative BT did not correlate significantly with perioperative bleeding. Of the indicators of bleeding risk, bleeding history correlated statistically significantly with prolonged BT, but medications, thrombocytopenia, increased creatinine levels, or prolonged prothrombin or activated partial thromboplastin times did not. There were no statistically significant correlations between any of the indicators of bleeding risk and perioperative bleeding. The BT did not correlate with blood product usage. In relation to perioperative bleeding, BT testing had a positive predictive value of 5%, a negative predictive value of 95%, and an efficiency of 50%.

Conclusions.—The poor predictive value and lack of association between indicators of bleeding risk and perioperative bleeding indicate that preoperative BT testing does not reliably indicate the risk of clinically significant perioperative bleeding.

▶ The BT has never been such a controversial preoperative test as it is now. This was a retrospective study and examined blood loss and blood product usage as a measure of bleeding. Anesthesiologists are more interested in using the BT as a means of assessment as to whether neural blockage should be undertaken. It is an operator-dependent labor-intensive test, and there is now a recognition that BT may not be a useful test for anesthesiologists.[1]

M. Wood, M.D.

Reference

1. O'Kelly SW, Lawes EG, Luntley JB: Bleeding time: Is it a useful clinical tool? *Br J Anaesth* 68:313–315, 1992.

Intraoperative Phrenic Nerve Monitoring in Cardiac Surgery

Mazzoni M, Solinas C, Sisillo E, et al (IRCCS Centro Cardiologico Fondazione Italo Monzino, Milano, Italy)

Chest 109:1455–1460, 1996

5–10

Objective.—Hypothermic arrest with cold crystalloid solutions is widely used to protect the heart during cardiac surgery. Further cooling sometimes is obtained by immersing the heart in ice-cold saline or crushed ice. Some patients undergoing hypothermic cardiopulmonary bypass sustain phrenic nerve damage leading to diaphragmatic paralysis. The cause of this complication is uncertain, but it may be related to cold injury to the phrenic nerve. Intraoperative monitoring of phrenic nerve conduction was evaluated for its feasibility, safety, and clinical utility.

Methods.—The study included 12 patients undergoing myocardial revascularization surgery using the left internal mammary artery. During and after surgery, all patients underwent monitoring of compound diaphragmatic action potentials (CDAPs) by transcutaneous stimulation of the phrenic nerves. In 6 patients (group 1), the only cardioplegic technique used was intracoronary administration of cold St. Thomas's solution. In the other 6 patients, topical cardiac cooling with iced saline solution slush also was used. The CDAP recordings were analyzed to observe phrenic nerve conduction changes, to define the factors causing them, and to determine whether monitoring aided in the clinical management of patients with postoperative hemidiaphragmatic paralysis.

Results.—The two groups were comparable in age, mean bypass time, and mean aortic cross-clamp time. All patients in group 1, who received intracoronary cardioplegia only, had continuous maintenance of phrenic nerve function during surgery. In contrast, 3 patients in group 2 had disappearance of phrenic nerve conduction after the heart was immersed in the ice-cold saline solution. The phrenic nerve conduction abnormality was bilateral in 2 patients and affected only the left phrenic nerve in 1. The action potential of the left hemidiaphragm was still absent at the end of surgery in 2 patients. In the other patient, nerve conduction potential returned when the patient was rewarmed.

Conclusions.—Intraoperative CDAP monitoring is a safe and simple technique that permits observation of changes occurring in phrenic nerve conduction during cold cardioplegia. Although cold injury of the phrenic nerve could account for these changes, nerve ischemia is still a possibility. Intraoperative CDAP monitoring can be used to predict which patients will have postoperative diaphragmatic dysfunction. It also can warn the surgeon when the pericardium and surrounding structures are being cooled too much, permitting preventive action.

▶ There is no question that the phrenic nerve can be injured during the cold temperatures used to "preserve" the myocardium during heart surgery. There also is mechanical pressure from packs, traction, and even ice. I am not sure how common phrenic nerve damage really is. Although the authors would have us believe that the complication is common, perhaps they have a vested interest. Intraoperative phrenic nerve monitoring will add complexity and expense, and we will have to decide whether it is worth same.

J.H. Tinker, M.D.

Monitoring Adequacy of α-Adrenoceptor Blockade Following Systemic Phentolamine Administration

Raja SN, Turnquist JL, Meleka S, et al (Johns Hopkins Hosp, Baltimore, Md)
Pain 64:197–204, 1996 5–11

Objective.—Although systemic IV administration of phentolamine has been suggested as a diagnostic test for patients with sympathetically maintained pain (SMP), the dose necessary to block peripheral α-adrenoceptor function is not known. The optimal dose of phentolamine and the safety of this dose in controlling SMP in patients with chronic extremity pain was evaluated in a dose-response study.

Methods.—A total of 130 phentolamine diagnostic tests using 0.5 mg/kg over 20 minutes (n=60) and/or 1 mg/kg over 10 minutes (n=59) were performed in 117 patients (30 men), aged 13 to 79 years, with pain of 1 to 184 months' duration. Eleven patients received no phentolamine. Patients who were given more than 1 phentolamine test received them on separate days. Blood pressure, heart rate, ECG, and skin temperature were monitored before, after, and every 5 minutes during infusion. In 17 patients, skin blood flow was measured using a laser Doppler blood flow monitor. Skin temperature was measured while patients inhaled deeply and held their breath for 5 seconds to elicit sympathetically mediated vasoconstrictor response (SMR).

Results.—Phentolamine caused a significant dose-related increase in skin temperature, with the 1-mg/kg group experiencing a significantly larger increase that either the 0.5-mg/kg group or the untreated group. Blood flow was nonsignificantly lower in the painful extremity compared with the nonpainful extremity. High-dose phentolamine only significantly increased skin blood flow. The change in blood flow was significantly correlated with the change in temperature. The increases in mean blood pressure and heart rate caused by phentolamine were not clinically significant. Both doses of phentolamine mediated, but did not completely relieve, SMR.

Conclusion.—In the phentolamine diagnostic test for SMR, phentolamine at 1 mg/kg over a 10-minute period blocked α-adrenoceptor pain more effectively than phentolamine at 0.5 mg/kg over a 20-minute period.

▶ Although this study enhances our understanding of the effects of IV phentolamine and improves the technical quality of the procedure, it fails to answer a critical question: Of what value is the procedure? Does it predict responses to subsequent therapeutic interventions, such as systemic medications, sympathetic blocks, or sympathectomy? Is it itself therapeutic? Is there a difference in the natural history of pain syndromes based on response to the test? Simply to learn whether a condition is sympathetically mediated is of no help unless the knowledge can direct our treatment toward more successful interventions. Future studies should concentrate on this issue.

S.E. Abram, M.D.

A New Method for Continuous Intramucosal P_{CO_2} Measurement in the Gastrointestinal Tract

Knichwitz G, Rötker J, Brüssel T, et al (Westfälische Wilhelms-Universität, Münster, Germany)

Anesth Analg 83:6–11, 1996 5–12

Introduction.—The problem of partial pressure of carbon dioxide (P_{CO_2}) instability in the tonometric fluid can be solved by finding the direct determination of P_{CO_2} using a fiberoptic P_{CO_2} sensor, which can continuously measure P_{CO_2} in blood. A fiberoptic P_{CO_2} sensor would determine the P_{CO_2} of certain fluid better than conventional tonometry. Such a sensor would determine P_{CO_2} continuously and avoid equilibration times. Variations in arterial and mesenteric venous P_{CO_2} would have good correlation to the intramucosal P_{CO_2} values.

Methods.—A thermocouple for determining temperature, a miniaturized Clark electrode for determining partial pressure of oxygen (P_{O_2}), and 2 modified optical fibers for measuring P_{CO_2} and pH are the components of the fiberoptic P_{CO_2} sensor. The device is 0.5 mm in diameter and has a length of 600 mm. The in vitro experiment determined the P_{CO_2} of water and humidified air with predefined P_{CO_2} values using the fiberoptic P_{CO_2} sensor and a nasogastric tonometer. The function of the fiberoptic P_{CO_2} sensor was determined in fluids comparable to the medium within the gastrointestinal tract in an in vitro experiment. The performance of the fiberoptic P_{CO_2} sensor was evaluated in the gastrointestinal tract of 6 female pigs in the in vivo experiment. Determinations were made on cardiac index, arterial P_{CO_2}, mesenteric venous P_{CO_2}, and intramucosal

TABLE 1.—Mean and 2 SD of Partial Pressure of Carbon Dioxide Differences After 30, 60, and 90 Minutes of Equilibration Time with Three Different Carbon Dioxide Concentrations

		P_{CO_2} difference (measured-predefined) (mean ± 2 SD in mm Hg)		
			Fiberoptic P_{CO_2} sensor	
Predefined P_{CO_2}*	Equilibration time (min)	Nasogastic tonometer	In water	In air
CO_2 5.0%, 34.8–35.6 mm Hg	30	−10.4 ± 2.6	0.0 ± 0.8	0.5 ± 0.4
	60	−6.7 ± 0.9	0.0 ± 0.8	0.5 ± 0.1
	90	−4.8 ± 1.6	0.1 ± 0.8	0.5 ± 0.2
CO_2 6.0%, 41.9–42.8 mm Hg	30	−10.3 ± 2.5	0.8 ± 0.4	1.0 ± 0.6
	60	−7.5 ± 0.4	0.9 ± 0.4	1.0 ± 0.5
	90	−5.2 ± 0.8	1.0 ± 0.4	0.9 ± 0.5
CO_2 7.0%, 48.8–50.1 mm Hg	30	−12.3 ± 3.9	0.9 ± 0.2	0.8 ± 0.4
	60	−8.5 ± 0.4	1.0 ± 0.4	0.9 ± 0.4
	90	−5.8 ± 0.7	1.0 ± 0.4	0.9 ± 0.3

Note: N = 4. Differences are measured minus predefined value.

*Predefined partial pressure of carbon dioxide values are calculated and corrected for water vapor saturation and actual barometric pressure.

Abbreviation: P_{CO_2}, partial pressure of carbon dioxide.

(Courtesy of Knichwitz G, Rötker J, Brüssel T, et al: A new method for continuous intramucosal P_{CO_2} measurements in the gastrointestinal tract. *Anesth Analg* 83:6–11, 1996.)

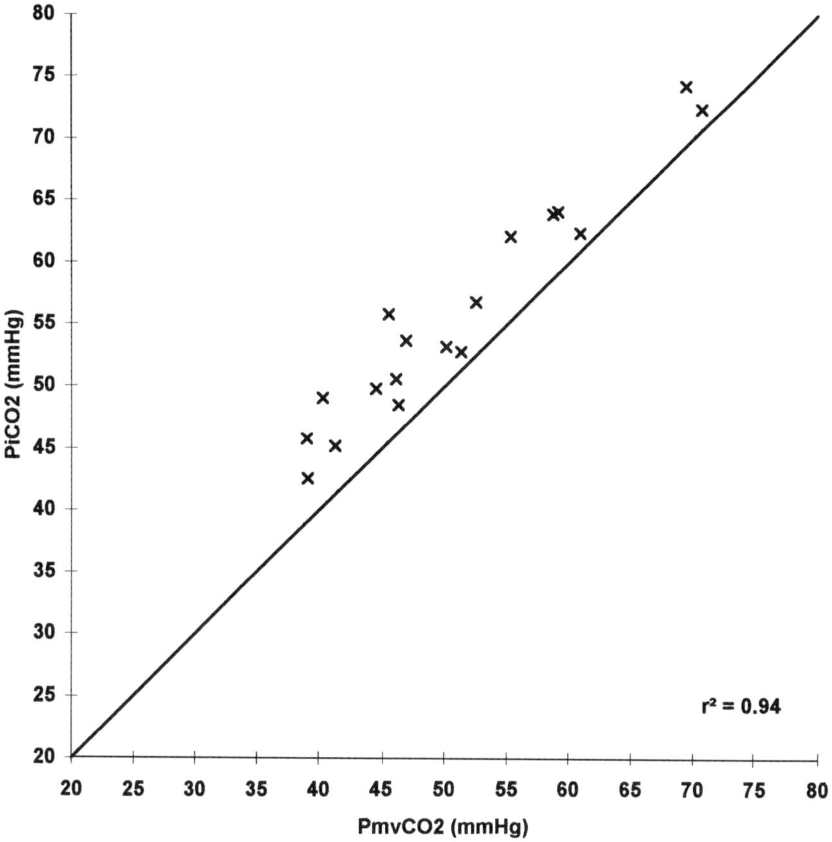

FIGURE 4.—Correlation between mesenteric venous P_{CO_2} (Pmvco2) and intramucosal P_{CO_2} (Pico2) after ventilatory changes ($r^2 = 0.94$). Abbreviation: P_{CO_2}, partial pressure of carbon dioxide. (Courtesy of Knichwitz G, Rötker J, Brüssel T, et al: A new method for continuous intramucosal P_{CO_2} measurements in the gastrointestinal tract. *Anesth Analg* 83:6–11, 1996.)

P_{CO_2} after preparation and 60 minutes of steady state conditions. Variables were also measured after 10 minutes of hypoventilation and after 10 minutes of hyperventilation.

Results.—After 30, 60, and 90 minutes of equilibration for the 3 different gas concentrations, absolute P_{CO_2} differences between predefined and measured P_{CO_2} values were made (Table 1). After 9 minutes of equilibration with a maximum deviation less than 3.5%, predefined carbon dioxide values of 35, 42, and 49 mm Hg could be assessed in water and humidified air. Tonometry P_{CO_2} had greater differences from the predefined P_{CO_2} than with the fiberoptic P_{CO_2} sensor. In the in vivo experiment during hypoventilation, the intramucosal P_{CO_2} increased from 53.8 ± 2.0 mm Hg to 66.5 ± 4.9 mm Hg. Arterial P_{CO_2} went from 39.8 ± 1.4 mm Hg to 52.7 ± 31. mm Hg. Mesenteric venous P_{CO_2} increased from 48.7 ± 2.7 mm Hg to 62.4 ± 5.7 mm. With hyperventilation, the intramucosal P_{CO_2} decreased to 46.8 ± 2.5 mm Hg. The coefficient of correlation was 0.82 between intramucosal PCO_2 and arterial PCO_2. It was 0.94 between intramucosal PCO_2 and mesenteric venous PCO_2 (Fig 4).

Conclusion.—Intramucosal PCO_2 can be determined in a precise and reliable manner with the fiberoptic PCO_2 sensor. Fast intraluminal changes of carbon dioxide in the ileum caused by ventilatory changes can be continuously recorded with this sensor. In the gastrointestinal tract, the fiberoptic PCO_2 sensor is the only method that reliably monitors intramucosal PCO_2.

▶ This article would appear to represent cutting edge technology in the field of gastric tonometry, eliminating calibration and equilibration error. I will anxiously await future clinical studies in critically ill patients.

D.M. Rothenberg, M.D.

Oscillometric Blood Pressure Measurements by Different Devices Are Not Interchangeable

Kaufmann MA, Pargger H, Drop LJ (Massachusetts Gen Hosp, Boston; Harvard Med School, Boston)

Anesth Analg 82:377–381, 1996 5–13

Introduction.—Blood pressure (BP) values measured by noninvasive blood pressure (NIBP) monitors may appear to be interchangeable. However, their concordance has not been established. A wide range of BP values were obtained by 3 different oscillometric NIBP devices in 25 consecutive patients admitted for electroconvulsive therapy (ECT) for major depression.

Methods.—All BP measurements were taken in the supine position. Blood pressure was measured simultaneously on the right and left arms. Dinamap (DIN), SpaceLabs (SpL), and Marquette (Marq) devices were used to measure BP with simultaneous measurements taken in 3 sets: DIN and DIN, SpL and DIN, and Marq and DIN. Agreement between devices was measured according to American Association for Advancement of Medical Instrumentation guidelines. Blood pressures were measured frequently during induction of anesthesia and after termination of ECT in 4 consecutive treatments.

Results.—In the DIN–DIN set, no significant differences existed for diastolic blood pressure (DBP), systolic blood pressure (SBP), and mean BP. Significant differences did exist in DBP, SBP, and mean BP for the SpL–DIN and Marq–DIN comparisons.

Conclusion.—Oscillometric BP measurements obtained by the 3 NIBP devices evaluated were not interchangeable. Which device was the most accurate was not determined. Comparisons were not made with a standard sphygmomanometer. The 3 different NIBP devices used were considered to track accurate perturbations in BP.

▶ The key points in measuring blood pressure are both the absolute levels and how accurately changes are measured. The authors show that one out of three of the times the systolic blood pressure is different by more than 10 mL of mercury, and even the mean blood pressure is different by 10 mL of mercury in 25% of situations with different diseases. Nevertheless, they say that the changes in blood pressure recorded by one device tracked with the changes recorded in the other. This seems to be a key point as most of us acutely measure the degree of stability or lack of stability by the change rather than the absolute level. Clearly, however, chronically taken blood pressure is very important. One wonders which was the accurate monitor, and how we know when the true blood pressure steps forward.

M.F. Roizen, M.D.

Anesthesia-Related Techniques

A Trigonometric Analysis of Needle Redirection and Needle Position During Neural Block

Horlocker TT (Mayo Clinic, Rochester, Minn)
Reg Anesth 21:30–34, 1996 5–14

Purpose.—Three-dimensional anatomical visualization is needed for successful regional anesthesia. If the needle is not placed correctly the first time, it may have to be withdrawn, redirected, and readvanced. A logical approach to needle redirection should be followed to minimize the number of readjustments. The relation between needle insertion angle and needle position was evaluated trigonometrically.

Methods.—A computer model was used to determine needle position during the advancement of 2-, 3.5-, and 5-inch needles. The model then calculated the change in needle position resulting from decreasing needle position from 90 degrees in 5- and 10-degree increments. The needle depths considered ranged from 0.5 to 11.0 cm.

Results.—A 5-degree redirection produced significantly less change in needle position than a 10-degree redirection. Needle depth and acute angle of needle insertion were strongly related to the change in needle position.

Conclusions.—In performing neural block, a 5-degree needle redirection produces about one half the change in needle position that a 10-degree redirection does. Thus, a 5-degree redirection permits a precise survey of neural structure and adjacent anatomy. In contrast, a 10-degree redirection may result in "walking over" the desired neural structure. To achieve appropriate needle exploration with minimal trauma, the shortest needle suited for the regional anesthetic procedure should be used.

► This article presents an interesting computer analysis of the degree of redirection one needs to get a particular degree of change in needle tip position. Those who frequently perform regional anesthesia are advised to read this study because it may help explain the change and angle you need in redirection.

M.F. Roizen, M.D.

Virtual Bronchoscopy

Virtual Bronchoscopy: Relationships of Virtual Reality Endobronchial Simulations to Actual Bronchoscopic Findings

Vining DJ, Liu K, Choplin RH, et al (Bowman-Gray School of Medicine, Winston-Salem, NC)

Chest 109:549–553, 1996 5–15

Purpose.—Computer technology is now available to convert helical chest CT imaging data into simulations of the internal and external tracheobronchial tree. The endobronchial view available with bronchoscopy can be reproduced using real-time three-dimensional (30) techniques; however, no previous reports have described the associations between the 3D images and the actual bronchoscopic results. The results of "virtual bronchoscopy" in simulating the tracheobronchial tree were compared with the actual anatomy of the airways, as viewed by videotaped bronchoscopy.

Methods.—The analysis included virtual bronchoscopic images created using helical CT data from 20 patients with various pathologic conditions. All CT images were scanned and transferred to a computer work station at which a 3D simulation of the tracheobronchial tree was made. The simulations were displayed in colors simulating the general appearance of the mucosa and as if the viewer were looking down the trachea. The viewer was able to change the perspective to that obtained when the position of the bronchoscope is moved within an actual airway. The simulations were compared with videotaped bronchoscopic examinations performed in

TABLE 1.—Bronchoscopically Confirmed Endobronchial Abnormalities Correctly Demonstrated by Virtual Bronchoscopy Simulations in 10 Patients

Right middle lobe obstruction by tumor (1)
Complete right upper lobe occlusion and eccentric narrowing, bronchus intermedius, by tumor (1)
Concentric narrowing, bronchus intermedius, with middle lobe narrowing by tumor (1)
Tracheal distortion, right upper lobe retraction and ectasia (previous tuberculosis) (1)
Two accessory bronchi, right upper lobe (1)
Right upper lobe compression, with crescentic narrowing due to calcified mediastinal lymph nodes (1)
Concentric narrowing, left upper lobe apical-posterior segment, by tumor (1)
Diffuse ectasia (both patients with previous granulomatous disease and bronchiectasis) (2)
Left mainstem bronchial narrowing, left upper lobe occlusion by tumor (1)

(Courtesy of Vining DJ, Liu K, Choplin RH, et al: Virtual bronchoscopy: Relationships of virtual reality endobronchial simulations to actual bronchoscopic findings. *Chest* 109:549–553, 1996.)

each patient. The comparison focused on the clinically significant abnormalities as well as the characteristic landmarks.

Results.—Acceptable simulations were achieved in 10 patients. A number of different endobronchial abnormalities were demonstrated by virtual bronchoscopy, including airway obstruction by tumor, tortuosity and ectasia of the tracheobronchial tree, and anatomical variants (Table 1). The results of virtual bronchoscopy were confirmed at actual bronchoscopy.

Conclusions.—Virtual bronchoscopy can provide excellent simulations of bronchial abnormalities, confirming the findings of actual clinically indicated bronchoscopic examinations. Although the economics and technology of virtual bronchoscopy are currently prohibitive, these problems will be overcome within the next decade. The speed of image data processing will be an important obstacle to overcome—the cases described in this study totaled about 100 megabytes.

▶ I imagine that having skills in virtual bronchoscopy will come in handy one day when, because of extraneous pressures on the field of anesthesiology, we will all be practicing "virtual anesthesia!"

D.M. Rothenberg, M.D.

Force of Laryngoscopy

Force and Torque Vary Between Laryngoscopists and Laryngoscope Blades

Hastings RH, Hon ED, Nghiem C, et al (Univ of California San Diego)
Anesth Analg 82:462–468, 1996 5–16

Background.—Although several researchers have studied the effects of patient characteristics on the force of laryngoscopy, few have investigated the importance of technique and equipment. Whether laryngoscopic force and torque vary significantly among different laryngoscopists was determined and the effects of laryngoscopic technique were documented.

Methods.—Fifty-eight adults scheduled for elective surgery requiring general anesthesia with endotracheal tube placement were studied. All were American Society of Anesthesiologists grade I or II. Force, torque, head extension, and view among laryngoscopists were studied, and force and torque using Macintosh 3 and Miller 2 blades were compared.

Findings.—When laryngoscopy was repeated by 1 individual, force, torque, head extension, and laryngeal view were highly reproducible. When different anesthetists were compared, however, force and torque varied greatly. Peak force, which varied over a range of 56 newtons among patients, also varied as much as 30 newtons among different anesthetists performing laryngoscopies on the same patient. Force and head extension with the Miller laryngoscope were 30% less than with the Macintosh.

Conclusions.—Laryngoscopic force, torque, and head extension vary according to technique and equipment. Additional research on force and torque may help improve techniques. The force-measuring laryngoscope may be useful in the teaching of laryngoscopy.

▶ I think the most important point here is that the force-measuring laryngoscope could be a useful tool in teaching anesthesia. It is clear to me that force and torque vary significantly between experienced laryngoscopists. For example, peak force differed as much as 3-fold between experienced laryngoscopists repeating laryngoscopy in the same patients; thus, one is compelled to conclude that force and torque depend on anesthesiologist technique and that the use of this versus the gentleness in handling tissue vary significantly even among experienced laryngoscopists. I guess that is the same as we see in surgeons, some of whom handle tissue gently and recovery is predictably quick and easy, and some of whom handle tissue roughly.

M.F. Roizen, M.D.

Ultrathin Endotracheal Tube

New Ultrathin-walled Endotracheal Tube With a Novel Laryngeal Seal Design: Long-term Evaluation in Sheep

Reali-Forster C, Kolobow T, Giacomini M, et al (Natl Heart, Lung, and Blood Inst, Bethesda, Md)

Anesthesiology 84:162–172, 1996 5–17

Introduction.—Tracheal stenosis, aspiration, and resistance to gas flow are among the serious adverse effects of tracheal intubation, especially prolonged intubation. A new ultrathin-walled 2-stage endotracheal tube (ETT) has been developed in an attempt to reduce these risks. The new tube replaces the tracheal cuff with a no-pressure sealing system positioned within the larynx that eliminates cuff pressure on the tracheal wall. The ETT segment within the glottis is oval-shaped, which is more consistent with the natural outline of the glottic opening (Fig 1). Finally, the tube's wall thickness is only 0.2 mm, which reduces flow resistance to levels comparable with those of the normal upper airway. The advantages of the new ultrathin-walled ETT were evaluated in a randomized study in sheep.

Methods.—Anesthetized, paralyzed sheep were randomized to mechanical ventilation with the new ETT or a standard ETT with hi–lo cuffs. The results were assessed in terms of airway leakage, aspiration, and adverse effects on the trachea and larynx.

Results.—Neither group showed any tracheal air leaks at 1 or 3 days of ventilation at peak inspiratory pressures of up to 40 cm H_2O. Short- and long-term studies showed no evidence of aspiration in animals with the new ETT, whereas signs of aspiration were present in some animals intubated with the standard ETT. Laryngotracheal erosion was noted in some sheep receiving the standard ETT for 1 day; those with the new ETT had only mucosal erythema or edema or both. Vocal cord edema was more common with the standard ETT. After 3 days of intubation, the trachea was better preserved with the new ETT. One day of intubation led to

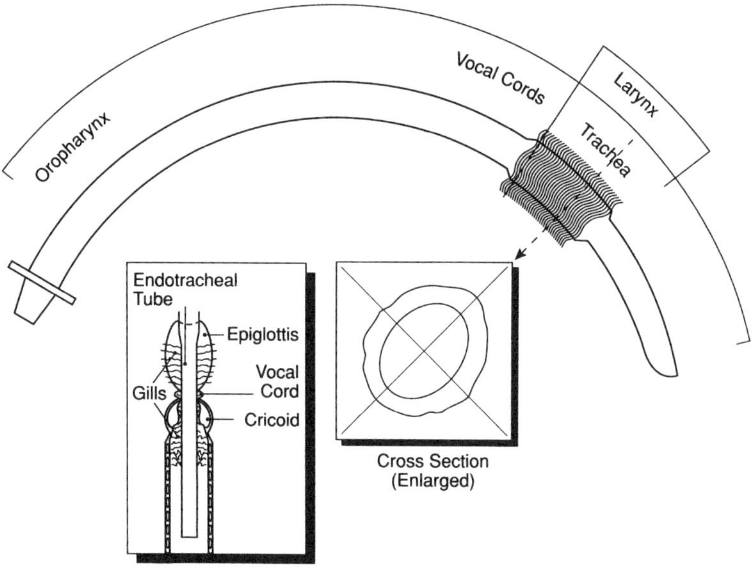

FIGURE 1.—The ultrathin-walled two-staged endotracheal tube (ETT). The approximate midsection of the ETT labeled "larynx" is positioned at the level of the glottic opening. Hence, some of the "gills" will be above and some will be below the level of the vocal cords; the optimal position is midway (*insert*). Gills that pass across the glottic opening commonly are somewhat folded. (Courtesy of Reali-Forster C, Kolobow T, Giacomini M, et al: New ultra-thin endotracheal tube with a novel laryngeal seal design. *Anesthesiology* 84:162–172, 1996.)

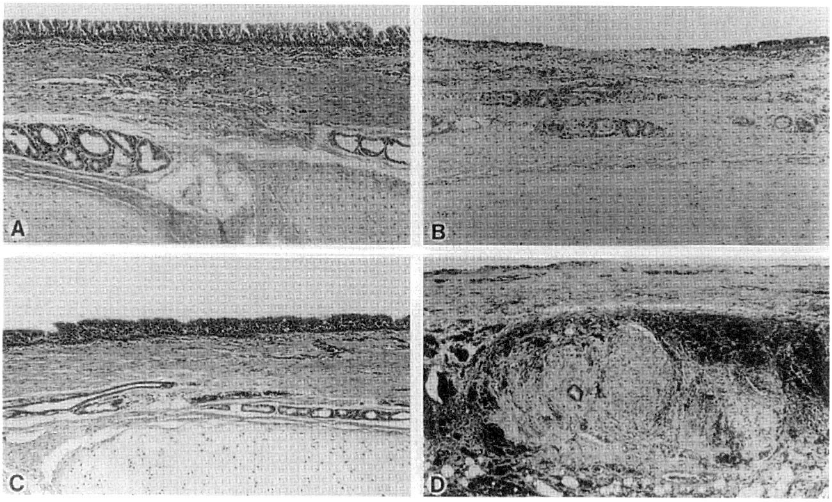

FIGURE 4.—Representative sections from trachea of sheep intubated with the new ETT or the standard ETT for 1 or 3 days; hematoxylin and esosin stain. Original magnification x160. **A,** 1-day intubation, new ETT. The epithelium is mostly intact. Tissue reaction is minimal. **B,** 1-day intubation, standard ETT. Widespread epithelial erosion is present with minimal tissue reaction. **C,** 3-day intubation, new ETT. Epithelium is intact. There is no submucosal hemorrhage or edema. **D,** 3-day intubation, standard ETT. Area in contact with the cuff shows wide epithelial erosion. Note severe submucosal hemorrhage. (Courtesy of Reali-Forster C, Kolobow T, Giacomini M. et al: New ultra-thin endotracheal tube with a novel laryngeal seal design. *Anesthesiology* 84:162–172, 1996.)

significantly milder tracheal epithelial injury with the ultrathin-walled ETT than with the standard ETT. The newer tube was associated with intact tracheal epithelium and no evidence of erosion, no edema or hemorrhage, and only mild to moderate neutrophil infiltration (Fig 4).

Conclusions.—The new ultrathin-walled ETT, with its no-pressure seal design, appears to prevent air leak and aspiration while reducing tracheal injury. Elimination of the tracheal cuff is the logical approach to reducing tracheal damage. The avoidance of aspiration should help reduce the occurrence of nosocomial pneumonia.

▶ This new ultrathin-walled, nonkinking, ETT was first described in 1994[1] with emphasis placed on its low-pressure sealing system (the so-called gills) designed to eliminate tracheal damage resulting from ETT cuff pressure. These gills may also decrease the incidence of nosocomial pneumonia by trapping bacterially infected secretions that are often silently aspirated. In addition, the thinner wall decreases intraluminal resistance to such an extent that it approximates the normal resistance of the upper airway. Although I'm greatly encouraged by the histopathologic results cited in this article, I do not believe that the authors have performed a true long-term study that can be extrapolated, as of yet, to patients in the ICU who often require more than 3 days of mechanical ventilation.

D.M. Rothenberg, M.D.

Reference

1. Kolobow T, Rossi N, Tsuno K, et al: Design and development of ultrathin-walled nonkinking endotracheal tubes of a new "no pressure" laryngeal seal design. *Anesthesiology* 81:1061–1067, 1994.

Spinal Needle Tip After Puncture

Microscopic Analysis of the Tips of Thin Spinal Needles After Subarachnoid Puncture

Rosenberg PH, Pitkänen MT, Hakala P, et al (Helsinki Univ)

Reg Anesth 21:35–40, 1996 5–18

Objective.—It has been suggested that particles from the skin and underlying tissues could pass into the subarachnoid space when spinal needles are used for subarachnoid puncture. Three different types of spinal needles are currently used: the Quincke-type tip with sharp cutting bevel, the sharp 2-zone bevel tip, and the pencil-point tip. These 3 types of needles were compared for adherence of foreign material after subarachnoid puncture.

Methods.—Subarachnoid puncture was performed in human cadavers using 3 types of spinal needles: a 27-gauge Quincke needle, a 26-gauge 2-zone bevel needle, and a 27-gauge Sprotte or pencil-point needle. After the subarachnoid space was penetrated, the needle types were cut through the open spinal canal. They were then prepared for fluorescence microscopy.

Results.—When the pencil-point needles were used without an introducer, considerably more strength had to be exerted to achieve skin puncture than with the other types of needles. Almost all needles of all 3 types showed fluorescence and attached small particles. Quincke needles showed the largest particles. Many needle tips—especially the 2-zone bevel needles—were bent or hooked after subarachnoid puncture. Bone or hard metal contacts occurring during needle insertion were not recorded. Both attached material and bent tips occurred least frequently with pencil-point needles. Nerve root perforation occurred in a few cases.

Conclusions.—Foreign material frequently adheres to spinal needles used for subarachnoid puncture. Bent needle tips also appear to be common. Both these findings may be least frequent with pencil-point needles. Occasional nerve root perforation also occurs, although neurologic sequelae of spinal puncture are rare.

▶ This study is ingenious. It is done in cadavers and highlights 2 potential problems of spinal needles: first, bending of the needles, and second, carrying by the needles of microscopic particles or foreign material into the subarachnoid space. We often wondered why some individuals are not very good at performing spinals—one reason may be because they use so much pressure that they bend the needles. This study would say that those who tend to have problems with spinal puncture might have better results with pencil-point needles. On the other hand, at least 6 of 8 of each of the needle tips carried microscopic particles into the spinal canal.

Perhaps the most interesting observation by these authors was that in 3 of the 24 needle insertions, a nerve root was perforated, indicating that easily passed sharp needles may puncture nervous tissue in humans. Does this happen, or is a cadaver different from freely floating nerves in spinal fluid, and do patient responses make this unlikely to happen in clinical practice? Like most good studies, this one raises more questions than it answers.

M.F. Roizen, M.D.

Metal Particles After Needle-Through-Needle

No Additional Metal Particle Formation Using the Needle-through-needle Combined Epidural/Spinal Technique

Herman N, Molin J, Knape KG (Univ of Texas Health Science Ctr, San Antonio)

Acta Anaesthesiol Scand 40:227–231, 1996 5–19

Background.—The needle-through-needle technique of combined epidural/spinal analgesia has gained popularity, especially for use in obstetrics. However, there is concern about whether metal fragments are deposited in the epidural space, considering the concave deformities occurring at the orifice of Tuohy needles after spinal passage. Whether metallic flecks are produced by the needle-through-needle technique was studied.

Methods.—Ten unused Tuohy and Hustead epidural needles were photomicrographed, then saline was flushed through each and into a single tissue culture well. A 120-mm, 24-gauge Sprotte needle was then single-passed through each now-dry epidural needle to maximal extension while the orifice was within another tissue culture well. The needles were flushed into a third well, then were re-examined microscopically. Microscopic examination for metallic particles was done on each of the wells.

Results.—Photomicrographs taken before and after the needle experiments were compared, revealing concave deformities at the orifice of all the needles tested. No metallic particles were observed in any of the wells. Inspection of unused Tuohy needles exposed to a magnetic field revealed that metal filings "stood up" along the bevel of every needle examined.

Conclusions.—All epidural needles appear to be contaminated with metal particles, although these particles appear adherent enough to resist dislodging with a saline flush. Their tendency to dislodge into tissue during needle placement is not known, but use of the needle-through-needle technique does not appear to confer any additional risk.

► This is a clever study documenting that 1 of our concerns—fragmentation of the Tuohy needle after spinal needle passage—is perhaps unfounded.

M.F. Roizen, M.D.

Anesthesia Technique Effects on CABG Recovery

The Effects of Anesthetic Technique on the Hemodynamic Response and Recovery Profile in Coronary Revascularization Patients

Mora CT, Dudek C, Torjman MC, et al (Emory Univ, Atlanta, Ga; Thomas Jefferson Univ, Philadelphia; Univ of Texas, Dallas)

Anesth Analg 81:900–910, 1995 5–20

Background.—Inhalation anesthetics have been proposed as the best strategy for achieving early extubation after cardiac surgery. Propofol is a rapid, short-acting IV sedative-hypnotic agent that may be an alternative to volatile inhalation agents for anesthesia during cardiac surgery. Recovery times and intraoperative hemodynamic stability were compared in patients receiving propofol or 1 of 3 other agents for maintenance of anesthesia during coronary artery revascularization surgery.

Methods.—Ninety patients undergoing elective coronary artery bypass grafting underwent anesthesia induction with fentanyl, after which anesthesia was maintained with 1 of 4 agents: enflurane, fentanyl, propofol, or thiopental. The study drugs were administered via the extracorporeal circuit and were titrated to maintain mean arterial pressure values within 10% of the baseline values or between 65 and 95 mm Hg. Systolic, diastolic, and mean systemic and pulmonary arterial pressures, as well as central venous pressure and heart rate values, were monitored continually perioperatively. Recovery was assessed by determining the time at which patients opened their eyes, responded to verbal communication, and responded correctly to specific commands.

Results.—No significant differences occurred among the groups in the amount of time required to re-establish blood pressure and heart rate control or the duration of hypotension. However, the propofol group experienced significantly shorter durations of intraoperative hypertension than the other 3 groups. Vasopressor support before cardiopulmonary bypass was required more frequently in the propofol and fentanyl groups, whereas the fentanyl group required the most vasoconstrictor therapy and the propofol group required the least frequent inotropic drug support before weaning from cardiopulmonary bypass. Patients in the propofol group opened their eyes before patients in the fentanyl and thiopental groups and responded to verbal stimuli and correctly responded to commands earlier than patients in all of the other 3 groups. Tracheal extubation occurred significantly sooner in the propofol and enflurane groups than in the fentanyl and thiopental groups.

Conclusions.—Maintenance anesthesia with propofol permits rapid increase in the depth of anesthesia and also facilitates rapid recovery after coronary artery revascularization without affecting intraoperative hemodynamic stability.

► The authors found that addition of propofol during anesthesia for coronary bypass allowed better "fast-tracking" of these patients and that the cost savings of fast-tracking might offset the increased costs of the propofol. When I see numbers less than $50 per case, and I read extensive and elegantly done studies comparing costs at this level, I believe that there must be a "500-pound gorilla" here somewhere, but I do not think it has much to do with costs at the $50 level.

The famed business strategist C.K. Prahalad talks about "denominator management," that is, cutting costs as ways of improving the bottom line, as opposed to "competing for the future," which means developing new products, new innovations, new markets, etc. This type of study strikes me as the epitome of the current fad, namely, let's cut costs, no matter how unimportant they might be, because there is immediate bottom-line benefit, however small. Maybe we could do outpatient open hearts? Just get the relatives to massage the chest tubes? Doesn't anybody out there but me believe that cost-cutting is boring and nonprogressive as long-term strategy?

J.H. Tinker, M.D.

Needle Comparisons: Leakage After Dural Puncture

An *In Vitro* Comparison of Fluid Leakage After Dural Puncture With Atraucan, Sprotte, Whitacre, and Quincke Needles

Morrison LMM, McCrae AF, Foo I, et al (St John's Hosp at Howden, Livingston, Scotland)

Reg Anesth 21:139–143, 1996 5–21

Background.—Postdural puncture headache appears to be related to the characteristics of the needle used to puncture the dura. Two new needle tip designs—the Sprotte and the Atraucan—have been described in the past 5

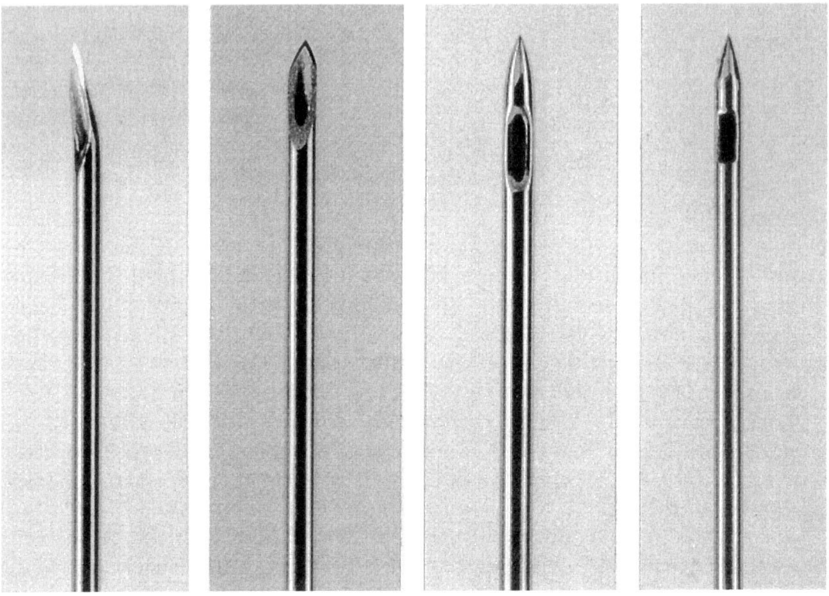

FIGURE 1.—From left to right the 4 needles tested are the Atraucan, Quincke, Sprotte, and Whitacre tip designs. (Courtesy of Morrison LMM, McCrae AF, Foo I, et al: An *in vitro* comparison of fluid leakage after dural puncture with Atraucan, Sprotte, Whitacre, and Quincke needles. *Reg Anesth* 21:139–143, 1996.)

years. The transdural leakage rates that have resulted from these new needle designs were compared.

Methods.—Sprotte (24- and 26-gauge), Atraucan (24- and 26-gauge), Quincke (26- and 29-gauge), and Whitacre (22- and 25-gauge) needles were tested in an in vitro model and fresh human lumbar dura (Fig 1). The

TABLE 1.—Transdural Fluid Leakage Rates

		Median (range) of Leakage Rates (mL/min)	
Needle	Gauge	Group 1 (CSF)	Group 2 (Saline)
Quincke	26	0.61 (0.00–6.11)	1.49 (0.00–5.90)
Quincke	29	0.06 (0.00–2.95)*	0.52 (0.00–3.40)*
Sprotte	24	0.65 (0.00–5.36)	0.93 (0.03–5.20)*
Sprotte	26	—	0.50 (0.00–3.20)
Whitacre	22	—	2.26 (0.02–6.80)*
Whitacre	25	—	0.68 (0.00–3.80)
Atraucan (long)	24	0.75 (0.00–11.05)	—
Atraucan (long)	26	0.17 (0.00–2.74)*	—
Atraucan (short)	26	0.33 (0.00–5.99)	—

*In group 1, the Quincke 29-gauge leaked significantly less than the Quincke 26-gauge ($P < 0.05$), and the 26-gauge long Atraucan leaked significantly less than the 24-gauge ($P < 0.05$). In group 2, the Quincke 29-gauge leaked significantly less than the Quincke 26-gauge ($P = 0.0023$), the 22-gauge Whitacre leaked significantly more than the 25-gauge Whitacre ($P = 0.001$), and the 24-gauge Sprotte leaked significantly more than the 26-gauge Sprotte ($P = 0.03$).

(Courtesy of Morrison LMM, McCrae AF, Foo I, et al: An *in vitro* comparison of fluid leakage after dural puncture with Atraucan, Sprotte, Whitacre, and Quincke needles. *Reg Anesth* 21:139–143, 1996.)

Sprotte is a modification of the Whitacre conical point design, and the Atraucan is a modified Huber point.

Findings.—The finer-gauge needles tended to result in less leakage. Traditional Quincke pattern bevels were associated with more leakage than pencil-point designs of the same diameter (Table 1).

Conclusions.—The rate of transdural fluid leakage in this in vitro model was associated with needle size and bevel design. These findings are consistent with observations on the incidence of postdural puncture headache in clinical practice. The leakage rate of the new Atraucan needle is comparable to that of pencil point needles. This needle design may also have other advantages.

▶ These authors constructed an innovative test apparatus in which human lumbar dura, obtained at autopsy, was stretched and mounted in a test frame that allowed leakage of liquid to be collected and measured carefully. The authors tested several of the fancy new needles, including 2 "pencil point" versions—the Sprotte and the Whitacre. The needle of most interest to the authors was called the Atraucan. I cannot find any evidence in this report that the study was sponsored by commercial interests in favor of the Atraucan needle, although the authors came down more or less in favor of the Atraucan. The data they report are confusing, to say the least. Suffice it to say that these new needles do leak a lot less than the Quincke of the past.

J.H. Tinker, M.D.

6 Complications, Mishaps, and Other Perioperative Trouble

Complications With Regional Anesthesia/Analgesia

High Sensory Block After Intrathecal Sufentanil for Labor Analgesia
Hamilton CL, Cohen SE (Stanford Univ, Calif)
Anesthesiology 83:1118–1121, 1995 6–1

Background.—Intrathecal opioids for labor analgesia have become popular. Few complications have been reported. Six women experiencing a high sensory "block" after intrathecal sufentanil for labor analgesia are discussed.

Case Reports.—The women were in active labor with a term, singleton, vertex fetus. Five patients were healthy, and 1 was obese with mild pregnancy-induced hypertension. Intrathecal sufentanil was administered to all women as part of a combined spinal-epidural procedure. The lumbar epidural space was identified in sitting patients with a loss-of-resistance technique using an 18-G Tuohy needle. Sufentanil, 10 µg, diluted to 1 or 2 mL with preservative-free saline, was injected intrathecally through a 120-mm or 127-mm 24-G pencil-point spinal needle in 5 women and a 120-mm 25-G Quincke needle in 1. The needles were introduced through the 18-G needle. After the spinal needle was withdrawn, a 20-G epidural catheter was threaded into the epidural space. Painless uterine contractions were achieved in all women soon after injection. Woman, 26, reported itching on her face and an inability to swallow ten minutes after injection. She was found to have a bilateral sensory block to cold and pinprick, from T3 to S3. By 35 minutes after injection, the sensory changes had stopped. Woman, 30, reported facial and lip tingling 10 minutes after injection; she had reduced sensation bilaterally to cold on her legs, abdomen, and thorax to a T4 level on the right and V3 on the left. Woman, 32, had mild hypertension and reported facial and upper arm numbness and difficulty swallowing 25 minutes after injection. Woman, 20, 2 minutes after infusion was begun, sat up abruptly and screamed that she could not breathe; she became agitated, the infusion was stopped, and oxygen was administered. Her airway was unobstructed, and there was no evidence of motor block. Sensory block was not checked. She was agitated for 10 minutes, when she reported dry throat and inability to swallow. Subsequently, her epidural catheter was removed and, at her request, was not replaced. Woman, 30, reported facial tingling with no other symptoms. Woman, 35, described unilateral facial numbness.

Conclusions.—Potent intrathecal opioids should be administered cautiously. Doses should not exceed those shown to be effective. Patients must be monitored carefully, especially in the first hour after intrathecal injection.

▶ Some anesthesiologists have embraced intrathecal opioid analgesia because of a belief that this technique results in fewer complications—and requires less vigilance—than epidural analgesia. This series of 6 cases suggests that such optimism is unfounded. There is a growing awareness that intrathecal opioid analgesia—even small doses of a lipid-soluble opioid—is not as innocuous as first thought. The authors of this series urged "caution when potent intrathecal opioids are administered for labor analgesia." They correctly emphasized: "Careful monitoring of patients is indicated, particularly in the first hour after injection."

D.H. Chestnut, M.D.

A Case of Coronary Artery Spasm During Spinal Anesthesia

Imamura M, Matsukawa T, Kashimoto S, et al (Yamanashi Med Univ, Japan)
J Clin Anesth 8:522–524, 1996 6–2

Introduction.—Although there have been many reports of coronary artery spasm during general anesthesia or general plus epidural anesthesia, this event is rare during spinal anesthesia. A case of coronary artery spasm was described that appears to have been induced by spinal anesthesia.

Case Report.—Man, 42, was admitted for treatment of a left testicular tumor. Laboratory findings were normal, as were the results of chest radiography, ECG, and physical examination. The patient was not premedicated before undergoing left testectomy. A spinal block was performed at the L2-3 interspace. The injected dose, 2.6 mL of a mixture of 0.24% dibucaine and 0.12% tetracaine solution, created a block extending to T8.

Coronary artery spasm was suspected about 50 minutes into the operation, when blood pressure (BP) suddenly fell to 80/48 mm

Hg, heart rate was 62 bpm, and ECG exhibited remarkable elevation of the ST segment in lead II. Within 5 minutes of treatment with oxygen, ephedrine, and a nitroglycerin infusion, BP and the ST segment elevation gradually returned to normal. The patient did not complain of chest pain during the episode, and postoperative studies ruled out myocardial infarction.

Discussion.—The previously reported case of coronary artery spasm attributed to spinal anesthesia involved a patient with primary hyperparathyroidism. In the present case, the patient had no pre-existing medical conditions that might have contributed to the event, and there were no perioperative complications. The episode was preceded by a complaint of upper back pain when the peritoneum was retracted. The coronary artery spasm may have resulted from a combination of activation of the parasympathetic nervous system by retraction of the peritoneum and spinal anesthesia. Anesthesiologists should be aware of the possibility of coronary artery spasm during spinal anesthesia and have ready access to nitroglycerin.

► There are several different kinds of episodic spasms that occur in clinical medicine, including migraine headaches, asthma, and coronary spasm. I happen to have some degree of asthma and have had asthma "attacks" at all hours of the day and night, during all kinds of activity or inactivity. I have long wondered why spasmodic attacks such as these occur when they do. The authors contend that retraction of the peritoneum in this case plus blockage of the sympathetic nervous system by the spinal anesthetic may well have triggered the coronary spasm. Who knows? All I know is that episodic spasmodic disease, as a part of the history, should raise various red flags up the pole for clinical anesthesiologists.

J.H. Tinker, M.D.

Paraplegia, Epidural Analgesia, and Thoracic Aneurysmectomy
Fitzgibbon DR, Glosten B, Wright I, et al (Univ of Washington, Seattle)
Anesthesiology 83:1355–1359, 1995 6–3

Objective.—The incidence of sustained neurologic deficits associated with epidural anesthesia is 1 in 11,000. The incidence of permanent paralysis or paresis in these patients has been reported to be 0.02%. A case of delayed permanent paraplegia in a patient who underwent thoracic aneurysmectomy was presented.

Case Report.—Man, 74, with radiating chest pain, a history of hypertension, and previous repair of an abdominal aortic aneurysm was found to have a 5-cm aneurysm extending from the 6th to the 10th thoracic vertebrae. His aneurysm was repaired uneventfully. After IV analgesia proved inadequate, a thoracic epidural catheter was placed using the loss of resistance to saline technique. The procedure was unremarkable. The administration of lidocaine diminished his pain. After 40 minutes, the patient reported warmth and heaviness in his legs, exhibited profound bilateral motor paresis, and experienced a decrease in his blood pressure and heart rate. An MRI T2 sequence study of the thoracic spine revealed hemorrhage around the cord. A repeated study 24 hours later showed significant spinal cord ischemia. After 5 months, the patient is unable to move his legs and has a neurogenic bowel and bladder.

Discussion.—The paraplegia was caused by spinal cord ischemia as a result of interrupted cord blood flow when the thoracic aorta was cross-clamped. The incidence of paraplegia after descending and thoracoabdominal aneurysmectomy has been estimated at 5% to 21% and is highest in patients with significant abdominal aortic disease. Direct trauma, infection, hematoma, neurotoxic reaction to the injected substance, ischemia followed by hypotension, local anesthetic, epinephrine, spinal artery spasm, or injury as a result of volume pressure may be contributing factors associated with epidural block. MRI was used to demonstrate spinal cord ischemia.

▶ This case report highlights the complications of epidural analgesia when it is performed during thoracic aneurysmectomy, and emphasizes the importance of early aggressive investigation of the cause of delayed paraplegia after a thoracic epidural block for control of postoperative pain. Magnetic resonance imaging was used to demonstrate spinal cord ischemia.

M. Wood, M.D.

Frequency and Severity of Headache After Lumbar Myelography Using a 25-Gauge Pencil-Point (Whitacre) Spinal Needle

Quaynor H, Tronstad A, Heldaas O (Kongsberg sykehus, Norway)

Neuroradiology 37:553–556, 1995 6–4

Background.—The rate of postdural-puncture headache after lumbar myelography with 20 to 22-gauge spinal needles is as high as 50%. The use of a new type of spinal needle, the pencil-point (Whitacre) spinal needle, has lowered the incidence of these headaches after lumbar puncture. These needles have not been used for lumbar myelography. The incidence and severity of postdural-puncture headaches after using the Whitacre pencil-point spinal needle for lumbar myelography were examined.

Methods.—Sixty-three patients underwent lumbar myelography. Patients were premedicated with oral diazepam 5 mg at 30–60 minutes before lumbar puncture. Within 2 weeks of the procedure, a questionnaire was distributed to all patients. There were 15 questions on postdural-puncture headache, including accompanying symptoms, site, time of onset, and severity of headaches. Postdural-puncture headaches were defined as headaches that were alleviated by lying down; exacerbated by an upright position or factors that alter intracranial pressure; and accompanied by visual symptoms, auditory symptoms, nausea, vomiting, or giddiness.

Results.—Questionnaires were returned by 61 of the 63 patients. There were 29 women and 32 men. Three patients reported postdural-puncture headache. The headaches were moderate in 2 patients and mild in 1 patient. All headaches were relieved by mild analgesics. No patient had a severe headache that required a blood-patch. Three patients had a postdural-puncture–related headache that was not postural. Four patients reported ordinary, mild headaches.

Discussion.—The prevalence of postdural-puncture headache in these patients was 4% to 7%, and the headaches were reported as mild to moderate. This is one of the lowest reported rates of this type of headache after myelography. Other reports of postdural-puncture headache range from 20% to 50% using a 20- to 22-gauge spinal needle. If CSF leakage contributes to postdural-puncture headaches, then small-bore needles should lower the risk of these headaches. The pencil-point shape of the Whitacre needles may also lower the risk of postdural-puncture headache because the dural fibers are separated, not cut.

▶ This study demonstrates what we in anesthesia know, that is, that the use of a Whitacre needle as opposed to standard spinal needles, whether for spinal anesthesia or for myelography, is associated with a reduction in headaches from 20% to 50% with the conventional 20- to 22-gauge needle down to, in this instance, 4.7% using an introducer and 25-gauge Whitacre needle. It would have been nice had this study been randomized, but it does confirm the same findings in a totally different set of patients than most anesthesiologists see and, thus, is an important article.

M.F. Roizen, M.D.

Rebound Hypertension and Acute Withdrawal Associated With Discontinuation of an Infusion of Epidural Clonidine

Fitzgibbon DR, Rapp SE, Butler SH, et al (Univ of Washington, Seattle; Swedish Hosp, Seattle)

Anesthesiology 84:729–731, 1996 6–5

Background.—Epidural clonidine has been shown to produce effective pain relief in patients with severe cancer pain refractory to other treatments. Although acute withdrawal and rebound hypertension is a recognized risk of suddenly withdrawn systemically administered clonidine, this effect has not been reported after abrupt cessation of epidurally administered clonidine. However, 1 patient experienced acute withdrawal and rebound hypertension after cessation of epidural clonidine.

Case Report.—Man, 49, with metastatic adenocarcinoma of the pancreas, had pain that could not be adequately controlled with morphine. With combined epidural infusion of bupivacaine and morphine, pain control was adequate for 6 weeks, after which pain control diminished and lower extremity motor impairment and postural hypotension developed. The addition of epidural clonidine resulted in satisfactory pain control and enabled the rapid reduction of bupivacaine and morphine concentrations. However, the tunneled catheter migrated and required replacement. Concerns about potential infection prompted removal of the tunneled catheter and prophylactic 24-hour administration of IV vancomycin.

Within 2 hours after cessation of epidural therapy, agitation developed, followed by progressive diaphoresis, hypertension, and a heart rate increase. An ECG revealed sinus tachycardia with new left bundle-branch block. After administration of orally administered clonidine and IV midazolam, the patient's anxiety was reduced, his blood pressure and heart rate normalized, and the left bundle-branch block resolved. Subsequently, the patient was treated with long-term epidural infusions of bupivacaine, morphine, and clonidine, resulting in satisfactory pain control and no further adverse effects of treatment.

Conclusions.—Epidural clonidine therapy, like orally administered clonidine therapy, should be discontinued cautiously, because of the risk of acute withdrawal and rebound hypertension. These effects occur substantially more quickly after cessation of epidural infusions than after cessation of systemically administered clonidine. Recommended treatment includes aggressive treatment of hypertension with IV phentolamine and the reinstitution of orally administered clonidine therapy.

▶ It is well known that acute withdrawal of systemically administered clonidine can lead to severe rebound hypertension, even myocardial infarction. This turns out to also be the case with sudden cessation of epidural clonidine used for pain relief.

J.H. Tinker, M.D.

Lidocaine Inhibits Blood Coagulation: Implications for Epidural Blood Patch

Tobias MD, Pilla MA, Rogers C, et al (Univ of Pennsylvania, Philadelphia; Massachusetts Gen Hosp, Cambridge; St Andrews College, Berrion Springs, Mich)

Anesth Analg 82:766–769, 1996 6–6

Background.—Through its inhibitory effects on coagulation, lidocaine in the epidural space may reduce the efficacy of epidural autologous blood patch (EBP). The effects of achievable epidural concentrations of lidocaine admixed with whole blood on coagulation and fibrinolysis were studied.

Methods and Findings.—Twenty patients with American Society of Anesthesiologists physical status I and II were included in the study. Computerized thromboelastography (TEG) was used to study ex vivo blood coagulation in whole blood. Each specimen was exposed to serial dilutions of lidocaine or saline, resulting in end concentrations of 0, 2.3, 4.6, 9.2, 18.5, and 36.9 mM lidocaine. Compared with control subjects, the 3 highest concentrations of lidocaine caused hypocoagulable and/or fibrinolytic changes.

Conclusions.—Lidocaine significantly changes coagulation and fibrinolysis in whole blood as assessed by TEG. These changes were observed at the 3 highest concentrations of lidocaine tested. When significant epidural lidocaine concentrations are suspected, clinicians should dilute the lidocaine with an epidural saline infusion or wait for dissipation of the block.

▶ The interference with coagulation by residual local anesthetic in the epidural space may play a role in the relative lack of efficacy of prophylactic epidural blood patch performed in the early postoperative period. Other factors, such as dilution of blood by large volumes of CSF in the epidural space, may be at work as well. A common dilemma in performing a blood patch after the onset of the headache is CSF return on entering the epidural space. If there is a question of possible subarachnoid position of the needle, I generally inject a test dosage of 3 mL 2% lidocaine. Given the results of this study, it would seem that this amount would be unlikely to interfere with coagulation appreciably, and the risks of injecting 15–20 mL of blood intrathecally are not trivial.

S.E. Abram, M.D.

Misplacement of Multihole Epidural Catheters: A Report of Two Cases

Sala-Blanch X, Martinez-Palli G, Agusti-Lasus M, et al (Hosp Clinic i Provincial de Barcelona)

Anaesthesia 51:386–388, 1996 6–7

Background.—The use of multihole epidural catheters for epidural anesthesia-analgesia has been associated with misplacement of 1 or more holes. Epiduro-subdural misplacement of a multihole epidural catheter was described.

Case Report.—Woman, 28, was admitted to the delivery suite. Epidural analgesia was offerred when she asked for pain relief. She was placed in the left lateral position, and an 18-gauge Touhy needle was inserted in the midline through the $L_{3–4}$ interspace by a loss-of-resistance method with saline. The epidural space was easily identified at a depth of 4 cm with the bevel of the needle in the cephalad direction. A multihole closed-end epidural catheter was then threaded 3 cm into the epidural space with no difficulty. A test dose of lignocaine was administered. Five minutes later, 6 mL of bupivacaine 0.25% was injected through the catheter. About 30 minutes later, a unilateral sensory block was noted on the right side, which extended to the T_4 level.

At this time the patient was in the second stage of labor. A forceps delivery was performed through the use of a pudendal block. Two hours later, 3 mL of a nonionic water-soluble radiographic contrast medium was injected through the catheter. On a lateral view radiograph, the classic railroad track appearance was seen, which indicated diffusion into the subdural space. A further injection of 5 mL of contrast medium demonstrated spread in the subdural space and unilateral spread in the epidural space. After another 10 mL of contrast medium was injected, the anteroposterior view of the spinal column showed contrast spread within the subdural space and bilateral spread in the epidural space. The patient was discharged from the hospital on day 3 with no sequelae.

Conclusions.—Multihole epidural catheters can come to rest in both epidural and subdural spaces. The unpredictable features of subdural block may be explained by the presence of local anesthetic in both spaces.

▶ The authors correctly noted that there are published reports of subdural block with both endhole and multihole epidural catheters. In each of these two cases, the authors demonstrated the "epiduro-subdural misplacement" of a multihole epidural catheter. However, it is unclear that subdural block occurs more frequently with multihole epidural catheters than with endhole catheters. Overall, I believe that the advantages of multihole epidural catheters outweigh the disadvantages.

D.H. Chestnut, M.D.

Coronary Artery Spasm After Ephedrine in a Patient With High Spinal Anesthesia

Hirabayashi Y, Saitoh K, Fukuda H, et al (Jichi Med School, Tochigi, Japan)
Anesthesiology 84:221–224, 1996 6–8

Introduction.—A few reports have described coronary artery spasm causing sudden circulatory collapse and death in patients undergoing regional anesthesia. A patient with ephedrine-induced coronary artery spasm during spinal anesthesia, in the absence of a history of ischemic heart disease, was described.

Case Report.—Man, 69, underwent high spinal anesthesia with hyperbaric tetracaine for transurethral resection of a bladder tumor. The patient had no history of hypertension, myocardial infarction, or angina pectoris. Shortly after the start of the operation, he had a sudden decline in blood pressure and heart rate that did not respond to atropine. Ephedrine 5 mg was given, resulting in increased heart rate and blood pressure. Premature ventricular contractions and marked ST-segment elevation appeared on the ECG, and the patient complained of chest pain. Intravenous nitroglycerin produced dramatic improvement in blood pressure, ST-segment elevation, and chest pain. The patient's hemodynamic condition remained stable for the rest of the operation. In the coronary care unit, echocardiography showed impaired left ventricular contraction and anteroseptal-apical-inferior wall dyskinesia. Specific markers of angina and myocardial infarction (i.e., ST-segment depression and increased creatine phosphokinase) were absent.

Twenty days after surgery, coronary angiography showed no stenosis in the coronary arteries at rest. However, hyperventilation caused a 50% stenosis in the distal left circumflex branch. When acetylcholine was administered into the left coronary artery, the response was chest pain and diffuse vasoconstriction of the left circumflex branches. Narrowing of the distal right coronary artery occurred when acetylcholine was administered into the right coronary artery. Intracoronary nitrate administration restored the coronary arteries to their normal size.

Conclusions.—The contribution of high spinal anesthesia to the onset of coronary artery spasm is unclear, but the administration of adrenergic agonists appears to play a role. Coronary artery spasm is fairly common during myocardial revascularization but rare during regional anesthesia.

▶ Spinal anesthesia is commonly administered to elderly patients undergoing transurethral operations, many of whom must have ischemic heart disease. The patient described in this case report did not have a history of ischemic heart disease. However, the authors very elegantly demonstrated that acetylcholine (a parasympathetic muscarinic agonist) induced spasm of the right coronary artery not accompanied by chest pain 3 weeks after surgery. Many factors theoretically may provoke perioperative coronary artery spasm, including excess α-adrenergic agonist activity (epinephrine) and parasympathetic nervous system stimulation. Thus, coronary artery spasm in this patient may have resulted from either the high spinal anesthesia with relative parasympathetic excess or the ephedrine. Note that the patient received diltiazem and aspirin postoperatively, the correct anti-anginal therapy for coronary artery vasospasm.

M. Wood, M.D.

Permanent Unilateral Vestibulocochlear Dysfunction After Spinal Anesthesia

Wemama J-P, Delecroix M, Nyarwaya J-B, et al (Universitaire de Lille, France)

Anesth Analg 82:406–408, 1996 6–9

Introduction.—Numerous cases of hearing loss, vertigo, and other signs of vestibulocochlear dysfunction have been reported after lumbar puncture. Most such cases are transient, although in 1 report hearing loss persisted for 7 months. A patient in whom unilateral vestibulocochlear dysfunction persisted for more than 2 years after spinal anesthesia is reported.

Case.—Man, 45, underwent technically successful spinal anesthesia for an ankle arthrodesis procedure. The day after surgery he vomited and reported vertigo with acute echoing in the left ear and a hearing deficit in the right ear. He had a 50-dB hearing loss at high frequencies in the right ear. After hemorrheologic therapy, including hemodilution with low-weight dextran and vasodilating drugs, the hearing loss improved to 30 dB. The patient continued taking vasodilators after hospital discharge. Over the following 9 months, the patient was seen repeatedly for a fluctuating hearing deficit with vertigo, which improved with betahistine dichlorohydrate treatment. Meniere's disease was suspected on the basis of the symptoms and audiogram. His condition was unimproved nearly 2 years after his operation.

Discussion.—Vestibulocochlear disturbances after spinal anesthesia can sometimes be permanent, as suggested by this case. The mechanism of this complication is uncertain, although it may have involved CSF leakage with partial or complete blockage of the right cochlear aqueduct. The result would have been decreased pressure-regulating capacity and loss of protection against pressure changes in the inner ear. The preoperative health history before spinal anesthesia should include vestibular function, and pencil-point spinal needles should be used. Treatment for patients with vestibulocochlear dysfunction after spinal anesthesia should include hemorrheologic therapy and measures to minimize the effects of CSF leakage.

▶ The fact that a 22-gauge "Quincke" needle was used here indicates, from an artificial model study using human dura, reported elsewhere in this issue of YEAR BOOK, that it was likely to result in maximal CSF leakage. I suppose this complication could be due to the rate as well as the total volume of CSF leakage. This does seem to be a bit of an advertisement for the new pencil-point–type needles.

J.H. Tinker, M.D.

Awareness

Recall of Awareness During Cardiac Anaesthesia: Influence of Feedback Information to the Anaesthesiologist

Ranta S, Jussila J, Hynynen M (Helsinki Univ)

Acta Anaesthesiol Scand 40:554–560, 1996 6–10

Background.—The incidence of awareness with recall during general surgery is reportedly about 0.2%. Few studies have investigated this complication in patients undergoing cardiac surgery. The incidence of intraoperative awareness during cardiac surgery was studied.

Methods and Findings.—Three hundred three patients were included. Initially, 99 patients were chosen randomly and interviewed. Four percent reported awareness and recall. The cardiac anesthesiologists were then told of the interview findings and were given general information on how to reduce awareness and recall during general anesthesia. Thereafter, 204 consecutive patients were interviewed, 1.5% of whom reported intraoperative awareness with recall. This reduction in incidence, however, was nonsignificant. The doses of the main anesthetic drugs had increased significantly between the 2 phases of the study. The dose of pancuronium, the principal muscle relaxant, had been reduced significantly. The number of anesthesias in patients undergoing continuous methods instead of bolus or noncontinuous dosing techniques also was significantly increased. The doses of anesthetic agents given did not differ between patients with awareness and recall and those without it. However, patients reporting awareness were significantly younger.

Conclusions.—The incidence of intraoperative awareness during cardiac anesthesia may be reduced through education and vigilance. The observed incidence of 1.5% in this study is comparable to previously reported incidences among patients undergoing cardiac surgery.

► I very much agree with the authors' title, in which they use the term "recall of awareness." This implies, correctly I think, that there is a difference between awareness and its recall. The authors reported between 1.5% and 4% of this "recall of awareness." This is consistent with other reports in the past. Cardiac and obstetric anesthesia seem to be the areas in which we find the largest incidence of this problem. If this is the incidence of "recall of awareness," then surely the incidence of "awareness" must be higher, not lower. If there is an incidence of awareness without its recall, the question arises whether there are any residual effects. In fact, residual effects of either awareness or recall of awareness are of considerable importance, medicolegally. It will be very interesting to see whether the latest generation of modified electroencephalographic monitoring, namely the so-called "bispectral analysis," will help lower this incidence and thereby provide more assurance to anesthesiology personnel.

J.H. Tinker, M.D.

Bleeding Problems

Parenteral Ketorolac and Risk of Gastrointestinal and Operative Site Bleeding: A Postmarketing Surveillance Study

Strom BL, Berlin JA, Kinman JL, et al (Univ of Pennsylvania, Philadelphia; Syntex (USA) Inc, Palo Alto, Calif; Univ of Medicine and Dentistry of New Jersey/Robert Wood Johnson Med School, New Brunswick)

JAMA 275:376–382, 1996 6–11

Background.—Ketorolac tromethamine, a nonsteroidal anti-inflammatory drug (NSAID) indicated for short-term analgesia in parenteral form, has been used widely in settings different from those in the initial clinical trials since it was first marketed in 1990. Case reports of deaths from gastrointestinal (GI) and surgical site bleeding have appeared in the literature. The risk of GI and operative site bleeding associated with parenteral ketorolac tromethamine was evaluated.

Methods.—Data on 10,272 courses of parenteral ketorolac treatment were compared with data on 10,247 courses of a parenteral opiate. Patients in the 2 groups were matched by hospital, admitting service, and date of study drug initiation.

Findings.—Compared with opiates, ketorolac had a multivariate adjusted odds ratio (OR) for GI bleeding of 1.3. For operative site bleeding, the OR was 1.02. In patients 75 years or older, the OR for GI bleeding was 1.66; for operative site bleeding, it was 1.12. A dose-response relationship between mean daily ketorolac dose and GI and surgical site bleeding was noted. When analgesic treatment was given for 5 days or fewer, ketorolac was correlated with only a small increased risk of GI bleeding. When treatment lasted beyond 5 days, the OR associated with ketorolac was 2.2. Operative site bleeding was not correlated with treatment duration.

Conclusions.—The overall relationship between ketorolac treatment and GI and operative site bleeding is minimal. However, when ketorolac is used in higher doses, in elderly patients, and for more than 5 days, the risk is greater and clinically important.

▶ This large multicenter study helps put the risk of bleeding after postoperative NSAID use in perspective, and helps us discuss risks with surgeons and patients. It would be difficult to assess the additional risk of a rare complication such as epidural hematoma. Ketorolac is a tempting adjunct to epidural opioids because there is additional risk of respiratory depression when epidural and systemic opioids are combined.

S.E. Abram, M.D.

Intravenous Ketorolac Tromethamine Worsens Platelet Function During Knee Arthroscopy Under Spinal Anesthesia

Thwaites BK, Nigus DB, Bouska GW, et al (Brooke Army Med Ctr, Fort Sam Houston, Tex)

Anesth Analg 82:1176–1181, 1996 6–12

Introduction.—Ketorolac is a potent, cyclooxygenase inhibitor with well-documented analgesic and opioid-sparing qualities. There is concern that it may induce excess surgical site bleeding. If administered orally or intramuscularly to nonanesthetized adults, it causes a modest prolongation of bleeding time and a marked reduction in platelet aggregation that does not disappear until the body is clear of the drug. In a recent report, it did not worsen bleeding time or platelet aggregation during general anesthesia for arthroscopic surgery of the knee. Platelet function changes were observed during a standardized spinal anesthetic and surgery, as well as after a single intraoperative dose of IV ketorolac.

Methods.—Thirty American Society of Anesthesiologists (ASA) physical status I patients were prospectively randomly assigned to receive either ketorolac, 60 mg IV 15 minutes after skin incision, or placebo IV during spinal anesthesia for knee arthroscopy. At 3 different times during the procedure (15 minutes before spinal anesthesia, 10 minutes after skin incision, and 45 minutes after administration of ketorolac or placebo), patients underwent platelet function testing consisting of bleeding time, platelet aggregometry, thromboelastography (TEG), and serum thromboxane B_2 (TxB_2) assays. There were no significant between-group differences in bleeding times at any collection time. In the placebo group, there were no changes in any platelet function variable at any time. There was a significant increase in bleeding time from postincision to poststudy drug points in the ketorolac group. However, all bleeding times were within normal limits of 2–9 minutes in the ketorolac group. There were no significant between-group differences for any of the TEG variables for any data points and no significant TEG changes with regard to time. Platelet aggregometry to collagen, but not adenosine diphosphate, was significantly decreased from preoperative to poststudy drug data points in the ketorolac group. Platelet TxB_2 production decreased significantly in the ketorolac group from preoperative to poststudy drug data points.

Conclusion.—Findings suggest that platelet function is not accentuated during spinal anesthesia like it is during general anesthesia. Platelet function is impaired (i.e., bleeding time and platelet aggregometry to collagen) during spinal anesthesia, but not general anesthesia, when a single intraoperative dose of IV ketorolac is administered. It is not known whether this is clinically important.

► There are two important messages in this study. The first is a reconfirmation of the notion that regional anesthesia appears to prevent the hypercoagulability seen after general anesthesia that is probably associated with metabolic/endocrine responses to stress and noxious stimulation. The second is that ketorolac produces a statistically significant reduction in platelet function as measured by several different tests. The effect of nonsteroidal anti-inflammatory drugs on platelet function may offset the enhanced platelet activity seen after general anesthesia. It is not clear whether the effect produced after regional blockade is of sufficient degree to produce adverse responses (gastrointestinal bleed, increased wound hemorrhage, epidural hematoma).

S.E. Abram, M.D.

Carotid Artery Puncture

Carotid Artery Puncture, Airway Obstruction and the Laryngeal Mask Airway in a Preeclamptic Patient

Garcia-Rodriguez CR, Yentis SM (Royal Brompton Hosp, London; Chelsea and Westminster Hosp, London)

Int J Obstet Anesth 5:194–197, 1996 6–13

Objective.—The laryngeal mask airway (LMA) has been used successfully to treat patients with acute respiratory obstruction. A case is presented of a patient with multiple factors leading to acute respiratory obstruction where LMA was lifesaving on 2 occasions.

Case.—A Pakistani woman, 27, who spoke only Urdu, was admitted at 35 weeks of pregnancy because of reduced fetal movements. A diagnosis of fetal distress with abruption was made, and a cesarian section was immediately planned. The patient was frightened and refused any procedures until her husband was contacted and persuaded her to have the operation. General anesthesia without preoxygenation was administered, she was intubated, and a live male child was delivered. She was extubated when she was awake. Her Spo_2 and pulse rate remained normal over the next 12 hours, but her blood pressure increased. Her urine output fell, and she had heavy proteinuria despite the administration of 2 L of crystalloid. Pre-eclampsia was diagnosed and she was given sublingual nifedipine, IV hydralazine, and 500 mL of colloid. A central venous pressure monitor was placed with difficulty into the right jugular vein via the Seldinger technique. When the dilator was removed, arterial bleeding was noted, her neck swelled, and she lost consciousness. Because the obstruction made ventilation impossible, an LMA was inserted, and her Spo_2 increased from 40% to 92%. After sedation and paralysis, an orotracheal tube was placed blindly, and she was ventilated. Over the next 2 days, she required ventilation again because of swelling. Because ventilation by face mask was not possible, the LMA was again used for ventilation. She recovered fully and was discharged on day 30.

Discussion.—The patient's respiratory arrest was possibly the result of hematoma formation in the neck that caused laryngeal edema. This case illustrates the critical situation that can result from a series of mostly avoidable small problems that are not recognized or corrected.

Internal Jugular Vein and Carotid Artery Anatomic Relation as Determined by Ultrasonography

Troianos CA, Kuwik RJ, Pasqual JR, et al (Mercy Hosp of Pittsburgh, Pa)
Anesthesiology 85:43–48, 1996 6–14

Introduction.—Because of its accessibility during surgery and predictable anatomical location, the internal jugular vein is a route commonly used to access the central circulation. Unintentional carotid arterty puncture has occurred because of an anatomical relationship in which the internal jugular vein overlies the carotid artery. The anatomical relationship of the right internal jugular vein and the carotid artery in the direction of the cannulating needle was identified with ultrasound. Patient characteristics associated with an overlying, rather than a laterally posititioned, internal jugular vein were determined.

Methods.—A prospective study was conducted with 1,136 patients admitted for surgery. Those with neck surgery were excluded. Ultrasound imaging of the right internal jugular vein was performed at the apex of the angle formed by the division of the sternocleidomastoid muscle with patients awake and in a supine position without a pillow and with heads rotated as far to the left as was comfortable (Fig 1). Photographs were scored with the following system: 0, internal jugular vein was positioned

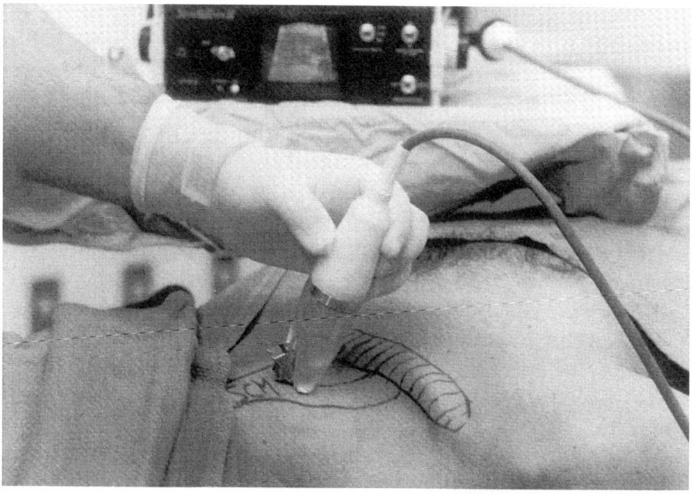

FIGURE 1.—Ultrasound probe placed on the neck in the direction of an attempted cannulation of the right internal jugular vein. The approach is at the apex of the angle formed by the division of the sternocleidomastoid muscle and directed toward the ipsilateral nipple. (Courtesy of Troianos CA, Kuwik RJ, Pasqual JR, et al: Internal jugular vein and carotid artery anatomic relation as determined by ultrasonography. *Anesthesiology* 85:43–48, 1996.)

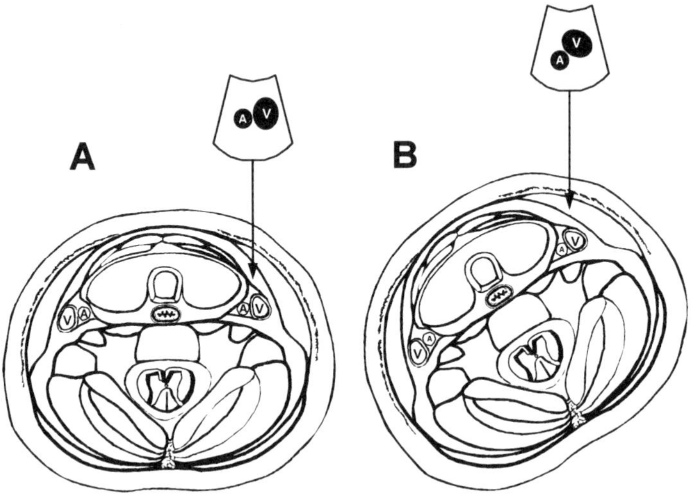

FIGURE 2.—Cross-sectional illustration of the neck that depicts the anatomical relationship of the carotid artery (*A*) and internal jugular vein (*V*). Quadrangles above the cross-sections illustrate the ultrasound images of the artery (*A*) and the vein (*V*). **A**, coronal approach, head facing anteriorly, representing the conventional anatomical approach. **B**, cannulating needle approach, head turned to left, representing actual operating conditions or "what the cannulating needle sees." (Courtesy of Troianos CA, Kuwik RJ, Pasqual JR, et al: Internal jugular vein and carotid artery anatomic relation as determined by ultrasonography. *Anesthesiology* 85:43–48, 1996.)

lateral to the carotid artery; 1, vein overlapped up to and including 25% of the diameter of the carotid artery; 2, vein overlapped more than 25% and up to and including 50% of the diameter of the carotid artery; 3, vein overlapped more than 50% and up to and including 75% of the diameter of the carotid artery; and 4, vein overlapped more than 75% of the diameter of the carotid artery.

Results.—Three investigators reviewed the photographs and if there was a disagreement in score by 2 or more investigators or if there was a poor image quality, the images were eliminated. Of the 1,009 patients remaining, 54% had a score of 4. Age was the only demographic datum predictive of score, with 64% of patients older than 60 years having a score of 4 or higher. Score was also related to vein size, both width and anteroposterior diameter.

Conclusion.—Classicially, the anatomical position of the internal jugular vein is described as lateral to the carotid artery. This is seen in the coronal plane but not in the directional plane of the cannulating needle with the head turned to the contralateral side (Fig 2). A greater proportion of patients than expected had an internal jugular vein positioned anterior to the carotid artery rather than lateral to it. Puncture of the carotid artery may result if the internal jugular vein is anterior to the carotid artery because undetected entry through a compressed internal jugular vein may occur.

Head Rotation During Internal Jugular Vein Cannulation and the Risk of Carotid Artery Puncture

Sulek CA, Gravenstein N, Blackshear RH, et al (Univ of Florida, Gainesville)
Anesth Analg 82:125–128, 1996 6–15

Introduction.—Accidental carotid artery puncture can be life threatening and can result in cerebrovascular accident, hemothorax, accidental intra-arterial cannulation, internal jugular vein carotid artery fistula, or airway compromise secondary to hematoma. By rotating the head, easier access is achieved for cannulating the internal jugular vein, with the amount of rotation ranging from 30 degrees to 90 degrees. Generally, the anatomical position of the internal jugular vein is lateral and anterior to the carotid artery. The influence of head position on the relative positions of the internal jugular vein and the carotid artery was examined.

Methods.—Twelve volunteers ranging in age from 18 to 60 years had internal jugular vein cannulation. They were placed in a 15-degree supine position, and ultrasound images were taken of the right and left sides of the neck at 2 and 4 cm from the clavicle along the lateral border of the sternal head of the sternocleidomastoid muscle. Images were also taken at 0 degrees, 40 degrees, and 80 degrees rotation of the head from midline. All imaging was done by 1 technician. Measurements were taken of the diameter of the internal jugular vein and the carotid artery and the percent overlap between the 2 vessels.

Results.—There was a significant increase of overlap of the carotid artery by the internal jugular vein when head rotation to the same side was increased to 40 degrees and then to 80 degrees, in comparison to head rotation of 0 degrees (Table 1) (Fig 2). There was no difference in data from 2 and 4 cm above the clavicle. With 80 degree of head rotation, the percent overlap was larger on the left than the right.

Conclusion.—The risk of inadvertent puncture of the carotid artery associated with the common occurrence of transfixion of the internal jugular vein before it is identified during needle withdrawal increases when

TABLE 1.—Percentage Overlap of Carotid Artery by Internal Jugular Vein at Three Different Degrees of Head Rotation

Side of neck	Overlap of vessels with different degrees of head rotation (%) 0°	40°	80°
Right	1.5 ± 0.8 (0–17.4)	6.5 ± 2.8 (0–48)	27.5 ± 7.4*† (0–100)
Left	5.2 ± 2.9 (0–54)	11.5 ± 4.9 (0–76.5)	44.7 ± 7.2*†‡ (0–100)

Note: Values are means ± standard error of the mean; range given in parentheses.
*$P < 0.05$ compared with 0 degrees rotation to same side of the neck.
†$P < 0.05$ compared with 40 degrees rotation to same side of the neck.
‡$P < 0.05$ compared with 80 degrees rotation to the right.
(Courtesy of Sulek CA, Gravenstein N, Blackshear RH, et al: Head rotation during internal jugular vein cannulation and the risk of carotid artery puncture. *Anesth Analg* 82:125–128, 1996.)

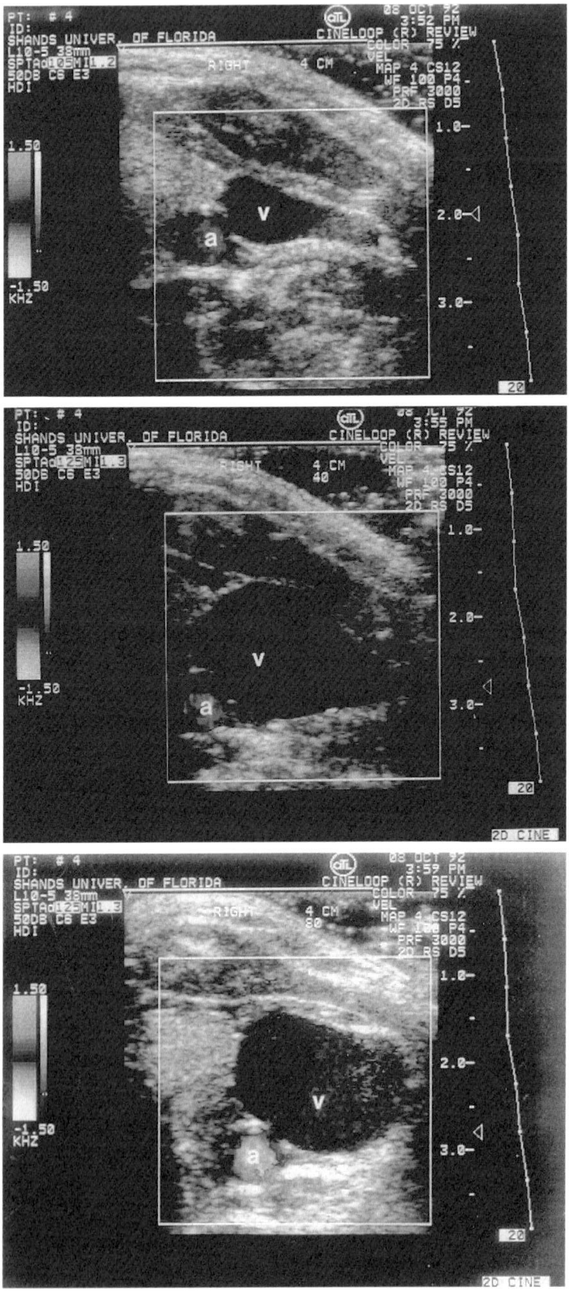

FIGURE 2.—Ultrasound images of the internal jugular vein (v) and the carotid artery (a) 4 cm above the clavicle on the right with evidence of substantial overlap at neutral head position (**top**) and even greater overlap with head rotation to 40 degrees (**middle**) and 80 degrees (**bottom**). (Courtesy of Sulek CA, Gravenstein N, Blackshear RH, et al: Head rotation during internal jugular vein cannulation and the risk of carotid artery puncture. *Anesth Analg* 82:125–128, 1996.)

the head is rotated more than 40 degrees. With needle insertion, the internal jugular vein frequently collapses, and this may result in puncture of the posterior wall of the vein and the artery when the 2 vessels overlap. During internal jugular vein cannulation, the head should be kept at less than 40 degrees rotation to decrease risk of puncture.

▶ This risk of accidental carotid artery puncture is well illustrated by the case report. (It is amazing that this particular patient ever survived her ordeal!). Although different approaches to the internal jugular vein (IJV) have been described to facilitate cannulation, none seem to minimize risk as well as methods that use ultrasonic guidance. Both clinical studies suggest that anatomical variation with a more medial location of the IJV may occur in 50% to 75% of patients. Extreme contralateral head rotation, advanced age, poor landmarks, and external needle compression may further alter the anatomy, thus making IJV cannulation more difficult and accidental carotid artery puncture more likely. In conditions in which accidental puncture may lead to airway obstruction (coagulopathy) or neurologic insult (significant carotid occlusive disease) or in surgery that may end up being canceled because of accidental carotid cannulation (coronary artery bypass graft or aortic aneurysm repair), the use of ultrasound-guided IJV catheter placement seems warranted and more than economically justified.

D.M. Rothenberg, M.D.

Latex Allergy

Anaesthesia for the Patient With Allergy to Latex

Spears FD, Littlewood KE, Liu DWH (Virginia Commonwealth Univ, Richmond)

Anaesth Intensive Care 23:623–625, 1995 6–16

Background.—Since the first systemic reactions to latex rubber were reported in 1987, severe Type I hypersensitivity reactions during surgery and anesthesia have been described with increasing frequency. The anesthetic management of several patients with a history of severe intraoperative anaphylactic reaction to latex rubber was reported.

Case Report.—Boy, 5, had confirmed latex allergy after a previous surgical procedure. Several precautions were taken before he underwent a dental restorative procedure under general anesthesia. Drugs were drawn up without the rubber tops, with direct aspiration from the glass bottle when necessary. Rubber injection ports in the IV line were taped to avoid use. To prevent airborne latex contamination, a microbial filter was placed between the reservoir bag and the anesthetic breathing system. The surgical staff wore latex-free gloves. Resuscitation drugs for use by bolus and infusion were made ready. All surgical and recovery room staff were informed of the patient's history of latex allergy. The boy was pretreated with IV ranitidine, chlorphenhydramine, and hydrocortisone. Anesthetic technique included preoxygenation, IV induction with fentanyl and thiopentone, and muscle relaxation with vecuronium. The trachea was intubated with a 5 mm clear plastic endotracheal tube. Anesthesia was maintained by manual ventilation with 70% nitrous oxide in oxygen and isoflurane 1%. The patient was monitored by ECG, noninvasive blood pressure, pulse oximetry, end-tidal carbon dioxide, temperature and train-of-four monitor. No adverse reactions occurred during the 2.5-hour procedure. The patient recovered uneventfully and was discharged home the same day.

Conclusions.—Latex allergy is likely to become more frequent in the future. Although patients may be pretreated with steroids and H_1 and H_2 receptor antagonists, avoidance of latex products is clearly the most important factor in the management of patients with latex sensitivity.

▶ Not long ago, when a case of latex allergy was presented at our mortality and morbidity conference, one of my colleagues commented that he thought that "latex allergy" was perhaps a "nursing disease." I am not sure whether his pejorative was related to his notion that this "disease" was discovered and/or promulgated by nursing personnel or whether he had implied that this disease was associated some kind of malingering or attempted "one upmanship," but he was not correct. This condition is real, dangerous, and has become more common or at least more commonly recognized. I think our readers would do well to read these case reports and become more aware of this problem.

J.H. Tinker, M.D.

Esophageal Perforation With Transesophageal Echocardiography

Gastroesophageal Perforation After Intraoperative Transesophageal Echocardiography
Kharasch ED, Sivarajan M (Univ of Washington, Seattle)
Anesthesiology 85:426–428, 1996 6–17

Introduction.—Complications are rare with the use of transesophageal echocardiography for intraoperative monitoring of cardiac function. An experience with perforation of the gastroesophageal junction in an anesthetized patient after an easy insertion of the echoprobe that provided good-quality transesophageal echocardiograms was reported.

Case Report.—Man, 66, underwent elective endoarterectomy of the left limb. A 5-MHz Omniplane transesophageal echoprobe was inserted after anesthesia to evaluate the cause of a V wave on the pulmonary artery catheter trace. The attending anethesiologist was well experienced. Echocardiographic examination revealed normal valvular anatomy. Several parameters of cardiac function were measured. When echocardiographic examination was not being performed, the acoustic power to the transducer was reduced to minimum level and the tip of the echoprobe was left in the unlocked position, free of any deflection. Because the patient was hemodynamically stable without evidence of mitral regurgitation, the echoprobe was removed after about 3 hours into the 8-hour surgery. At 4 AM the morning after the operation, the patient complained of nausea, followed by severe abdominal pain 2 hours later and an episode of coffee ground emesis. A nasogastric tube was inserted and 600 mL of coffee ground gastric contents was aspirated. The patient experienced tachypnea, hypotension, tachycardia, agitation, and arterial hemoglobin oxygen desaturation, despite high-flow oxygen administered by face mask. The patient's condition continued to worsen and a left thoracoabdominal esophagogastrectomy was performed the afternoon of the first postoperative day. Pathologic examination of the excised specimen revealed a large, 1.2 × 0.7–cm, hemorrhagic perforation of the gastroesophageal junction next to a smaller hole measuring 2 mm in diameter. There was gross and microscopic evidence of a thermally burned lateral edge and evidence of acid injury. Chronic gastritis and esophageal perforation, with ulceration, necrosis, and suppurative inflammation, was determined on pathologic examination. The postoperative course was complicated by sepsis, coagulopathy, and multiple organ system failure. The patient died on the 7th postoperative day. Postmortem examination showed extensive abdominal aortic atherosclerosis, congested firm spleen, and ischemic necrosis of the lower esophagus. The pathologic impression was that the esophagus was not able to endure the pressure of the echoprobe during its retention, which led to necrosis and perforation.

Conclusion.—The chance of echoprobe complications should be considered in patients with severe occlusive disease of the aorta and upper gastrointestinal tract ischemia.

▶ I selected this article to highlight the fact that, although transesophageal echocardiography has become a useful tool in the operating room, it is not without complication.

M. Wood, M.D.

Lung Injury During Cardiopulmonary Bypass

Acute Lung Injury During Cardiopulmonary Bypass: Are the Neutrophils Responsible?
Tönz M, Mihaljevic T, von Segesser LK, et al (Univ Hosp Zurich, Switzerland)
Chest 108:1551–1556, 1995 6–18

Introduction.—Cardiopulmonary bypass (CPB) is a recognized cause of acute respiratory distress syndrome (ARDS), and as in ARDS, there is increasing evidence that lung injury during CPB is related to the activity of neutrophils. The relation between neutrophil activation and pulmonary dysfunction after CPB and the potential influence of CPB temperature on cellular activation were evaluated in patients undergoing elective coronary artery bypass.

Methods.—Thirty-eight patients were enrolled in the study. Nineteen were randomly assigned to normothermic CPB (warm group) and 19 to hypothermic CPB (cold group). Blood temperature in the cold group was cooled to 26° to 28°C; patients in the warm group had temperature maintained at 36° to 37°C. Blood samples were obtained after induction of anesthesia, during and at the end of CPB, after weaning from CPB, and on the first postoperative day for determinations of the differential white blood cell count and plasma elastase concentrations.

Results.—With the exception of a lower prevalence of diabetic patients and a higher volume of transfused packed red blood cells in the cold group, the 2 groups were similar in preoperative risk factors and operative characteristics. Leukocyte counts and neutrophil counts increased significantly in the warm group during the first 30 minutes of CPB, but both remained unchanged in the cold group. Overall, the cellular response to the extracorporeal circulation was significantly delayed in the hypothermic group. The onset of neutrophilia and an increase in plasma elastase levels both occurred later in the cold group. Independent of bypass temperature, there was a significant deterioration in lung function after CPB, as assessed by respiratory index, alveolar-arterial oxygen gradient, and intrapulmonary shunt. Postoperative respiratory index and intrapulmonary shunt were positively correlated with peak elastase concentrations. Average period of intubation after CPB was 13.3 hours in the normothermic group and 16.4 hours in the hypothermic group.

Discussion.—Hypothermia during CPB delayed cellular activation but did not influence total activation of neutrophils or postoperative pulmonary dysfunction. Active rewarming appears to provoke a burst of cellular activation at the end of bypass. Manipulation of neutrophils may be a means of reducing postoperative lung injury.

► For years, we talked about "pump lung" and more or less assumed that there was pulmonary injury that occurred during CPB. These authors are implicating neutrophils and generation by them of increased plasma elastase levels as a possible culprit. I selected this paper because I think it is a solid start in understanding the mechanism of a common problem in clinical cardiovascular anesthesia, although I still do not understand how much contribution there is by the lack of pulmonary artery blood flow.

J.H. Tinker, M.D.

Bronchoconstriction With Lidocaine

Prevention of Lidocaine Aerosol-Induced Bronchconstriction With Intravenous Lidocaine

Bulut Y, Hirshman CA, Brown RH (Johns Hopkins Med Insts, Baltimore, Md)
Anesthesiology 85:853–859, 1996 6–19

Introduction.—Lidocaine administered as an aerosol produces little effect on pulmonary mechanics in healthy persons, but can cause bronchoconstriction in persons with hyperreactive airway disease. The effects of IV and aerosol lidocaine on baseline airway tone were compared in 5 Basenji-Greyhound dogs. The effect of pretreatment with IV lidocaine in preventing histamine-induced bronchoconstriction also was evaluated.

Methods.—Each dog acted as its own control. Animals were pretreated on separate days with IV lidocaine, aerosol lidocaine, or neither, followed by histamine aerosol challenge. High-resolution CT was used to assess airway caliber at 3 different times. Venous blood was drawn to determine serum lidocaine concentrations.

Results.—The airway area was decreased by 32% with the administration of histamine. Histamine-induced bronchoconstriction was significantly inhibited with the administration of IV or aerosol lidocaine. The airway area decreased by only 7% and 10%, respectively, of baseline after pretreatment with IV and aerosol lidocaine. This difference in treatment routes was nonsignificant. The administration of IV lidocaine had no significant effect on baseline airway caliber. When it was administered by aerosol at baseline, the airway area was significantly decreased by 27%. This decrease in airway area lasted less than 10 minutes. The airway caliber always returned to baseline before aerosol administration of histamine. Lidocaine aerosol–induced bronchoconstriction was prevented by the infusion of IV lidocaine. The combination of IV and aerosol lidocaine dilated airways by a significant 20%, compared to controls. The mean serum lidocaine concentrations were 3.0, 0.7, and 2.5 mg/L, respectively, in dogs treated with IV lidocaine, aerosol lidocaine, and IV lidocaine followed by aerosol lidocaine.

Conclusion.—An initial bronchoconstriction is caused by lidocaine given as an aerosol at a dose that blocks histamine-induced bronchoconstriction. The bronchoconstriction that results from the aerosol administration of lidocaine can be prevented by pretreatment with IV lidocaine.

► I selected this article to illustrate that, although there is a trend away from whole-animal physiologic studies, elegant studies of importance to clinical practice are still required in animal models such as the Basenji-Greyhound dog that has been used to study bronchoconstriction.

M. Wood, M.D.

Suction-induced Hemolysis

Suction-induced Hemolysis at Various Vacuum Pressures: Implications for Intraoperative Blood Salvage

Gregoretti S (Univ of Alabama, Birmingham)

Transfusion 36:57–60, 1996 6–20

Background.—Salvaged blood during surgery often has higher concentrations of plasma-free hemoglobin, attributable to the destruction of red cells during suction. To minimize hemolysis, a suction vacuum pressure of 150 mm Hg or less is recommended. When this cannot maintain a clear surgical field, it is recommended that an alternative suction connected to a high-vacuum pressure source be used and the blood discarded. However, there is little information to support these recommendations. Whether suction vacuum pressures above the recommended limit cause unacceptable hemolysis was investigated in an experimental study.

Methods.—Hemolysis caused by various suction vacuum pressures in a suction system was measured. For each test, blood with a hematocrit of 30% to 35% was prepared by mixing outdated units of red cells, fresh frozen plasma, and saline. Aliquots were suctioned at vacuum pressures of 150, 200, 250, and 300 mm Hg with or without maximal air entrainment. Measurements of total hemoglobin, hematocrit, red cell count, plasma-free hemoglobin, and serum potassium were taken.

Results.—Greater hemolysis occurred with the suction of blood mixed with air than with the suction of blood alone. When the vacuum pressure was raised from 150 to 300 mm Hg, hemolysis increased from 0.14% to 0.32% when blood alone was aspirated; hemolysis increased from 1.45% to 2.85% when blood was suctioned with air. Red cell count, hematocrit, and serum potassium did not change significantly with the different vacuum pressures tested.

Conclusions.—Hemolysis depends on the vacuum pressure and the amount of blood and air mixing. Vacuum pressures higher than 150 mm Hg were not associated with excessive hemolysis. The lowest vacuum pressure that allows a clear surgical field should be used. Suctioning of air should be avoided.

▶ Intraoperative blood salvage has become a routine procedure, but hemolysis can occur, especially if the suction vacuum pressure is high. These authors suggest that higher pressures can be used during hemorrhage and rapid blood loss than previously thought. Whether blood salvage should be continued or alternative methods used depends on the risk-benefit ratio for each individual patient and is a decision requiring clinical judgment.

M. Wood, M.D.

Paradoxical Cerebral Embolism

Fatal Paradoxical Cerebral Embolization During Bilateral Knee Arthroplasty

Weiss SJ, Cheung AT, Stecker MM, et al (Univ of Pennsylvania, Philadelphia)
Anesthesiology 84:721–723, 1996 6–21

Background.—Knee and hip arthroplasty are associated with neurologic complications that range from mild delirium to coma and death. The pathogenesis and operative events that lead to such injury are not completely understood. They are thought to be a consequence of the fat embolism syndrome. Intraoperative hemodynamic monitoring, carotid artery ultrasound, and electroencephalogram (EEG) were used to identify the sequence of events that led to a paradoxical cerebral embolization that caused fatal neurologic injury to a patient during bilateral knee arthroplasty.

Case Report.—Woman, 84, was scheduled to undergo bilateral total knee arthroplasty for rheumatoid arthritis. She also had hypertension treated with pindolol and captopril and left ventricular hypertrophy. General anesthesia was induced with fentanyl, thiopental, and pancuronium and maintained with desflurane, nitrous oxide, epidural bupivacaine, and epidural fentanyl. Extensive monitoring was used. Single-stage bilateral knee arthroplasty was performed. The first tourniquet was deflated after the first arthroplasty; increases were then noted in the pulmonary artery pressure, central venous pressure, and pulmonary vascular resistance. There were no changes in the EEG waveforms or carotid ultrasound examination. After the second tourniquet was deflated on the contralateral knee, pulmonary artery pressure, central venous pressure, and pulmonary vascular resistance increased further. Echogenic debris appeared in the lumen of the right carotid artery, and high-frequency activity on the EEG waveforms decreased. The maximum amount of debris traveling cephalad in the carotid artery occurred between 2 and 4 minutes after tourniquet release and persisted for more than 15 minutes. Within 2 minutes, EEG slowing was detected, which reached a nadir at 4 minutes after tourniquet deflation. The patient was extubated after she resumed spontaneous ventilation and responded to simple commands. Postoperative laboratory tests showed an increased alveolar-to-arterial oxygen gradient, anemia, thrombocytopenia, and coagulopathy. Chest radiographs were normal. Six hours after surgery, the patient became progressively obtunded. Her trachea was reintubated. On neurologic assessment, she was responsive only to painful stimulation, had no corneal reflexes, and showed intermittent decerebrate posturing. Postoperative EEG demonstrated severe diffuse slowing. Computed tomography scans of the head showed periventricular and subcortical lucencies consistent with multifocal regions of cerebral ischemia or infarction. Right ventricular and atrial dilation with moderate tricuspid regurgitation were observed on transesophageal echocardiography. The presence of an atrial septal defect and right-to-left intracardiac shunting was seen on a transesophageal echocardiography echocontrast and color flow Doppler study. The patient's condition worsened, and her family requested a "do not resuscitate" order. The patient died 3 days after surgery. Postmortem assessment confirmed the presence of a patent foramen ovale and diffuse embolic infarcts throughout the brain.

Conclusions.—These findings support the hypothesis that paradoxical cerebral embolization can result from the transit of venous emboli across the interatrial septum at the site of fossa ovalis. The risk of paradoxical embolization may be increased in patients with a patent foramen ovale or atrial septal defect. This abnormality is common, and occurs in about 27% of the population. Preoperative screening may be useful when a single-stage bilateral knee arthroplasty is considered.

▶ I have been involved in several cases in which the most reasonable diagnosis for the death of a patient was paradoxical embolism. The fact that probe-patent foramen ovale exists in approximately 27% of patients at autopsy does not seem very satisfying to either us or our legal colleagues when it comes as an explanation for a tragic event or outcome. I suppose the reason it is unsatisfying is because it is often viewed as "convenient." Nonetheless, it happens. These authors elegantly demonstrated that it was the correct diagnosis in this case.

J.H. Tinker, M.D.

Closed System: Foreign Gases

Accumulation of Foreign Gases During Closed-System Anaesthesia
Versichelen L, Rolly G, Vermeulen H (Univ Hosp, Ghent, Belgium)
Br J Anaesth 76:668–672, 1996 6–22

Background.—Previous research has demonstrated the presence of methane accumulation at the end of closed-system ventilation. The recent availability of on-line analysis of gas concentrations enabled an examination of the progressive increase in concentrations of methane, carbon monoxide, and acetone under modern, closed-system conditions and their influence on infrared halothane analysis.

Methods.—A computer-controlled closed-system anesthesia apparatus was used for ventilation during total IV anesthesia for gynecologic laparoscopy in 26 nonpregnant women. Every 15 minutes, methane, carbon monoxide, and acetone concentrations were analyzed in a photoacoustic infrared monitor and halothane concentrations were evaluated by built-in infrared spectrometry.

Findings.—After 105 minutes, mean methane concentrations progressively increased to 941 ppm. However, carbon monoxide and acetone concentrations did not increase significantly. The infrared measure incorrectly indicated 0.79% "halothane" after 1 hour in 18 patients, but the other 8 had no reading.

Conclusions.—Methane appears to accumulate progressively under strict closed-system conditions in greater concentrations than reported previously. It resulted in false "halothane" readings in two thirds of the patients.

► This fascinating report of the accumulation of methane during anesthesia needs to be tested to see whether it is of any clinical import. In this study, methane seems to have interfered with halothane readings during "computer-controlled closed-system anesthesia." Since I have never been an advocate of closed-system anesthesia, because of its complexity and the fact that the above-mentioned complexity ought to render it less safe, this is one of those papers where I get to shake my finger at the closed-system *evangelistas* and, perhaps, get to say just a little of "I told you so."

J.H. Tinker, M.D

Pulmonary Embolism: Pneumatic Stockings

The Efficacy of Pneumatic Compression Stockings in the Prevention of Pulmonary Embolism After Cardiac Surgery

Ramos R, Salem BI, de Pawlikowski MP, et al (St Luke's Hosp, Chesterfield, Mo)

Chest 109:82–85, 1996 6–23

Objective.—It has been suggested that the prophylactic use of pneumatic compression stockings (PCSs) in conjunction with subcutaneous heparin (SCH) would lower the risk of postoperative thromboembolism. The prophylactic use of bilateral PCSs in addition to SCH was evaluated for efficacy in reducing the incidence of pulmonary embolism (PE) in patients undergoing cardiac surgery.

Methods.—Between 1984 and 1995, 2,786 patients (769 women) undergoing open heart surgery received either prophylactic SCH, 5,000 U every 12 hours, (group A) or a combination of prophylactic SCH, 5,000 U every 12 hours, and PCSs extending from the ankle to the thigh and compressed to a peak pressure of 35 to 40 mm Hg for 11 seconds every 60 minutes (group B) for 4 to 5 days after surgery.

Results.—Postoperative PE developed in 69 patients, 48 in Group A and 21 in group B. The combined method reduced the risk of PE significantly by 62%.

Conclusion.—Although a connection between deep-vein thrombosis and pulmonary embolism is assumed, the 2.5% absolute risk reduction of the combined method compared with heparin prophylaxis alone is clinically significant.

▶ This well-designed, randomized outcome study shows the benefit of PCSs in the prevention of PE after cardiac surgery. The addition of PCSs to SCH prophylaxis led to a 1.5% incidence of PE compared to a 4% incidence with SCH alone. This absolute risk reduction of 2.5% is clinically significant. This study was performed in patients who underwent cardiac surgery; thus, they also received large doses of heparin and the superficial veins of their legs were operated on to perform coronary artery bypass grafting. The number of patients studied was large.

M. Wood, M.D.

Vent Problems After Laparoscopy

Acute Ventilatory Complications During Laparoscopic Upper Abdominal Surgery

Wahba RWM, Tessler MJ, Kleiman SJ (McGill Univ, Montreal)

Can J Anaesth 43:77–83, 1996 6–24

Background.—Serious complications can be expected to result from the increased number of patients undergoing laparoscopic upper abdominal surgery and the variety of operations performed. Published reports of subcutaneous emphysema, pneumothorax, and carbon dioxide (CO_2) embolism during laparoscopic upper abdominal surgery were reviewed.

Methods.—A Medline search of the literature was performed. In addition, the annual meeting supplements of several anesthesiology journals were perused.

Findings.—The first sign of subcutaneous emphysema and pneumothorax is a sudden increase in end-tidal CO_2 tension ($P_{ET}CO_2$). Pneumothorax and bronchial intubation are associated with desaturation and increased airway pressure, which do not occur with subcutaneous emphysema alone. Pneumothorax initially is diagnosed on the basis of the tube position, swelling and crepitus on physical examination, and auscultation for air entry. The diagnosis is confirmed by chest radiography and paracentesis. Pneumothorax often occurs with subcutaneous emphysema, but is rarely of the tension type. Although there have been no reports of pulmonary embolism caused by CO_2 during laparoscopic upper abdominal surgery, data suggest that small, hemodynamically inconsequential CO_2 embolism occurs without a change in $P_{ET}CO_2$. Massive embolism can occur, substantially reducing $P_{ET}CO_2$, arterial O_2 saturation, and blood pressure (Fig 2).

Conclusions.—A marked, sudden increase in $P_{ET}CO_2$ is the first sign of subcutaneous emphysema and pneumothorax. Increased $P_{ET}CO_2$ also may indicate an increased CO_2 load or cardic output. Simultaneous desaturation and hypotension indicate a tension pneumothorax. If either complication should occur, insufflation should be discontinued temporarily, the pneumothorax should be relieved by chest tube drainage, and minute

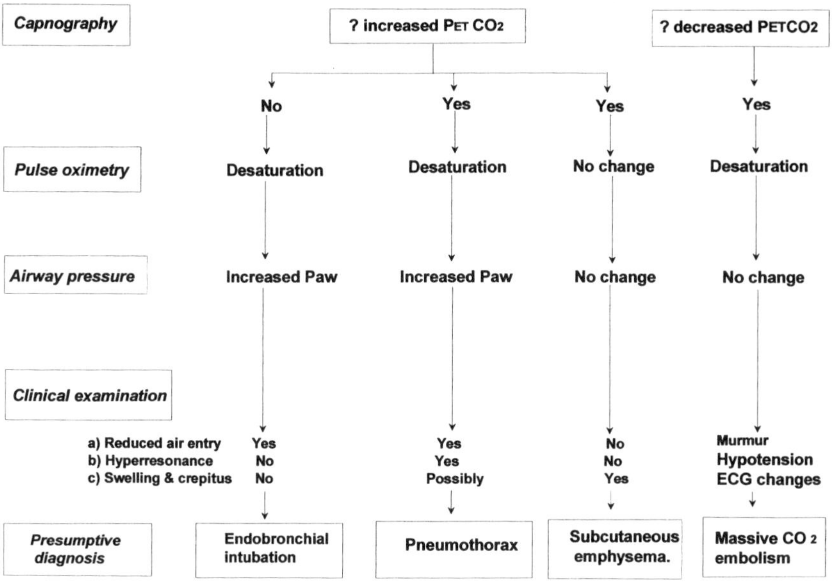

FIGURE 2.—Algorithm: acute ventilatory complications during laparoscopic upper abdominal surgery. (Courtesy of Wahba RWM, Tessler MJ, Kleiman SJ: Acute ventilatory complications during laparoscopic upper abdominal surgery. *Can J Anaesth* 43:77–83, 1996.)

ventilation should be increased. Small CO_2 emboli can occur during laparoscopic upper abdominal surgery. These microemboli, which may increase $P_{ET}CO_2$, can be detected by transesophageal echocardiographic monitoring. Carbon dioxide embolism after laparoscopy can have fatal consequences.

► I chose this article because it defines the major acute ventilatory complications of laparoscopic upper abdominal surgery reported in the literature and provides a scheme for their recognition and differential diagnosis, which I think will be very useful for the practicing anesthesiologist.

M. Wood, M.D.

Interference With CO_2 Analysis

Interference of Volatile Anaesthetics With Infrared Analysis of Carbon Dioxide and Nitrous Oxide Tested in the Dräger Cicero EM Using Sevoflurane

Wilkes AR, Mapleson WW (Univ of Wales, Cardiff)

Br J Anaesth 76:737–739, 1996 6–25

Background.—Concentrations of gases used during anesthesia—including carbon dioxide, nitrous oxide, and volatile anesthetics—are commonly measured using infrared absorption. However, if an infrared multigas analyzer is set to measure a volatile anesthetic different from that in the sampled gas mixture, the result might be interference with carbon dioxide and nitrous oxide readings. This theory was evaluated in the course of testing an anesthetic workstation.

Methods and Results.—The device under testing was the Dräger Cicero EM anesthetic workstation, which includes the ANDROS 4610 gas analyzer. The manufacturer claimed that the analyzer would compensate for the cross-sensitivity of carbon dioxide, nitrous oxide, and volatile anesthetic to ensure that the displayed concentrations were accurate. Testing showed that setting the analyzer for a different anesthetic than the one present in the sampled gas mixture did cause interference with the readings. The effect was most apparent when the analyzer was set to measure isoflurane but the gas mixture contained sevoflurane instead. Under these conditions, with a gas mixture containing 6% sevoflurane, the carbon dioxide reading decreased from 5.0% to 3.6% and the nitrous oxide reading increased from 0% to 8%. This situation would not have escaped clinical notice, however, because the isoflurane reading was 9.0%.

Conclusions.—When using an infrared multigas analyzer, the anesthetist should ensure that the device is set to measure the anesthetic that is actually being used and that the system does not contain a mixture of volatile anesthetics. Otherwise, readings for carbon dioxide, nitrous oxide, and the anesthetic may be incorrect. The Cicero EM anesthetic workstation is automatically set to measure the correct anesthetic when used with a Vapor vaporizer.

► In this elegant study, an infrared multigas analyzer set to measure end-tidal concentrations of a particular volatile anesthetic that doesn't happen to be the one in use in the circuit, can produce overlapping erroneous readings for carbon dioxide. In other words, the analyzer needs to "know" which volatile anesthetic is actually present to offset this problem. That's all fine and good, but in candor, a major reason that I included this paper in the Year Book is because it is authored by W.W. Mapleson. Dr. Mapleson's name will be forever revered in anesthesia circles, and other circuits, pun intended. Dr. Mapleson is a true legend in our specialty. I included this report to salute his great career.

J.H. Tinker, M.D.

Problems With Sublingual Nifedipine

Should a Moratorium Be Placed on Sublingual Nifedipine Capsules Given for Hypertensive Emergencies and Pseudoemergencies?

Grossman E, Messerli FH, Grodzicki T, et al (Chaim Sheba Med Ctr, Tel-Hashomer, Israel; Ochsner Clinic and Alton Ochsner Med Found, New Orleans, La; Univ School of Medicine, Kraków, Poland)

JAMA 276:1328–1331, 1996 6–26

Objective.—Although sublingual nifedipine is commonly used to treat hypertensive emergencies, numerous adverse events have been reported and sublingual absorption of the medication has been shown to be negligible. The literature on the use of sublingual nifedipine for hypertensive emergencies was reviewed.

Antihypertensive Efficacy.—Nifedipine is a quick-acting calcium antagonist that lowers arterial blood pressure by peripheral vasodilation. The effect peaks in 30–60 minutes and lasts about 6 hours. Monitoring of the drug, equally effective in both sexes and all ages, was not recommended initially because blood pressure lowering was thought to be proportional to initial readings and adverse effects were not thought to be life-threatening.

Administration and Absorption.—Sublingual absorption is negligible but intestinal absorption is faster and results in plasma levels 8 times higher than those achieved with buccal absorption.

Adverse Effects.—The adverse effect of buccal or oral nifedipine is an abrupt decrease in arterial pressure, resulting in neurologic deficits. The effects are exacerbated by hypovolemia and the use of other antihypertensive drugs.

Comment.—The Food and Drug Administration (FDA) has concluded after a review of the literature that dose-response and outcome data on oral nifedipine use are lacking. Nifedipine has not been approved for use in hypertension. The effect of nifedipine is primarily cosmetic. It has been used mainly in pseudoemergencies. In legitimate emergencies, nifedipine use is risky because of its unpredictability. These concerns apply to the short-acting form of the drug, rather than the sustained-release form.

Conclusion.—Data show that buccal absorption of nifedipine is poor, its effect on blood pressure lowering is unpredictable, it is not approved by the FDA for treatment of hypertension, and it is mainly being used in pseudoemergencies.

► The use of sublingual nifedipine seems to be a less popular technique in managing perioperative hypertension than it was 5 or 10 years ago. This is most likely because of the introduction of such IV agents as the calcium-channel antagonist nicardipine and the IV angiotensin-converting enzyme inhibitor enalapril. Nonetheless, sublingual nifedipine continues to be prescribed with very little data to support its safety and efficacy. It would behoove anesthesiologists who choose to administer this drug in sublingual form to reassess their practice in light of this report.

D.M. Rothenberg, M.D.

7 Critical Care Issues

Mechanical Ventilation Issues

Initial Experience With Partial Liquid Ventilation in Adult Patients With the Acute Respiratory Distress Syndrome
Hirschl RB, Pranikoff T, Wise C, et al (Univ of Michigan, Ann Arbor)
JAMA 275:383–389, 1996 7–1

Background.—The initial animal reports of spontaneous liquid breathing of perfluorocarbon appeared in 1966. More recently, laboratory studies of partial liquid ventilation (PLV), in which the lungs are filled with perfluorocarbon and mechanically ventilated, to improve gas exchange in acute respiratory distress syndrome (ARDS) have been reported. An initial clinical experience with PLV in adult patients with ARDS is described.

Methods.—The uncontrolled, phase I study included 10 consecutive patients who required extracorporeal life support (ECLS) for severe respiratory failure. The predicted survival for this category of patients was 10% to 20% without ECLS and 50% to 60% with ECLS. The patients were started on PLV 1–11 days after the start of ECLS. The dependent zone of the lung was filled with perflubron by tracheal instillation, followed by gas ventilation of the lung. As the alveolar gas/perfluorocarbon oxygen tensions increased, oxygen gas was distributed through the airways into alveoli. As alveolar gas/perfluorocarbon CO_2 levels decreased, CO_2 elimination occurred. The patients underwent volatilized perflubron replacement each day for 1–7 days; the median cumulative dose was 38 mL/kg. The results of PLV were assessed in terms of physiologic shunt and static pulmonary compliance.

Results.—Chest radiographs showed diffuse opacification and aeration of the lungs immediately after perflubron administration. The median physiologic shunt decreased from 0.72 to 0.46 in the 72 hours after PLV started. At the same time, the median static pulmonary compliance corrected for patient weight increased from 0.16 to 0.27 mL/cm H_2O/kg. Half of the patients survived. There was 1 case of pneumothorax and 1 case of mucus plug formation that may have been related to PLV.

Conclusions.—No gain in survival is demonstrated yet by PLV, as expected in a group of patients with such severe lung injury. However, the safety of administering perflubron into the lungs of patients receiving ECLS while maintaining gas exchange is demonstrated. The authors are conducting phase III studies of PLV for patients with respiratory insufficiency who are not receiving ECLS.

Initial Experience With Partial Liquid Ventilation in Pediatric Patients With the Acute Respiratory Distress Syndrome

Gauger PG, Pranikoff T, Schreiner RJ, et al (Univ of Michigan, Ann Arbor)

Crit Care Med 24:16–22, 1996 7–2

Introduction.—There have been no previous reports of liquid ventilation with perfluorocarbon in nonnewborn pediatric patients with respiratory failure. The use of partial liquid ventilation in 6 infants and children with acute respiratory distress syndrome (ARDS) who were receiving extracorporeal life support is reported.

Methods.—The patients, all older than 1 month, received partial liquid ventilation 2–9 days after the start of extracorporeal support. Perflubron administration started at a mean dose of 13 mL/kg. Extracorporeal life support flow was stopped for assessment of physiologic data, and bronchoscopy and chest radiography were repeated. The results were assessed in terms of alveolar–arterial oxygen gradient, static pulmonary compliance, and physiologic measures, determined each day at baseline and after perfluorocarbon administration.

Results.—In the 96 hours after the first dose of perfluorocarbon, mean PaO_2 increased from 39 to 92 mm Hg, and average alveolar–arterial oxygen gradient decreased from 635 to 499 mm Hg. During the same period, mean static pulmonary compliance normalized for weight increased from 0.12 to 0.28 mL/cm H_2O/kg (Fig 3). All 6 patients lived; 2 had pneumothoraces as complications of partial liquid ventilation.

Conclusions.—An experience with perfluorocarbon partial liquid ventilation for ARDS in children beyond the newborn period is reported. The safety of intratracheal perfluorocarbon administration in this group of patients is established. The treatment tends to improve lung gas exchange and pulmonary compliance.

▶ In the 1994 YEAR BOOK OF ANESTHESIOLOGY (Abstract 101-94-21–4, pp 338–340) a study was presented describing intratracheal perfluorocarbon in an experimental model of respiratory distress syndrome. Three years later, these 2 initial clinical studies, 1 in adults and 1 in children, show the relative safety of the use of the so-called liquid oxygen as a means to wean patients from extracorporeal life support (ECLS). Partial liquid ventilation with perfluorocarbon may reduce physiologic shunt and improve compliance while obviating the need for high levels of positive end-expiratory pressure. By lowering peak airway pressures and allowing for oxygenation at lower tidal volumes, barotrauma and volutrauma may be diminished. Because of its unique physical qualities, this agent may also allow for pulmonary lavage, which conceivably may alter the inflammatory cascade of adult respiratory distress syndrome. Perfluorocarbon may, because of its density (1.9 g/mL),

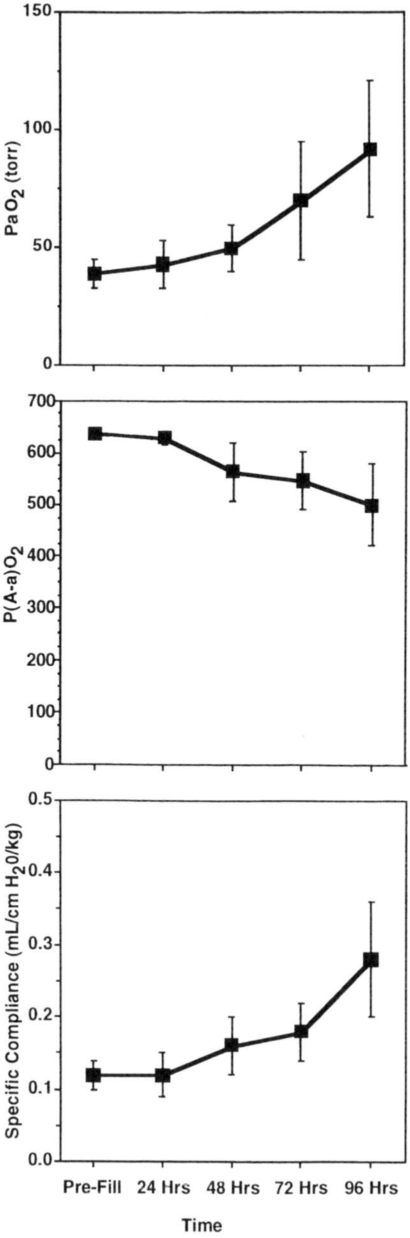

FIGURE 3.—**A**, mean PaO_2 during the initial 96 hours of partial liquid ventilation. **B**, mean alveolar-arterial oxygen gradient $P(A\text{-}a)O_2$, during the initial 96 hours of partial liquid ventilation. **C**, mean specific pulmonary compliance during the initial 96 hours of partial liquid ventilation. Data are expressed as mean plus or minus standard error of the mean. (Courtesy of Gauger PG, Pranikoff T, Schreiner RJ, et al: Initial experience with partial liquid ventilation in pediatric patients with the acute respiratory distress syndrome. *Crit Care Med* 24:16–22, 1996.)

cause pneumothoraces and is also associated with mucus plug formation that often requires frequent bronchoscopic suctioning. Whether patients with ARDS not receiving ECLS will benefit from intratracheal perfluorocarbon remains to be seen, but further studies will be anticipated with great interest.

D.M. Rothenberg, M.D.

Lung Aeration: The Effect of Pre-oxygenation and Hyperoxygenation During Total Intravenous Anesthesia

Reber A, Engberg G, Wegenius G, et al (Univ Hosp, Uppsala, Sweden)

Anaesthesia 51:733–737, 1996 7–3

Background.—Early atelectasis formation and pulmonary shunt during general anesthesia with mechanical ventilation is being recognized increasingly. The use of a lower oxygen concentration than is the current standard may prevent atelectasis formation. The effects of preoxygenation and hyperoxygenation on aeration and atelectasis formation in the lungs during total IV anesthesia were investigated.

Methods.—By random assignment, 27 consecutive patients received preoxygenation (group 1), no preoxygenation (group 2), or hyperoxygenation (group 3). Spiral CT was used to determine lung aeration. The aeration of lung regions on CT scans was classified as overaeration, normal aeration, reduced aeration, poor aeration, or atelectasis formation.

Findings.—Larger areas of atelectasis were found in the basal parts of the lungs in group 1 patients than in group 2 patients. Patients in group 3 had a significant increase in atelectatic regions and a corresponding decrease in regions with reduced aeration in the bases of the lungs.

Conclusions.—Atelectasis was markedly increased during preoxygenation and appeared rapidly during hyperoxygenation, suggesting that these procedures should be used cautiously. Pure oxygen should be delivered only when hypoxemia is overt or anticipated.

► This paper is interesting because it challenges our long-held and cherished concept of preoxygenation as being something "good." These authors studied, by CT, patients who were undergoing total intravenous anesthesia and decided that preoxygenation promoted atelectasis. How much clinical relevance this has is not yet obvious. This is interesting, but I doubt that it will change our practice.

J.H. Tinker, M.D.

Partial Liquid Ventilation With Perflubron in Premature Infants With Severe Respiratory Distress Syndrome

Leach CL, for the LiquiVent Study Group (State Univ of New York, Buffalo; Jefferson Med College, Philadelphia; Temple Univ, Philadelphia; et al)

N Engl J Med 335:761–767, 1996 7–4

Objective.—Ventilation with perfluorocarbon liquids has been used successfully to treat lung dysfunction in premature neonates with surfactant deficiency. The safety and efficacy of partial liquid ventilation, in which perfluorocarbon liquid is introduced into the lungs during continuous positive-pressure gas ventilation, were evaluated in premature infants with severe respiratory distress syndrome; in addition, perfluorocarbon was compared with other treatments.

Methods.—Perflubron was instilled at the rate of 1 mL/kg/min into the lungs of 13 at-risk-of-death, premature infants less than 5 days old with arterial oxygen tension less than 60 mm Hg or arterial carbon dioxide tension greater than 60 mm Hg. Mechanical ventilation maintained at an end-expiratory pressure of 4 cm H_2O was continued throughout the instillation, and partial liquid ventilation was continued for a minimum of 24 hours. New medical conditions, developmental progress, changes in arterial tension, dynamic compliance, ventilatory requirements, oxygenation index (fraction of inspired oxygen × mean airway pressure × 100 divided by arterial oxygen tension), and survival were monitored.

Results.—The 10 infants who completed the study were ventilated for an average of 42 hours. Gas exchange and lung mechanics improved, and arterial oxygen tension increased from 60 mm Hg at baseline to 143 mm Hg after 1 hour of ventilation. Within 24 hours, the fraction of inspired oxygen was significantly reduced, and the arterial carbon dioxide tension normalized. The oxygenation index decreased significantly from 49 at baseline to 9 at 24 hours. The procedure was well tolerated. Adverse events included endotracheal tube obstruction (n = 5), hypoxic episodes (n = 2), intracranial hemorrhage (n = 3), pneumothorax (n = 1), and upper gastrointestinal hemorrhage (n = 1). There were 5 deaths, 2 from respiratory distress syndrome, 2 from intracranial hemorrhage, and 1 from pneumonia and sepsis.

Conclusion.—Partial liquid ventilation results in clinical improvement and increased survival in premature neonates with respiratory distress syndrome.

▶ Safety studies in both adults and infants and now premature neonates have shown that partial liquid ventilation with perfluorocarbon is relatively free of systemic toxicity. Encouraging results in preliminary studies such as the one presented necessitate the need for persistent clinical research into this exciting new area of therapy for both respiratory distress syndrome and adult respiratory distress syndrome.

D.M. Rothenberg, M.D.

▶ Many new exciting therapies are available in the neonatal nursery: high frequency ventilation, extracorporal membrane oxygenation (ECMO) inhaled nitric oxide and surfactant treatment. Partial liquid ventilation–perfluorocarbon associated gas exchange in combination with mechanical ventilation–is a new form of therapy that is now being studied in infants with congenital diaphragmatic hernia, pulmonary hypertension and respiratory distress syndrome of prematurity.

M. Wood, M.D.

Volume-controlled Ventilation Is Made Possible in Infants by Using Compliant Breathing Circuits With Large Compression Volume

Badgwell JM, Swan J, Foster AC (Texas Tech Univ Health Sciences Ctr, Lubbock)

Anesth Analg 82:719–723, 1996 7–5

Objective.—Smaller infants ventilated using volume-limited ventilators and circle breathing systems require a higher preset tidal volume (VTset) to make up for the compression volume of compliant breathing circuits. However, it is uncertain what the VTset should be, on a milligram-per-kilogram basis. Many clinicians simply start with a low tidal volume and increase it gradually to reach appropriate chest expansion, peak inspiratory pressure (PIP), $ETCO_2$, and SpO_2. The weight dependency of VTset was studied in infants and children receiving mechanical ventilation with a variety of breathing circuits.

Methods.—The study included 80 infants undergoing anesthesia for major or minor surgical procedures, including abdominal, thoracic, and neurosurgical procedures. Premature infants, newborns, and previously premature infants all were represented. Neuromuscular blockade was administered, and the infants were intubated. They then were ventilated with an Ohmeda 7800 volume-limited ventilator and a pediatric circle

TABLE 1.—Weight, Age, and Respiratory Measurements With Different Breathing Circuit Combinations

Breathing system	*n*	Weight (kg)	Age (mo)	PIP (cm H_2O)	$ETCO_2$ (mm Hg)	SpO_2 (%)
ACAB	11	11.2 ± 5.3*	21.7 ± 16.9*	19.3 ± 3.5	35.2 ± 5.0	99.0 ± 1.6
ACPB	17	6.2 ± 4.1	9.1 ± 10.0	22.6 ± 4.0	30.7 ± 5.5	99.1 ± 1.5
BaPB	16	3.7 ± 2.5	3.2 ± 4.2	22.2 ± 4.0	32.6 ± 7.7	98.3 ± 2.9
PCAB	7	6.8 ± 4.0	8.4 ± 8.0	20.9 ± 1.3	34.0 ± 5.0	98.3 ± 2.3
PCPB	29	3.5 ± 2.9	3.7 ± 8.2	22.3 ± 3.7	29.8 ± 8.3	98.7 ± 1.8

Abbreviations: ACAB, adult circle/adult-sized bellows; *ACPB,* adult circle/pediatric-sized bellows; *BaPB,* Bain circuit/pediatric-sized bellows; *PCAB,* pediatric circle/adult-sized bellows; *PCPB,* pediatric circle/pediatric-sized bellows.
(Courtesy of Badgwell JM, Swan J, Foster AC: Volume-controlled ventilation is made possible in infants by using compliant breathing circuits with large compression volume. *Anesth Analg* 82:719–723, 1996.)

(PC) or adult circle (AC) breathing system, or a Bain circuit (Ba) and a pediatric- or adult-sized bellows (PB or AB).

Results.—The various groups were similar in terms of body weight, age, PIP, $ETCO_2$, and SpO_2, except for larger and older infants in the ACAB group (Table 1). All circuits were associated with substantial compression volume loss. The curvilinear relation describing the weight-related variation in VTset per kilogram was $y = 175.02x^{-0.087}$; $r^2 = 0.87$, where y represents volume added and x represents PIP. By this relation, VTset was about 150 to 200 mL/kg for a 1-kg infant and about 25 mL/kg for infants weighing 10 kg or more. Poor pulmonary compliance caused problems in 1 patient; the rest were adequately ventilated.

Conclusions.—Volume-controlled ventilators can be used in small infants, given the large compression volumes associated with compliant breathing systems. Data on the weight dependency of VTset in this situation were determined. The guidelines may not be suitable for use in infants with very poorly compliant lungs or with noncompliant pediatric breathing circuits.

► This is a very controversial topic; however, it is important to recognize that this type of experiment does not apply to small infants with poorly compliant lungs. If alternative equipment is not readily available, using modified adult equipment may not be safe. I, for one, would not like to throw away my Jackson-Rees circuit!

M. Wood, M.D.

The Use of an Endotracheal Ventilation Catheter in the Management of Difficult Extubations

Cooper RM (Toronto Hosp)
Can J Anaesth 43:90–93, 1996 7–6

Objective.—Recent guidelines state that the anesthetists should have a plan for extubation of the difficult airway. This strategy should account for the need for reintubation, which is difficult to predict. An experience with the endotracheal ventilation catheter (ETVC), a device designed to maintain airway access after extubation, is described.

Methods.—The ETVC, designed after the "jet stylet," is a 65-cm long semirigid polyurethane catheter with a distal end hole and several side holes (Fig). It was approved at the author's institution for use in patients who had elective orthognathic surgery and who were expected to have a restricted postoperative mouth opening.

> *Technique.*—For tracheal extubation, the trachea and oropharynx are suctioned, and the ETVC is introduced through the patient's endotracheal tube. After the proximal connector on the ETVC is removed, the tracheal cuff is deflated, and the endotra-

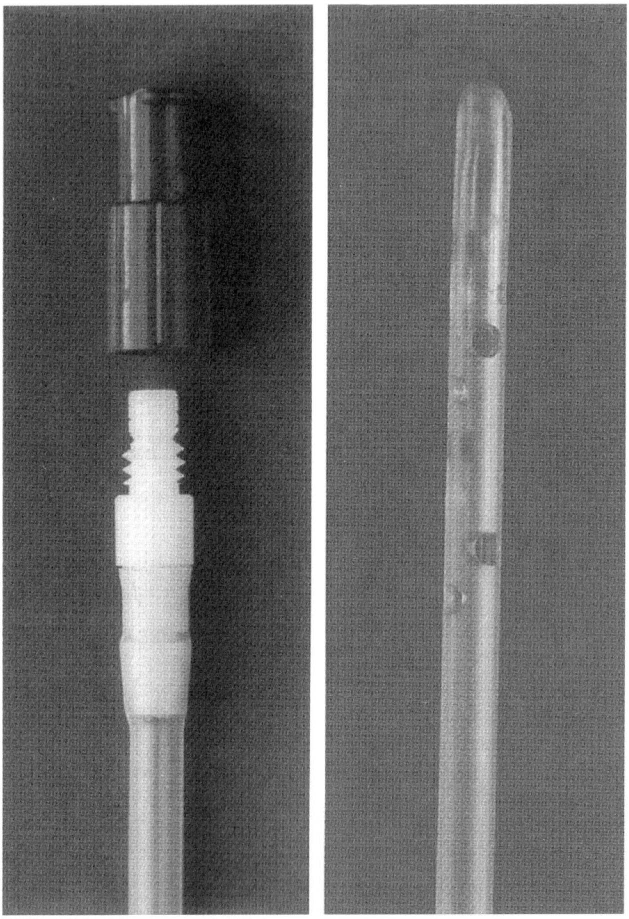

FIGURE.—**A**, Close up of the distal end of the endotracheal ventilation catheter (CardioMed Supplies, Inc.). Eight helically arranged side holes and an end hole are present. **B**, the proximal end. A conical male connector is welded into the catheter and a removable luer-lock jet adaptor can be threaded onto the catheter. This can be attached to a jet injector, oxygen tubing for insufflation, or a capnograph for respiratory monitoring. (From Cooper RM: The use of an endotracheal ventilation catheter in the management of difficult extubations. *Can J Anaesth* 43:90–93, 1996, and Cooper RM, Cohen DR: The use of an endotracheal ventilation catheter for jet ventilation during a difficult intubation. *Can J Anaesth* 41:1196–1199, 1994.)

cheal tube is withdrawn over the ETVC. Maintenance of the ETVC at the desired depth is ensured by aligning its distance markers with those of the endotracheal tube. The ETVC is secured and left in place until there is no longer any concern about the potential need for reintubation.

Results.—The ETVC was used in 202 patients, most often to maintain airway access. Patients with this indication tended to have airways requiring multiple attempts, various techniques, or fiberoptic intubation. There was no need for supplemental analgesia, local anesthesia, or sedation. When the patient coughed, it was often a sign that the catheter had been placed too far distal. Discomfort occurred in only 5 patients, in whom it was managed by catheter removal or lidocaine instillation.

Conclusions.—The ETVC appears to provide an effective new technique for preserving airway access in difficult extubations. The new device is effective even in patients whose glottis cannot be visualized. More patients must be studied to establish the reliability of the ETVC.

► The ETVC is unique in that patients appear to tolerate this foreign body passed through their vocal cords without coughing or respiratory distress. Indeed, 3 patients tolerated this catheter for 48–72 hours without any apparent respiratory compromise. This catheter may be ideal for use in patients in whom upper airway obstruction is suspected and in whom success of extubation is often unpredictable.[1]

D.M. Rothenberg, M.D.

Reference

1. 1996 Year Book of Anesthesiology and Pain Management, p 379.

Oxygen Consumption

Comparison Between Oxygen Consumption Calculated by Fick's Principle Using a Continuous Thermodilution Technique and Measured by Indirect Calorimetry

Bizouarn P, Blanloeil Y, Pinaud M (Hôpital G et R Laënnec, Nantes, France; Hôtel Dieu, Nantes, France)

Br J Anaesth 75:719–723, 1995 7–7

Background.—The reverse Fick principle traditionally is used to determine oxygen consumption. However, measuring cardiac output by thermodilution may be erroneous. Recently, a thermodilution method was described for measuring cardiac output continuously, in which a combination of thermal indicator dilution and stochastic system identification techniques is used. Oxygen consumption as calculated by the Fick principle using a continuous thermodilution method was compared with that using indirect calorimetry.

Methods and Findings.—Nine patients who were stable after cardiac surgery were studied. Six successive measures of continuous cardiac output and gas exchange were made during 5 minutes at 10-minute intervals in each patient. The average difference between estimates was 15 mL/ min^{-1}/m^2. The relative error of the continuous cardiac output method was 5% and that of the gas exchange method was 4%. The repeatability of the new cardiac output technology was good compared with direct measurement.

Conclusions.—The Fick principle using a continuous cardiac output thermodilution method did not accurately predict oxygen consumption by a gas exchange method. However, the repeatability of calculating oxygen consumption was good compared with direct measurement, probably because the precision of continuous cardiac output measures is good.

▶ Continuous thermodilution cardiac output measurement has been around for some time now. These authors used it to calculate oxygen consumption by the Fick principle, in comparison with a relatively standard gas exchange method for $\dot{V}O_2$. I think this paper shows, as have others, that the continuous thermodilution technique is an elegant and accurate method of measuring cardiac output. The problem is that you still need a pulmonary artery catheter! The right ventricle still pounds itself into subendocardial hemorrhage against the catheter and the valves on the right side of the heart are still in jeopardy over time. As I have ranted and raved on these pages before, we have an aorta, 1 inch in diameter or so, just a few centimeters below the sternum, with about 5 L or more per minute flow of iron-containing particles in it and we still cannot measure the flow in that pipe continuously and noninvasively! Even though this is a legitimate and reasonable advance, pulmonary artery catheter technology is more than 30 years old now and has recently come into yet another round of cost/efficacy/safety criticism. I continue to believe that we need to learn how to measure cardiac output continuously but noninvasively.

J.H. Tinker, M.D.

Oxygen Consumption Calculated From the Fick Equation Has Limited Utility

Stock MC, Ryan ME (Emory Univ, Atlanta, Ga)

Crit Care Med 24:86–90, 1996 7–8

Introduction.—The hemodynamic and ventilatory support provided to critically ill patients depends on accurate assessment of their oxygen transport and oxygen consumption ($\dot{V}O_2$). The $\dot{V}O_2$ is commonly calculated using the Fick relationship (calculated $\dot{V}O_2$). Although $\dot{V}O_2$ can be directly measured with a water-sealed spirometer, this method is impractical for use outside the research setting. The capability of the Fick-calculated $\dot{V}O_2$ to determine the true total body $\dot{V}O_2$ precisely enough for clinical use was evaluated in a laboratory study.

Methods.—Thirteen adult Yucatan minipigs underwent anesthesia and vascular cannulation. The animals breathed through a closed circuit including a CO_2 absorber; 2 large-diameter, low-resistance, unidirectional valves; and a spirometer. After the pigs breathed on their own for 30 minutes, physiologic data on their cardiac output, spirometry $\dot{V}O_2$ and arterial and mixed venous blood gases, pH, and oxyhemoglobin saturation were measured (normal lungs/normal heart). They were then given IV esmolol to induce heart failure, and the measurements were repeated. Acute lung injury was induced with oleic acid administered via the right atrial port of the pulmonary artery catheter, and the measurements were repeated again. For the last set of measurements, heart failure was super-

TABLE 2.—Difference Between Spirometry Oxygen Consumption ($\dot{V}O_2$) and Fick-calculated $\dot{V}O_2$ for All Physiologic Conditions (Mean ± SD)

Physiology: Lungs	Physiology: Heart	N	Spirometry $\dot{V}O_2$-Calculated $\dot{V}O_2$ (mL O_2/min) Bias ± Precision	Minimum Difference (mL O_2/min)	Maximum Difference (mL O_2/min)
Normal	Normal	13	+126 ± 28	+62	+177
Normal	Failure	13	+85 ± 87	−80	+296
Injured	Normal	13	+105 ± 44	0	+161
Injured	Failure	13	+64 ± 48	−42	+147
Pooled data		52	+95 ± 59	−80	+296

Note: Mean difference is bias; mean SD is precision.
Abbreviations: N, sample size or number in sample; *SD*, standard deviation.
(Courtesy of Stock MC, Ryan ME: Oxygen consumption calculated from the Fick equation has limited utility. *Crit Care Med* 24:86–90, 1996.)

imposed over acute lung injury with IV esmolol. The mean spirometry $\dot{V}O_2$ values were compared with the calculated $\dot{V}O_2$ values, derived from the equation

$$\dot{V}O_2 = CO \times (CaO_2 - C\bar{v}O_2)$$

where CO is thermodilution cardiac output.

Results.—There were significant differences between the mean spirometry and calculated $\dot{V}O_2$ in all 4 physiologic states and on analysis of the pooled data. A large positive bias was noted, and consistent underestimation of spirometry $\dot{V}O_2$ by calculated $\dot{V}O_2$ occurred. The mean bias in the pooled data was 95 mL O_2/min) (Table 2). The slopes created on linear regression of the 4 physiologic subgroups and the pooled data were indistinguishable from 1.0.

Conclusions.—The calculated $\dot{V}O_2$, as calculated using the Fick relationship, consistently underestimates the "true" $\dot{V}O_2$ as measured by spirometry. The reason for the bias noted may be that the Fick method excludes intrapulmonary $\dot{V}O_2$, which may extend as high as 15% of total body $\dot{V}O_2$ in metabolically active or infected lungs. Although a change in calculated $\dot{V}O_2$ probably reflects the direction of a change in true $\dot{V}O_2$, an error of 20% to 25% of the absolute value should be expected. The imprecision of calculated $\dot{V}O_2$ should be taken into account in clinical practice.

Spirometric Versus Fick-derived Oxygen Consumption: Which Method Is Better?

Thrush DN (Univ of South Florida, Tampa)
Crit Care Med 24:91–95, 1996 7–9

Introduction.—The Fick equation is commonly used to assess oxygen consumption ($\dot{V}O_2$) in critically ill patients. However, the accuracy of these calculations compared with independent measurements of $\dot{V}O_2$ has been questioned. The $\dot{V}O_2$ values calculated by the Fick equation and measured by a spirometer were compared in an experimental study.

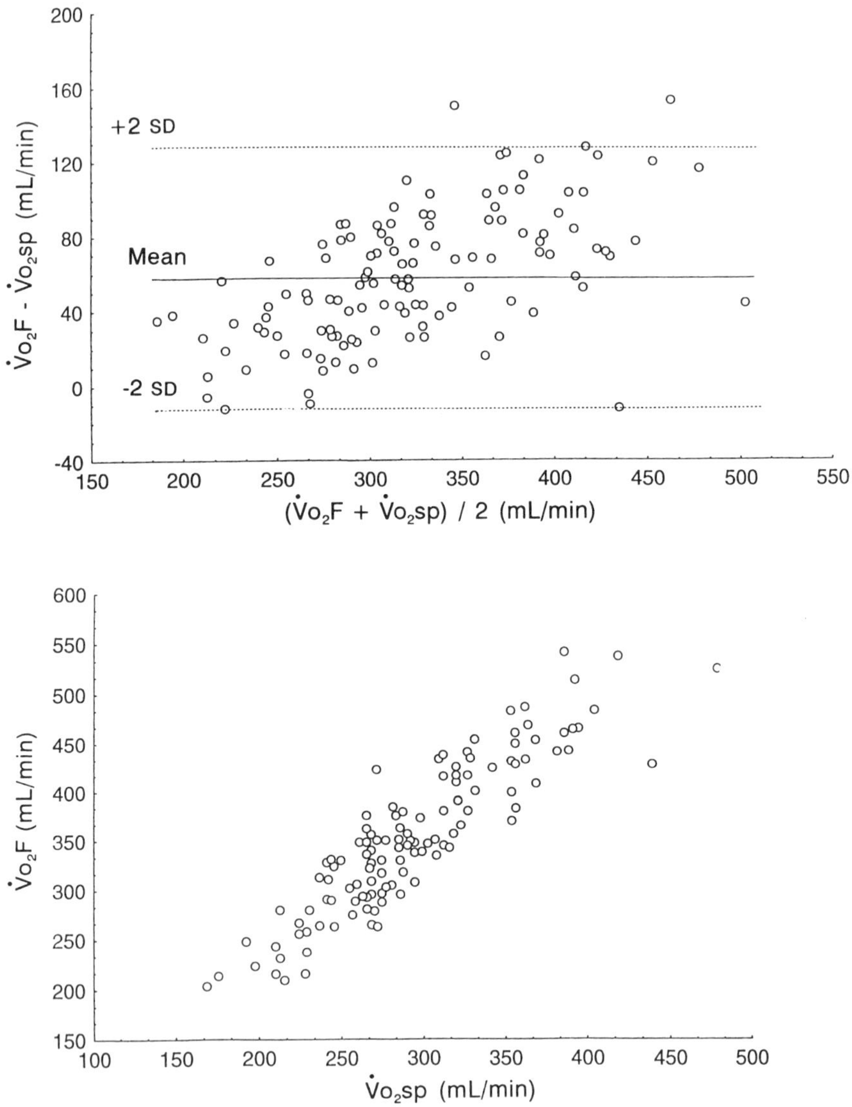

FIGURE 1.—**A**, bias plot of Fick-derived minus spirometrically measured oxygen consumption ($\dot{V}O_2F - \dot{V}O_2sp$) shows differences between the two methods. **B**, scattergram plot of Fick-derived ($\dot{V}O_2F$) and spirometrically measured ($\dot{V}O_2sp$) oxygen consumption. Although the correlation, 0.90, and the coefficient of variation, 0.82, are high, the bias plot in **A** demonstrates poor agreement between methods. (Courtesy of Thrush DN: Spirometric versus Fick-derived oxygen consumption: Which method is better? *Crit Care Med* 24:91–95, 1996.)

Methods.—Nineteen instrumented pigs were studied while breathing spontaneously through a closed circuit, including a CO_2 absorber, unidirectional valves, and a water-sealed spirometer. The slope of the end-expiratory volume during 6 consecutive 1-minute recordings was used to measure $\dot{V}O_2$. The Fick method was also used to calculate $\dot{V}O_2$ as cardiac output multiplied by the arterial-venous oxygen content difference. Triplicate bolus-thermodilution measurements were made at random moments of the respiratory cycle, and the results were averaged. Data were collected at baseline, during and after IV dobutamine infusion to increase spirometrically measured $\dot{V}O_2$ by 50% to 75%, and during and after labetalol infusion to decrease spirometrically measured $\dot{V}O_2$ by 50% to 75%.

Results.—Mean $\dot{V}O_2$ was 294 ± 55 mL/min as measured by spirometry and 352 ± 75 mL/min as calculated by the Fick equation. The bias and precision between the 2 values was 58 ± 35 mL/min (Fig 1). Despite the high correlation and coefficient of variation values between the 2 techniques, agreement was poor.

Conclusions.—Use of the Fick calculation produces significantly greater $\dot{V}O_2$ values than spirometer measurement of $\dot{V}O_2$ in pigs. The differences persist even with efforts to reduce measurement error. Fick-derived $\dot{V}O_2$ values must be used cautiously in the clinical setting.

▶ These experimental studies conclude (although in totally opposite fashion) that calculated oxygen consumption as derived from the Fick equation is an imprecise measurement with limited research utility. Although it would make sense that Fick-derived oxygen consumption underestimated "true" oxygen consumption because of the failure to take into account oxygen consumption of the lung, there does not appear to be a clear-cut answer as to why Fick-derived oxygen consumption would overestimate spirometrically-derived oxygen consumption ($\dot{V}O_2sp$) as was seen in the second study. Methodological error could conceivably cause such a discrepancy but this does not seem readily apparent. Indeed, both studies were similar with the exception of CaO_2 measurements, which were calculated in the Stock study (using 1.34 mL of O_2/gHb as oxygen-binding capacity) and directly measured using a galvanic fuel cell method in the Thrush study. This would not appear to be a significant enough variance in experimental protocol to explain such differences in bias and precision data. Although I am at a loss to explain the divergent data in these 2 studies (could it be that $\dot{V}O_2sp$ isn't such a "gold standard"?), the data do call into question results of prior studies that have attempted to direct therapy and improve outcome in critically ill patients by targeting supernormal changes in oxygen delivery and calculated oxygen consumption with the use of vasopressors and ionotropic therapy.

D.M. Rothenberg, M.D.

Stress Ulcers in Critical Care

Stress Ulcer Prophylaxis in Critically Ill Patients: Resolving Discordant Meta-analyses

Cook DJ, Reeve BK, Guyatt GH, et al (McMaster Univ, Hamilton, Ontario, Canada; Univ Hosp Bergmannsheil, Bochum, Germany)
JAMA 275:308–314, 1996 7–10

Purpose.—Stress ulcer prophylaxis has been the subject of several systematic reviews. However, these studies have produced some inconsistent results. An updated review of stress ulcer prophylaxis in the critical care unit is presented, including a meta-analysis performed to resolve previous inconsistencies.

Methods.—The review included randomized clinical trials comparing the use of various prophylactic drugs—including antacids, histamine$_2$-receptor antagonists, or sucralfate—with each other or with no treatment. Only studies of critically ill adults using gastrointestional (GI) bleeding or pneumonia as outcome measures were included. The analysis included 57 unique trials representing 7,218 critically ill patients with a wide range of medical and surgical diagnoses.

Results.—Histamine$_2$-receptor antagonist treatment reduced the risk of overt GI bleeding and clinically important bleeding. In addition, antacids tended to decrease the risk of overt bleeding compared with no treatment. The rate of clinically important bleeding tended to be lower with histamine$_2$-receptor antagonists and antacids than with sucralfate. However, histamine$_2$-receptor antagonists tended to increase the risk of pneumonia compared with no prophylaxis. In addition to reducing the nosocomial pneumonia rate, sucralfate was also associated with a lower mortality than antacids or histamine$_2$-receptor antagonists.

Conclusions.—An up-to-date review of the evidence suggests that histamine$_2$-receptor antagonist treatment decreases the rate of clinically important GI bleeding in critically ill adults. Sucralfate may be just as effective in reducing the bleeding rate while also reducing the risk of nosocomial pneumonia and death. The net effect of sucralfate vs. no prophylaxis remains to be determined.

► Although neither of these meta-analyses clarify whether there is an increased incidence in nosocomial pneumonia with histamine$_2$-blockers or a decreased incidence in nosocomial pneumonia with sucralfate, there can be no question that a tremendous amount of money is wasted by administering these expensive agents to patients who have no risk factors for GI hemorrhage.

D.M. Rothenberg, M.D.

Prophylaxis for Stress-Related Gastrointestinal Hemorrhage: A Cost Effectiveness Analysis

Ben-Menachem T, McCarthy BD, Fogel R, et al (Henry Ford Hosp and Health Sciences Ctr, Detroit)

Crit Care Med 24:338–345, 1996 7–11

Objective.—The prevention of stress-related gastrointestinal (GI) hemorrhage in the ICU has potentially important economic implications. However, there have been no cost-effectiveness analyses of routine prophylaxis for stress-related hemorrhage. The cost-effectiveness of pharmacologic prophylaxis for stress-related GI hemorrhage was evaluated using decision analysis techniques.

Methods.—The decision model used in the analysis addressed the cost and efficacy of 2 drugs commonly used for prevention of stress-related GI hemorrhage: sucralfate and cimetidine (Fig 1). Outcome data were drawn from published studies, and cost data were from the authors' institution. As a base, the study assumed a 6% risk of stress-related hemorrhage and a 50% reduction of risk as a result of prophylaxis (Table 2).

Results.—Given the base case assumptions, sucralfate prophylaxis cost $1,144 per each episode of bleeding prevented. The risk of hemorrhage was the main factor affecting this cost, whereas the efficacy of sucralfate prophylaxis made a lesser contribution. The cost per episode of bleeding prevented ranged as high as $104,000 for patients at low risk for bleeding. For those at very high risk, sucralfate treatment saved money. When the

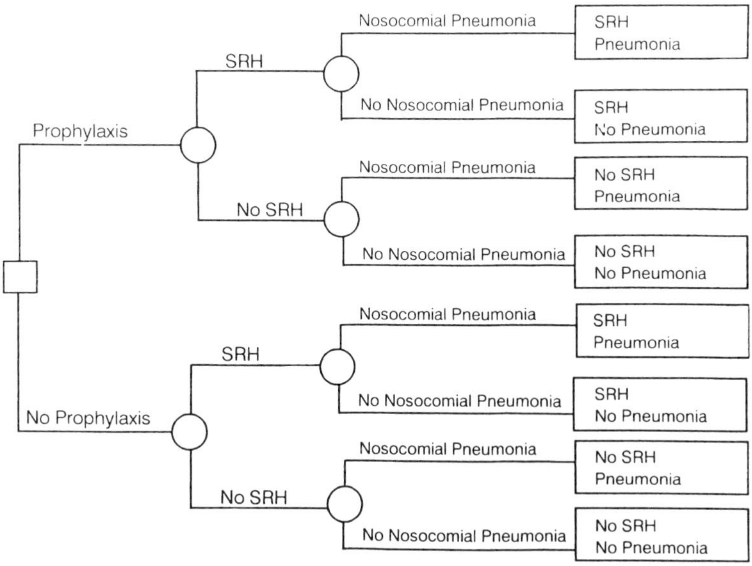

FIGURE 1.—Schematic representation of the decision tree used in the analysis. The single, square "decision node" represents the treatment choice: to use, or not to use prophylaxis. The 2 round "chance nodes" represent the major clinical outcomes: stress-related hemorrhage (SRH) and nosocomial pneumonia. (Courtesy of Ben-Menachem T, McCarthy BD, Fogel R, et al: Prophylaxis for stress-related gastrointestinal hemorrhage: A cost effectiveness analysis. *Crit Care Med* 24:338–345, 1996.)

TABLE 2.—Model Assumptions

	Baseline	Range
Outcomes Estimates		
Risk of stress-related hemorrhage (4, 8–21)	6%	0.1–33%
Risk reduction due to prophylaxis (4, 8–21)	50%	10–90%
Risk of nosocomial pneumonia* (13, 19, 20, 34–38)	0%	0–10%
Cost Estimates†		
Prophylactic Medications‡		
Sucralfate	$52	
Cimetidine	$244	
Treatment of Stress-Related Hemorrhage		
Esophagogastroduodenoscopy	$297	
Serial hematocrit determinations	$27	
Cimetidine therapy	$152	
Blood transfusions	$119	
Total	$595	
Treatment of Nosocomial Pneumonia		
Diagnosis and initial work-up	$193	
Antibiotics	$932	
Additional ICU length of stay	$8,937	
Total	$10,062	

*Attributable risk increase (absolute increase in risk of nosocomial pneumonia).
†Based on cost at Henry Ford Hospital.
‡Per patient, per 7 days average ICU stay.
(Courtesy of Ben-Menachem T, McCarthy BD, Fogel R, et al: Prophylaxis for stres-related gastrointestinal hemorrhage: A cost effectiveness analysis. *Crit Care Med* 24:338–345, 1996.)

risk of nosocomial pneumonia was considered as well, the cost to prevent an episode of bleeding increased significantly. Patients at low risk for GI bleeding showed a greater effect in terms of preventing pneumonia. Assuming that cimetidine and sucralfate were equally effective, the cost per episode of bleeding prevented was 6.5-fold higher with cimetidine.

Conclusions.—Prophylaxis against stress-related GI hemorrhage in the ICU is expensive, and the cost may be prohibitive for patients at low risk for bleeding. It is not possible to make standard recommendations until the risk and severity of stress-related GI bleeding in different ICU patient populations are known, along with the effects of prophylaxis on the risk of nosocomial pneumonia. This cost-effectiveness analysis likely underestimated the costs associated with treating nosocomial pneumonia.

Nitric Oxide Issues

Inhaled Nitric Oxide for High-altitude Pulmonary Edema

Scherrer U, Vollenweider L, Delabays A, et al (Centre Hospitalier Universitaire Vaudois, Lausanne, Switzerland; Inst of Physiology, Lausanne, Switzerland; Univ Hosp, Berne, Switzerland; et al)
N Engl J Med 334:624–629, 1996 7–12

Purpose.—A key aspect of high-altitude pulmonary edema is pulmonary hypertension, which may play a pathogenetic role. The endothelium-derived relaxing factor nitric oxide, given by inhalation, can reduce the pulmonary vasoconstriction resulting from short-term hypoxia. Its effects on pulmonary artery pressure and arterial oxygenation were studied in mountaineers who were susceptible and resistant to the effects of high-altitude pulmonary edema.

Methods.—The study included 18 mountaineers who had documented high-altitude pulmonary edema during the previous 4 years and another 18 mountaineers with no history of high-altitude pulmonary edema or acute mountain sickness. The research subjects were studied at baseline and after rapid ascent to a high-altitude research laboratory. Nitric oxide was given by face mask at a nitric oxide concentration of 40 parts per million in room air. The effects of nitric oxide inhalation on pulmonary artery pressure and arterial oxygenation were assessed. A subset of research subjects underwent lung perfusion scanning before and after nitric oxide inhalation at altitude to gain insight into its mechanisms of action.

Results.—Radiographic evidence of pulmonary edema developed within 18–36 hours at altitude in 55% of research subjects susceptible to high-altitude pulmonary edema versus none of the nonsusceptible controls. The mean mountain-sickness score in the susceptible group was 7.5. These research subjects had more severe hypoxemia and pulmonary hypertension than the controls. When given nitric oxide, the susceptible group had a much greater decrease in pulmonary artery pressure, which was directly correlated with the severity of their pulmonary hypertension. Arterial oxygenation improved rapidly with nitric oxide, despite a slight decline in the fraction of inspired oxygen. For the research subjects with no history of high-altitude pulmonary edema, nitric oxide impaired arterial oxygenation as it reduced pulmonary artery pressure. Four susceptible research subjects experienced pulmonary edema and underwent lung perfusion studies. When they inhaled nitric oxide at altitude, the blood flow in their lungs was redistributed away from edematous segments and toward nonedematous segments.

Conclusions.—Inhaled nitric oxide has beneficial effects in research subjects with high-altitude pulmonary edema; it decreases pulmonary artery pressure while it improves arterial oxygenation. It impairs rather than improves arterial oxygenation in research subjects with high-altitude pulmonary vasoconstriction alone, however. The pathogenesis of high-altitude pulmonary edema may involve a defect in nitric oxide synthesis.

▶ For those of you who enjoy recreational skiing or mountain-climbing and who, like myself, have suffered some of the ill-effects of high altitudes, this is an interesting article from both a design and result perspective. The high-altitude research laboratory located at an altitude of 4,559 m in the Swiss–Italian Alps is truly remarkable with regard to its location (I'm sure this is where they coined the term *breathtaking*) and to the technology available there to the researchers. The results of the study would suggest that inhaled nitric oxide may be a benefit in improving oxygenation in those who suffer high-altitude pulmonary edema and who cannot be quickly transported to a lower altitude. It would have been interesting to see also whether these mountaineers' improvement was relative to their high-altitude sickness scores; however, these data were not provided.

D.M. Rothenberg, M.D.

Nitric Oxide Synthase Inhibition Versus Norepinephrine for the Treatment of Hyperdynamic Sepsis in Sheep

Booke M, Hinder F, McGuire R, et al (Univ of Texas, Galveston)

Crit Care Med 24:835–844, 1996 7–13

Background.—Because a reduction in mean arterial pressure (MAP) correlates with mortality in patients who have sepsis, efficient correction of hypotension is crucial. Norepinephrine has been the treatment agent of choice in patients who have severe vasodilation, but responsiveness to it is reduced in patients who have sepsis. Because nitric oxide is the final common mediator for vasodilation in sepsis, treatment with nitric oxide synthase inhibitors can be effective. The effects of norepinephrine and N^{ω}-monomethyl-L-arginine (L-NMMA), a nitric oxide synthase inhibitor, were compared in a model of hyperdynamic ovine sepsis.

Methods.—Ultrasonic flow probes were placed on the carotid, left renal, and superior mesenteric arteries and the infrarenal aorta in 25 healthy, adult, female sheep for continuous monitoring. The sheep were continuously infused with live *Pseudomonas aeruginosa*. After 24 hours of sepsis, the sheep were given 1 of 3 infusions: L-NMMA (8 sheep), norepinephrine (8 sheep), or vehicle alone (9 sheep). The sheep in the norepinephrine group were each matched with a sheep in the L-NMMA group, and the dosage of norepinephrine was continuously adjusted to produce the same increase in MAP that occurred in the matched sheep that were receiving L-NMMA.

Results.—Within 24 hours after infusion of *P. aeruginosa*, all sheep had hyperdynamic sepsis, with intense vasodilation, increased cardiac index, reduced MAP, and reduced systemic vascular resistance index. Treatment with L-NMMA resulted in an immediate increase in MAP to baseline values, decreased cardiac index, and increased systemic vasuclar resistance index, thereby reversing the hyperdynamic state. Treatment with norepinephrine resulted in a similar increase in MAP, but continuously increasing dosages were needed to maintain increases in MAP (Fig 4); the same values could be achieved, however, with steady doses of L-NMMA. Norepinephrine produced no changes in either cardiac index or systemic vascular resistance index. Neither treatment affected renal blood flow, and both substantially improved urine output. There were no differences in the 3 groups in pulmonary bacteria clearance or in blood concentrations of bacteria.

Conclusion.—Both L-NMMA and norepinephrine were effective in increasing MAP and in improving renal function. Neither agent caused excessive vasoconstriction or produced adverse effects on cardiac index or

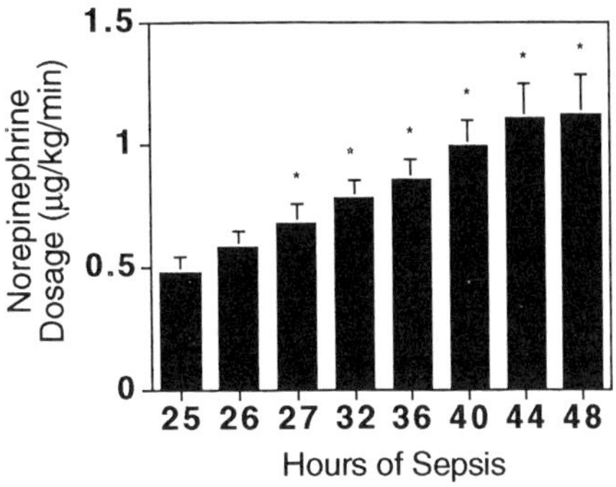

FIGURE 4.—The norepinephrine dosage in the norepinephrine group had to be continuously increased during the course of sepsis, which reflects the reduced vascular responsiveness to catecholamines during sepsis. $^*P \leq .05$ vs. 25 hours. Data are mean ± standard error of mean. (Courtesy of Booke M, Hinder F, McGuire R, et al: Nitric oxide synthase inhibition versus norepinephrine for the treatment of hyperdynamic sepsis in sheep. *Crit Care Med* 24(5):835–844, 1996.)

vital organ blood flow. Further study is recommended to examine the effects of combined norepinephrine and L-NMMA on sepsis.

▶ The use of a nitric oxide synthase inhibitor is another in a long line of novel approaches designed to counteract the mediators of sepsis. So-called magic bullets, such as monoclonal antibodies directed against interleukins, tumor necrosis factor, and other "evil humors," have been experimentally and clinically assessed over the past few years with limited success. Although these previous trials have failed to establish an improved outcome with mediator-specific therapy in patients who have sepsis, agents that target the support of end-organ perfusion, such as L-NMMA, may prove to be more beneficial.

Results of this study lend credence to the theory of downregulation of vascular-catecholamine receptors (see Fig 4), thus justifying the use of nitric oxide synthase inhibitors, agents that should restore vasculature responsiveness.

This study also shows the lack of any detrimental effects of L-NMMA or norepinephrine on regional blood flow, particularly to the gut or the kidney. Perhaps the use of these 2 agents together (similar to but more pathophysiologically oriented than the use of norepinephrine and low-dose dopamine) will be an ideal method of improving tissue perfusion for patients who have sepsis.

D.M. Rothenberg, M.D.

Comparison of Two Administration Techniques of Inhaled Nitric Oxide on Nitrogen Dioxide Production
Dubé L, Francoeur M, Troncy E, et al (Univ of Montreal)
Can J Anaesth 42:922–927, 1995 7–14

Background.—A new injection device, which enables direct injection of NO-N_2 into the inspiratory line of the ventilator circuit, is hypothesized to reduce NO_2 formation (by reducing contact time between O_2 and NO) relative to the classic method (introduction of the NO-N_2 mixture at the air inlet of the ventilator).

Methods.—A chemiluminescence analyzer was used to measure levels of NO and NO_2. The effect on NO_2 of 2 fraction of inspired oxygen FIO_2 and NO concentrations was determined. With the new injection system, NO injection is cyclic and occurs only during the inspiratory phase of the mechanical ventilator.

Results.—The amount of NO_2 produced was 8.9 ppm with the classic system and 4.4 ppm with the new system for an FIO_2 of 0.90 and a NO of 90 ppm. With an NO of 60 ppm, NO_2 produced measured 4.5 ppm with the classic method and 2.1 ppm with the new method. However, no difference occurred in amount of NO_2 produced between systems when the FIO_2 was 0.21.

Conclusions.—When high FIO_2 and NO concentrations are used, the new NO injection system seems to considerably reduce the concentration of inhaled NO_2 relative to the classic system.

▶ At low FIO_2's, no difference in NO_2 was found between the 2 NO delivery systems. However, with higher FIO_2's there appears to be a greater difference, with the difference being augmented when the parts per million of NO exceeds 20. Because clinical effectiveness of NO is now determined to be at much less than 20 in most patients, I doubt that a system that is riskier for delivery of NO—that is, the new system proposed—merits the slight benefit that would accrue. I remain an amateur in this field; however, I wait to be persuaded that this increased risk is worth the benefit.

M.F. Roizen, M.D.

Renal Function Issues

Preoperative α_2-Adrenergic Receptor Agonists Prevent the Deterioration of Renal Function After Cardiac Surgery: Results of a Randomized, Controlled Trial
Kulka PJ, Tryba M, Zenz M (Univ Hosp Bergmannsheil, Bochum, Germany)
Crit Care Med 24:947–952, 1996 7–15

Background.—The death rate associated with cardiac surgery ranges from 1% to 2%. Renal function impairment is an important determinant of outcome. Because renal function regulation and sympathetic nervous system function are closely related, the effect of preoperative clonidine administration on postoperative renal function was assessed in patients who underwent coronary artery bypass graft (CABG) surgery.

Methods.—Forty-eight patients at normal risk with no evidence of preexisting renal dysfunction were included in the prospective, double-blind, randomized, placebo-controlled trial. Clonidine, 4 µg/kg, or placebo was administered intravenously 1 hour before anesthesia was induced.

Findings.—Patients given clonidine had a significantly shorter duration of extracorporeal circulation. The 2 groups were comparable in fluid administration and blood loss during anesthesia and in the first 12 hours after surgery. Mean creatinine clearance declined the first night after surgery from 98 to 68 mL/min in patients given placebo. On the third night after surgery, creatinine clearance rose to 75 mL/min. Creatinine clearance remained at about 90 mL/min at all measurements in the clonidine-treated patients.

Conclusion.—Preoperative clonidine treatment prevented renal function deterioration after CABG surgery in these patients. This may have resulted from a clonidine-induced decrease in the sympathetic nervous system response to CABG surgery.

▶ Despite the authors' contention that clonidine imparts renal protection to patients who undergo CABG, this study merely shows that shorter bypass times result in improved postoperative glomerular filtration rates. In addition, it is unclear from the data presented as to how perioperative hemodynamic changes and/or the administration of vasopressors such as epinephrine or norepinephrine influenced the overall results. Finally, previous studies that examined the influence of epidural anesthesia-induced α-adrenergic blockade in patients who underwent major vascular surgery did not show any significant improvement in postoperative renal function. Therefore, I remain unconvinced that this line of therapy will offer any realistic hope to patients with preoperative renal insufficiency who are at the greatest risk to have post-CABG renal failure.

D.M. Rothenberg, M.D.

Renal Hemodynamics During Norepinephrine and Low-dose Dopamine Infusions in Man

Richer M, Robert S, Lebel M (Université Laval, Québec, Canada; L'Hôtel-Dieu de Québec Hosp, Canada)

Crit Care Med 24:1150–1156, 1996 7–16

Background.—Severe hypotension in patients who are in septic or cardiogenic shock is generally treated with vasopressors, particularly norepinephrine. Because of the risk of renal vasoconstriction with norepinephrine, dopamine is commonly used in combination with the norepinephrine to increase the glomerular filtration rate, renal blood flow, and excretion of sodium. Although this approach is a common management strategy, its benefits have not been adequately studied. The effects of combined nor-

TABLE 1.—Hemodynamic Parameters in 6 Healthy Volunteers (Mean ± Standard Deviation)

Variable	Treatment: Sodium Chloride	Norepinephrine	Dopamine	Norepinephrine/ Dopamine
MAP* (mm Hg)	80 ± 4[†, ‡]	101 ± 5[‡, §, ‖]	78 ± 7[†, ‡]	94 ± 7[†, §, ‖]
HR* (beats/min)	57 ± 5[¶, **]	50 ± 4[¶, ††]	65 ± 7[**, ††, ‡‡]	55 ± 5[¶]
GFR (mL/min/1.73 m²)	95 ± 9	99 ± 8	100 ± 11	98 ± 11
ERBF* (mL/min/1.73 m²)	1241 ± 208[¶, **]	922 ± 143[¶, ††, ‡‡]	1781 ± 84[**, ††, ‡‡]	1191 ± 175[¶, **]

*$P < 0.0001$ (analysis of variance).

$P = 0.0008$ (Tukey's procedure): † vs. norepinephrine; ‡ vs. norepinephrine/dopamine; § vs. sodium chloride; ‖ vs. dopamine.

$P = 0.03$ (Tukey's procedure): ¶ vs. dopamine; ** vs. norepinephrine; †† vs. sodium chloride; ‡‡ vs. norepinephrine/dopamine.

Abbreviations: MAP, mean arterial pressure; *HR*, heart rate; *GFR*, glomerular filtration rate; *ERBF*, effective renal blood flow.

(Courtesy of Richer M, Robert S, Lebel M: Renal hemodynamics during norepinephrine and low-dose dopamine infusions in man. *Crit Care Med* 24(7):1150–1156, 1996.)

epinephrine and low-dose dopamine on renal hemodynamics were therefore evaluated in healthy volunteers.

Methods.—Six healthy adult men underwent each of 4 treatments, which consisted of 180-minute infusions of the following: 0.9% sodium chloride (control); pressor doses of norepinephrine (the dose required to produce an increase of approximately 20 mm Hg in mean arterial pressure), 3 µg/kg/min of dopamine, and pressor doses of norepinephrine plus 3 µg/kg/min of dopamine. The study infusions were begun 60 minutes after the administration of an inulin–para-aminohippurate infusion. Blood pressure and heart rate were monitored. Clearances of inulin and para-aminohippurate were measured to determine glomerular filtration rates and effective renal blood flow. Urine electrolyte clearances were also determined.

Results.—The mean pressor dose of norepinephrine alone was 118 ng/kg/min. When the pressor dose of norepinephrine was combined with dopamine, the mean increase in mean arterial pressure was reduced from 22 to 15 mm Hg. The effective renal blood flow was decreased with norepinephrine from 1,241 to 922 mL/min/1.73 m² but returned to 1,191 mL/min/1.73 m² with the addition of dopamine (Table 1). There were no significant differences in urine output or glomerular filtration rate with the 4 treatments (Fig 2). Urine sodium clearance was increased by 82% with dopamine alone. It decreased by 42% with norepinephrine alone and by 48% with the combination.

Conclusion.—The improvement in renal blood flow produced by combining dopamine with norepinephrine was confirmed in these healthy volunteers. There was no effect of any treatment on urine output and glomerular filtration rate, however, which suggests that these are not

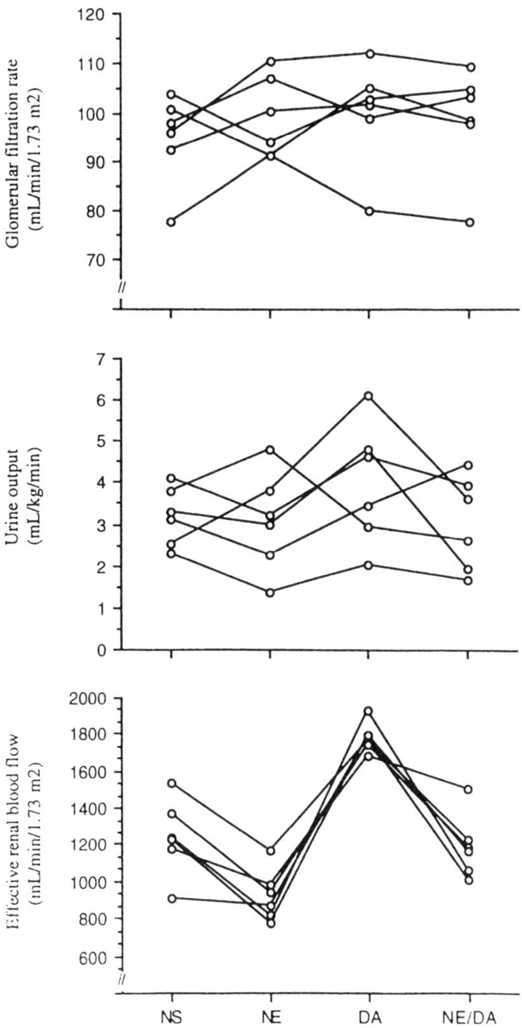

FIGURE 2.—Individual changes in glomerular filtration rate, urine output, and effective renal blood flow for the 6 individuals during control (*NS*) and infusions of norepinephrine (*NE*), dopamine (*DA*), and norepinephrine plus dopamine (*NE/DA*). Each *line* represents a participant. (Courtesy of Richer M, Robert S, Lebel M: Renal hemodynamics during norepinephrine and low-dose dopamine infusions in man. *Crit Care Med* 24(7):1150–1156, 1996.)

reliable indicators of the effects of these drugs on renal function. Further studies are needed to confirm these results in critically ill patients, whose baseline renal function and renal hemodynamics may be altered.

▶ This study attempts to show the beneficial effects on renal blood flow when low-dose dopamine is administered to patients who are receiving infusions of norepinephrine (NE). Although this study has numerous design faults (e.g., failure to use a NE-saline group to decrease bias, failure to monitor cardiac output noninvasively with bioimpedance of transthoracic echocardiography to rule out an inotropic effect of dopamine, and failure to use 1 or 2-hour creatinine clearances to assess the clinical correlation of these measurements with the less clinically applicable inulin clearance), it does tend to support prior experimental and clinical data, particularly in patients with sepsis, thereby showing the attenuation of deleterious renal effects of NE in patients who are receiving low-dose dopamine. Although inulin and para-aminohippurate clearances are not clinically relevant parameters of glomerular filtration rate and renal blow flow, this study emphasizes the clinical irrelevancy of urine output as a measurement of renal function, a concept that is often unappreciated by medical students, residents, and practicing anesthesiologists alike.

D.M. Rothenberg, M.D.

Prolonged Motor Weakness

Economic Impact of Prolonged Motor Weakness Complicating Neuromuscular Blockade in the Intensive Care Unit
Rudis MI, Guslits BJ, Peterson EL, et al (Henry Ford Hosp, Detroit)
Crit Care Med 24:1749–1756, 1996 7–17

Introduction.—In critically ill patients, the neuromuscular weakness syndrome has been associated with pharmacologic paralysis with nondepolarizing neuromuscular blocking agents. In ICU patients who have received continuous neuromuscular blockade, neuromuscular weakness is an important cause of prolonged morbidity and may influence outcome. In terms of ICU and hospital resource utilization, this may have a significant impact economically. A case series of patients with neuromuscular weakness after neuromuscular blockade was studied to quantify the economic outcomes that can be attributed to the neuromuscular weakness. Patient charges and costs were compared with case-controls who were paralyzed, but who did not have prolonged motor weakness.

Methods.—A retrospective review was conducted of the medical and accounting records of 10 patients with neuromuscular weakness. The records were reviewed for exposure to neuromuscular blocking agents, nature of neuropathy, demographic data, associated morbidities, and rate and extent of recovery. The review compared these patients with controls with regard to use of paralytic drug, morbidities associated with neuromuscular weakness, development of prolonged paralysis, length of ICU and hospital stays, number of days requiring mechanical ventilation, neurologic studies, and physical therapy.

Results.—Patients who had neuromuscular weakness had median hospital charges of $91,476, which included charges for continuous mechanical ventilation, neuromuscular blocking agents, neurologic studies, ICU and hospital beds, and physical therapy. Median charges were $22,191 for the controls. The cost differential was a median of $66,713 (Table 4). There were significant differences for full costs, patient charges, mechan-

TABLE 4.—Comparison of Hospital Charges, Full Costs, and Marginal Costs for the Outcome Parameters Evaluated in 10 Patients With Neuromuscular Weakness vs. 10 Controls

Parameter	Patient Charges ($)	Full Cost ($)	Marginal Cost ($)
Medication	−501 (−2063, 2315)	−306 (−1258, 1412)	−119 (−488, 547)
MV*	18,052 (6550, 43885)	3,610 (1310, 8777)	1,234 (448, 2999)
EMG†	524 (10, 665)	199 (4, 253)	181 (3, 229)
Rehabilitation	138 (0, 3069)	30 (0, 675)	26 (0, 568)
Location			
ICU*	23,170 (8275, 53319)	18,304 (6537, 42122)	4,668 (1667, 10741)
IMU‡	15,990 (4920, 52890)	10,394 (3198, 34379)	2,862 (881, 9468)
IPD	0 (0, 4576)	0 (0, 3112)	0 (0, 809)
Total§	66, 713 (23485, 189214)	39, 021 (15817, 116667)	10,597 (3802, 31551)

Note: The median estimated cost difference and its 95% confidence interval are presented for each outcome parameter and their total sum. The following represent significant differences in estimated cost for the patients with neuromuscular weakness: $^{*}P = 0.002$; $^{\dagger}P = 0.014$; $^{\ddagger}P = 0.003$; $^{\S}P = 0.001$.

Abbreviations: Medication, nondepolarizing neuromuscular blocking agent; *MV*, mechanical ventilation; *EMG*, electromyographic studies; *ICU*, intensive care unit bed; *IMU*, intermediate medical care unit bed; *IPD*, inpatient bed.

(Courtesy of Rudis MI, Guslits BJ, Peterson EL, et al: Economic impact of prolonged motor weakness complicating neuromuscular blockade in the intensive care unit. *Crit Care Med* 24:1749–1756, 1996.)

ical ventilation, marginal costs, ICU and hospital stays, and neurologic studies.

Conclusion.—An increase in ICU and hospital stays, mechanical ventilation, and disproportionate health care expenditures in excess of $66,000 per patient were associated with the development of motor weakness. This was a small group of 10 of 183 patients paralyzed for more than 24 hours in the ICU, representing a prevalence of 5.5% of patients having neuromuscular weakness after neuromuscular blockade. In asthmatic patients receiving vecuronium and corticosteroids, the incidence may be as high as 24%. A prospective study of the prevalence of neuromuscular weakness after neuromuscular blockade and the resulting costs to the health care system is needed.

▶ Although this article offers compelling economic reasons to avoid the use of nondepolarizing neuromuscular blocking agents in the ICU, it also brings into question how 8 patients in only 3 months' time could develop this syndrome of prolonged motor weakness. It cannot be ascertained from these data, though it does not seem to be too far fetched to assume, that had train-of-four monitoring or more optimal use of sedative and analgesic agents been employed, this complication could have been prevented or avoided.

D.M. Rothenberg, M.D.

Magnesium Repletion in Critical Care

Magnesium Repletion and Its Effect on Potassium Homeostasis in Critically Ill Adults: Results of a Double-blind, Randomized, Controlled Trial

Hamill-Ruth RJ, McGory R (Univ of Virginia, Charlottesville)

Crit Care Med 24:38–45, 1996 7–18

Objective.—It may be difficult to treat hypokalemia in patients with coexisting hypomagnesemia. Potassium replacement therapy in these patients may lead to increased urine potassium excretion and a backward trend in serum potassium concentration. The effects of an aggressive magnesium replacement regimen on potassium retention in critically ill patients with hypokalemia were evaluated in a prospective, randomized, double-blind, placebo-controlled trial.

Methods.—The individuals were 32 adult surgical patients in the ICU with circulating potassium concentrations of less than 3.5 mmol/L. Patients were assigned to receive active treatment—magnesium sulfate, 2 g in 50 mL of 5% dextrose in water during 30 min every 6 hours for 8 doses—or placebo given by the same schedule. Standard potassium and magnesium replacement therapy continued in both groups, as indicated for a serum potassium concentration of less than 3.5 mmol/L or a serum magnesium concentration of less than 1.8 mg/dL. Colorimetric and potentiometric assays were used to evaluate the serum and urine magnesium and potassium concentrations.

Results.—The 2 groups were similar in their baseline serum magnesium and potassium concentrations. Six hours after the start of the study, just 12% of patients in the active treatment group had their test dose withheld because of a magnesium concentration exceeding 2.8 mg/dL. After 36 and 42 hours, half of the patients had this dose withheld. The 2 groups received similar total amounts of potassium, including replacement infusions, IV solutions, and parenteral nutrition. However, mean potassium excretion in 48 hours was 418 mmol in the control group vs. 173 mmol in the active treatment group (Fig 3). Clinically significant ventricular ectopy was noted in 3 patients in the active treatment group within the first 12 hours of the study compared with 5 patients in the control group. None of the patients required treatment for dysrhythmias, and there were no complications of magnesium therapy.

Conclusions.—In the ICU, hypokalemia identifies a group of patients who are likely to have magnesium deficiency. The aggressive magnesium sulfate regimen used in this study safely increases circulating magnesium concentration, enhances magnesium retention, and improves potassium homeostasis.

▶ This study confirms that magnesium replacement should invariably occur in the setting of hypokalemia. In patients receiving digoxin and furosemide, it is especially important to administer potassium and magnesium supplements to prevent or treat atrial and ventricular dysrhythmias. Although

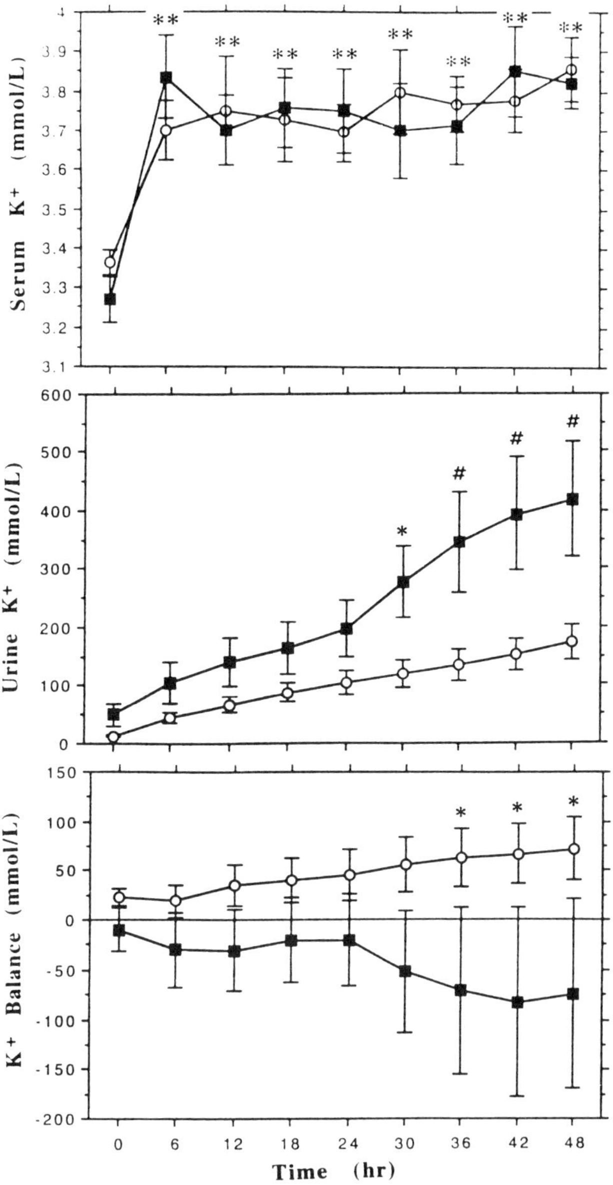

FIGURE 3.—Serum potassium (K^+) (mmol/L) values and millimoles excreted in the urine over time. Potassium balance represents the cumulative difference between millimoles of potassium administered and that amount excreted in the urine. *Open circles*, treatment group; *solid squares*, control group. $*P < 0.05$; $**P < 0.01$; $\#P < 0.005$. Values are expressed as mean plus or minus standard error of the mean. (Courtesy of Hamill-Ruth RJ, McGory R: Magnesium repletion and its effect on potassium homeostasis in critically ill adults: Results of a double-blind, randomized, controlled trial. *Crit Care Med* 24:38–45, 1996.)

magnesium has been shown to be directly efficacious in the treatment of ventricular tachycardia and digoxin toxicity, its use may also prevent these disorders by indirectly improving potassium reabsorption.

D.M. Rothenberg, M.D.

Psychiatric Illness and Serotonin Syndrome

Psychiatric Illness and the Serotonin Syndrome: An Emerging Adverse Drug Effect Leading to Intensive Care Unit Admission

Nijhawan PK, Katz G, Winter S (Yale Univ, New Haven, Conn)

Crit Care Med 24:1086–1089, 1996 7–19

Background.—Patients who have refractory obsessive-compulsive disorder are increasingly being treated with combination therapy, including 2 or 3 serotonin-potentiating agents. The serotonin syndrome, which consists of behavioral, neuromuscular, and autonomic changes, may result from an elevated serotonin availability in the CNS. Although few cases of the serotonin syndrome as an adverse drug reaction have been reported, the incidence may increase with the increasing therapeutic use of serotonin-potentiating agents. A case of serotonin syndrome that required ICU admission was reported.

Case Report.—Man, 48, was brought to the emergency department with loss of consciousness, diaphoresis, and myoclonus. The patient had fallen and injured his head several hours earlier. He had a history of obsessive-compulsive disorder and alcoholism. Two weeks earlier, he had been prescribed an increased dose of clomipramine (to 250 mg daily) plus buspirone and fluoxetine.

Physical examination revealed responsiveness with decerebrate posturing only to noxious stimuli. He was also tachycardic, hypertensive, tachypneic, tremulous, diaphoretic, and febrile. He demonstrated a preferential left lateral gaze and had dilated reactive pupils. His lower extremities were rigid, with substantially increased tone. A CT scan showed contusion and shear injuries sustained during his fall. His chemical profile revealed recent ingestion of alcohol. There were no electroencephalographic abnormalities.

The patient was treated with supportive measures, including sodium nitroprusside to control his nitroprusside and fluids and urine alkalization for his rhabdomyolysis. His episodic shivering, myoclonus, and diaphoresis decreased gradually over 4 days, when he was released to a rehabilitation facility.

Discussion.—Diagnosis of serotonin syndrome is challenging in a patient who has traumatic head injuries and possible alcohol use. The syndrome may also be confused for neuroleptic malignant syndrome or tricyclic overdose (Table 1). The increased brain concentrations of serotonin

TABLE 1.—Differential Diagnosis of the Serotonin Syndrome

	Serotonin Syndrome	Alcohol Withdrawal	Tricylic Overdose
Neurologic	Confusion Restlessness Tremor Myoclonus Hyperreflexia Nystagmus Ataxia	Confusion Agitation Tremor Hallucinations Delusions Seizures	Confusion Agitation Hallucinations Stupor Coma Seizures
Cardiovascular	Tachycardia Hypertension	Tachycardia Hypertension Vascular collapse	Tachycardia Hypotension
Miscellaneous	Diaphoresis Euthermia Diarrhea Rhabdomyolysis Shivering Teeth chattering	Diaphoresis Fever	Dry mucus membranes Fever or hypothermia Constipation/ileus Urinary retention Mydriasis/blurred vision

(Courtesy of Nijhawan PK, Katz G, Winter S: Psychiatric illness and the serotonin syndrome: An emerging adverse drug effect leading to intensive care unit admission. *Crit Care Med* 24(6): 1086–1089, 1996.)

that cause the serotonin syndrome may be associated with several mechanisms, including enhanced serotonin synthesis, serotonin-receptor agonism, increased serotonin release, decreased serotonin reuptake, and inhibition of serotonin breakdown. The mechanism involved depends on the agent used, and combinations of agents may involve multiple mechanisms. The syndrome is generally treated with the withdrawal of all suspected medications and supportive care. Resolution usually occurs within 1–7 days.

▶ This case report is presented to enlighten the reader to a relatively new syndrome that may become prevalent in the critical care setting, presumably because of the more frequent prescribing of serotonin-potentiating drugs. The decrease in serotonin reuptake and the increased serotonin release that occurs with meperidine add further merit to the recommendation that this drug should not be administered to critically ill patients.[1]

D.M. Rothenberg, M.D.

Reference

1. Shapiro BA, Warren J, et al: Practice parameters for intravenous analgesia and sedation for adult patients in the intensive care unit: An executive summary. *Crit Care Med* 23:1596–1600, 1995.

Right Heart Catheter in Critical Care

The Effectiveness of Right Heart Catheterization in the Initial Care of Critically Ill Patients

Connors AF Jr, for the SUPPORT Investigators (Case Western Reserve Univ, Cleveland, Ohio)

JAMA 276:889–897, 1996 7–20

Introduction.—The popularity of right heart catheterization and the widespread belief that it is beneficial make the performance of a randomized, controlled trial difficult, even though the benefit of right heart catheterization has not been fully demonstrated. The variety of factors that influence the selection of patients for right heart catheterziation have not been adjusted comprehensively by existing studies. The association of right heart catheterization performed during the initial 24 hours of an ICU stay with length of stay, subsequent survival, intensity of care, and cost of care was evaluated using the propensity technique, a powerful method of accounting for factors and adjusting for treatment selection bias.

Methods.—There were 5,735 Study to Understand Prognoses and Preferences for Outcomes and Risks of Treatments (SUPPORT) patients from 5 centers who were in an ICU for 1 of 9 prespecified disease categories. All patients were followed for 180 days to track date of death or survival. Other outcome measures included hospital and ICU length of stay and total hospital charges. The propensity score was calculated by a panel of 7 specialists in critical care who specified the variables that related significantly to the decision to use a right heart catheter. A multivariable logistic regression analysis was used on these variables. Patients with and without right heart catheterization were matched.

Results.—There was an increased 30-day mortality rate among the 2,184 partients managed with right heart catheterization in the first 24 hours, compared with the 3,551 managed without right heart catheterization. For those with right heart catheterization, the mean cost per hospital stay was $49,300, and for those without right heart catheterization, the mean cost was $35,700. For those with right heart catheterization, the mean length of stay in the ICU was 14.8 days, and for those without right heart catheterization, the mean length of stay was 13 days. There was no patient group or site associated with improved outcomes for right heart catheterization. The highest relative risk of death following right heart catheterization was among patients with higher baseline probability of surviving 2 months.

Conclusion.—Increased mortality and increased utilization of resources were associated with right heart catheterization; the cause is unclear. Other observational studies should be conducted to confirm the results of this analysis. A randomized, controlled trial of right heart catheterization is justified.

▶ This article focuses on the possibility that right heart catheterization may lead to increased mortality in extremely ill patients. The authors' highly sophisticated statistical techniques make it difficult to dismiss this article outright merely on the basis of their retrospective analysis. Unfortunately, one is left to speculate, along with the authors of the study, as to how right heart catheterization itself was directly hazardous to patient care. I, for one, can certainly believe that interpretation of inaccurate data,[1, 2] or misinterpretation of accurate data could lead to inappropriate clinical decisions and, therefore, poor outcome.

I am intrigued by the notion that critically ill postoperative patients were found to be in a subgroup that is at greatest risk. Could it be that those of us who practice in surgical ICUs are less skilled and knowledgeable than our counterparts in internal medicine? Perhaps important clinical decisions are made "over-the-phone" from the operating room without physical observation and corroboration of the right heart catheterization data. Irrespective of the findings put forth in this study, there can be no quarreling with the fact that right heart catheterization is no panacea and when used improperly, can be detrimental to patient care. The accompanying editorial[3] calling for either a randomized, controlled trial to assess the benefits of right heart catheterization or an immediate moratorium on its use was, unfortunately, applying "chicken little" reasoning to a complex problem that requires a far more calm and rational scientific approach.

D.M. Rothenberg, M.D.

References

1. Iberti TJ, Fischer EP, Leibowitz AB, et al: A multicenter study of physicians' knowledge of the pulmonary artery catheter. The Pulmonary Artery Catheter Study Group. *JAMA* 264:2928, 1990.
2. Iberti TJ, Daily EK, Leibowitz AB, et al: Assessment of critical care nurses' knowledge of the pulmonary artery catheter. The Pulmonary Artery Catheter Study Group. *Crit Care Med* 22:1674, 1994.
3. Dalen JE, Bone RC: Is it time to pull the pulmonary artery catheter? *JAMA* 276:916, 1996.

Heatstroke: Endothelial Injury

Evidence for Endothelial Cell Activation/Injury in Heatstroke

Bouchama A, Hammami MM, Haq A, et al (King Faisal Specialist Hosp and Research Centre, Riyadh, Saudi Arabia)

Crit Care Med 24:1173–1178, 1996 7–21

Background.—Heatstroke has been associated with endotoxemia and elevated levels of tumor necrosis factor (TNF)-α, interleukin (IL)-1, IL-6, and interferon-γ. The infusion of TNF-α and/or IL-1 causes pathophysiologic and morphologic changes in animal models that closely resemble the changes observed in heatstroke. In addition, recent in vitro studies have shown that endotoxin and proinflammatory cytokines can activate the vascular endothelium, which increases adhesiveness of leukocytes to the endothelium and the release of vasoconstrictor and procoagulant peptides, and thus promote vasoconstriction and thrombosis, respectively. Whether the plasma levels of endothelial cell activation/injury markers, circulating intercellular adhesion molecule-1 (ICAM-1), endothelin, and von Willebrand factor-antigen are increased in heatstroke was determined. Their relationships with the pathologic manifestations and the severity of heatstroke were also examined.

Methods and Findings.—Twenty-two patients seen at a heatstroke center in Makkah, Saudi Arabia, were included in the prospective analysis. Before they were cooled, circulating levels of endothelin were increased in 100% of the patients, circulating ICAM-1 in 80%, and von Willebrand factor-antigen in 77%. Average endothelin levels were similar in patients with and without renal dysfunction. Mean von Willebrand factor-antigen levels were comparable in patients with and without lung injury or disseminated intravascular coagulation. After cooling, the mean levels of circulation ICAM-1 and endothelin declined significantly. However, the mean von Willebrand factor-antigen level rose.

Conclusion.—Circulating levels of ICAM-1, endothelin, and von Willebrand factor-antigen are increased significantly in patients with heatstroke, which suggests endothelial cell activation or injury. Further research is needed to determine whether these markers can mediate certain aspects of the pathophysiology of heatstroke.

► In July, 1995 the citizens of Chicago suffered through a record heat wave that claimed over 700 predominantly elderly and bedridden people. Whereas epidemiologic reports stratify the risks for heat-related death,[1] very little in the way of treatment modalities, other than active cooling and supportive measures, are available to prevent the severe organ injury that often ensues. Studies such as this may help define the pathways that lead to heat-induced tissue necrosis and may thereby direct therapy in the future toward cytokine or other inflammatory mediator modulation.

D.M. Rothenberg, M.D.

Reference

1. Semenza JC, Rubin CH, Falter KH, et al.: Heat-related death during the July 1995 heat wave in Chicago. *N Engl J Med* 335:84–90, 1996.

Use of the Nasal Bridle

Nasal Bridle Revisited: An Improvement in the Technique to Prevent Unintentional Removal of Small-bore Nasoenteric Feeding Tubes

Popovich MJ, Lockrem JD, Zivot JB (Cleveland Clinic Found, Ohio; Univ of Colorado, Denver)
Crit Care Med 24:429–431, 1996 7–22

Background.—At some time during enteral feeding, unplanned tube dislodgement occurs in 58% to 100% of patients. The likelihood of this

TABLE 1.—Equipment Needed for Placement of a Bridle to Anchor a Nasoenteric Feeding Tube

One-eighth inch umbilical tape
Bacitracin ointment
Red rubber suction catheter (or 10-Fr nasogastric tube)
Tongue depressor
Penlight
Magill forceps
3-0 silk suture
Unused central venous catheter fastener

(Courtesy of Popovich MJ, Lockrem JD, Zivot JB: Nasal bridle revisited: An improvement in the technique to prevent unintentional removal of small-bore nasoenteric feeding tubes. *Crit Care Med* 24:429–431, 1996.)

occurrence can be reduced by anchoring the tube to the nasal septum with a bridle. The safety and efficacy of a new version of the nasal bridle were reported.

Methods.—Twenty-six critically ill patients who had removed or were at risk for removing properly placed nasoenteric feeding tubes were studied. None of the patients had nasotracheal tubes, facial trauma, or fractures. The procedure consisted of looping a 3.2-mm umbilical tape around the nasal septum and vomer by serially attaching the umbilical tape ends to a suction catheter, passing the catheter through the nostrils into the oropharynx, and retrieving the ends from the oropharynx. The feeding tube was anchored to the umbilical tape with the use of a central venous catheter fastener clamp (Table 1; Fig 1).

Findings.—Patients who could communicate reported no discomfort. No episodes of bleeding, infection, sinusitis, or nasal septal trauma resulted from the use of the bridle. The bridle remained in place for more than 30 days in 5 patients. Only 2 patients were able to remove the feeding tube. In 1 of these, the fastener clamp anchor had failed, but the same bridle and tube had been in place for 170 days.

Conclusions.—The use of an umbilical tape bridle with a central venous catheter fastener clamp anchor is recommended for confused or uncooperative critically ill patients. This method is safe and prevents unplanned removal of nasoenteric feeding tubes.

▶ Although this article does not represent a new idea in caring for patients with nasoenteric feeding tubes, it does offer a new technique that appears to be simple and reliable. Concerns about epistaxis and infection, in addition to the time necessary to replace inadvertently removed enteral feeding tubes, are reasons enough to consider the "nasal bridle" in a select group of critically ill patients.

D.M. Rothenberg, M.D.

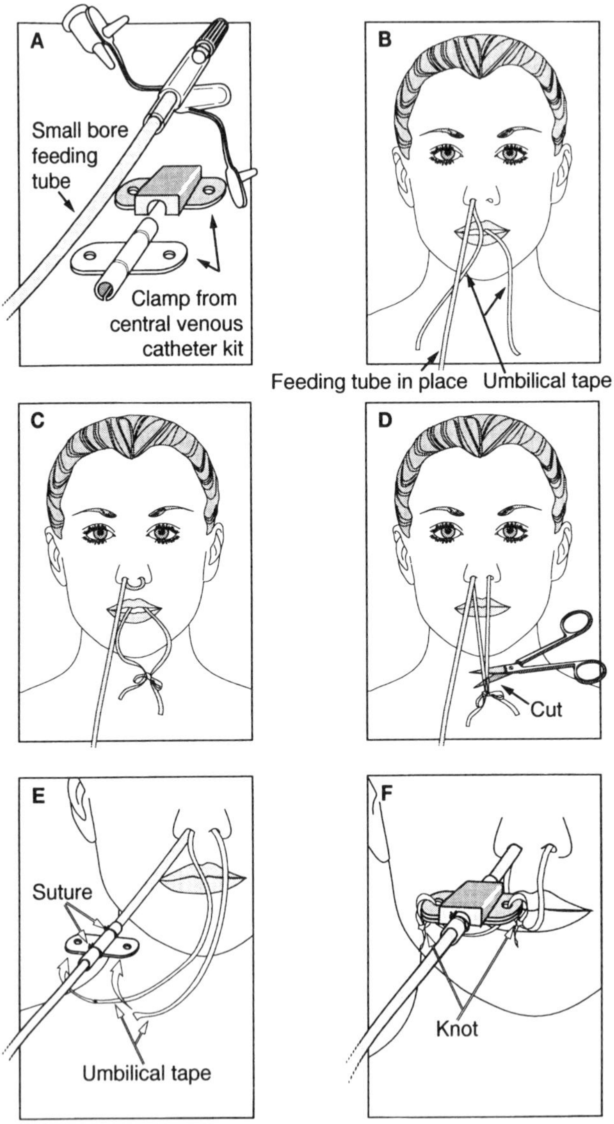

FIGURE 1.—Placement of umbilical tape for nasal bridle and attachment of central venous catheter anchor. The unused fastener from a central venous catheter kit (**A**) permits a reliable anchor between a properly positioned small-bore feeding tube and the umbilical tape and nasal bridle. Bacitracin-coated umbilical tape is inserted with a suction catheter into one nostril. The umbilical tape is retrieved from the oropharynx, and the suction catheter is removed (**B**). This procedure is then repeated using the end of the tape protruding from the nostril. The tape ends are tied (**C**), and the knot is pulled out through a nostril and cut off (**D**). The central venous catheter fastener is then sutured and clamped to the feeding tube (**E**), and the bridle is tied to the side wings of the fastener clamp (**F**). (Courtesy of Popovich MJ, Lockrem JD, Zivot JB: Nasal bridle revisited: An improvement in the technique to prevent unintentional removal of small-bore nasoenteric feeding tubes. *Crit Care Med* 24:429–431, 1996.)

Gastric Intramucosal pH vs. Abdominal Pressure

Intraabdominal Pressure and Gastric Intramucosal pH: Is There an Association?

Sugrue M, Jones F, Lee A, et al (Liverpool Hosp, Sydney, Australia)
World J Surg 20:988–991, 1996 7–23

Introduction.—Gastric tonometry is an important indicator of visceral perfusion. Visceral and renal perfusion is influenced by intra-abdominal pressure. Little is known about whether there is an association between gastric intramucosal pH and intra-abdominal pressure. In a sample of surgical ICU patients, the association between intra-abdominal pressure and gastric intramucosal pH was evaluated.

Methods.—A prospective study was conducted with 73 patients who had major abdominal surgery in a 9-month period. Surgery included upper gastrointestinal tract surgery, lower gastrointestinal tract surgery, and aortic surgery; 44 of the patients had emergency surgery. Three times daily, all had intravesical intra-abdominal pressure measurements and gastric tonometry. Readings of an intra-abdominal pressure of more than 20 mm Hg and a gastric intramucosal pH of more than 7.32 were considered abnormal. Documentation of complications included hypotension, abdominal sepsis, renal impairment, and death.

Results.—Abnormal gastric intramucosal pH occurred in 36 patients while they were in the ICU. Twenty-eight patients had an intra-abdominal pressure reading of more than 20 mm Hg, and 79% of these had abnormal gastric intramucosal pH readings. Patients with an abnormal gastric intramucosal pH were 11.3 times more likely to have an increased intra-abdominal pressure than patients with normal gastric intramucosal pH. Hypotension, sepsis, renal impairment, repeat laparotomy, and death were significantly associated with abnormal gastric intramucosal pH. Of the 13 deaths, 12 had abnormal gastric intramucosal pH. Nine patients needed repeat laparotomy, 8 of them for intra-abdominal sepsis. In patients with abnormal gastric intramucosal pH, renal impairment was significantly greater.

Conclusion.—There was a significant clinical association found between poor outcome and abnormally low gastric intramucosal pH, which may be an indicator of increased risk of death and a predictor of major complications.

▶ The majority of abnormally low intramucosal pH and abnormally high intra-abdominal pressure (IAP) readings were seen early in the patient's admission to the ICU suggesting poor resuscitation intraoperatively. This may be attributable to a poor correlation with intraoperative measurements of *global* perfusion such as mixed venous oxygen saturation, cardiac index, and urinary output with *regional* hypoperfusion. The intraoperative use of gastric tonometry in conjunction with the postoperative use of IAP readings may be a more effective means of assessing visceral and renal perfusion. Questions remain from this study, however, as to how or if changes in intramucosal pH or IAP altered therapy.

D.M. Rothenberg, M.D.

8 Pain Management

Acute Pain Management

Pre-emptive Effect of Pre-incisional Versus Post-incisional Infiltration of Local Anaesthesia on Children Undergoing Hernioplasty

Dahl V, Raeder JC, Ernø PE, et al (Bærum Hosp, Norway)

Acta Anaesthesiol Scand 40:847–851, 1996 8–1

Introduction.—Reports vary regarding the clinical efficacy of pre-emptive analgesia. To determine which approach provided the best long-lasting pain relief, the clinical efficacy of wound infiltration before and after surgery in 50 children undergoing hernioplasty was compared. Also studied was whether preoperative local anesthesia could influence the need for concomitant general anesthetics and the recovery of the children.

Methods.—The age range of the children was 2 to 10 years. Twenty-eight children randomly assigned to group 1 received infiltration of bupivacaine 2.5 mg/mL, 1 mg of the drug per kilogram after induction of general anesthesia and 0.9% of the same volume of saline after surgery. Twenty-two group 2 patients received these infiltrations in reverse order in double-blind fashion. Both groups of patients underwent anesthesia induction with thiopenthone and were maintained with N_2O and halothane, adjusted to sustain stable hemodynamic measurements. All children received 15–20 mg paracetamol per kilogram rectally on admission to the recovery room. Pain scores and need for analgesics were recorded. At discharge, parents were given a questionnaire to be completed after 48 hours at home to evaluate activity level, amount and quality of sleep, appetite, pain in general, pain during defecation, and need for analgesia. Parents were interviewed by telephone at 1 week regarding pain and activity levels and appetite during the first week.

Results.—Group 2 patients required a significantly higher mean concentration of halothane, compared with group 1 patients. Group 1 patients tended to awaken more quickly and had a significantly lower pain score 30 minutes after surgery, compared with group 2 patients. There were no between-group differences in measures for additional analgesia, activity level, appetite, or quality of sleep. The need for opioid analgesics was low in both patient groups.

Conclusion.—The need for general anesthesia was reduced in children who received wound infiltration of local anesthetics before surgery. Patients in the pre- and post-incisional infiltration groups had a rapid and smooth recovery with little discomfort or pain. It was not possible to show a pre-emptive effect of preoperative infiltration of bupivacaine in this short procedure of hernia repair.

► So far only 1 study has shown a significant advantage to presurgical vs. postsurgical wound infiltration with local anesthetic. There is theoretical and at least some experimental evidence that initiation of regional anesthetic techniques before surgery provides better postoperative analgesia than those initiated postoperatively. In practical terms, the differences for most patients are small. However, there may be occasional patients who are at risk for development of chronic postoperative pain, such as those with a history of reflex sympathetic dystrophy or chronic neuropathic pain, or patients undergoing lateral thoracotomy, carpal tunnel release, or amputation, for whom pre-emptive initiation of regional anesthesia may represent a major advantage.

S.E. Abram, M.D.

A Comparison of Intrathecal Morphine-6-Glucuronide and Intrathecal Morphine Sulfate as Analgesics for Total Hip Replacement

Grace D, Fee JPH (Queen's Univ of Belfast, Northern Ireland)

Anesth Analg 83:1055–1059, 1996 8–2

Introduction.—Morphine-6-glucuronide (M6G) is a potent active metabolite of morphine that has been extensively tested parenterally and intrathecally in healthy volunteers and patients with chronic cancer pain. The effects of M6G administered intrathecally for postoperative analgesia have not been investigated adequately. The postoperative analgesia and the incidence of adverse events were compared after intrathecal administration of M6G and morphine sulfate in this randomized, controlled, double-blind trial of 75 patients undergoing elective total hip replacement during spinal anesthesia.

Methods.—Patients received preoperative instructions in use of a 10-cm visual analogue scale (VAS) and a patient-controlled analgesia (PCA) system. Twenty-five patients each were randomly assigned to receive 500 μg preservative free morphine sulfate (group MS), 100 μg preservative free M6G (group M6G100), or 125 μg preservative free M6G (group M6G125); the first 2 groups also received 0.9% sodium chloride. The time to first PCA demand, total number of PCA demands, number of doses delivered, and use of supplemental boluses of meperidine for analgesia were recorded. Patients recorded VAS at rest and on movement at 1, 2, 4, 6, 8, 10, 12, and 24 hours after surgery. The incidence of nausea, vomiting, use of anti-emetics, pruritus, and respiratory depression was recorded.

Results.—All 3 groups were similar in patient characteristics; rate of onset, extent, and duration of sensory and motor block; and postoperative analgesia as assessed by PCA demand. The VAS pain scores at rest and on movement were very low for all 3 groups at all recording times. The only significant difference was observed at 10 hours with VAS with movement. Patients in both M6G groups had a median score of 0, and patients in the morphine group had a third-quartile score of 1.0. Significantly fewer patients in group MS recorded pain as 0 at 6 and 10 hours, compared with patients in group M6G125 and at 24 hours compared with patients in group M6G100. Nausea and vomiting occurred frequently in all 3 groups: nausea in 88% and vomiting in 76% in group MS, nausea in 76% and vomiting in 64% in group M6G100, and nausea in 88% and vomiting in 60% in group M6G125. The rate of pruritus was 36% for all groups, and similar numbers of patients in each group were treated for adverse effects. Two patients in group M6G100 and 3 in group M6G125 became excessively sedated and experienced reductions in the respiratory rate to less than 8 breaths per minute. They required treatment with naloxone.

Conclusions.—All 3 drugs administered intrathecally provided excellent analgesia after total hip replacement. Analgesia was similar for all groups at all recorded times, except at 6 and 10 hours significantly more patients in group M6G125 recorded that they were completely pain free than patients in group MS. A type II error may explain why significantly more patients in group M6G100 than patients in group M6G125 recorded they were pain free at 24 hours, compared with patients in group MS. The incidence of nausea, vomiting, and pruritus was similar in all 3 groups. Two patients in group M6G100 and 3 patients in group M6G125 required naloxone for respiratory depression. Smaller doses of M6G may reduce the incidence of adverse effects while still maintaining effective analgesia.

▶ Although it is somewhat disappointing that M6G did not provide a better therapeutic index than morphine when administered spinally, this study provides some insight into the mechanism of action of intrathecally administered morphine.

S.E. Abram, M.D.

A Comparison of Variable-dose Patient-controlled Analgesia With Fixed-dose Patient-controlled Analgesia

Love DR, Owen H, Ilsley AH, et al (Flinders Med Centre, Bedford Park, South Australia)

Anesth Analg 83:1060–1064, 1996 8–3

Background.—The potential of patient-controlled analgesia (PCA) continues to be limited by variability in analgesic needs and adverse effects. These problems may be addressed by increasing the patient control component of PCA—by giving patients some control over dose size and the interval between demands. In a preliminary study, patients were able to understand the concept of and use "a variable-dose" PCA (VDPCA). Pain relief, adverse effects, and patient satisfaction with VDPCA were compared with those of fixed-dose PCA (FDPCA) in a follow-up study.

Methods.—Sixty patients undergoing major abdominal gynecologic surgery or hip or knee arthroplasty were included in the study. By random assignment, 1 group used VDPCA and the other, FDPCA. Patients in the VDPCA group had a 3-button hand piece to select a 0.5-, 1.0-, or 1.5-mg bolus dose of morphine. A modified Graseby 3400 Anaesthesia Pump controlled by a Toshiba T1900 computer was used. The FDPCA group received the conventional fixed dose of 1 mg of morphine delivered by a Graseby 3300 PCA Pump. Both groups had a 5-minute lockout period.

Findings.—The groups were similar in duration of PCA treatment, total morphine use, and time spent with mild or severe oxyhemoglobin desaturation. The groups also did not differ in ease of or satisfaction with pain control, occurrence of pain on movement, quality of sleep, severity of nausea, or incidence of vomiting.

Conclusions.—Adequate postoperative pain relief can be achieved with the more complex VDPCA system. However, this system does not appear to be better than conventional FDPCA.

▶ Although variable dose PCA may not offer advantages for opiate-naive patients, it may be a useful tool for patients receiving long-term opiate therapy. These patients have enormous variability in their opiate requirements, and the variable-dose device may eliminate the need for frequent reprogramming in such cases.

S.E. Abram, M.D.

Epidural Ropivacaine Infusion for Postoperative Analgesia After Major Lower Abdominal Surgery: A Dose Finding Study

Scott DA, Chamley DM, Mooney PH, et al (St Vincent's Hosp, Melbourne, Australia; Middlemore Hosp, Auckland, New Zealand; Astra Pain Control AB, Södertälje, Sweden)

Anesth Analg 81:982–986, 1995 8–4

Background.—Because ropivacaine is less cardiotoxic and causes less motor block than equianalgesic doses of bupivacaine, it may be well suited for epidural infusion for postoperative analgesia. Three concentrations of epidural ropivacaine infused for postoperative analgesia were compared in their ability to attenuate opioid analgesia needs and to minimize motor block.

Methods.—Forty patients in ASA I through III completed the double-blind study. All were undergoing major lower abdominal surgery. By random assignment, 10 patients in group 1 received epidural 0.1% ropivacaine; 10 in group 2, 0.2% ropivacaine; 10 in group 3, epidural 0.3% ropivacaine; and 10 in group S, epidural saline. In the recovery room, epidural infusions were administered at 10 mL/hr for 21 hours. Patients used IV patient-controlled analgesia (PCA) devices as needed for supplemental analgesia.

Findings.—During the 21-hour period, group S used more PCA morphine than any of the 3 ropivacaine groups. The difference between group S and group 2 was significant. Compared with the control group scores, visual analogue scale scores for coughing were significantly lower in all ropivacaine groups after 4 hours of infusion and also in groups 2 and 3 after 8 hours of infusion. A dose-related increase in amount of motor block was observed. Group 3 had significantly more motor block than all other groups at 4 and 8 hours.

Conclusions.—Epidural infusions of ropivacaine, 0.2% and 0.3%, with PCA provided better postoperative analgesia than PCA alone in these patients. Infusion of 0.2% ropivacaine resulted in the best balance of analgesia and minimal motor block.

Continuous Epidural Infusion of Ropivacaine for the Prevention of Postoperative Pain After Major Orthopaedic Surgery: A Dose-finding Study

Badner NH, Reid D, Sullivan P, et al (Univ Hosp, London, Ont, Canada; Ottawa Gen Hosp, Ont, Canada; Ottawa Civic Hosp, Ont, Canada)

Can J Anaesth 43:17–22, 1996 8–5

Background.—Some studies of epidural bupivacaine for postoperative analgesia have reported potentially toxic systemic concentrations. Ropivacaine, a new amide local anesthetic that is structurally similar to bupivacaine but with a propyl substitution for the butyl side chain, should, in theory, minimize this risk of toxicity. The effects of varying concentrations of epidural ropivacaine infusions in postoperative analgesia after major orthopedic surgery were studied.

Methods.—Forty-four patients completed the randomized, double-blind study. Surgery was done with a combination of a lumbar epidural block with 0.5% ropivacaine and a standardized general anesthetic. After surgery, an epidural infusion of saline or ropivacaine (0.1%, 0.2%, or 0.3%) was begun at the rate of 10 mL/hr and continued for 21 hours. Analgesia was supplemented with morphine delivered by a patient-controlled analgesia (PCA) device.

Findings.—The patients receiving ropivacaine needed less morphine during the 21 hours in the postanesthesia care unit than the patients receiving saline. Pain scores were also lower in the groups given ropivacaine. Compared with the saline group, the ropivacaine groups maintained sensory anesthesia to pinprick. At all assessments, the motor block in the 0.3% group was significantly greater than that in the saline group. In addition, motor block in this ropivacaine group was greater than in the 0.1% group at 8 hours. The 0.2% group had higher Bromage scores than the saline group at 4 and 21 hours.

Conclusions.—Continuous epidural infusions of ropivacaine 0.1%, 0.2%, and 0.3% at 10 mL/hr improved postoperative pain relief and reduced PCA morphine use in these patients undergoing major orthopedic surgery. Sensory anesthesia was similar at the 0.1% and 0.2% concentrations. Motor blockade at these levels was significantly less than at the 0.3% concentration.

► Ropivacaine has 2 potential advantages over bupivacaine when used as an epidural infusion for postoperative pain. The first is that it may have less motor-blocking effect for a given degree of analgesia, and the second is that it may have less potential for cardiac arrhythmias in the event of a drug overdose. Although these studies demonstrate that optimal doses of ropivacaine were associated with an opioid-sparing effect with minimal motor blockade, they do not establish whether ropivacaine offers any advantage over bupivacaine. It seems unlikely that there would be a substantial safety difference between ropivacaine and bupivacaine when used for this application. I know of no serious arrhythmias associated with low-dose bupivacaine infusion. Nearly every case of life-threatening bupivacaine- or etidocaine-induced arrhythmia reported has been associated with accidental intravascular injection. The practice of intermittent injection of partial doses has reduced the incidence of that complication to very low levels.

S.E. Abram, M.D.

Oral Clonidine Premedication Reduces Postoperative Pain in Children

Mikawa K, Nishina K, Maekawa N, et al (Kobe Univ, Japan)

Anesth Analg 82:225–230, 1996 8–6

Objective.—Although the postoperative analgesic properties of caudal clonidine in children have been demonstrated in 1 study, the pre-anesthetic effects of oral clonidine have not been studied. Postoperative pain was compared in children who were premedicated with oral clonidine and children who received placebo.

Methods.—The analgesic effects of 2 or 4 µg/kg of oral clonidine or placebo were studied in 3 groups of 30 children, aged 5 to 12 years, who were undergoing minor surgery. Clonidine or placebo was administered 105 minutes before the induction of anesthesia. Atropine (0.03 mg/kg orally) was administered 60 minutes before the induction of anesthesia with halothane and 60% nitrous oxide in oxygen. Postoperative pain was assessed at intervals for 12 hours by a blinded observer using the objective pain scale (OPS), with 0 indicating no pain and 10 indicating severe maximum pain.

Results.—Clonidine at 4 µg/kg provided the best preoperative sedation, although 6 patients in this group had postoperative bradycardia compared with 1 in the 2-µg/kg group and none in the placebo group. Patients who received clonidine at 4 µg/kg had the best postoperative OPS score over the 12-hour test period, and fewer required rescue analgesics. Patients who received clonidine did not experience severe postoperative hypotension, rebound hypertension, bradycardia, respiratory depression, or desaturation.

Conclusion.—Premedication with oral clonidine at 4 μg/kg provides effective postoperative analgesia for children undergoing minor surgery.

▶ There are several issues regarding the mechanism of analgesic action of clonidine that are not yet known. First, it is unclear whether neuraxial administration is more effective than systemic administration. A few clinical studies suggest it is not. It seems worthwhile, therefore, to explore the potential benefits of oral, transdermal, and IV use of clonidine in the perioperative period. Although the authors speculate about a possible preemptive effect of the drug, there are no animal or human data to either confirm or rule out such an effect.

S.E. Abram, M.D.

Comparison of the Effects of Adrenaline, Clonidine and Ketamine on the Duration of Caudal Analgesia Produced by Bupivacaine in Children

Cook B, Grubb DJ, Aldridge LA, et al (Royal Hosp for Sick Children, Edinburgh, Scotland; Royal Infirmary of Edinburgh, Scotland)

Br J Anaesth 75:698–701, 1995 8–7

Background.—Performing a caudal block with local anesthetic is one of the most common analgesic techniques used in pediatric anesthesia. However, the duration of analgesia provided by the single caudal injection is limited to the duration of action of the anesthetic, typically bupivacaine (2–4 hours). To prolong the duration of caudal analgesia, other agents, most commonly adrenaline, have been added to the local anesthetic mixture. Other potentially useful prolonging agents are ketamine and clonidine. The effects of these 3 agents on the duration of caudal block produced by bupivacaine were compared.

Methods.—Sixty boys aged 1–10 years undergoing unilateral orchiopexy were studied. Twenty patients each were randomly selected to receive either adrenaline (group A), clonidine (group C), or ketamine (group K) in addition to bupivacaine in a caudal injection. The intervals between discontinuation of anesthesia to spontaneous eye opening, leg movement, and first micturition were noted. Sedation was assessed at 1 and 4 hours postoperatively. Parents assessed postoperative pain and analgesic requirement for 24 hours after discharge, using the modified objective pain score, which quantitatively assesses crying, agitation, movement, posture, and localization of pain.

Results.—The first dose of postoperative analgesia was required at 12.5 hours in group K, 5.8 hours in group C, and 3.2 hours in group A, all significant differences (Fig 1). Similarly, patients in group A required significantly more doses of postoperative analgesics than did patients in the other 2 groups. There were no significant differences between the 3 groups in the intervals between the cessation of anesthesia and spontaneous eye opening, spontaneous leg movements, and first micturition. In addition,

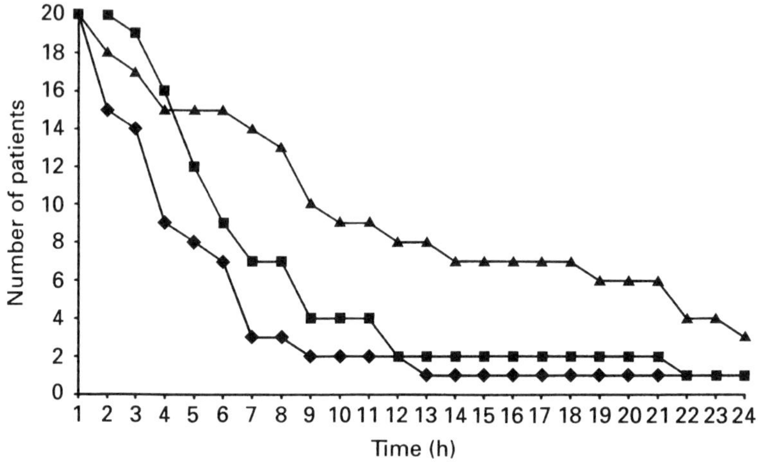

FIGURE 1.—Duration of caudal analgesia in groups A (*diamonds*), C (*squares*), and K (*triangles*). (Courtesy of Cook B, Grubb DJ, Aldridge LA, et al: Comparison of the effects of adrenaline, clonidine and ketamine on the duration of caudal analgesia produced by bupivacaine in children. *Br J Anaesth* 75:698–701, 1995.)

the median sedation scores were similar in the 3 groups at 4 hours after surgery.

Conclusions.—The addition of ketamine or clonidine to bupivacaine provides better prolongation of the caudal block, without prolonging the motor block, than does the addition of adrenaline to bupivacaine.

▶ Although several previous studies have evaluated the efficacy of epidural ketamine in providing postoperative analgesia, none have examined the effect of the drug when given before the onset of the surgical stimulus. Because those studies showed a short-duration effect (about 3 hours) whereas the ketamine group in this study had a much more prolonged effect, suggests that the preincisional administration of spinal or epidural N-methyl-D-aspartate (NMDA) antagonists may indeed be a beneficial technique.

S.E. Abram, M.D.

Pain Relief With Low-dose Intravenous Clonidine in a Child With Severe Burns

Lyons B, Casey W, Doherty P, et al (Our Lady's Hosp for Sick Children, Dublin)

Intensive Care Med 22:249–251, 1996 8–8

Background.—The pain associated with severe burns is intense, especially during wound dressing. There currently is no good alternative to potent opioid analgesics for patients with severe burns. One patient who experienced severe side effects from the large doses of morphine used for analgesia was described.

> *Case Report.*—Boy, 11 years, had second and third degree burns to 78% of his body after being doused with gasoline and set on fire. When admitted to the hospital, the patient was intubated and ventilated. Morphine and midazolam infusions were started for sedation and analgesia. The boy's clinical condition was stable for the first 4 days, after which it began to deteriorate. Tachycardia, pyrexia, leukocytosis, and progressive hypoxia were followed by organ failure, mainly affecting the respiratory and renal systems. Broad-spectrum antibiotics, dopamine, and vecuronium were adminsitered. By the ninth day, gas exchange had improved enough to stop vecuronium infusion. However, the high dose of morphine needed for analgesia produced several serious adverse effects. Gastrointestinal (GI) motility was impaired, with consequent nausea, constipation, and poor tolerance of enteral feeding. This resulted in poor nutritional status. The boy also had bouts of extreme agitation, sweating, anxiety, and nightmares. An IV lignocaine infusion was started on day 11 in an attempt to decrease the amount of morphine needed. The initial 0.3 mg $kg^{-1}h^{-1}$ was gradually decreased to 1.2 mg $kg^{-1}h^{-1}$. The initial reduction in morphine consumption could not be sustained. Failure to wean the patient from morphine infusion was paralleled by a failure to wean him from the ventilator. Morphine requirements were increased after debridement. Clonidine, given intravenously at a rate of 7.5 µg every 4 hours, was begun. On the following day, this rate was increased to 10 µg without adversely affecting hemodynamic parameters. Despite frequent surgical interventions, morphine requirements were greatly reduced after clonidine was introduced, permitting successful extubation within 7 days. Tolerance of enteral feeding was improved, and psychological disturbances were eliminated.

Conclusions.—In this case of a boy with severe burns, large morphine doses resulted in ventilatory dependence, GI impairment, and psychological disturbance. The addition of low-dose IV clonidine precipitated a dramatic decrease in morphine consumption, with attendant improvement in ventilatory, GI, and psychological functioning.

► Systemically administered α-2 adrenergic agonists provide analgesia through non-opioid mechanisms that seems at least additive when combined with opioids. This feature, plus a different side effect profile, makes this a logical combination. It remains to be determined whether the addition of α-2 adrenergic agonists can slow the development of tolerance to opioids.

S.E. Abram, M.D.

Ketorolac Does Not Decrease Postoperative Pain in Elderly Men After Transvesical Prostatectomy

Fredman B, Olsfanger D, Flor P, et al (Meir Hosp, Kfar Sava, Israel; Tel Aviv Univ, Israel)

Can J Anaesth 43:438–441, 1996 8–9

Background.—Ketorolac has become increasingly common in the treatment of postoperative pain. Its analgesic properties and lack of opioid-induced adverse effects may make this agent particularly useful in elderly patients. However, few researchers have investigated ketorolac-induced analgesia in elderly individuals.

Methods.—Sixty men (age range, 60–88 years) were enrolled in the randomized, placebo-controlled, double-blind trial. All were undergoing transvesical prostactectomy and were American Society of Anesthesiologists physical status I to III. A standard general anesthetic was given; 30 minutes before the end of surgery, 60 mg ketorolac or an equal volume of saline was administered intramuscularly. Pain was assessed every hour for 6 hours after surgery by visual analog scale and treated with morphine via patient-controlled analgesia (PCA) device.

Findings.—The administration of ketorolac did not affect hourly PCA demands, actual morphine delivered, or patient-rated pain scores. The total PCA morphine delivered was 11.9 mg in patients receiving saline and 10.8 in those receiving ketorolac.

Conclusions.—In these men, a single intraoperative dose of 60 mg ketorolac did not improve analgesia or affect actual morphine delivered after transvesical prostatectomy. Neither objective nor subjective indicators of pain were improved during recovery.

▶ Apparently, word of the efficacy of ketorolac has reached the urology literature, and urologists often object to our use of postoperative epidural analgesia after open prostatectomy, citing the benefits of ketorolac. This study suggests that the analgesic efficacy of this drug may have been overstated, at least in the elderly population.

S.E. Abram, M.D.

Ketorolac and Spinal Morphine for Postcesarean Analgesia

Cohen SE, Desai JB, Ratner EF, et al (Stanford Univ, Calif)

Int J Obstet Anesth 5:14–18, 1996 8–10

Introduction.—Spinal morphine (SM) is an effective postcesarean analgesic, but nausea, pruritus, and the risk of respiratory depression limit its usefulness. The prostaglandin synthetase inhibition of the nonsteroidal anti-inflammatory drug ketorolac (K) may give effective analgesia alone or in combination with epidural opioids. The postcesarean analgesia and side effects of SM and K alone and in combination with each other were compared in 48 women.

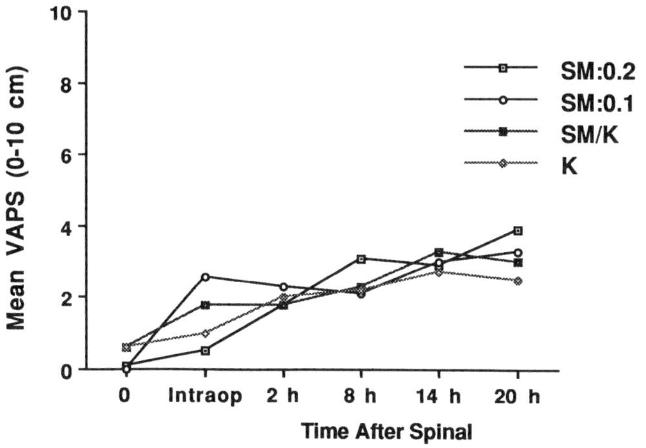

FIGURE 1.—Mean visual analogue pain scores (0–10 cm) during the first 20 hours after spinal morphine (*SM*), 0.2; SM, 0.1; SM/ketorolac (*K*); and K. (Courtesy of Cohen SE, Desai JB, Ratner EF: Ketorolac and spinal morphine for postcesarean analgesia. *Int J Obstet Anesth* 5:14–18, 1996.)

Methods.—In double-blind fashion, patients were randomly assigned to receive 12 mg of hyperbaric bupivacaine and 1 of the following: SM 0.1 mg or SM 0.2 mg and saline placebo but no K; SM 0.1 mg plus K 60 mg IV 1 hour after spinal injection and 30 mg IV every 6 hours for 3 doses; or IV K dosed as previously described plus saline placebo but no SM. Pain, pruritus, nausea, and sedation were assessed at several perioperative intervals using visual analogue scales.

Results.—Mean pain scores were similar postoperatively for all groups at all evaluation periods (Fig 1). Patients receiving K alone had significantly lower pruritus scores, compared with patients receiving morphine

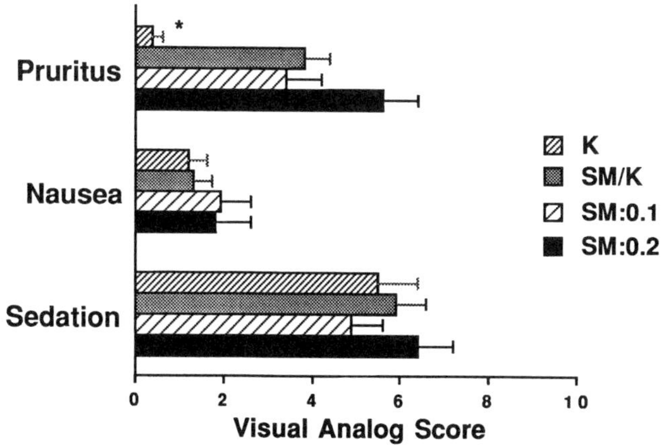

FIGURE 2.—Mean maximum visual analogue scores (0–10 cm, where 0 = no symptom and 10 = worst possible symptom) for pruritus, nausea, and sedation after each treatment during the first 20 hours. *Bars* represent standard errors. (Courtesy of Cohen SE, Desai JB, Ratner EF: Ketorolac and spinal morphine for postcesarean analgesia. *Int J Obstet Anesth* 5:14–18, 1996.)

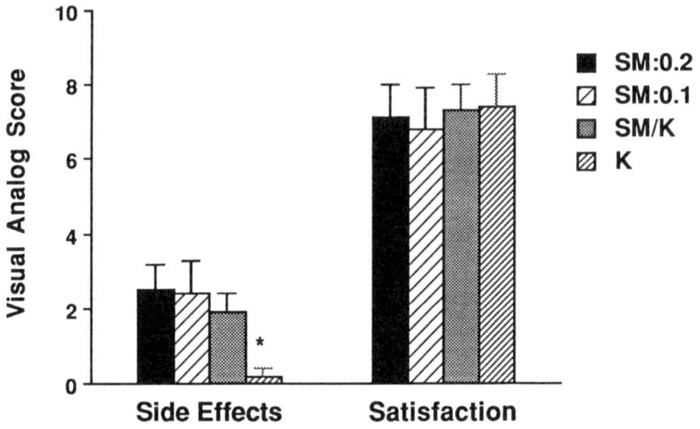

FIGURE 3.—Patients' overall evaluation of the severity of side effects and overall rating of their satisfaction with their postoperative analgesia (visual analogue scores of 0–10 cm, assessed 24 hours after delivery). Mean standard error. (Courtesy of Cohen SE, Desai JB, Ratner EF: Ketorolac and spinal morphine for postcesarean analgesia. *Int J Obstet Anesth* 5:14–18, 1996.)

alone or in combination with K (Fig 2). Two patients dropped out of the group that received SM 0.2 mg because of severe pruritus. There were no between-group differences in the incidence of nausea (see Fig 2). Patients in the K group had a nonsignificant lower incidence of vomiting, compared with groups receiving morphine alone or in combination with K. The overall score for severity of side effects was lowest in patients receiving K alone (Fig 3). Sedation was similar for all patient groups. At 24 hours postoperatively, patients in all groups reported similarly high satisfaction scores (see Fig 3). No patients had overt respiratory depression or slow respiratory rate. One patient in the group that received SM 0.1 mg had a transient decrease in oxygen saturation.

Conclusion.—Patients receiving SM had a higher incidence of pruritus, compared with patients receiving K alone. Pain relief and patient satisfaction with sedation were similarly high in all patient groups.

▶ In 1995, the manufacturer of ketorolac issued a statement that ketorolac is "contraindicated in nursing mothers because of the potential adverse effects of prostaglandin-inhibiting drugs on neonates." The manufacturer issued this warning despite the fact that other nonsteroidal anti-inflammatory drugs with similar antiprostaglandin effects are widely used as analgesics in postpartum patients. I am skeptical that maternal administration of modest doses of ketorolac is hazardous to healthy neonates. However, the authors of this study correctly noted that "further studies are needed to determine whether maternal ketorolac therapy poses a risk to healthy neonates via the milk."

D.H. Chestnut, M.D.

A Comparison of Morphine, Pethidine and Fentanyl in the Postsurgical Patient-controlled Analgesia Environment

Woodhouse A, Hobbes AFT, Mather LE, et al (Univ of Sydney, Australia; Royal North Shore Hosp, St Leonards, Australia)

Pain 64:115–121, 1996 8–11

Background.—Because only the patient can judge the efficacy of opioids used in patient-controlled analgesia (PCA) systems, it is essential to evaluate patients' reactions to the analgesic agents used. It was determined whether patients have preferences for any of 3 commonly used opioids, what such preferences are based on, and whether clinicians should prefer any of these opioids.

Methods.—Fifty-five patients aged 20–70 years were studied. Most had undergone orthopedic, abdominal, vascular, or gynecologic surgery. Morphine, pethidine, and fentanyl were the PCA opioids assessed.

Findings.—Patients receiving morphine had more pruritus than patients in the other 2 groups, but the incidence of other adverse effects did not differ significantly among the groups. Patients with vomiting or pruritus had a greater intensity of these effects with morphine and fentanyl compared with pethidine. Most patients said they were very satisfied with their postoperative pain management and with PCA. Reported satisfaction did not vary significantly among the groups.

Conclusions.—From the patient's perspective, any of these 3 agents delivered by PCA can be equally effective in relieving postoperative pain. Although pethidine appeared to have some advantages over morphine and fentanyl, no single agent was clearly better for PCA. The possibility of norpethidine-related toxicity, although not occurring in this study, should be considered, especially when prescribing a PCA analgesic for patients with renal abnormalities.

▶ Experimental animal data exist that show very potent opioids, such as fentanyl and sufentanil, provide more effective analgesia than less potent drugs, such as meperidine or morphine, under circumstances of opiate tolerance or extremely intense noxious stimulation. Likewise, there are 2 human studies that indicate improved postoperative analgesia with the use of more potent opioids in patients who are receiving chronic opioid administration preoperatively.[1, 2] However, under the conditions of this study—i.e., opiate naive patients undergoing elective surgery—there appears to be no significant benefit to using fentanyl as opposed to meperidine or morphine.

S.E. Abram, M.D.

References

1. Paix A, Coleman A, Lees J, et al: Subcutaneous fentanyl and sufentanil infusion substitution for morphine intolerance in cancer pain management. *Pain* 63:263–269, 1995.

2. de Leon-Casasola OA, Myers DP, Donaparthi S, et al: A comparison of postoperative epidural analgesia between patients with chronic cancer taking high doses of oral opioids versus opioid-naive patients. *Anesth Analg* 76:302–307, 1993.

Sufentanil Does Not Preempt Pain After Abdominal Hysterectomy

Sarantopoulos C, Fassoulaki A (St Savas Hosp, Athens, Greece)

Pain 65:273–276, 1996 8–12

Background.—Preemptive analgesia has been controversial in studies of postoperative pain. The hypothesis that sufentanil administered before skin incision would provide more effective postoperative pain relief than intraoperatively administered sufentanil in patients undergoing total abdominal hysterectomy was tested in a prospective, double-blind, placebo-controlled trial.

Methods.—Forty women undergoing elective abdominal hysterectomy were randomly assigned to receive 1 μg of sufentanil per kilogram either 5 minutes before induction of anesthesia or when the round ligaments of the uterus were ligated, with normal saline administered at the other time point. All patients underwent general anesthesia induction with midazolam, thiopental, and vecuronium, and maintenance with isoflurane and N_2O in oxygen. Postoperatively, propoxyphene and paracetamol were given on request for pain relief, with pethidine given for overnight or for the management of unrelieved pain. Pain at rest was assessed with visual analogue scales and verbal rating scales immediately before the first analgesic administration and every 4 hours thereafter for 24 hours.

Results.—The 2 groups had no differences in consumption of propoxyphene, paracetamol, and pethidine and no differences in either visual analogue scale or verbal rating scale scores at any time point.

Conclusions.—There were no differences in pain relief or analgesic requirements between patients receiving systemic sufentanil preoperatively and patients receiving sufentanil intraoperatively. Therefore, IV sufentanil failed to show a preemptive effect.

▶ The findings of this study are in agreement with studies in experimental animals that fail to show blockade of spinal sensitization by pre-injury systemic opioids. On the other hand, there is experimental evidence that intrathecal opioids exert at least a modest preemptive effect.

S.E. Abram, M.D.

Comparison of Intravenous Nalbuphine Infusion Versus Saline as an Adjuvant for Epidural Morphine

Wang J-J, Ho S-T, Hu OY-P (Natl Defense Med Ctr/Tri-Service Gen Hosp, Taipei, Taiwan, Republic of China)

Reg Anesth 21:214–218, 1996 8–13

Background.—Radical hemorrhoidectomy may require aggressive pain management. The analgesic efficacy and side effects of IV nalbuphine infusion used as an adjuvant to epidural morphine were investigated.

Methods.—Sixty patients were enrolled in the randomized, double-blind trial. Epidural morphine, 4 mg, was given at the end of surgery, and for the next 48 hours, morphine dosages of 2 and 3 mg were administered epidurally at 8 p.m. and 8 a.m., respectively. In addition, patients assigned to group 1 were given an adjuvant IV infusion of nalbuphine 15 µg/kg/hr. Patients in group 2 received IV saline only. Intramuscular meperidine 40 mg every 4 hours was available as a rescue analgesic.

Findings.—Postoperative pain relief was adequate in all patients. Analgesic requirements at 48 hours were similar. During that period, $PaCO_2$ exceeded 45 mm Hg in 1 patient in group 1 and 6 in group 2. None of the patients had an SaO_2 of less than 90%. Thirteen percent of group 1 patients and 62% of group 2 patients reported nausea and/or vomiting. Pruritus occurred in 7% of the patients in group 1, compared with 62% of those in group 2 (Table 4).

Conclusions.—Intravenous nalbuphine infusion is a useful adjuvant to epidural morphine in patients undergoing radical hemorrhoidectomy. This

TABLE 4.—Incidence of Side Effects*

Effect/Time	Nalbuphine Group (n = 30)	Saline Group (n = 26)	*P*‡
Respiratory depression†			
2 hr	1	6	< .05
8 hr	0	0	NS
Nausea/ vomiting			
0–12 hr	1	10	< .01
12–24 hr	2	8	< .05
24–48 hr	1	2	NS
0–48 hr	4	16	< .01
Pruritus			
0–12 hr	0	5	< .05
12–24 hr	2	12	< .01
24–48 hr	0	2	NS
0–48 hr	2	16	< .01

*Data represented as numbers of patients with symptoms in each observation period.
†Respiratory depression is defined as a $PaCO_2$ > 45 mm Hg.
‡Fisher's exact test.
Abbreviation: NS, not significant.
(Courtesy of Wang J-J, Ho S-T, Hu OY-P: Comparison of intravenous nalbuphine infusion versus saline as an adjuvant for epidural morphine. *Reg Anesth* 21:214–218, 1996.)

agent decreases the incidence of adverse effects without reducing the quality of pain relief.

► The incidence of nausea and pruritus after epidural morphine previously has been shown to be reversible or preventable through the use of opioid antagonists. Because the incidence of delayed respiratory depression is low, it is difficult to demonstrate conclusively that any technique is capable of reducing that incidence. This study provides convincing evidence that nalbuphine reduces the incidence of nausea and pruritus, but it does not seem to provide any additional analgesia. Because there was no documented delayed respiratory depression in either group, it is not possible to assess its ability to prevent that complication.

S.E. Abram, M.D.

Intra-operative Epidural Morphine, Fentanyl, and Droperidol for Control of Pain After Spinal Surgery: A Prospective, Randomized, Placebo-controlled, and Double-blind Trial

Rainov NG, Gutjahr T, Burkert W (Martin-Luther-Univ Halle-Wittenberg, Federal Republic of Germany)

Acta Neurochir (Wien) 138:33–39, 1996 8–14

Background.—Controlling postoperative pain is essential in the management of patients who have undergone spinal surgery. The analgesic effects of intraoperative epidural morphine were investigated in patients having surgery for lumbar disc disease.

Methods.—Sixty-eight patients (age range, 16–70 years) were enrolled in the double-blind study. By random assignment, patients received 5 mg morphine and 2.5 mg dehydrobenzperidol (DHB) in 10 mL physiologic saline, 5 mg morphine and 0.1 mg fentanyl in the same amount of saline, or saline only. Solutions were injected epidurally through a catheter after hemostasis and before wound closure.

Findings.—Analgesia associated with the morphine-fentanyl and morphine-droperidol combinations was significantly better than that associated with placebo. The duration and quality of analgesia and the occurrence of adverse effects were comparable in the 2 morphine groups. The side effects in the morphine groups were minimal and not significantly different from the placebo group. Additional epidural fentanyl did not significantly improve postoperative analgesia.

Conclusions.—The intraoperative use of 5 mg epidural morphine in spinal surgery is recommended. Single doses of epidural opioids administered by the surgeon under direct visual control may also be useful in postoperative analgesia for major spinal interventions, such as instrumental scoliosis correction and stabilization.

► Unfortunately, this study did not include a group that received epidural morphine alone to determine whether there is any benefit from the addition of either fentanyl or droperidol. The fact that droperidol has been used in a previous human study does not justify its ongoing use. To my knowledge, little if any safety data exists for neuraxial administration of this drug.

S.E. Abram, M.D.

Postoperative Analgesia With Continuous Epidural Sufentanil and Bupivacaine: A Prospective Study in 614 Patients

Broekema AA, Gielen MJM, Hennis PJ (Univ Hosps, Groningen, The Netherlands; Univ Hosps, Nijmegen, The Netherlands)

Anesth Analg 82:754–759, 1996 8–15

Background.—The use of continuous epidural analgesia on surgical wards is controversial because of the risk of respiratory depression. Early respiratory depression has been reported after a single dose of 50 µg epidural sufentanil. The effect of bupivacaine added to continuous epidural sufentanil infusion was investigated.

Methods.—Six hundred fourteen patients (age range, 13–90 years) undergoing major surgery were enrolled in the prospective study. Most patients were American Society of Anesthesiologists class II or III. An initial dose of 50 µg sufentanil in 6 to 10 mL bupivacaine 0.125% was administered by lumbar or thoracic catheter before surgical incision. Continuous infusion with 50 µg sufentanil in 60 mL bupivacaine 0.125% at 6 to 10 mL/hr was begun 1 hour later and continued for 1 to 5 days or more after surgery.

Findings.—Most patients had adequate pain relief at rest and during movement. Three patients had late respiratory depression. Adverse effects were minor in most patients. Technical complications occurred in 4% of epidural punctures and in 3% of catheter insertions.

Conclusions.—In most patients undergoing major surgery, postoperative analgesia for 1 to 5 days with continuous epidural sufentanil and bupivacaine infusion was effective at rest and during movement. Most side effects were minor.

▶ This study indicates that epidural infusion of bupivacaine plus sufentanil provides satisfactory analgesia and a reasonable side effect profile after thoracic, abdominal, and lower extremity surgery. It does not address the question of whether this technique provides analgesia that is superior to other epidural drugs for the average surgical patient. de Leon-Casasola et al. demonstrated improved analgesia with this technique, compared with bupivacaine-morphine in opioid-tolerant patients,[1] but it is not clear whether there is any benefit for opioid-naive individuals.

It still has not been shown definitively that epidural sufentanil infusion differs qualitatively from intravenous sufentanil infusion. (It has been shown that no such difference exists for fentanyl.) The only evidence the authors cite for a spinal site of action for sufentanil comes from a study of epidural sufentanil administration for cancer pain in which postmortem studies showed highest spinal cord levels at sites adjacent to the catheter tip.

It is not clear whether the delayed respiratory depression seen in 3 patients was related to gradual systemic accumulation or to intracranial spread via the CSF. Given the low water solubility of the drug, I suspect the former explanation is the case.

S.E. Abram, M.D.

Reference

1. de Leon-Casasola OA, Lema MJ: Epidural bupivacaine/sufentanil therapy for post-operative pain control in patients tolerant to opioid and unresponsive to epidural bupivacaine/morphine. *Anesthesiology* 80:2,303–309, 1994.

A Multidimensional Comparison of Morphine and Hydromorphone Patient-controlled Analgesia

Rapp SE, Egan KJ, Ross BK, et al (Univ of Washington, Seattle)
Anesth Analg 82:1043–1048, 1996 8–16

Background.—Patient-controlled analgesia (PCA) pumps have been used for more than 10 years. However, the most effective PCA analgesic has not been established. The relative efficacy and side effects of morphine and hydromorphone PCA were investigated.

Methods.—Sixty-one opioid-naive patients were enrolled in the double-blind trial. All were adults scheduled for lower abdominal surgery. Analgesic efficacy was assessed by verbal rating scores and medication use. Cognitive functioning and affective states were also evaluated.

Findings.—Morphine and hydromorphone both provided adequate analgesia. Side effects were comparable. Patients receiving hydromorphone had poorer cognitive performance but also reported less anger/hostility and generally better mood elevations than patients receiving morphine.

Conclusions.—Morphine and hydromorphone provide comparable analgesia with similar dosing. Hydromorphone may be an alternative to morphine and meperidine, particularly in patients sensitive to morphine. Hydromorphone results in greater problems in cognitive functioning but improved mood.

► To date, there has been very little evidence that some opioids are better than others when given by PCA. This study suggests there may be subtle differences in side effects, but it does not seem that the differences are sufficient to justify choosing one drug over another. It would, however, be interesting to determine whether more potent drugs, which have a lower fraction of receptor occupancy (i.e., they need to occupy fewer opioid receptors to achieve a given effect), are more effective in opioid-tolerant individuals.

S.E. Abram, M.D.

Thoracic Versus Lumbar Administration of Fentanyl Using Patient-controlled Epidural After Thoracotomy

Bouchard F, Drolet P (Univ of Montreal)

Reg Anesth 20:385–388, 1995 8–17

Purpose.—Epidural injection of fentanyl has been shown to provide analgesia for patients who have undergone thoracotomy. However, there is still uncertainty as to whether the catheter should be inserted in the lumbar or the thoracic epidural space. The 2 sites were compared for their effects on postoperative analgesia in patients using patient-controlled analgesia (PCEA) with fentanyl.

Methods.—The randomized study included 30 patients undergoing pulmonary resection. The patients received either a lumbar or thoracic epidural catheter for PCEA with fentanyl, 10 μg/mL. The PCEA pump was programmed to deliver a 25 μg bolus with a 10-minute lockout interval and no continuous infusion. Postoperative pain was measured on a 10-cm visual analogue scale (VAS), and fentanyl requirements were assessed. In addition, plasma fentanyl levels were assessed at 8 and 16 hours postoperatively.

Results.—At no time were there any differences between groups in VAS scores or fentanyl requirements. In the patients with lumbar catheters, VAS scores were higher at 0 and 4 hours than at 12, 16, and 20 hours. Eight-hour plasma fentanyl levels were 0.26 ng/mL in the lumbar group and 0.22 ng/mL in the thoracic group. Sixteen-hour values were also similar: 0.36 and 0.44 ng/mL, respectively (Fig 1).

Conclusions.—In patients who have undergone thoracotomy and are receiving PCEA with fentanyl, thoracic vs. lumbar catheter placement

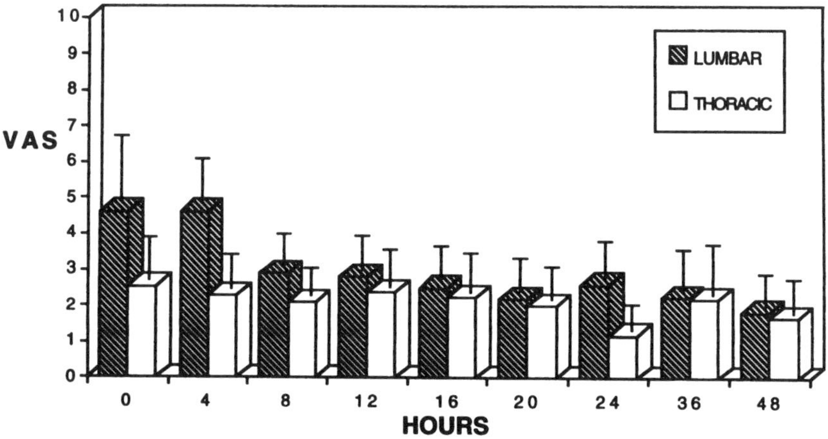

FIGURE 1.—Mean visual analogue pain scores (VAS) in cm during the first 48 postoperative hours for lumbar vs. thoracic epidural catheters. There were no significant differences between groups. Scores at 0 and 4 hours in the lumbar group are significantly higher than scores at 12 (P = .04), 16 (P = .02), and 20 hours (P = .01) in the same group. (Courtesy of Bouchard F, Drolet P: Thoracic versus lumbar administration of fentanyl using patient-controlled epidural after thoracotomy. *Reg Anesth* 20:385–388, 1995.)

appears to offer little or no advantage. Both techniques offer the same degree of analgesia, with few side effects.

► It is not surprising that this study failed to show a difference between lumbar and thoracic fentanyl delivery, inasmuch as there is overwhelming evidence that, at least with continuous administration, the predominant effect of epidurally administered fentanyl is not related to direct spinal effects. It is interesting, however, that there is a trend toward better analgesia for the thoracic group in the early hours after bolus epidural injection (2 μg/kg). Perhaps there is a transient spinal effect if a sufficient bolus dose is administered. There is experimental evidence to support this speculation.

S.E. Abram, M.D.

Comparison of Morphine and Morphine With Ketamine for Postoperative Analgesia

Javery KB, Ussery TW, Steger HG, et al (Univ of Kentucky, Lexington)
Can J Anaesth 43:212–215, 1996 8–18

Background.—Ketamine has been used as an IV anesthetic for acute and chronic pain. Ketamine does not suppress cardiovascular function or laryngeal protective reflexes; it depresses ventilation less than opioids or nonopioids, and may stimulate respiration. Adverse effects include tolerance, accumulation of metabolites, malaise, cardiovascular excitation, and psychomimetic effects. Results of studies of morphine and ketamine combined have been varied. Levels of postoperative analgesia provided by morphine alone and by morphine with sub-anesthetic doses of ketamine were compared.

Methods.—There were 42 patients aged 21 to 55 years who underwent lumbar microdiscectomy who were American Society of Anesthesiologists level 1 and 2. Either morphine 1 mg/mL^{-1} or morphine with ketamine 1 mg/mL^{-1} each was administered by patient-controlled analgesia. Patient-reported pain scores and side effects were evaluated.

Results.—Pain scores were lower for patients who received morphine with ketamine than for patients who received morphine alone. Patients given morphine with ketamine reported less nausea, pruritus, and urinary retention. There were few reports of dysphoria. Patients given morphine alone received almost twice as much opioid as those given morphine plus ketamine.

Conclusions.—Morphine combined with ketamine provided better pain relief than morphine alone. Patients who received morphine with ketamine experienced fewer side effects and required lower doses of morphine. Morphine plus ketamine is a safe alternative to morphine alone for postoperative analgesia.

▶ Although this study describes a potentially useful technique, the study design fails to examine what may be the most efficient use of ketamine, that is, pre-emptive administration. Because ketamine is an effective *N*-methyl-D-aspartate antagonist, pre-incisional initiation of ketamine administration may produce profound suppression of nociception-induced spinal hyperalgesia.

S.E. Abram, M.D.

Double-blind Randomized Evaluation of Intercostal Nerve Blocks as an Adjuvant to Subarachnoid Administered Morphine for Post-thoracotomy Analgesia

Liu M, Rock P, Grass JA, et al (Johns Hopkins Med Insts, Baltimore, Md)

Reg Anesth 20:418–425, 1995 8–19

Background.—Thoracotomy is associated with pain, pulmonary complications, and reduced lung function. Pain relief can result in better pulmonary function, less hypercarbia and hypoxia, and better patient comfort. Intercostal nerve blocks can provide 6 hours of analgesia, and subarachnoid morphine has been used after thoracotomy to provide up to 24 hours of analgesia. Intercostal nerve blocks and subarachnoid morphine block the pain pathways at 2 different sites. The analgesic effect of intercostal nerve blocks combined with subarachnoid morphine after thoracotomy was investigated.

Methods.—Twenty patients underwent lateral thoracotomy for pulmonary resection. The patients were randomly assigned to receive intercostal nerve blocks with 0.5% bupivacaine or saline before wound closure. All patients were given 0.5 mg of subarachnoid morphine before surgical incision. Pain scores, 1-second forced expiratory volume, 1 forced vital capacity, and use of opioids were measured at intervals for up to 72 hours after surgery.

Results.—Patients given subarachnoid morphine and bupivacaine had better values for 1-second forced expiratory volume and forced vital capacity, and had less pain at rest and with cough. At 24 hours, however, 1-second forced expiratory volume decreased in these patients to values lower than in patients given subarachnoid morphine and saline. Pain scores at rest for patients given bupivacaine were significantly lower at 4 hours, but were similar for both groups beyond 4 hours. Use of opioids during the first 24 hours was similar for both groups.

Conclusions.—The benefits of added intercostal nerve blocks to subarachnoid morphine are transient for post-thoracotomy analgesia. In some cases, intercostal nerve blocks may be associated with hypotension. The addition of intercostal nerve blocks to subarachnoid morphine, 0.5 mg, is not recommended.

▶ The authors did not explore the possibility that pre-incisional blocks might have been more effective than blocks instituted at the end of surgery. In addition, the profound analgesia afforded by intrathecal morphine, which was administered before surgery, may have obscured any potential benefit of the regional blocks. It would be worthwhile to compare pre-incisional blocks, postoperative blocks, and no blocks in patients receiving no analgesic techniques except postoperative systemic opioids.

S.E. Abram, M.D.

Reduction of Nausea and Vomiting From Epidural Opioids by Adding Droperidol to the Infusate in Home-bound Patients

Aldrete JA (North West Florida Comunity Hosp, Chipley)

J Pain Symptom Manage 10:544–547, 1995 8–20

Objective.—Droperidol reduces nausea and vomiting in hospitalized patients receiving epidural infusions of opioids. The antiemetic effects of droperidol added to an infusate containing an opioid and a local anesthetic were evaluated in ambulatory patients.

Methods.—A total of 184 postlaminectomy patients (101 men), aged 35 to 62 years, received an epidural infusate of either 92 mL of 0.25% bupivacaine, 600 μg fentanyl, and 5 mg of droperidol (group A) or 92 mL of 0.25% bupivacaine, 600 μg fentanyl, and 2 mL of 0.9% sodium chloride (group B) at rates of 0.5 to 2 mL/hr. Patients were followed up by home care workers for 2 to 55 days. Patients could turn pumps on or off depending on their pain.

Results.—All patients had excellent pain relief, and only 3 needed permanently implanted pain relief devices. Group B patients experienced significantly more nausea and vomiting than did Group A patients.

Conclusion.—Droperidol, added to epidural infusates, significantly reduces nausea and vomiting in ambulatory postlaminectomy patients receiving fentanyl and bupivacaine.

▶ The use of injectable, FDA approved drugs for nonindicated spinal and epidural applications is being reported with increasing frequency. Whereas the development of existing drugs for new indications is an important means for expanding our therapeutic options, the ability to bypass the usual regulatory processes may place patients at risk. Very little preclinical animal testing of neuraxial droperidol has been done. What is particularly distressing about this report is its failure to indicate institutions research board approval by the hospital and the failure to cite previous studies of safety in animals. Preclinical studies should incorporate multiple species and behavioral, histopathologic and spinal cord blood flow studies. Human studies that fail to cite evidence of safety or IRB approval should not be accepted for publication. Although the addition of droperidol to epidural opioids may be a safe and efficacious technique, we must abide by the processes that safeguard patient well-being when evaluating new spinal and epidural injection techniques.

S.E. Abram, M.D.

Other Acute Pain Management Studies

Intrathecal Steroids to Reduce Pain After Lumbar Disc Surgery: A Double-blind, Placebo-controlled Prospective Study

Langmayr JJ, Obwegeser AA, Schwarz AB, et al (Universitätsklinik für Neurochirurgie, Innsbruck, Austria; Institut für Biostatistik, Innsbruck, Austria)

Pain 62:357–361, 1995 8–21

Objective.—Whether the use of steroids can reduce radicular pain after lumbar disc surgery is controversial. The effect on postoperative and long-term radicular pain of intrathecal administration of betamethasone was determined in a double-blind, placebo-controlled, prospective study in patients undergoing discectomy for lumbar disc herniation.

Methods.—A total of 26 patients, with preoperative pain of 14 to 150 days' duration, resistant to nonsurgical treatment, received a discectomy. Before wound closure, 13 (3 females) received intrathecal betamethasone and 13 (3 females) received saline. Patients graded pain intensity on a 100-mm visual analogue scale 1 day before surgery, on the day of discharge, and at 6-month follow-up. Consumption of nonsteroidal anti-inflammatory drugs (NSAIDs) was monitored.

Results.—Preoperative pain levels were similar for both groups (55 and 54 mm). For the placebo group, pain declined slowly after surgery from days 1 to 4 and 8 (39, 29, 24, 20, and 10 mm). For the steroid group, pain declined rapidly from days 1 to 4 and 8 (15, 15, 11, 8, and 5 mm). Analysis of variance showed that the effect of time ($P < 0.001$) and steroid application ($P = 0.014$) was significant, as was the interaction between time and steroid use ($P = 0.042$). The use of NSAIDs was similar between groups. At follow-up, radicular pain was rated similarly by both groups.

Conclusion.—Intrathecal administration of corticosteroids after discectomy provides significant short-term postoperative pain relief.

► Studies done in the 1960s demonstrated that water-soluble steroid preparations injected intrathecally were cleared from the CSF quite rapidly. Within about 30 minutes, there was equilibration between CSF and blood levels. It is not surprising, therefore, that substantial lasting benefit was not seen with soluble betamethasone in this study. There is sufficient controversy associated with the intrathecal use of insoluble steroid suspensions to preclude their use in such a study.

S.E. Abram, M.D.

Absence of an Early Pre-emptive Effect After Thoracic Extradural Bupivacaine in Thoracic Surgery

Aguilar JL, Rincón R, Domingo V, et al (Hosp Universitario Germans Trias i Pujol, Barcelona)

Br J Anaesth 76:72–76, 1996 8–22

Objective.—Whereas standard doses of oral nonsteroidal anti-inflammatory drugs before surgery do not show an early benefit, some pre-emptive field block or extradural block studies using local anesthetics or opioids show a positive effect on pain intensity. Whether an extradural thoracic block with local anesthetic before surgical incision has a pre-emptive effect on postoperative pain intensity was determined using a double-blind, placebo-controlled, crossover design study.

Methods.—The 45 patients undergoing posterolateral thoracotomy for lung resection were randomly assigned to 1 of 3 groups: group 1 received 8 mL of 0.5% bupivacaine containing 5 µg/mL of adrenaline (B+E) through a thoracic extradural catheter 30 minutes before incision and 8 mL of saline 15 minutes after incision; group 2 received 8 mL of saline extradurally before and 8 mL of B+E after incision; and group 3 received 8 mL of saline extradurally before and after incision. Patients received propofol, alfentanil, and atracurium by infusion as anesthesia. Before chest closure, alfentanil infusion was stopped, and 50 µg of fentanyl in saline was administered extradurally. In the recovery room, patient-controlled extradural analgesia (PCEA) included 0.125% bupivacaine with adrenaline 1/400,000 and 6 µg/mL of fentanyl administered extradurally at 2 mL/hr with boluses of 0.5 mL with a 6-minute lock-out time during the 48-hour postoperative period. Side effects, verbal rating scale (VRS) reports, and visual analogue scale (VAS) pain scores during arm movement and cough were recorded at 1, 3, 7, 11, 19, and 43 hours after surgery.

Results.—Use of PCEA and scores on the VAS and VRS did not differ between groups.

Conclusion.—No pre-emptive effect of epidural anesthesia was demonstrated.

▶ The design of this study may preclude detection of a pre-emptive effect. There is evidence that parenteral opioids given before the onset of a noxious stimulus reduce the *N*-methyl-D-aspartate receptor-mediated sensitization of dorsal horn neurons. Therefore, the pre-emptive use of alfentanil may have limited the potential of this study to demonstrate an effect.

Although some experimental models have demonstrated the ability of regional anesthesia to block spinal-mediated hyperalgesia, several studies have failed to demonstrate pre-emptive effects clinically in the perioperative setting. This may be due to the ability of afferent impulses from injured tissues to induce wind-up in the postoperative period, after the block has worn off. Studies that compare pre-incisional to postoperative effects of regional blockade also may fail to demonstrate differences in subsequent pain levels if the post-incisional block produces intense analgesia, allowing the sensitized state of CNS neurons to return to their premorbid condition.

Another reason this study failed to demonstrate a pre-emptive effect of epidural anesthesia may be related to the relatively small dose of local anesthetic used. It now appears likely that a dense block is required to produce a pre-emptive effect and to abolish the endocrine/metabolic consequences of surgery. Studies that use regional block without general anesthesia are more effective at blocking endocrine/metabolic responses than those that use a combined approach, probably because the block is, by necessity, more profound. A partial block is theoretically capable of enhancing pain perception by inhibiting activity in the superficially located dorsolateral funiculus, which contains descending inhibitory fibers.

S.E. Abram, M.D.

Thoracic Epidural Anesthesia Via the Lumbar Approach in Infants and Children

Blanco D, Llamazares J, Rincón R, et al (Hosp Universitari "Germans Trías i Pujol," Barcelona)

Anesthesiology 84:1312–1316, 1996 8–23

Introduction.—The total dose of local anesthetic can be reduced in upper abdominal or chest surgery using the segmental approach to the

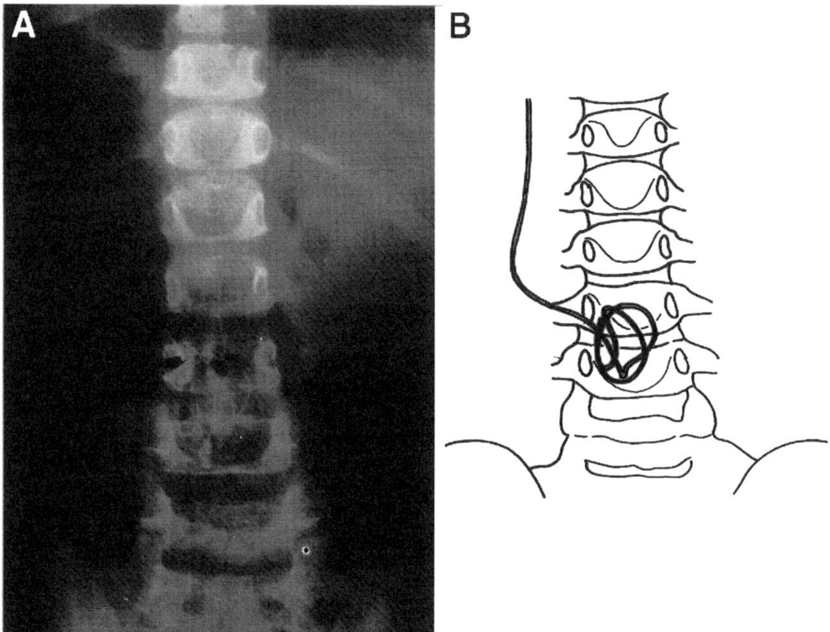

FIGURE 1.—A and B, common placement of catheter tip. (Courtesy of Blanco D, Llamazares J, Rincón R: Thoracic epidural anesthesia via the lumbar approach in infants and children. *Anesthesiology* 84:1312–1316, 1996.)

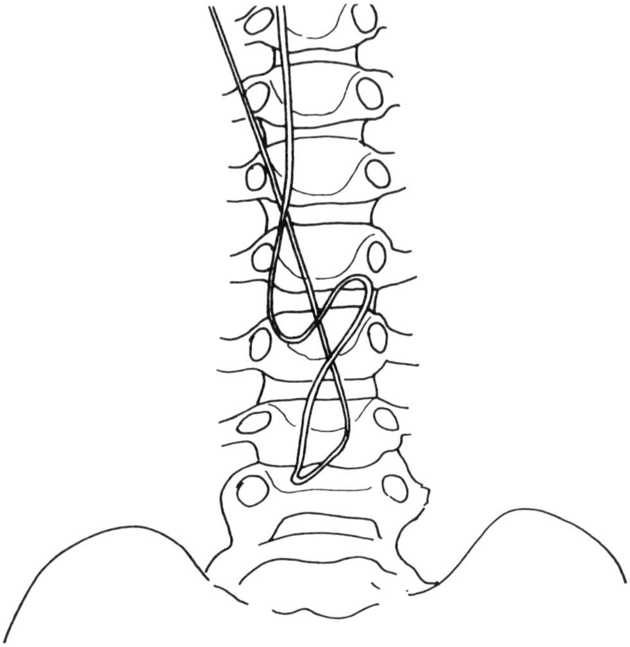

FIGURE 3, B.—The distal tip of the catheter is well above the insertion point. (Courtesy of Blanco D, Llamazares J, Rincón R: Thoracic epidural anesthesia via the lumbar approach in infants and children. *Anesthesiology* 84:1312–1316, 1996.)

thoracic epidural space. Even with a highly experienced anesthesiologist performing this procedure, there is a risk of neurologic damage or dural puncture. The risk of spinal cord damage and contamination could be reduced with the introduction and advancement of a catheter from the lumbar epidural space to the thoracic level. This has not been described in a pediatric population. The success and degree of difficulty in advancing a 19-gauge catheter from the lumbar epidural space to the thoracic level were evaluated in 39 children aged 96 months or younger.

Methods.—Patients were placed in the lateral decubitus position to measure the cutaneous distance between the L4-5 and T10-11 interspaces. That distance was marked on a 19-gauge multiorifice catheter, and the entire length of the catheter was inserted through an 18-gauge Tuohy needle with the bevel directed cephalad at the L4-5 level. The difficulty in advancing the catheter was classified as easy, difficult, or impossible. Catheter tips were located radiologically.

Results.—There were 3 main positions in which the catheters appeared in the epidural space: (1) the catheter circled itself near the point of entrance without advancing in any direction (Fig 1); (2) it formed a figure 8; and (3) the distal tip in the epidural space was well above the insertion point, although the catheter formed a wavy line below (Fig 3, B). Catheters were difficult to insert at the L4-5 level in 8 patients (Table 1). The level actually reached was T10–T12 in 7 patients, L2 in 1 patient, L3 in 8

TABLE 1.—Degree of Difficulty in Advancing the Catheter and the Location of the Tip in the Epidural Space

	T10–T12	T12–L1	L1–L2	L2–L3	L3–L4	L4–L5
Easy	7	0	0	1	8	15
Difficult	0	0	0	0	0	8
Impossible	0	0	0	0	0	0

Note: Values are the number of the catheters reaching the space named.
(Courtesy of Blanco D, Llamazares J, Rincón R: Thoracic epidural anesthesia via the lumbar approach in infants and children. *Anesthesiology* 84:1312–1316, 1996.)

patients, and L4-5 in 23 patients. All catheters were removed easily. There was no relationship between easy advance of the catheter and success in reaching the T10–T12 level. There were no dural punctures, but there was an intravascular insertion in 1 patient.

Conclusion.—The insertion of a 19-gauge unstiffened catheter at the lumbar level is a poor technique for reaching the thoracic epidural space. Tip placement must be verified by radiograph if this approach is used. An unstiffened catheter should not be advanced further than 2–3 cm to avoid potential knotting. Easy advancement of the catheter was not associated with desired catheter placement.

► A previous study[1] documented that it is relatively easy to place thoracic epidural catheters via the caudal route in neonates but not in older children. This study showed a low success rate for thoracic placement via the lumbar epidural route in neonates as well as older children. This is an important issue because some anesthesiologists feel that the risk of placing thoracic epidural catheters in anesthetized patients is not justified, since contact of the needle with the spinal cord would not be recognized.

S.E. Abram, M.D.

Reference

1. Bösenberg AT, Bland BAR, Schulte-Steinberg O, et al: Thoracic epidural anesthesia via caudal route in infants. *Anesthesiology* 1988; 69:265–269.

Evaluation of Intrapleural Analgesia in the Management of Blunt Traumatic Chest Wall Pain: A Clinical Trial

Short K, Scheeres D, Mlakar J, et al (Butterworth Hosp, Grand Rapids, Mich; Michigan State Univ, Grand Rapids)
Am Surg 62:488–493, 1996 8–24

Background.—Previous studies of the use of intrapleural analgesia (IPA) to relieve chest wall pain have yielded conflicting findings. Many of these studies have been criticized for design flaws. In theory, the incidence of respiratory and circulatory depression is lower with IPA, suggesting significant advantages over epidural analgesia. The value of IPA in chest wall pain relief was studied in a prospective, randomized, double-blind, crossover, placebo-controlled trial.

Methods.—Sixteen patients (age range, 35–80 years) with rib fractures who were admitted to a trauma service during a 2-year period were studied. None of these patients were intubated or had significant trauma outside the chest wall. A standardized technique was used to place the intrapleural catheters. The patients received a saline solution placebo or a combination of bupivacaine/lidocaine in a blinded, crossover fashion for two 24-hour periods.

Findings.—No complications resulted from catheter placement or anesthetic toxicity. Opposite trends occurred in mean pain ratings from patients and nurses. Mean values for supplemental narcotic use, P_{CO_2}, P_{O_2}, forced vital capacity, and forced expiratory volume did not differ significantly between groups.

Conclusions.—In these patients with blunt chest injuries, IPA was not beneficial in managing chest wall pain. The crossover design of this study should have enabled clinically significant differences to emerge, even though the number of patients studied was small.

▶ This study suggests that the failure of this technique to achieve widespread use in patients who have had chest wall injuries or thoracic surgery may be related to a relative lack of efficacy compared with more conventional techniques. The lack of benefit in these patients may be related to dilution of anesthetic by pleural fluid or blood.

S.E. Abram, M.D.

Age Is the Best Predictor of Postoperative Morphine Requirements

Macintyre PE, Jarvis DA (Univ of Adelaide, North Terrace, Australia)

Pain 64:357–364, 1995 8–25

Background.—The opioid dose prescribed for postoperative pain relief has traditionally been based on the patient's weight. Although dose reductions are often considered in elderly patients, age-related dose changes are generally not considered in younger patients. The factors that best predict the amount of morphine used in the first 24 hours after surgery were determined.

Methods.—The medical records of 1,010 patients younger than 70 years of age were reviewed. All had been prescribed morphine in a patient-controlled analgesia (PCA) system after major surgery. Variables studied were patient age, sex, weight, operative site, verbal numeric pain score, and a nausea/vomiting score (Fig 2). The effects of intraoperative and recovery room doses of opioid were analyzed in a subgroup of 78 patients.

Findings.—Interpatient variability in PCA morphine doses was great, with differences of as high as 10-fold in each age group. However, the best predictor of PCA morphine requirement in the first 24 hours postoperatively was patient age. For patients older than 20 years of age, these

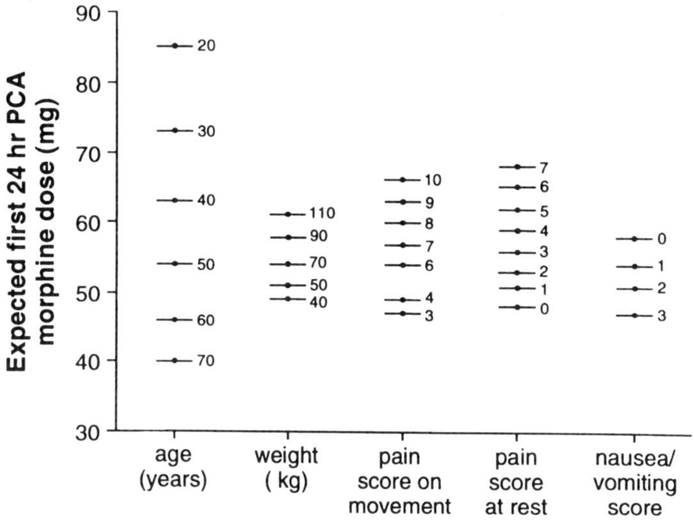

FIGURE 2.—Influence of each variable on the expected first 24 hour patient-controlled analgesia (*PCA*) morphine dose with all other variables held at their mean value for the sample. (Reprinted from Macintyre PE, Jarvis DA: Age is the best predictor of postoperative morphine requirements. *Pain* 64:357–364, 1995. With kind permission from Elsevier Science—NL, Sara Burgerhartstraat 25, 1055 KV Amsterdam, The Netherlands.)

requirements could be estimated by the formula: *average first 24 hour morphine requirement (mg) = 100 − age.*

Conclusions.—Previous studies have reported a correlation between patient age and the amount of opioid needed. In the current study, this association was quantified and provided a guideline for opioid dosing (Table 5). Prescriptions for conventional analgesic regimens should include a dose range centered on values from the formula above to allow for the wide variation among patients in each age group. The initial morphine

TABLE 5.—Guide for the Prescription of Initial Morphine Doses for Intermittent IM or Subcutaneous Injection (in Opioid Naive Patients)

Patient age (yrs)	Morphine dose range (mg)
20–29	7.5–12.5
30–39	7.5–12.5
40–49	5.0–10.0
50–59	5.0–10.0
60–69	2.5– 7.5
70–79	2.5– 5.0
80–89	2.5– 5.0
> 89	2.0– 3.0

Note: These dose ranges are ordered 2 hourly as necessary.

(Reprinted from Macintyre PE, Jarvis DA: Age is the best predictor of postoperative morphine requirements. *Pain* 64:357–364, 1995, with kind permission from Elsevier Science - NL, Sara Burgerhartstraat 25, 1055 KV Amsterdam, The Netherlands.)

dose should be determined according to patient age and not weight, but subsequent doses must be titrated based on effect.

▶ This study is a good example of how well-designed outcome studies can produce useful practical information for common clinical situations. This type of data should be incorporated into standard protocols for PCA and opioid ordering as necessary.

S.E. Abram, M.D.

Chronic Pain Management

Long-term Use of Subarachnoid Clonidine for Analgesia in Refractory Reflex Sympathetic Dystrophy: Case Report

Kabeer AA, Hardy PAJ (Gloucestershire Royal Hosp, England)

Reg Anesth 21:249–252, 1996 8–26

Background.—Clonidine has been used for short periods to relieve postoperative pain, severe neurogenic pain, and intractable pain from cancer. Recently, a report suggested that patients with intractable reflex sympathetic dystrophy (RSD) could also benefit from clonidine administration. There is very little information about the prolonged use of clonidine in humans. The long-term use of subarachnoid clonidine in a patient with RSD unresponsive to other treatments was described.

Case Report.—Man, 49, sought treatment at a pain clinic for right knee pain of long duration. Pain onset had occurred after a football injury. He had all the classic signs of RSD. Despite several treatment attempts, his pain progressed. Within 2 years he was dependent on elbow crutches or a wheelchair. Eventually, an infusion of clonidine in an initial dose of 300 μg daily was administered, completely relieving both his continuous pain, allodynia, and limb coldness. The symptoms returned within 1–2 hours after the infusion was stopped. An intraspinal catheter was implanted for continuous clonidine treatment. The initial dosage was 75 μg twice a day. The patient and his wife were carefully educated in injection technique and dose incrementation. At a dosage of 150 μg twice a day, the patient was stable and comfortable, and he began to mobilize. His condition remained satisfactory for 1 year, at which time a "foreign body reaction" to the catheter developed. A new system was inserted. Eighteen months after the beginning of clonidine treatment, the patient continues to be comfortable.

Conclusions.—In this patient with RSD, twice-daily subarachnoid clonidine delivered through an implanted drug delivery system successfully alleviated the symptoms. No signs of tolerance or toxicity have occurred during the more than 18 months of therapy.

► There are several interesting issues associated with this report. First is the ability of spinally administered nonopioid analgesics to provide long-term pain relief in opioid-tolerant individuals. Clonidine appears to be effective in the face of opioid tolerance. Whether substantial tolerance develops to the analgesic activity of clonidine remains to be seen. There is a reduction of antihypertensive efficacy after long-term clonidine administration and rebound hypertension after its abrupt discontinuation, suggesting receptor downregulation. There has also been a report of the loss of efficacy of intrathecal clonidine over time in a patient with intractable cancer pain.[1] This, however, may be associated with increased tumor spread as opposed to tolerance development.

A thorny ethical issue is associated with the institution of long-term spinal infusions for patients whose life expectancy is many years and whose pain is expected to continue indefinitely. The likelihood of infectious and technical complications occurring during such prolonged periods is fairly high. The institution of such therapy implies a willingness on the part of the treating physician to manage that patient's pain problem indefinitely. I have seen examples of these devices being placed (at considerable expense) and, after failure to provide adequate relief, the patient is referred to another center for continued care.

S.E. Abram, M.D.

Reference

1. Coombs DW, Saunders R, Lachance D, et al: Intrathecal morphine tolerance: Use of intrathecal clonidine, DADLE, and intraventricular morphine. *Anesthesiology* 62:358–363, 1985.

Reflex Sympathetic Dystrophy: Skin Blood Flow, Sympathetic Vasoconstrictor Reflexes and Pain Before and After Surgical Sympathectomy

Baron R, Maier C (Christian-Albrechts-Universität Kiel, Germany)
Pain 67:317–326, 1996 8–27

Introduction.—Reflex sympathetic dystrophy (RSD) may develop after trauma affecting the limbs. Although clinical signs and symptoms vary considerably, 3 major components have been distinguished: sensory abnormalities, vascular and sweating abnormalities, and motor abnormalities. Some studies suggest that patients with RSD are characterized by sympathetic overactivity in the affected limb. To better understand the mechanisms of vascular disturbances in RSD and the role of the sympathetic nervous system, 12 patients were studied with laser Doppler flowmetry.

Methods.—Study participants were 12 consecutive patients referred for evaluation of RSD of the hand. Eleven recalled a previous trauma to the affected limb. Controls were 12 healthy volunteers. Cutaneous blood flow, skin resistance, and skin temperature were measured at the affected and contralateral hands. To measure the function of sympathetic vasoconstrictor fibers, autonomic reflexes were examined after deep inspiration. Eleven patients were treated with local anesthetic stellate ganglion blocks, regional guanethidine blocks, or both. One experienced long-term relief, 5 had temporary relief, and 4 did not respond to sympathetic blocks. Four of those who had temporary relief underwent surgical sympathectomy.

Results.—In 10 patients, both blood flow and skin temperature were considerably lower after acclimatization in a cold environment (18°C or less), indicating vasoconstriction of cutaneous vessels. No additional vasoconstrictor reflexes were elicited ipsilaterally under these conditions. In a warm (22°C to 24°C) environment, blood flow and skin temperature showed no significant side differences. Sympathetic vasoconstrictor responses to deep inspiration were also quantitatively the same on both sides in a warm environment. Vasoconstrictor reflexes were absent after sympathectomy and skin resistance was considerably higher on the affected hand. For 4 weeks after the procedure, the affected hand was warmer and blood flow higher when compared with the unaffected hand. There was a subsequent, slow decrease in skin temperature and perfusion, and the affected hand turned from warm to cold. The 2 patients who experienced long-term pain relief had postsympathectomy skin temperature and blood flow values that were only slightly less in the affected hand than in the normal hand.

Conclusion.—Side differences in patients with RSD must be interpreted with care because skin temperature and blood flow vary according to changes in environmental temperature. Vascular disturbances do not result from constant overactivity of sympathetic vasoconstrictor neurons. Some patients experience a relapse of pain after sympathectomy, perhaps because of denervation supersensitivity of blood vessels and vasomotion.

▶ It is hoped that this article will discourage the temptation to perform surgical sympathectomies on the many patients who experience transient relief from local anesthetic sympathetic blocks. There are many reasons that pain is relieved by sympathetic blocks, most of which have nothing to do with sympathetic denervation. These include placebo effect, pharmacologic effect of systemically absorbed local anesthetic, spread of anesthetic to somatic structures, and blockade of somatic and visceral afferent fibers that pass through the sympathetic chain.

The variable response to sympathectomy seen by the authors is typical of most authors' experience with patients who undergo sympathectomy for RSD (complex regional pain syndromes type I). There is little evidence to support the hypothesis that the pathophysiology of this condition is related to abnormally high sympathetic tone. Microneurographic studies have failed to show increases in sympathetic outflow, even in patients with persistent vasoconstriction. Likewise, catecholamine levels are not elevated in the venous blood draining affected limbs. The reason that some patients with RSD experience persistent relief from surgical sympathectomy remains unclear.

S.E. Abram, M.D.

Long-term Results of Peripheral Nerve Stimulation for Reflex Sympathetic Dystrophy

Hassenbusch SJ, Stanton-Hicks M, Schoppa D, et al (MD Anderson Cancer Ctr, Houston; Cleveland Clinic Found, Ohio)

J Neurosurg 84:415–423, 1996 8–28

Background.—Reflex sympathetic dystrophy (RSD) is typically managed successfully with medication, blocks, or infusions. However, peripheral nerve stimulation (PNS) is a treatment strategy that has been used with some success in patients with severe RSD. Its efficacy in patients with severe RSD with symptoms related to the distribution of just 1 major peripheral nerve was assessed prospectively.

Methods.—A 2-day trial of PNS was offered to patients with pain related to PNS entirely or mainly in the distribution of 1 major peripheral nerve that was refractory to other conservative RSD treatments. A permanent, implanted generator connected to the electrode was programmed in patients experiencing at least 50% reductions in pain and objective improvements in the physical examination categories of vasomotor tone, trophic changes, and somatic motor changes. The patients were seen for follow-up assessments at intervals of 2–6 weeks. Results were considered good if pain was reduced by at least 50% and there were improvements in at least 2 physical categories, fair if pain was reduced by at least 50% and there was improvement in no more than 1 physical category, or if pain was reduced by at least 25% and there was improvement in at least 1 physical category.

Results.—Thirty-two patients underwent the 2-day trial, and the permanent generator was placed in 30 patients. Of these 30 patients, PNS was successful in 19 (63%), with 10 having consistently good results and 9 having fair relief, with a follow-up of more than 2 years. In the patients with successful treatment, the mean pain score was reduced from 8.3 to 3.5. There was marked improvement in vasomotor tone, but there were less significant improvements in motor weakness and trophic changes. Activity levels increased substantially, with improvements in working ability as well as sleeping, motor strength, and driving. Treatment failures occurred at a mean of 1.3 years after treatment began, with a reversal of pain relief and no significant improvements in the physical categories or activity levels. Complications included the need for electrode implantation revision in 8 patients (27%), with generators detaching from the anchoring sutures in 2 patients, and cosmetic revisions in 2.

Conclusions.—Peripheral nerve stimulation can be highly effective in the treatment of RSD localized in the distribution of just 1 major peripheral nerve that is refractory to conservative management. A comparative study is needed to determine the relative efficacy of PNS and spinal cord stimulation in these patients.

▶ Because spinal cord stimulation appears to be effective for many patients with RSD or chronic regional pain syndrome type 1 (CRPS-1), it would be useful to compare efficacy of spinal and PNS techniques. Percutaneous trial stimulation may be a useful technique for determining the better procedure for a given patient. One potential drawback to PNS is that manipulation of the already injured nerve may at least temporarily aggravate symptoms.

S.E. Abram, M.D.

High-dose Oral Morphine in Cancer Pain Management: A Report of Twelve Cases

Radbruch L, Grond S, Zech DJ, et al (Univ of Cologne, Germany)
J Clin Anesth 8:144–150, 1996 8–29

Introduction.—Seventy-four percent of patients with advanced cancer experience pain. The use of morphine in cancer pain has been thoroughly investigated, but not much has been published regarding the high-dose range of this analgesic. The efficacy and side effects of high-dose orally administered morphine was evaluated in 12 patients with cancer pain.

Methods.—Of 705 patients treated at a pain clinic for advanced cancer from various sites, the mean orally administered morphine dose for this cohort was 120 mg/day. Fourteen of these patients received more than 600 mg/day of morphine. Twelve patients were followed up until their death. Patients were evaluated for pain etiology, type, localization, and intensity on admission to the pain clinic. Pain types included nociceptive pain (periosteum/bone, visceral, and soft-tissue pain) and neuropathic pain (compression or infiltration of nerve structures). Patients used a 6-step verbal rating scale or a numeric rating scale to assess pain intensity. Patients were given analgesic treatment according to the analgesic ladder recommended by the World Health Organization. The efficacy and side effects of orally administered morphine and other methods of pain relief were assessed regularly.

Results.—None of the 12 patients receiving high-dose morphine experienced serious side effects. Even with the frequent combination of morphine with hypnotics, patients did not experience respiratory depression. Morphine doses had to be individualized for each patient to achieve adequate pain relief. Ten of 12 patients had adequate pain relief with lower morphine doses for varying lengths of time. When the administration mode needed to be altered, the conversion factors were: 2 patients—oral to IV 2:1, 1 patient—oral to epidural 10:1, and 1 patient—oral doses required for adequate analgesia were ninefold those required subcutaneously or IV. Two patients were changed to transdermal fentanyl to counteract the development of tolerance. This change provided good pain relief for 1 patient and no improvement for the other. Low patient compliance lengthened dose titration, with intermittent prescription of excessive doses without adequate pain relief in 1 patient. Morphine-related side effects were more frequent in periods of low compliance in this patient. The major reason for dose increases seemed to be disease progression and not tolerance.

Conclusions.—There do not seem to be any specific pain syndromes that could be considered opioid resistant. Most patients with inadequate analgesia with opioid administration alone were treated adequately with a combination of morphine and non-opioids or supplemented with co-analgesics. Advanced cancer disease was the most common reason for dose increases. Orally administered morphine may be considered a safe analgesic in the high-dose range. The side effects of morphine therapy are not more prevalent with increasing doses, and symptomatic relief of side effects may be treated with adjuvant medications. The absence of respiratory depression with high doses of morphine supports the contention that the presence of pain is an antagonist to respiratory depression.

► The authors' message that cancer pain often can be controlled well with escalation of orally administered morphine doses to levels that are manyfold higher than required for opiate-naive patients is certainly an important one. However, their comment that nearly all patients with pain from advanced cancer can be adequately managed on such a regimen is misleading. Most palliative care services encounter patients whose pain is poorly controlled or whose side effects are excessive when they are using orally or parenterally administered morphine. Many of these patients can be made much more comfortable by changing to other opioids or by initiating neuraxial drug infusions or neurolytic blocks. The message expressed in this article may lead to undertreatment of those patients whose pain problems are the most desperate.

S.E. Abram, M.D.

Direct Conversion From Oral Morphine to Transdermal Fentanyl: A Multicenter Study in Patients With Cancer Pain

Donner B, Zenz M, Tryba M, et al (Univ Hosp Bergmannsheil, Germany)

Pain 64:527–534, 1996 8–30

Background.—Transdermal fentanyl is a new method of administering long-term opioid therapy that has recently been investigated for use in management of cancer pain. Direct conversion to transdermal fentanyl has not been studied for patients receiving constant pain relief through conventional therapy with long-acting opioids. The feasibility of a calculation table for the conversion from oral morphine (sustained-release morphine [SRM]) to transdermal fentanyl with a ratio of 100:1 was investigated.

Methods.—Participants included 98 adults with stable and low levels of cancer pain who required 600 mg or less of SRM per day. Patients received continuous SRM medication during the 6-day prestudy phase. The conversion table (oral morphine to transdermal fentanyl, 100:1) was then used to calculate initial fentanyl dosage, and the 15-day study phase was begun. The transdermal system was changed every 72 hours and the dose of fentanyl was adjusted in accordance with the patient's needs, as deter-

TABLE 4.—Dosage of Sustained-Release Morphine and Transdermal Fentanyl

	Mean	Range
Sustained-release morphine dosage (mg/day)	138.6	25 – 600
Fentanyl TTs dosage on day 0 (mg/day)	1.4	0.6 – 6
Fentanyl TTS dosage on day 15 (mg/day)	2.4	0.6 – 12

(Reprinted from Donner B, Zenz M, Tryba M, et al: Direct conversion from oral morphine to transdermal fentanyl: A multicenter study in patients with cancer pain. *Pain* 64:527–534, 1996, with kind permission of Elsevier Science - NL, Sara Burgerhartstraat 25, 1055 KV Amsterdam, The Netherlands.)

mined by visual analogue pain scale scores and requirement for liquid morphine.

Results.—A mean morphine/transdermal fentanyl ratio of 70:1 was revealed by regression analysis (Table 4). Pain relief during treatment was identical between forms of analgesia, and the number of patients suffering from pain attacks did not increase with transdermal fentanyl. However, significantly more patients required supplemental medication with liquid morphine when they received transdermal fentanyl. Most side effects and vital signs were identical between forms of therapy, but patients showed less constipation and laxative use when receiving fentanyl. Morphine withdrawal syndrome occurred in 3 patients within the first 24 hours of fentanyl therapy. Approximately 95% of participants chose to continue transdermal fentanyl therapy because of its better performance relative to oral morphine.

Conclusions.—Use of a calculation table for the conversion of oral morphine to transdermal fentanyl with a ratio of 100:1 seems safe and effective. This ratio is slightly low; a true ratio of 70:1 was determined, implying a sufficient margin of safety. Supplementation with liquid morphine may be needed to meet the patient's analgesic needs for the first few days of the transition. The transdermal system may provide a useful alternative method of opioid administration for patients with chronic pain who are sensitive to opioids.

▶ There are considerable animal data to suggest that the more potent lipid-soluble opioids such as fentanyl and sufentanil may have some pharmacological advantages over less potent opioids such as morphine or meperidine. The more potent agents have a higher intrinsic activity; i.e., they require a lower fraction of receptor occupancy to achieve the same degree of analgesia compared with less potent agents. Therefore, under conditions of intense nociceptor activity or opioid tolerance, they are able to provide continued effect with less dose increase. As tolerance develops and nociceptor activity increases, as is typical in terminal cancer, less potent agents may begin to act as partial agonists, and increasing doses of meperidine or morphine may produce increasing side effects but no improvement in analgesia. Paronis and Holtzman showed that in rats fentanyl maintained its efficacy much better than morphine or meperidine in animals that had been made tolerant to morphine.[1] In addition, they showed that there was less development of tolerance to opioids during fentanyl infusions than during either morphine or meperidine infusions. There is now growing clinical evidence for these observations. Paix et al. demonstrated improved analgesia and reduced side effects in patients with cancer pain who were switched from morphine to sufentanil infusions,[2] and de Leon-Casasola and Lema demonstrated improvement in analgesia in cancer patients who were switched from epidural bupivacaine/morphine to epidural bupivacaine/sufentanil.[3] Whereas this study failed to show improved analgesia after the change to fentanyl, there was some improvement in constipation.

S.E. Abram, M.D.

References

1. Paronis CA, Holtzman SG: Development of tolerance to the analgesic activity of μ agonists after continuous infusion of morphine, meperidine, or fentanyl in rats. *J Pharmacol Exp Ther* 262:1–9, 1992.
2. Paix A, Coleman A, Lees J: Subcutaneous fentanyl and sufentanil infusion substitution for morphine intolerance in cancer pain management. *Pain* 63:263–269, 1995.
3. de Leon-Casasola OA, Lema MJ: Epidural bupivacaine/sufentanil therapy for postoperative pain control in patients tolerant to opioid and unresponsive to epidural bupivacaine/morphine. *Anesthesiology* 80:303–309, 1994.

Intrathecal Ketamine Reduces Morphine Requirements in Patients With Terminal Cancer Pain

Yang C-Y, Wong C-S, Chang J-Y, et al (Tri-Service Gen Hosp, Taipei, Taiwan, Republic of China)

Can J Anaesth 43:379–383, 1996 8–31

Background.—Although intrathecal morphine has been used to control cancer pain, its use is associated with many undesirable side effects. Whether the intrathecal administration of ketamine can potentiate that of morphine, decreasing the side effects, was investigated.

Methods.—Twenty hospitalized patients with terminal cancer pain participated in the double-blind crossover study. In phase M, patients received intrathecal morphine twice daily at an initial dose of 0.05 mg; daily incremental increases in dose were given until adequate analgesia was achieved. In phase M+K, patients received morphine as in phase M plus 1.0 mg ketamine with benzethonium chloride as preservative twice daily. Pain relief was considered acceptable when numeric rating scales of pain (0–10) were less than or equal to 3 and when the rescue dose of intramuscular morphine required after each intrathecal administration was less than 5 mg for 2 days. Patients received the crossover treatment with no washout period after experiencing 48 hours of acceptable analgesia with the first regimen.

Results.—During phase M, the effective dose of intrathecal morphine was 0.38 mg/day; during phase M+K, the effective dose was 0.17 mg/day (Table 2). Pain scales averaged 7.95 before intrathecal drug administration, decreasing to 2.2 in phase M and 1.95 in phase M+K after an

TABLE 2.—Intrathecal and Rescue Morphine Requirements and Frequency of Intrathecal Morphine Titration in Phase M and Phase M+K

	Phase M	*Phase M+K*
Effective dose of intrathecal morphine (mg)	0.38 ± 0.04	0.17 ± 0.02*
Total dose of intrathecal morphine during treatment (mg)	1.32 ± 0.19	0.38 ± 0.08*
Total dose of rescue morphine during treatment (mg)	33.25 ± 7.40	9.00 ± 3.58*
Frequency of intrathecal morphine titration	9.10 ± 0.51	5.00 ± 0.40*

Note: Values are mean ± SEM, n=20. Phase M, intrathecal morphine only; phase M+K, coadministered ketamine 1 mg with morphine.

*$P < 0.05$ vs. Phase M.

(Courtesy of Yang C-Y, Wong C-S, Chang J-Y, et al: Intrathecal ketamine reduces morphine requirements in patients with terminal cancer pain. *Can J Anaesth* 43:379–383, 1996.)

effective dose of morphine was reached (Fig 1). No serious side effects were noted.

Conclusions.—The coadministration of 1 mg of ketamine with intrathecal morphine decreases the dose of morphine needed to manage cancer pain, and the combination seems as effective as intrathecal morphine alone.

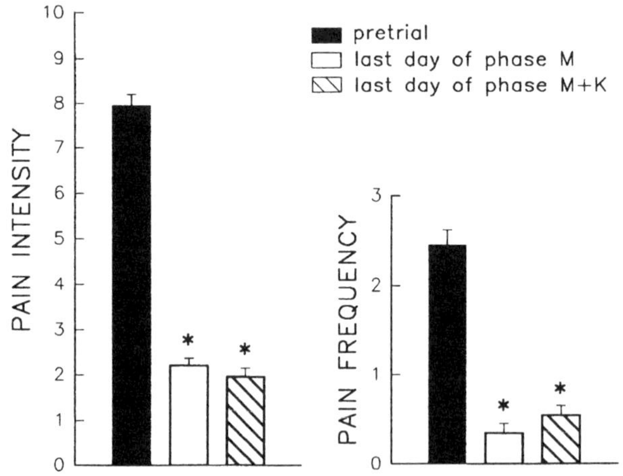

FIGURE 1.—Pain intensity (numeric rating scale) and frequency (4-point verbal ordinal scale) on the day before intrathecal administration and on the last day of the 2 phases. Values are mean ± SEM, n =20. Phase M, intrathecal morphine only; phase M+K, coadministered ketamine 1 mg with morphine. *$P < 0.05$ vs. before intrathecal administration. (Courtesy of Yang C-Y, Wong C-S, Chang J-Y, et al: Intrathecal ketamine reduces morphine requirements in patients with terminal cancer pain. *Can J Anaesth* 43:379–383, 1996.)

► The addition of an *N*-methyl-D-aspartate antagonist to spinally administered morphine for the treatment of cancer pain is theoretically appealing because it may add a dimension of analgesia (ie, the blockade or reversal of nociceptor-induced spinal sensitization). In addition, it may block the development of tolerance to morphine. I have some concerns, however, about the use of the preparation that is commercially available in the United States, which contains the preservative benzethonium chloride. Although this preparation was shown not to be neurotoxic in primate models,[1] the combination of ketamine and this preservative were shown to be neurotoxic in a rabbit model.[2] As Coombs et al showed recently,[3] a drug that may seem benign over a short term of intrathecal administration (in this case, high concentration morphine) may produce neurotoxicity whin administerd for a longer period.

S.E. Abram, M.D.

References

1. Brock-Utne JG, Kallichurum S, Mankowitz E, et al: Intrathecal ketamine with preservative—histological effects on spinal nerve roots of baboons. *S Afr Med J* 61:360–361 and 440–441, 1982.
2. Malinovsky JM, Cozian A, Lepage JY, et al: Ketamine and midazolam neurotoxicity in the rabbit [see comments]. *Anesthesiology* 75:91–97, 1991.
3. Coombs DW, Colburn RW, DeLeo JA, et al: Comparative spinal neuropathology of hydromorphine and morphine after 9- and 30-day epidural administration in sheep. *Anesth Analg* 78:674–681, 1994.

Acute Pain After Thoracic Surgery Predicts Long-term Post-thoracotomy Pain

Katz J, Jackson M, Kavanagh BP, et al (Toronto Hosp; Univ of Toronto)
Clin J Pain 12:50–55, 1996 8–32

Background.—Post-thoracotomy pain syndrome, which is pain that persists or recurs along a thoracotomy scar more than 2 months after surgery, occurs in about half of all patients still alive 1 to 2 years after thoracotomy. Little is known about the factors contributing to the development of this chronic, pathologic pain. In an attempt to identify predictors of post-thoracotomy pain syndrome, the significance of early postoperative pain was evaluated.

Methods.—Thirty patients participated in a prospective study evaluating preemptive multimodal analgesia after thoracotomy. Follow-up contact was attempted about 1.5 years after thoracotomy, during which a questionnaire was administered to assess current thoracotomy pain. Acute pain was assessed on the first postoperative day with a visual analogue scale (VAS) and on the first 2 postoperative days with the McGill Pain Questionnaire (MPQ). Analgesic requirements from a patient-controlled analgesia infusion pump during the first 72 hours after surgery were recorded. Patients were assessed for psychiatric variables before surgery.

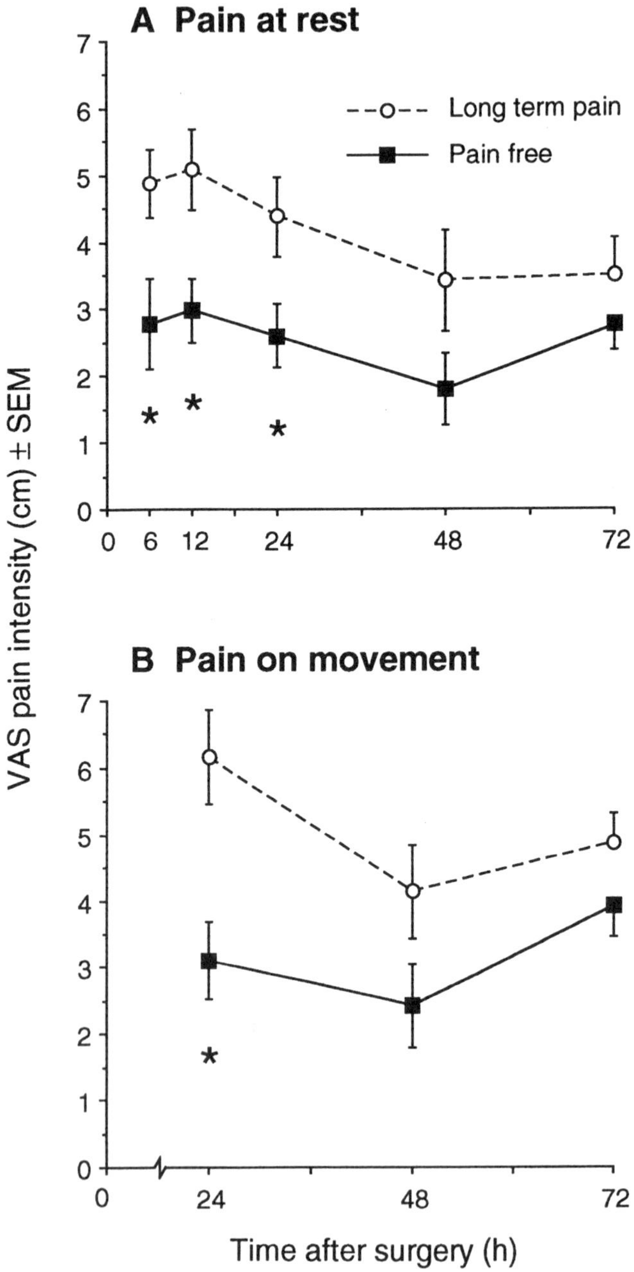

FIGURE 1.—Visual analogue scale (vas) pain scores at rest (**A**) and after movement (**B**) on postoperative days 1 to 3 shown for patients with and without long-term post-thoracotomy pain. *$P < .03$. (Courtesy of Katz J, Jackson M, Kavanagh BP, et al: Acute pain after thoracic surgery predicts long-term post-thoracotomy pain. *Clin J Pain* 12:50–55, 1996.)

Correlations between post-thoracotomy pain and early postoperative pain, as well as demographic and clinical variables, were analyzed.

Results.—Of the 30 patients, 23 could be interviewed at the 1.5-year follow-up. Of these 23 patients, 11 were pain-free and 12 had post-thoracotomy pain. The patients with long-term pain had significantly greater VAS scores for pain both at rest and after movement and higher MPQ scores than the patients without long-term pain (Fig 1). The 2 groups had identical cumulative morphine consumption and comparable scores on all the psychological scales. There were no differences between the groups in preoperative and postoperative pain thresholds. There were no significant correlations between post-thoracotomy pain and any demographic or clinical variables.

Conclusions.—Post-thoracotomy pain is predicted by pain intensity within the first day after surgery. Aggressive management of acute postoperative pain may be useful in preventing chronic pain by disrupting the peripheral and central neural processes that maintain nociception.

► Although this study identifies a relation between severe early postoperative pain and long-term pain, it was not designed to answer the question of whether aggressive intraoperative and postoperative analgesic management will reduce the risk of persistent pain. Given the high incidence of chronic post-thoracotomy pain identified by this study, this is an important question that may have substantial economic implications.

S.E. Abram, M.D.

Continuous Co-administration of Dextromethorphan or MK-801 With Morphine: Attenuation of Morphine Dependence and Naloxone-reversible Attenuation of Morphine Tolerance

Manning BH, Mao J, Frenk H, et al (Virginia Commonwealth Univ, Richmond; Tel Aviv Univ, Ramat Aviv, Israel)

Pain 67:79–88, 1996

8–33

Background.—Research has shown that *N*-methyl-D-aspartate (NMDA) receptor antagonists attenuate the development of opiate tolerance and dependence in rodents. Several unanswered questions about morphine tolerance were addressed in a study of rats.

Methods.—The ability of continuous systemic infusion of MK-801 (a noncompetitive NMDA antagonist) and dextromethorphan (DM; a clinically available antitussive agent with NMDA antagonist properties) to prolong the antinociceptive effect of continuous systemic morphine administration in rats was evaluated. In addition, the capacity of rats for unimpaired locomotor activity after continuous administration of different dose combinations of morphine plus DM or morphine plus MK-801 was assessed quantitatively. Whether the prolonged antinociception that occurs after continuous co-administration of morphine plus DM or morphine plus MK-801 is naloxone-reversible also was determined.

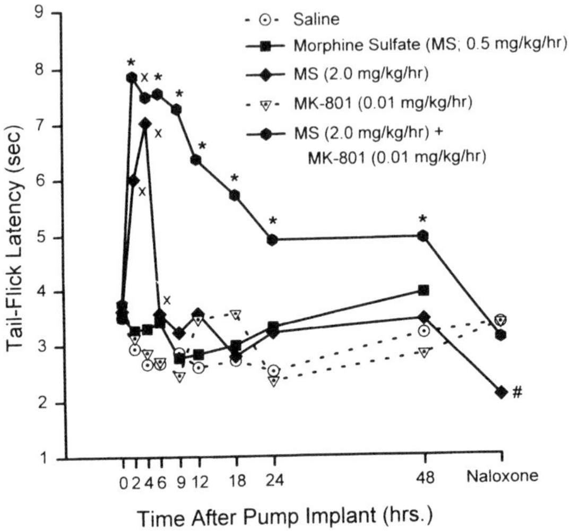

FIGURE 1.—Mean tail-flick latencies (TFLs) of rats receiving continuous subcutaneous infusion of saline alone, morphine alone, or MK-801 alone are compared with TFLs of rats receiving continuous subcutaneous co-infusion of morphine sulfate (*MS*) and MK-801. Continuous subcutaneous infusion of MK-801 alone did not result in reliably higher TFLs than saline at any point. When MK-801 was continuously co-infused with MS, however, the antinociceptive effects of MS were both potentiated (at time points when infusion of MS alone was still antinociceptive) and prolonged. This prolonged antinociception was completely reversed by naloxone. Furthermore, the hyperalgesia that occurred after administration of naloxone to rats treated with MS alone (i.e., morphine-tolerant rats) was not apparent after naloxone administration to rats having received co-infusion of MK-801 with MS. **P* <.05, Waller-Duncan *K*-ratio *t*-test (WD), as compared with rats receiving continuous subcutaneous infusion of saline alone *or* rats receiving continuous subcutaneous infusion of MS alone. Comparisons are across the same time point. [x]P<.05 (WD) as compared with rats receiving continuous subcutaneous infusion of saline alone. Comparisons are across the same time point. [#]*P*<.05, Waller-Duncan *K*-ratio *t*-test (WD) as compared with rats treated with naloxone after continuous (48-hour) subcutaneous infusion of saline alone. (Reprinted from Manning BH, Mao J, Frenk H, et al: Continuous co-administration of dextromethorphan or MK-801 with morphine: Attenuation of morphine dependence and naloxone-reversible attenuation of morphine tolerance. *Pain* 67:79–88, copyright 1996, with kind permission from Elsevier Science—NL, Sara Burgerhartstraat 25, 1055 KV Amsterdam, The Netherlands.)

Findings.—The continuous subcutaneous infusion of MK-801 or DM reliably prolonged the antinociceptive effect of continuous subcutaneous infusion of morphine sulfate. This indicates attenuation of the development of morphine tolerance. Naloxone completely reversed this prolonged antinociception. MK-801 and DM doses that attenuated morphine tolerance equally well were found to have different effect profiles on locomotor activity and naloxone-precipitated abstinence/withdrawal symptoms. Rats given continuous subcutaneous infusion of morphine sulfate and MK-801 but not those given morphine sulfate and DM had a reliable, striking increase in locomotor activity compared with those given morphine alone. Continuous subcutaneous co-infusion of MK-801 or DM with morphine attenuated naloxone-precipitated hyperalgesia compared with rats given morphine alone. However, MK-801 was more effective than DM in decreasing other naloxone-precipitated withdrawal symptoms. The effects of MK-801 on all withdrawal symptoms, however, were confounded by the

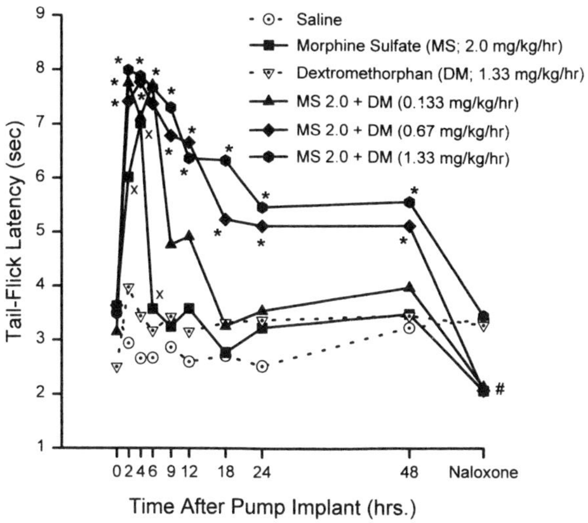

FIGURE 2.—Mean tail-flick latencies (TFLs) of rats receiving continuous subcutaneous infusion of saline alone, morphine sulfate (*MS*) alone, or dextromethorphan (*DM*) alone are compared with TFLs of rats receiving continuous subcutaneous co-infusion of MS and DM. Continuous subcutaneous infusion of DM alone did not result in reliably higher TFLs than saline at any time point. When DM was continuously co-infused with MS, however, the antinociceptive effects of MS were potentiated (at time points when infusion of MS alone was still antinociceptive) and prolonged (compare with Fig. 1). This prolonged antinociception was completely reversed by naloxone. Furthermore, the hyperalgesia that occurred after administration of naloxone to rats treated with MS alone (i.e., morphine-tolerant rats) was not apparent after naloxone administration to rats having received co-infusion of the highest dose of DM with MS (compare with Fig. 1). **P*<.05, Waller-Duncan *K*-ratio *t*-test (WD), as compared with rats receiving continuous subcutaneous infusion of saline alone or rats receiving continuous subcutaneous infusion of MS alone. Comparisons are across the same time point. ^X^*P*<.05 (WD) as compared with rats receiving continuous subcutaneous infusion of saline alone. Comparisons are across the same time point. ^#^*P*<.05, Waller-Duncan *K*-ratio *t*-test (WD) as compared with rats treated with naloxone after continuous (46-hour) subcutaneous infusion of saline alone. (Reprinted from Manning BH, Mao J, Frenk H, et al: Continuous co-administration of dextromethorphan or MK-801 with morphine: Attenuation of morphine dependence and naloxone-reversible attenuation of morphine tolerance. *Pain* 67:79–88, copyright 1996, with kind permission from Elsevier Science—NL, Sara Burgerhartstraat 25, 1055 KV Amsterdam, The Netherlands.)

occurrence of flaccidity after naloxone administration to animals given MK-801 and morphine (Figs 1 and 2).

Conclusions.—The prolonged antinociception that occurs after the co-administration of morphine and an NMDA antagonist is completely reversible by naloxone, which supports the notion that this antinociception reflects a prolongation of an opioid receptor-mediated effect. However, the different profiles of side effects observed with MK-801 and DM suggest that attenuation of naloxone-precipitated withdrawal symptoms by MK-801 may be an artifact of toxicity and that DM may be useful clinically for preventing morphine tolerance, considering its lack of observable side effects when co-administered with morphine to rats.

▶ There is now clear evidence that the long-term administration of exogenous opioids leads to enhanced sensitivity of excitatory amino acid receptors (e.g., the NMDA receptor) as well as reduced responsiveness of the opioid receptor. In addition, prolonged release of excitatory amino acids at the primary afferent nerve terminal, as occurs with peripheral neuropathic pain, leads to reduced response to exogenously administered opioids. It has been proposed that both these mechanisms are mediated by the activation of protein kinases that enhance NMDA receptor response and reduce opioid receptor response. Understanding of these mechanisms has dramatic implications. First, we now have the potential to develop pharmacologic tools, such as NMDA antagonists, that modify these untoward responses. Second, we are able to comprehend why certain patients obtain little relief from opioids and may actually improve clinically when they are discontinued, because continued opiate receptor stimulation may actually lead to a pharmacologically mediated hyperalgesic state. This knowledge adds a new dimension to the debate over the advisability of initiating long-term opioid therapy for chronic non-cancer pain.

S.E. Abram, M.D.

The Utility of Comparative Local Anesthetic Blocks Versus Placebo-Controlled Blocks for the Diagnosis of Cervical Zygapophysial Joint Pain

Lord SM, Barnsley L, Bogduk N (Univ of Newcastle, Callaghan, Australia)
Clin J Pain 11:208–213, 1995 8–34

Background.—Subjective patient responses to local anesthetic blocks may be influenced by the placebo effect. To help eliminate the confounding of results by this effect, the paradigm of comparative local anesthetic blocks was developed. With this technique, 2 local anesthetics with different durations of action are applied; only patients obtaining reproducible relief and correctly identifying the longer-acting agent are considered "true positive" responders (as opposed to placebo responders). The reliability of comparative blocks was examined through blocks of the medial branches of the cervical dorsal rami for diagnosis of pain of the cervical zygapophysial joint.

Methods.—Participating in the study were 50 consecutive patients (mean age, 41 years) who had been in motor vehicle accidents and suffered neck pain for more than 3 months afterward. Patients received 3 blocks of 3 different agents (0.5 mL of solution each), administered on separate occasions under double-blind conditions. Each patient was first given either the short-acting local anesthetic 2% lignocaine or the longer-acting local anesthetic 0.5% bupivacaine. Positive responses were followed by administration of the opposite anesthetic and of normal saline in random order. Diagnostic decisions made based on the comparative blocks alone were compared with those based on the criterion standard of placebo-controlled, double-blind, randomized blocks.

Results.—Analysis of comparative blocks offered a specificity of 88%, but a sensitivity of only 54%. These blocks result in few false positive diagnoses but more false negative diagnoses. If the comparative block diagnostic criteria are altered to include patients with reproducible relief regardless of duration, sensitivity is increased to 100%, but specificity decreases to 65%. If diagnoses are based solely on comparative blocks, 46% of patients who are not placebo responders are incorrectly categorized as such.

Discussion.—Comparative blocks fail to identify a large proportion of patients who have the condition but are not placebo responders. Comparative blocks may suffice if relatively innocuous therapies are to be prescribed based on a positive diagnosis. If, however, diagnostic certainty is critical, triple blocks incorporating placebo controls are advised.

► Given the high placebo response rate among patients with chronic pain, it is imperative that diagnostic block protocols include at least 1 placebo injection. The addition of the comparative block technique, (ie, the comparison of results using anesthetics of differing durations) adds to the reliability of the conclusions of the test. However, as the authors point out, such a rigorous paradigm may produce false positives. It is obvious that diagnostic blocks should be considered as one of multiple techniques used to assess the mechanism of an individual patient's pain. Even when all of the diagnostic interventions point to a common source of pain, there may still be high failure rates in treating the problem. A diagnostic procedure is useful if it provides information that directs treatment to an effective modality or treatment program.

S.E. Abram, M.D.

Intrathecal Infusion Systems for Treatment of Chronic Low Back and Leg Pain of Noncancer Origin

Tutak U, Doleys DM (HealthSouth Med Ctr, Birmingham, Ala; Pain and Rehabilitation Inst, Birmingham, Ala)

South Med J 89:295–300, 1996 8–35

Background.—Intrathecal and epidural treatment with morphine sulfate has been used successfully in the treatment of intractable chronic cancer pain. This method of administration has advantages such as minimal cerebral, brain stem, and systemic side effects and possible delayed tolerance. The development of implantable, programmable continuous drug delivery systems and preservative free morphine sulfate solutions has expanded the uses of intraspinal morphine. Its effectiveness in patients with intractable, chronic noncancer pain was evaluated.

Methods.—Twenty-six patients with severe, chronic low back and leg pain unresponsive to other medical and surgical treatments received implantable infusion systems after an epidural morphine trial provided at least 50% pain relief and increased or more comfortable activity. All patients also were evaluated to rule out significant psychopathology. The dose of morphine was adjusted postoperatively and re-assessed at 2 and 4 weeks after discharge. The patients were followed up for an average of 23 months, with assessments of pain, function, activity level, satisfaction, oral narcotic use, and complications.

Results.—Average pain scores (on a 10-point scale) were reduced from 8.9 before implantation to 5.5 at 6 months and 4.9 at 12 months postimplantation. Functional scores (on a 6-point scale) improved from 4.0 to 2.8. The patients reported a 50% average improvement in daily functioning. Oral morphine use decreased from 289 mg/day to 175 mg/day. The overall satisfaction level (on a 4-point scale) was 3.2 for patients and 2.3 for spouses. Physicians or clinic nurses rated overall improvement as excellent in 19% and good in 81%. The average daily dose of intrathecal morphine increased gradually over time.

Eight patients had adverse side effects, including pruritus, nausea and vomiting, urinary retention, decreased libido, sweating, and weakness. Catheter-related complications requiring surgical correction occurred in 9 patients.

Conclusions.—Intrathecal administration of morphine sulfate with an implantable infusion system is effective in the management of noncancer pain, but it requires monitoring and adjustment and is not without complications. Careful patient selection, including a trial to confirm narcotic responsiveness and a behavioral/psychological evaluation, is important. Tolerance does occur, but it may possibly be moderated by using local anesthetics in combination with the narcotics. Because increased activity also may cause dose escalation, physical reconditioning and rehabilitation therapy may be helpful for these patients.

▶ Of note is that more than half of the patients had tetracaine added to the intrathecal infusion regimen, yet no mention was made of the dose or side effects of the local anesthetic. It is also noteworthy that, although all of the patients received opioids before spinal implantation, there was no mention of trials of reduction or discontinuation of these agents. Among patients with neuropathic or radiculopathic pain, opioids may be relatively ineffective or frankly detrimental. There is growing evidence that exogenous opioids may lead to increased sensitivity of dorsal horn neurons with resultant hyperalgesia mediated through an increase in intracellular protein kinase C. It is not unusual for such patients to experience improvement in pain and function when opioids are weaned and discontinued. This would seem a reasonable first step before initiation of a technique whose benefits are less than stunning and whose complications and side effects are substantial.

S.E. Abram, M.D.

A Meta-analysis on the Efficacy of Epidural Corticosteroids in the Treatment of Sciatica

Watts RW, Silagy CA (Flinders Univ, Bedford Park, South Australia)

Anaesth Intensive Care 23:564–569, 1995 8–36

Background.—Low back pain and sciatica are frequently treated with epidural corticosteroid agents. However, studies of its efficacy have generally been too small to report statistically significant effects. A meta-analysis of all randomized trials of epidural steroids was performed to evaluate their efficacy in the treatment of sciatica.

Methods.—Eleven randomized trials of epidural treatment for sciatica were identified from a Medline search and were assessed for methodologic quality. Data on diagnosis, duration of symptoms, randomization process, epidural technique, corticosteroid used, additional treatments, control, and the number of patients involved were extracted and analyzed. Relief of pain was the main measure of efficacy.

Results.—The 11 placebo-controlled trials involved 907 patients and had generally good quality. The pooled odds ratio for at least 75% pain relief was 2.61 and for near-complete relief was 2.79 (Fig 1). The efficacy appears to be independent of injection route, with odds ratios of 3.80 for caudal epidural steroids and 2.43 for lumbar epidural steroids. The odds ratio was 3.59 for short-term relief and 1.87 for long-term relief (Fig 2). There was significant variation between studies in short-term, but not long-term, pain relief, suggesting that patient selection and response assessment influenced short-term efficacy. Adverse events were rare and included dural taps, transient headache, transient pain increase, and irregular periods.

Conclusions.—Pooled data from randomized trials provided evidence of the efficacy of caudal or lumbar epidural steroid treatment of lumbosacral radicular pain.

Trial reference	Responders / No. Entered Treatment	Control	OR [FE] (95% CI)		
Beliveau 1971	18/24	16/24	1.48	0.43	5.09
Breivik 1976	9/16	5/19	3.36	0.88	12.80
Bush 1991	8/12	2/11	6.60	1.31	33.16
Cuckler 1985	12/42	8/31	1.15	0.41	3.22
Dilke 1973	21/35	11/36	3.23	1.28	8.17
Klenerman 1984	15/19	32/44	1.38	0.41	4.71
Mathews 1987	14/21	18/32	1.53	0.50	4.67
Popiolek 1991	18/28	8/30	4.46	1.60	12.45
Ridley 1988	17/19	3/16	16.53	4.40	62.17
Snoek 1977	8/27	5/24	1.57	0.45	5.49
▪ TOTAL (95% CI)	140/243	108/267	2.61	1.80	3.77

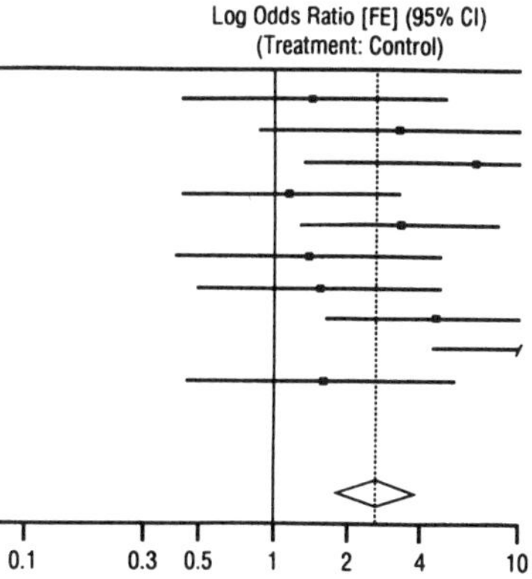

Between trial test for heterogeneity: X^2 (df = 9) = 15.89

FIGURE 1.—The efficacy of epidural corticosteroids vs. placebo in patients with sciatica in the short term (less than 60 days). (Courtesy of Watts RW, Silagy CA: *Anaesth Intensive Care* 23:564–569, 1995.)

Trial reference	Responders / No. Entered Treatment	Control	OR [FE] (95% CI)		
Bush 1991	10/12	7/11	2.66	0.43	16.43
Cuckler 1985	11/46	4/27	1.73	0.54	5.57
Dilke 1973	16/43	8/38	2.15	0.83	5.56
Mathews 1987	9/23	14/34	0.92	0.32	2.68
Swerdlow 1970	76/117	98/208	2.04	1.30	3.22
▪ TOTAL (95% CI)	122/241	131/318	1.87	1.31	2.68

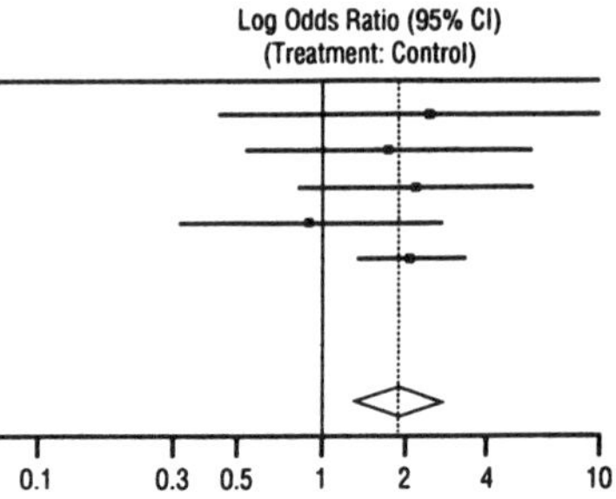

Between trial test for heterogeneity: X^2 (df = 4) = 2.08

FIGURE 2.—The efficacy of epidural steroids vs. placebo in patients with sciatica in the long term (up to 12 months). (Courtesy of Watts RW, Silagy CA: *Anaesth Intensive Care* 23:564–569, 1995.)

▶ This is an important study that was meticulous in its methodology and selection process. It should be noted that the investigators were not anesthesiologists and cannot be accused of creating a study design to serve their financial purposes. It is noteworthy that the 95% confidence intervals for the odds ratios did not extend below 1 for caudal or lumbar injections, for short- or long-term improvement, or when partial relief or near-complete relief were selected as outcomes. Only 5 of the 13 studies selected demonstrated significant benefit from treatment, but all but 1 study achieved odds ratios greater than 1 for treatment success. Thus, the technique of meta-analysis allowed the investigators to apply statistical analysis to a group large enough to reveal an effect. As the authors point out, however, this methodology is no substitute for a large, well-conducted clinical trial.

S.E. Abram, M.D.

Evaluation of Continuous Intraspinal Narcotic Analgesia for Chronic Pain From Benign Causes

Yoshida GM, Nelson RW, Capen DA, et al (Univ of California, Los Angeles; USC-Rancho Los Amigos Med Ctr, Downey, Calif; Advanced Orthopedic Care Associates, Las Vegas, Nev; et al)
Am J Orthop 25:693–694, 1996 8–37

Introduction.—Continuous intraspinal narcotic analgesia (INA) has gained popularity with spine surgeons and pain management physicians, but this modality appears to be more successful in the management of patients with chronic cancer pain than in those with chronic pain of benign causes. A retrospective study evaluated the benefits of the morphine pump when used for patients with failed back syndrome or arachnoiditis.

Methods.—Study participants were 18 patients with intractable and debilitating pain that was unrelieved by conventional means. Before the pump was implanted, all had reported relief of significant duration from a trial of morphine—either 1 to 2 mg injected intrathecally or 5 mg/day via epidural injection. The patients were studied for 2 years to determine whether continuous INA enabled them to regain an active lifestyle or to reduce or eliminate their need for orally administered narcotics.

Results.—Two patients were lost to follow-up, 8 had to have the pump removed or turned off because of complications or lack of efficacy, and 8 still had the pump functioning. Five patients who retained the pump said they would have the procedure repeated, but only 4 of 8 had objective evidence of benefit from INA. Three of these patients had a reduced need for orally administered narcotics and 1 was able to return to work. Twenty-two complications were recorded overall, including 5 cases of deep infection and 7 instances of catheter kinks requiring revision.

Discussion.—In patients with chronic cancer pain, INA has a reported success rate of 80% and better. Despite careful preoperative screening, however, only 25% of these patients with chronic pain of benign cause experienced any benefit from the morphine pump. The risks of pump insertion far outweigh the benefits gained by patients with failed back syndrome.

▶ With new technologies, there is always a tendency to initially overestimate the potential benefits. This study suggests that the ultra-long-term benefits of this very labor-intensive technology may be very low in patients with chronic pain. The chances of an implanted pump system working flawlessly for many years is probably quite low, even if the technology is excellent. Catheters break, batteries fail, and pumps shift positions. In addition, the development of tolerance or resistance to the effects of the drugs administered is likely to limit efficacy in patients in whom technical problems do not develop.

S.E. Abram, M.D.

Long-term Intraspinal Infusions of Opioids in the Treatment of Neuropathic Pain

Hassenbusch SJ, Stanton-Hicks M, Covington EC, et al (MD Anderson Cancer Ctr, Houston; Cleveland Clinic Found, Ohio)

J Pain Symptom Manage 10:527–543, 1995 8–38

Objective.—Longterm intraspinal infusions of opioids have been used to treat noncancer patients with chronic intractable neuropathic pain. There is a lack of information regarding patients who fail to get relief from pain. Success and failure rates for pain relief and technical problems of such infusions were determined in a prospective study of a consecutive series of patients with neuropathic pain.

Methods.—During a 5-year period, 18 noncancer patients with no other treatment options received implanted pumps and were administered intrathecal morphine sulfate (0.05 mg/hr) or sufentanil citrate (0.05 μg/hr) for 2–5 days. Pain severity was graded on a numerical rating scale (NRS) with 0 being no pain and 10 being the worst pain imaginable. Only those patients with a 25% or less NRS pain reduction with Schedule III opioids

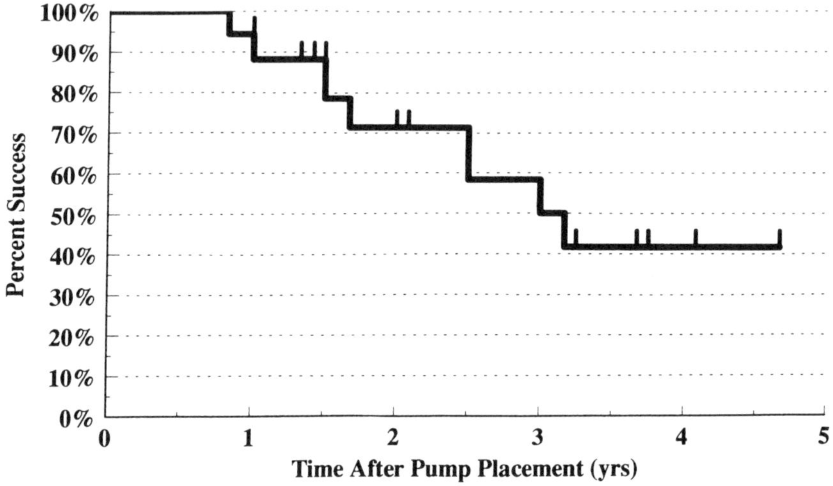

FIGURE 1.—Kaplan-Meyer–type analysis of patient outcome where success is a final "good" or "fair" rating and failure is a "poor" or "no relief" rating. The *tick marks* (or "blips") on the line indicate length of follow-up time at last evaluation for successful patients. *Down steps* in the line indicate follow-up time at which individual patients became treatment failures. (Reprinted by permission of Elsevier Science, Inc., courtesy of Hassenbusch SJ, Stanton-Hicks M, Covington EC, et al: Long-term intraspinal infusions of opioids in the treatment of neuropathic pain. *J Pain Symptom Manage* 10:527–543. Copyright 1995 by the U.S. Cancer Pain Relief Committee.)

without intolerable side effects were admitted to the study. Dosages of morphine sulfate and sufentanil citrate were increased every 12 hours until significant pain relief had been achieved, side effects became intolerable, or a dosage of 2.0 mg/hr or 2.0 μg/hr respectively, had been attained. If greater than 50% pain relief was achieved, a permanent infusion pump and intrathecal infusion catheter were implanted.

Results.—The average prestudy NRS was 8.1. Patients were followed for an average of 2.4 years. Pain reduction and improvement in activity were evaluated by both the patient and a third party. Eleven patients (61%) had good or fair pain relief. There was a significant pain reduction averaging 39% in these patients. In 5 patients, opioid doses could be decreased to 12–24 mg/day of morphine. In the remaining 6 patients, dosages were increased to more than 34 mg/day of morphine. Seven patients (39%) failed to obtain long-term relief of pain (Fig 1). Six patients required reoperation for preventable problems.

Conclusion.—Intraspinal infusions of opioids for pain control in noncancer patients have strengths and weaknesses. Before their proper role can be determined, more studies need to be done.

▶ This is a helpful discussion that provides much greater perspective of this topic than the usual anecdotal report of a few dramatic treatment successes. It provides some evidence that there are certain patients for whom the intrathecal route provides more effective pain relief than the systemic route (this evidence would have been more convincing had there been better documentation of daily systemic vs. intrathecal opioid requirements). It also documents that there are treatment failures and technical complications as well as the failure to eliminate or reduce systemic opioid use in nearly half of the "success" patients.

With a technique that requires long-term and very labor-intensive follow-up, it is critical that its use be restricted to centers that have an active multidisciplinary pain management center with those services needed for pump maintenance and surveillance, as well as services needed should the device fail. The practice of placing an implanted infusion pump and referring to another facility when that treatment fails should be condemned. Physicians using this technique must be aware that there is an implied long-term commitment to the patient. If the device is effective, it may need to be managed for decades.

S.E. Abram, M.D.

Performance of Local Anesthetic and Placebo Splanchnic Blocks Via Indwelling Catheters to Predict Benefit From Thoracoscopic Splanchnicectomy in a Patient With Intractable Pancreatic Pain

Strickland TC, Ditta TL, Riopelle JM (Louisiana State Univ, New Orleans)

Anesthesiology 84:980–983, 1996 8–39

Background.—The development of a thoracoscopic technique for performing operative splanchnicectomy has renewed interest in this method of relieving intractable pancreatic pain.

Case Report.—Man, 33, was referred to the pain service with an 18-year history of recurrent, excruciating upper abdominal pain thought to be of pancreatic origin. His pain, nausea, and vomiting had become so severe that he could not eat or drink, prompting hospitalization. After a thorough evaluation, a series of diagnostic splanchnic blocks was recommended, to be followed by thoracoscopic splanchnicectomy if the pharmacologic block relief was much better than relief provided by saline placebo injections. Catheters were inserted while the patient was under local anesthesia and minimal nonanalgesic sedation using biplane fluoroscopy. After the splanchnic block, the patient reported that the abdominal pain had completely abated, and he was able to drink without nausea, vomiting, or pain for the first time in recent memory. During the next 5 days, 4 bupivacaine injections and 2 saline injections were administered after abdominal pain returned. The bupivacaine injections resulted in good or very good pain relief, lasting 1–2 days. The saline injections resulted in no or fair relief of pain lasting 0–1 day. Surgical splanchnicectomy was then done. Postoperatively, the patient reported complete relief of abdominal pain and was able to tolerate a normal diet. Right hypochondrial dysesthesia persisted for several months, possibly resulting from an electrocautery injury to an intercostal nerve. At 25 months after surgery, the patient remained asymptomatic. He takes no medication and has gained 20 kg.

Conclusions.—The usefulness of prognostic blocks in the selection of patients for splanchnicectomy was validated experimentally. However, before recommending pancreatic denervation rather than alternative methods of providing analgesia, clinicians must consider relevant medical information as well as the patient's response to local anesthetic and placebo splanchnic blocks.

Persistent Pain Associated With Long-term Intrathecal Morphine Administration

Parris WCV, Janicki PK, Johnson B Jr, et al (Vanderbilt Univ, Nashville, Tenn)

South Med J 89:417–419, 1996 8–40

Introduction.—Although intrathecal administration of morphine is usually highly effective in the management of acute and chronic pain, some patients unresponsive to morphine have been reported. Quantitative differences in the levels of the active morphine metabolites may contribute to morphine resistance. The levels of morphine and its metabolites were measured in the plasma and urine of a patient with chronic, morphine-resistant pain.

Case Report.—Man, 32, was referred for the management of chronic, intractable right lower extremity pain. His pain had not been satisfactorily relieved by lumbar epidural steroids, orally administered opioids, intrathecal morphine therapy, and several neurosurgical procedures. There were no remarkable neurologic findings, and psychological tests were normal. The patient was managed with training in pain management coping and relaxation skills, goal setting, and behavioral modification; family systems and individual therapy; 4 right sciatic nerve blocks; and detoxification with methadone. This management strategy reduced his pain by 60%. Morphine, its metabolites, and hydrocodone were measured in the patient's plasma and urine before medication changes were made. The plasma concentrations were as follows: morphine, 109 ng/mL; hydrocodone, 345 ng/mL; M3G, 680.8 ng/mL; M6G, 82 ng/mL; and M3G:M6G ratio, 8.3:1. The 24-hour urine concentrations were as follows: morphine, 1.8 mg; hydrocodone, 3.4 mg; M3G, 15.9 mg; M6G, 1.5 mg; and M3G:M6G ratio, 10.6:1.

Discussion.—The M3G and M6G metabolites are both pharmacologically active, with M6G acting as a potent analgesic and M3G acting as an antagonist of the analgesic activity of both morphine and M6G. The high M3G:M6G ratio in this patient suggests that this imbalance may be at least partially responsible for morphine resistance. Further study is needed to examine interindividual differences and the normal range of the ratio in opioid-naive individuals.

► The accumulation of the M3G metabolite may not be the only cause of morphine-induced hyperalgesia. Exogenous opioids are known to increase the intracellular levels of protein kinases, which phosphorylate the *N*-methyl-D-aspartate receptor, leading to enhanced calcium entry and the development of long-term potentiation. Drug holidays therefore make good sense in patients receiving either systemic or neuraxial opioids, because some patients are likely to experience improvement in painful symptoms when opioids are discontinued.

S.E. Abram, M.D.

Epidurograms in the Management of Patients With Long-term Epidural Catheters: Case Report

Du Pen SL, Williams AR, Feldman RK (Univ of Washington, Seattle)
Reg Anesth 21:61–67, 1996 8–41

Objective.—Because of the increased use of indwelling epidural catheters for relief of chronic pain or extended postoperative analgesia, there is a need for improved diagnostic tools to assist in catheter placement. The role of epidurograms in differential diagnosis, a discussion of the procedure, and 2 cases were presented.

Epidurogram Procedure and Report.—The standard procedure uses serial epidurograms from T1 through L4 to verify placement of the catheter and record epidural flow of nonionic dye. The report should include information about the condition of the catheter and its location, limits of dye spread and flow, abnormalities of the epidural space or vertebrae, and extravasation of dye.

Study Interpretation.—Analysis of dye dispersion and volume flow permit the radiologist to determine any obstructions or restrictions and assist in treatment planning.

Differential Diagnosis and Review of Repeated Epidurograms.— Acute loss of analgesia can indicate sudden disease progression, catheter dislodgement, or abnormality of the epidural space. Repeated epidurograms can reveal tip withdrawal, infection, catheter encapsulation or obstruction, or disease progression.

Case 1.—A film of the lumbar spine of a patient with breast cancer who had acute loss of analgesia revealed "pooling" of injectate at the tip of the catheter and "tracking out" with pain of a second injectate consistent with an epidural abscess. After antibiotic therapy, the catheter was replaced.

Case 2.—Woman, 68, with multiple myeloma, had increasing pain not relieved by dose elevations of morphine and bupivacaine. An epidurogram revealed a dramatic curvature of the catheter tip. Dye injection revealed a compromised epidural space with mechanical obstruction resulting from bony destruction. Her infusion was reconcentrated to restore analgesia, and sublingual morphine was prescribed for breakthrough pain.

Conclusion.—A review of repeated epidurograms is a valuable diagnostic and treatment planning tool and is very useful for determining abnormalities associated with the epidural space or the catheter itself. The standard technique provides differential diagnostic data, is relatively inexpensive, and gives accurate information about catheter placement.

▶ Epidurography would appear to provide information that is useful in guiding ongoing continuous epidural drug therapy. The technique also is being used to provide diagnostic information for patients with chronic low back pain who are not receiving continuous epidural analgesia. Its diagnostic utility for that application is unproven, and it probably provides little, if any, information that is not obtainable with more conventional imaging procedures.

S.E. Abram, M.D.

Lidocaine Patch: Double-blind Controlled Study of a New Treatment Method for Post-herpetic Neuralgia

Rowbotham MC, Davies PS, Verkempinck C, et al (Univ of California, San Francisco)

Pain 65:39–44, 1996 8–42

Background.—Post-herpetic neuralgia (PHN) is a neuropathic pain syndrome that is often difficult to manage. Uncontrolled studies have reported pain relief with subcutaneous lidocaine infiltration of the painful area and with topical local anesthetics. The efficacy of 5% lidocaine gel in a nonwoven polyethylene adhesive patch was evaluated in a randomized, double-blind, controlled study.

Methods.—Forty patients with PHN underwent 4 12-hour study sessions, consisting of the application of a lidocaine patch twice, a vehicle patch once, and observation only once. The sessions were performed in random order and were separated by 3 to 7 days. Pain intensity and pain relief were assessed at 30 minutes and 1, 2, 4, 6, 9, and 12 hours. Side effects were rated at the same time points. Blood samples were obtained at 1, 4, and 6 hours after patch application and assayed for lidocaine concentration.

Results.—Of the 40 patients, 35 completed the study. With the lidocaine patch, pain intensity was significantly reduced at all time points when compared to observation only and was significantly reduced at 4, 6, 9, and

12 hours when compared to vehicle patch. Pain relief was significantly greater at all time points with the lidocaine patch than with either the vehicle patch or observation only. No new symptoms occurred during any study session. The highest level of lidocaine concentration in the blood was 104 ng/mL, occurring at 6 hours after application. This concentration is significantly lower than the minimum venous antiarrhythmic lidocaine level of 1,000 ng/mL.

Conclusions.—The topical 5% lidocaine patch significantly reduces the pain of PHN while allowing minimal systemic lidocaine absorption. Topical lidocaine patches offer several advantages, including ease of application and removal, comfort, the ability to custom fit the patch to the area of pain, and the absence of systemic side effects.

▶ This study demonstrates that topical lidocaine has local rather than systemic analgesic effects. EMLA cream is helpful for some patients with severe allodynia, but probably is not as convenient as the technique described.

S.E. Abram, M.D.

9 Anesthesia Mechanisms/Basic Science

Nitric Oxide–related Issues

Pregnancy and Ephedrine Increase the Release of Nitric Oxide in Ovine Uterine Arteries
Li P, Tong C, Eisenach JC (Wake Forest Univ, Winston-Salem, NC)
Anesth Analg 82:288–293, 1996 9–1

Background.—In obstetric patients who have received epidural and spinal anesthesia, ephedrine is the agent of choice to treat subsequent hypotension because it is better able to preserve uterine perfusion compared with pure α-adrenergic agonists. Previous studies investigating vascular rings in vitro suggest that direct uterine vasoconstriction from ephedrine is decreased during pregnancy. The aim of this study was to determine whether nitric oxide synthase (NOS) is up-regulated in uterine arteries during pregnancy, and whether ephedrine causes NOS to release nitric oxide (NO) and reduce direct vasoconstriction.

Methods.—Twelve pregnant and 9 nonpregnant ewes were used in the study. Uterine arteries were obtained and vessel tension was evaluated in vitro in conjunction with increasing concentrations of ephedrine or metaraminol. In some experiments, vascular endothelium was mechanically removed, and in others, antagonist of NO synthase, NO diffusion, or guanylate cyclase (N^w-nitro-L-arginine methyl ester [L-NAME], hemoglobin [Hgb], and methylene blue [MB], respectively) were included. In additional experiments, solutions containing ephedrine were superfused over uterine arteries from pregnant ewes onto uterine arteries from nonpregnant ewes. Uterine arteries from pregnant and nonpregnant ewes also were evaluated for NOS activity, as demonstrated by ^{14}C-citrulline production.

Results.—Concentration-dependent constriction of uterine artery rings was noted in both pregnant and nonpregnant ewes with application of ephedrine and metaraminol. In pregnant animals, ephedrine reduced maximum constriction more than metaraminol. A greater increase in ephedrine-induced constriction also was noted in uterine arteries from pregnant animals treated to lessen the effects of NO (L-NAME, Hgb, MB, endothelium removal). In uterine arteries from nonpregnant ewes, ephedrine-induced constriction was decreased when it was superfused over uterine arteries for pregnant animals. Compared with nonpregnant animals, NOS activity was increased in uterine arteries from pregnant ewes.

Conclusions.—During pregnancy, ephedrine results in decreased direct uterine arterial vasoconstriction. This decrease is caused by an increased release of an endogenous vasodilator (NO) from either the vascular endothelium or the vessel wall.

▶ Ephedrine, a mixed α- and β-agonist is the preferred vasopressor for most cases of hypotension in obstetric patients, largely because it preserves uteroplacental perfusion better than pure α-adrenergic agonists. Using state-of-the-art methodology, the authors of the present study observed that ephedrine results in release of a nonprostaglandin vasodilator from uterine arteries in pregnant ewes, and that this vasodilator reduces vasoconstriction in response to ephedrine. The pharmacology of the vasodilator is consistent with that of NO. The present study provides further laboratory support for ephedrine as the vasopressor of choice for most cases of hypotension in clinical obstetric anesthesia practice.

D.H. Chestnut, M.D.

Inhaled Nitric Oxide Does Not Alter Endotoxin-induced Nitric Oxide Synthase Activity During Rat Lung Perfusion

Kurrek MM, Castillo L, Bloch KD, et al (Massachusetts Gen Hosp, Boston; Harvard Med School, Boston; Massachusetts Inst of Technology, Cambridge)

J Physiol 79:1088–1092, 1995 9–2

Background.—Research has shown that nitric oxide (NO) reduces its own synthesis in tissue preparations. Exogenous NO may decrease endogenous NO synthesis induced by lipopolysaccharides (LPS) during isolated lung perfusion. This possibility was investigated in a rat model.

Methods.—Rat lungs were harvested 48 hours after pretreatment with LPS or saline. To determine NO synthase activity, conversion of L-[^{14}C]-arginine to L-[^{14}C]citrulline was assessed during 90 minutes of perfusion. The ventilating gas used during lung perfusion in 1 group of control or LPS-treated rats contained 100 ppm of NO. Another group of control or LPS-treated rats received 100 ppm of NO for 48 hours before lung harvest and 100 ppm in the ventilating gas during lung perfusion.

Findings.—Control lungs showed minimal conversion of L-[^{14}C]arginine to L-[^{14}C]citrulline, whereas LPS pretreatment was associated with an increased response. The rate of L-[^{14}C]citrulline production was not affected by NO in the ventilating gas during the 90 minutes of ex vivo perfusion.

Conclusions.—In the isolated perfused rat lung, LPS pretreatment substantially increases L-[^{14}C]arginine to L-[^{14}C]citrulline conversion. However, neither acute exposure of the lung to NO nor up to 2 days of breathing exogenous NO at 100 ppm inhibited this high rate of conversion. Thus, NO withdrawal–induced pulmonary vasoconstriction and hypertension in mammals probably is not caused by inducible NO synthase feedback inhibition by inhaled NO.

▶ Nitric oxide is produced from L-arginine under the influence of the enzyme NO synthase. It has been suggested that NO might exert a negative feedback mechanism, decreasing its own synthesis by decreasing the activity of inducible NO synthase (iNOS). This could mean that clinically, inhaled NO might prevent endogenous pulmonary vascular NO production, with adverse effects in patients with pulmonary hypertension and the adult respiratory distress syndrome. This elegant study shows that if NO withdrawal–induced pulmonary vasoconstriction occurs, it is not likely to be due to iNOS feedback inhibition.

M. Wood, M.D.

Opioid Mechanisms

Comparison of the Spinal Actions of the μ-Opioid Remifentanil With Alfentanil and Morphine in the Rat

Buerkle H, Yaksh TL (Univ of California, San Diego)

Anesthesiology 84:94–102, 1996 9–3

Background.—Remifentanil is a μ-opioid agonist metabolized by plasma and tissue esterases. Systemic remifentanil in humans produces analgesia, sedation, muscle rigidity, nausea, and respiratory depression; these can be reversed by naloxone. Pharmacokinetics may alter these supraspinal side effects. The antinociceptive effects and supraspinal side effects of intrathecal and intraperitoneal remifentanil, morphine, and alfentanil were compared.

Methods.—Remifentanil, alfentanil, and morphine were administered intrathecally and intraperitoneally in rats. Antinociceptive effects were determined by measuring hind paw thermal withdrawal latency. An index of supraspinal effects was used consisting of 4 parameters shown to be blocked by opioids in a dose-dependent manner.

Results.—Intrathecal administration of all opioids produced a dose-dependent analgesic response. The rank order of antinociceptive potency (intrathecal ED_{50} in μg) was remifentanil (0.7) > morphine (12) > alfentanil (16.3) > GR90291, the principal remifentanil metabolite (> 810 μg). Rank order of time to analgesic onset was morphine > remifentanil = alfentanil. The opioids were matched for analgesic effect, and the rank order of relative duration of action was morphine >> alfentanil > remifentanil. A dose-dependent increase was shown by the supraspinal index for all opioids. Dose-dependent increases in antinociception were shown by all intraperitoneal opioids; the rank order of potency (intraperitoneal ED_{50} in μg)

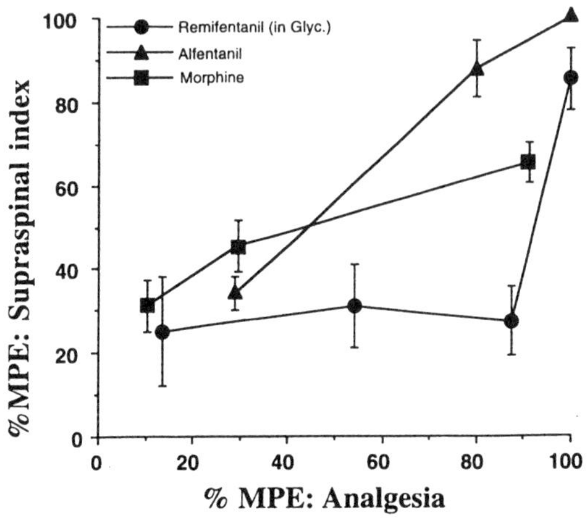

FIGURE 3.—Data present the comparison of intrathecally administered opioids over increasing doses and their percent maximum possible effect (*MPE*) of the supraspinal index vs. percent MPE of analgesia, assessed with the thermal withdrawal test. Each data point represents the mean ± SEM of 5 to 8 animals. (Courtesy of Buerkle H, Yaksh TL: Comparison of the spinal actions of the μ-opioid remifentanil with alfentanil and morphine in the rat. *Anesthesiology* 84:94–102, 1996.)

of remifentanil (4.3) > alfentanil (24.4) > morphine (262). Intrathecal and intraperitoneal ratios for supraspinal side effects and analgesia were determined (supraspinal index ED_{50}/analgesia ED_{50}); that of remifentanil was greatest when administered intrathecally (Fig 3): remifentanil (4 intrathecal, 1.4 intraperitoneal); alfentanil (0.7 intrathecal, 1.5 intraperitoneal); and morphine (1 intrathecal, 5.6 intraperitoneal).

Conclusions.—Remifentanil produces strong spinal opioid action. Both remifentanil and alfentanil have an early onset, but remifentanil has a shorter duration of action. The spinal therapeutic ratio of remifentanil is significant in spite of its lipid solubility. These findings may reflect the quick inactivation of agents systemically redistributed by plasma esterases.

► This study may portend an important clinical effect. The short-acting lipid-soluble opioids presently available (fentanyl, sufentanil, and alfentanil) show only modest increases in potency and duration when used intrathecally. There is minimal clinical difference between epidural and parenteral administration of these drugs. Epidural infusions tend to produce respiratory depression related to vascular absorption. However, neuraxial administration of remifentanil may provide a spinal analgesic effect with minimal systemic side effects because of the rapid hydrolysis of drug that reaches the systemic circulation.

S.E. Abram, M.D.

Differential Effects of Pre-treatment With Intrathecal or Intravenous Morphine on the Prevention of Spinal Cord Hyperexcitability Following Sciatic Nerve Section in the Rat

Luo L, Wiesenfeld-Hallin Z (Huddinge Univ, Sweden)

Acta Anaesthesiol Scand 40:91–95, 1996 9–4

Background.—Studies suggest that tissue damage results in long-term changes in the way in which nociceptive information in the nervous system is processed. Pre-emptive analgesia may reduce postoperative pain and prevent spinal hyperexcitability by blocking the central effect of afferent discharge resulting from injured peripheral axons. Prolonged hyperexcitability of the spinal cord in rats results from section of the sciatic nerve and can be reduced by intrathecal morphine before axotomy. The effect of intrathecal and IV morphine on spinal flexor reflex hyperexcitability after nerve section was determined.

Methods.—Unilateral section of the sciatic nerve was performed in 31 decerebrate, spinalized, unanesthetized rats. Intrathecal (3 or 10 µg) or IV (0.2, 1, or 10 mg/kg) morphine was administered before nerve section. The hamstring flexor reflex response to the activation of afferents was determined by recording the electromyogram from the posterior biceps femoris/semitendinosus muscles.

Results.—Section of the sciatic nerve resulted in a biphasic, prolonged hyperexcitability of the flexor reflex. The flexor reflex was significantly suppressed by all doses of morphine. The less intense, prolonged second component of reflex hyperexcitability also was eliminated by all doses of morphine. The first phase of spinal cord sensitization was significantly depressed by 1 and 10 mg/kg of IV morphine. Spinal cord hyperexcitability was more significantly suppressed by 3 and 10 µg of intrathecal morphine than by IV morphine.

Conclusions.—Intrathecal morphine is more effective in preventing spinal cord sensitization after sciatic nerve section than even very high doses of IV morphine. This may result from low spinal concentrations after systemic administration. Spinally injected morphine may be more effective than IV morphine in reducing postoperative pain.

▶ Several animal studies indicate that spinally administered morphine is more effective at blocking spinal sensitization than equianalgesic systemic doses of morphine. The phenomenon may be related to the ability of spinal, but not systemic, opioids to block the release of excitatory amino acids and substance P from primary afferent nerve terminals. The benefits of preemptive spinal opioids in the perioperative period remain to be proven.

S.E. Abram, M.D.

Intravenous Opioids Stimulate Norepinephrine and Acetylcholine Release in Spinal Cord Dorsal Horn: Systematic Studies in Sheep and an Observation in a Human

Bouaziz H, Tong C, Yoon Y, et al (Wake Forest Univ, Winston-Salem, NC)

Anesthesiology 84:143–154, 1996 9–5

Background.—Opioids provide analgesia by direct effects in the brain, spinal cord, and periphery, and by various interactions among these sites. There is little information on spinal norepinephrine release by systemic opioids in nonanesthetized whole animals, or on the relation between IV opioids and CSF norepinephrine and acetylcholine levels. The effect of IV morphine-induced opioid stimulation on CSF concentrations of norepinephrine and acetylcholine was evaluated.

Methods.—Intravenous morphine or saline was administered to 10 sheep; 5 animals also received naloxone and 5 animals also received idazoxan. Cerebrospinal fluid samples were obtained at intervals and tested for norepinephrine and acetylcholine. Spinal cord microdialysis was performed in another 10 sheep. Intravenous fentanyl or morphine was administered to 6 sheep; 3 animals also received naloxone. Transection of the cervical spinal cord was performed in 1 sheep.

Results.—Dose-dependent increases in CSF norepinephrine and acetylcholine levels were produced by IV morphine; similar increases were not seen in epinephrine or dopamine levels. Peak concentrations of CSF norepinephrine did not differ from baseline concentrations. Intravenous naloxone and intrathecal idazoxan blocked the effect of morphine. Spinal cord microdialysis showed that IV morphine increased concentrations of norepinephrine and acetylcholine in the dorsal horn, but did not increase concentrations of epinephrine or dopamine. Intravenous morphine had no effect on the monoamines in the ventral horn. Intravenous naloxone and cervical cord transection both blocked the effect of morphine on norepinephrine in the dorsal horn.

Conclusions.—Increased concentrations of lumbar CSF norepinephrine and acetylcholine resulted from IV morphine in a naloxone-reversible manner. These increases may reflect local release of these neurotransmitters from the dorsal horn because of bulbospinal pathway activation. Opioid-induced activation of descending noradrenergic pathways in sheep and humans is supported. It is not clear whether increased spinal cholinergic activity after the administration of morphine results from the activation of descending pathways or norepinephrine-induced activation of spinal cholinergic interneurons.

► This study adds to our understanding of the mechanisms of action of systemic vs. neuraxial morphine administration and explains some of the qualitative differences between routes of administration. The fact that some patients experience profound analgesia with spinal, but not systemic, morphine may be explained by differences in the spinal mechanisms of the 2 techniques. The authors' findings also help to explain the synergy between intracerebroventricular and spinal morphine, and the synergy between spinal morphine and clonidine and spinal morphine and cholinergic agonists. A working knowledge of these mechanisms is likely to lead to improvements in our selection of therapeutic options in patients with acute or chronic pain that is difficult to control with conventional techniques.

S.E. Abram, M.D.

Halothane Hepatotoxicity

Halothane Hepatotoxicity and Hepatic Free Radical Metabolism in Guinea Pigs: The Effects of Vitamin E

Durak I, Güven T, Birey M, et al (Ankara Univ, Turkey; Numune Hosps, Ankara, Turkey; Gazi Univ, Ankara, Turkey)

Can J Anaesth 43:741–748, 1996 9–6

Introduction.—Halothane can cause toxic effects on the liver, and this hepatotoxicity has been experimentally produced in guinea pigs. It has been suggested that free radicals generated by the reductive pathway in the course of halothane metabolism could be the main cause of halothane hepatotoxicity. The possible link between halothane hepatotoxicity and hepatic free radical metabolism was investigated, including an assessment of the possible protective effect of vitamin E.

Methods.—Guinea pigs were treated with halothane, 1.5% v/v in 100% oxygen for 90 min/day over 3 days. Some of the animals were pretreated with IM vitamin E, 3,000 mg/kg/day for 3 days. Two days after the last halothane treatment, the guinea pigs were killed and their livers were prepared for examination.

Results.—Compared with livers from control animals, the livers of guinea pigs treated with halothane showed decreased activities of superoxide dismutase and glutathione peroxidase. Catalase activity and malondialdehyde concentration both were increased after halothane treatment. On electron spin resonance analysis, a peak of CF_3CHCl·radical was observed in the halothane-exposed livers. Ultrastructural changes of the hepatic cells also were seen, regardless of whether the animals had received vitamin E.

Conclusions.—By interfering with the hepatic antioxidant defense system and accelerating peroxidation reactions, halothane can cause ultrastructural changes in hepatic tissue. The peroxidative damage is prevented by vitamin E treatment, but the ultrastructural changes occur nevertheless. Halothane hepatotoxicity is caused by impairment of the hepatic antioxidant defense system, as well as by other, unidentified factors.

► I could not resist including this paper because the hepatic antioxidant system, with lipid and other free radical peroxidation mechanisms, has been implicated in halothane hepatotoxicity for more than 20 years! The authors turn their results around in an interesting, although problematic (for me), way. Although they found some ultrastructural changes that occurred during halothane use, they did not find that vitamin E prevented either the hepatic peroxidative damage or the ultrastructural changes. Despite these negative findings, they do not hesitate to conclude that "halothane toxicity results *not only* [italics added] from impaired hepatic antioxidant defense systems but also from other unknown causes." I do not believe that the authors have shown at all, with this merely associative linkage, that halothane hepatotoxicity results even in part from impaired antioxidant systems. As you can see, I am not high on this paper, but it does indicate continued interest in an old, still unresolved problem.

J.H. Tinker, M.D.

Inflammatory Pain Mechanisms

Intrathecal Amitriptyline Acts as an N-Methyl-D-Aspartate Receptor Antagonist in the Presence of Inflammatory Hyperalgesia in Rats

Eisenach JC, Gebhart GF (Wake Forest Univ, Winston-Salem, NC; Univ of Iowa, Iowa City)
Anesthesiology 83:1046–1054, 1995 9–7

Background.—Amitriptyline and other tricyclic antidepressants demonstrate high-affinity binding to *N*-methyl-D-aspartate (NMDA) receptors in vitro. They also inhibit NMDA receptor activation–induced neuroplasticity in hippocampal slices. Spinal NMDA receptor activation is thought to be central to the generation and maintenance of hyperalgesic pain. Whether intrathecal amitriptyline decreases inflammation-induced hyperalgesia in rats was determined.

Methods.—Rats were prepared with chronic lumbar intrathecal and femoral IV catheters. Nociceptive threshold was determined by hind paw withdrawal to a radiant heart stimulus. Rats were injected with carrageenin in 1 hind paw. Thermal paw withdrawal testing was done 3 hours later. Intrathecal amitriptyline and/or IV morphine injection followed. In other groups of rats, either intrathecal saline or 60 µg of amitriptyline was injected before intrathecal NMDA injection.

Findings.—Intrathecal amitriptyline reversed thermal hyperalgesia in a dose-dependent fashion. However, it did not affect withdrawal latency of the contralateral, uninjected paw. Intrathecal phentolamine plus methysergide did not change the effect of amitriptyline except in the lowest dose. In both inflamed and control paws, IV morphine increased paw withdrawal latency in a dose-dependent manner. Morphine interacted with intrathecal amitriptyline in an additive manner to reverse hyperalgesia. Intrathecal amitriptyline completely antagonized thermal hyperalgesia induced by NMDA.

Conclusions.—Intrathecal administration of amitriptyline and other tricyclic antidepressants may have a more profound effect on pain than when administered systemically. In this rat model, amitriptyline reversed hyperalgesia by a mechanism unassociated with monoamine reuptake inhibition. Most likely, this effect is caused by NMDA receptor antagonism.

▶ It has been difficult to explain why tricyclic antidepressants often provide analgesic effects in certain painful conditions, whereas other monoamine reuptake inhibitors, such as the selective serotonin reuptake inhibitors, generally do not. The NMDA receptor antagonism demonstrated for amitriptyline may help to explain the efficacy of tricyclics in conditions that are unaffected by conventional analgesic agents. Both systemic and spinally administered NMDA antagonists are analgesic in rat mononeuropathy pain models, and tricyclics are often effective for postherpetic neuralgia and other neuropathic pain states.

S.E. Abram, M.D.

Postaortic Occlusion Shock Mechanisms

Xanthine Oxidase Inactivation Attenuates Postocclusion Shock After Descending Thoracic Aorta Occlusion and Reperfusion in Rabbits
Nielsen VG, McCammon AT, Tan S, et al (Univ of Alabama, Birmingham)
J Thorac Cardiovasc Surg 110:715–722, 1995 9–8

Objective.—"Declamping shock" is a pathologic condition that occurs after aortic cross-clamping. Affected patients have hypotension and hypovolemia, along with treatment-refractory metabolic acidosis. Previous reports have suggested that oxidants play a key role in declamping shock. A rabbit model of declamping shock was used to assess the impact of oxidants derived from the hepatocellular enzyme xanthine oxidase (XO) and the therapeutic value of tungstate in inactivating XO.

Methods.—In the rabbit model, the descending thoracic aorta was occluded for 40 minutes by balloon catheter inflation. Sham-operated rabbits were studied as control subjects. The resuscitative interventions needed to maintain baseline hemodynamic and acid–base status were assessed. Systemic injury was assessed by the release of lactate dehydrogenase and alkaline phosphatase. Some rabbits in each group were fed a tungstate diet before aortic occlusion.

Results.—After reperfusion, rabbits who had received the tungstate diet required 28% less Ringer's solution, 68% less phenylephrine, and 30% less sodium bicarbonate. Tungstate pretreatment also was associated with lower lactate dehydrogenase and alkaline phosphatase levels. In the control group, plasma XO activities were lower in the tungstate-pretreated animals.

Conclusions.—This and previous studies support the hypothesis that circulating oxidants are involved in the clinical manifestations of declamping shock after occlusion of the thoracic aorta. Xanthine dehydrogenase and XO, along with high concentrations of purine substrates, may be released from the perfused hepatic and intestinal tissues after the descending thoracic aorta is unclamped. Free radicals may cause vascular endothelial cell injury, leading to declamping shock and the release of cytosolic enzymes. Tungstate or other treatments may be able to inactivate xanthine dehydrogenase and XO, reducing resuscitative requirements and the systemic injury associated with declamping syndrome.

► The authors of this article make a case both with biochemical measurements and through inhibition of enzymes that reperfusion after 2 hours of thoracic aortic occlusion leads to the "declamping syndrome," at least in part because of the production of oxidative intermediates and free radicals. Although the data statistically support their point of view, it is clear that this is not the only cause of the declamping syndrome, and may not even be a very important one. Nevertheless, one conclusion does clearly emanate from this—the faster your surgeon, the less likely you are to have declamping hypotension. Perhaps we should encourage everyone to do studies on what educational process it takes to promote faster surgery, and what is needed to get patients to select surgeons who do this procedure with a shorter time of temporary occlusion of the aorta. This once again confirms the adage that a great surgeon deserves a great anesthesiologist, whereas a barely adequate surgeon requires one.

M.F. Roizen, M.D.

Dexmedetomidine Mechanisms

Antisense Technology Reveals the α_{2A} Adrenoceptor to Be the Subtype Mediating the Hypnotic Response to the Highly Selective Agonist, Dexmedetomidine, in the Locus Coeruleus of the Rat
Mizobe T, Maghsoudi K, Sitwala K, et al (Stanford Univ, Calif)
J Clin Invest 98:1076–1080, 1996 9–9

Introduction.—The α_2-adrenergic agonists have useful sedative/hypnotic effects in anesthesia. However, the α_2-adrenoreceptor subtype by which these effects occur has not been identified. Four subtypes are known: α_{2A}, α_{2B}, α_{2C}, and α_{2D}, the latter being a species homologue of α_{2A}. Gene targeting studies were done to identify which adrenoreceptor subtypes are involved in the hypnotic action of an α_2-adrenergic agonist.

Methods.—The study used stably transfected cell lines for rat α_{2A} and α_{2B} adrenoreceptors. The cells were exposed to 5 μM antisense oligodeoxynucleotides (ODNs) for these α_2-receptor subtypes for 3 days. Radiolabeled ligand binding was done to assess individual receptor subtype expression, which was selectively decreased only by the appropriate antisense ODNs. Rats were then treated with these antisense ODNs, by cannula administration into the locus coeruleus, on 3 occasions on alternate days. The animals' hypnotic response to the highly selective α_2-adrenergic agonist dexmedetomidine was then assessed.

Results.—Only α_{2A} antisense ODNs—not α_{2C} antisense ODNs nor α_{2A} scrambled ODNs—altered the hypnotic response to dexmedetomidine. Treatment with α_2 antisense ODNs increased the latency to the loss of the righting reflex, and decreased the duration of that loss. Eight days after ODN treatment was stopped, the hypnotic response normalized.

Conclusions.—At least in the rat locus coeruleus, α_{2A} is the adrenoreceptor subtype involved in the hypnotic action of dexmedetomidine. In the future, it may be possible to synthesize new ligands specific for the beneficial anesthetic effects of α_2-adrenergic agonists while avoiding the side effects. These studies should focus on the α_{2A}-receptor subtype.

► Molecular cloning techniques have shown that 3 α_2-adrenergic subtypes exist: α_{2A}, α_{2B}, and α_{2A}. However, we do not know the precise pharmacologic role that these receptors play. Clonidine, a nonselective α_2-agonist, is considered to be an analgesic adjuvant in addition to possessing well-recognized cardiovascular effects. It would be interesting to develop an α_2-agonist devoid of cardiovascular effects but possessing anesthetic/analgesic effects. Thus, the development of a subtype-selective drug might have direct clinical relevance. In the past, receptor subtypes have been identified using selective antagonists and agonists (e.g., dexmedetomidine). Antisense technology, whereby antisense oligodeoxynucleotides are administered to reduce receptor density in cell lines, has been used to inhibit receptor expression and represents a new way to look at receptor function. Mervyn Maze and his group have shown that it is the α_{2A} subtype that is responsible for the hypnotic response to dexmedetomidine.

I chose this article to illustrate how basic science experiments might in the future change clinical anesthesia. At the moment, we are a long way from that point, but it is an exciting concept.

M. Wood, M.D.

Dorsal Root Cell Pain Studies

Abnormal Spontaneous Activity and Responses to Norepinephrine in Dissociated Dorsal Root Ganglion Cells After Chronic Nerve Constriction

Petersen M, Zhang J, Zhang J-M, et al (Univ Wuerzburg, Germany; Yale Univ, New Haven, Conn)

Pain 67:391–397, 1996 9–10

Objective.—The effects of a peripheral nerve injury on the responses of dissociated dorsal root ganglion (DRG) cells to norepinephrine (NE) was examined in an experimental study. In previous studies of nerve injury in rats, abnormal spontaneous nerve impulses and abnormal response to NE were able to be generated from the DRG as well as at the site of injury.

Methods.—The right sciatic nerve of male Sprague-Dawley rats was exposed and 4 chromic gut ligatures were tied loosely around the nerve. In a smaller number of animals, the nerve was tightly ligated. The ganglia L4 and L5 were excised 11 to 25 days after ligation and shortly after the rats were killed. Control animals without previous injury also had L4 and L5 removed. Whole-cell patch-clamp recordings under current clamp were obtained from L4 and L5 DRG cells. Small to medium-sized cells from uninjured and loosely ligated nerves were tested with NE.

Results.—Of 15 DRG cells from uninjured nerves, 1 responded to NE; the highest NE dose tested (500 μmol) elicited a small depolarization without action potentials. Many cells from injured nerves, however, responded to NE with a membrane depolarization, and in some cases this response was accompanied by generation of action potentials. The response rate was 52% with the highest NE dose (500 μmol) but considerably less with lower doses (26% of cells with 100 μmol NE and 14% of cells with 10 μmol NE). Cells that responded to NE also responded to capsaicin. Spontaneous activities was absent in all cells from uninjured nerves but occurred in 14% of cells from loosely ligated nerves and in 21% of cells from tightly ligated nerves. The discharge patterns were irregular in the loose ligation group and irregular or bursting in the tight ligation group.

Conclusions.—After injury of the sciatic nerve, the somata of certain peripheral nerve fibers appear to develop spontaneous discharges and abnormal responses to NE. Because the cells were dissociated and unlikely to be in communication with each other, the underlying mechanisms are intrinsic to the somata. The abnormal phenomena seen in injured cells occurred only rarely in cells from normal, uninjured nerve. Development of sensitivity to NE after peripheral axonal injury may contribute to sympathetically maintained pain.

▶ There is now considerable evidence that the DRG is an important site of ectopic impulse generation and that sympathetic nerve activity can augment spontaneous activity arising from DRG cells. Adrenergic fibers were shown to innervate DRG cells more than 30 years ago.[1] Recently, sprouting of new adrenergic fibers was shown in response to peripheral nerve injury.

S.E. Abram, M.D.

Reference

1. Owman C, Santini M: Adrenergic nerves in spinal ganglion of the cat. *Acta Physiol Scand* 68:127–128 , 1966.

Temperature Threshold Studies

Enflurane Decreases the Threshold for Vasoconstriction More Than Isoflurane or Halothane

Nebbia SP, Bissonnette B, Sessler DI (Univ of Toronto; Univ of California, San Francisco; Univ of Vienna)

Anesth Analg 83:595–599, 1996 9–11

Introduction.—The main cause of intraoperative hypothermia is the anesthetic's effect in inhibiting tonic thermoregulatory vasoconstriction. When body temperature drops below a certain point, peripheral vasoconstriction occurs, preventing further core hypothermia. The various volatile anesthetics all have been tested for their thermoregulatory effects, but there have been no direct comparisons of different anesthetics. Thermoregulatory responses to enflurane, isoflurane, and halothane were compared in surgical patients.

Methods.—The study included 27 children undergoing intra-abdominal surgery, mainly bilateral ureteral implantation. Each received anesthesia with halothane, isoflurane, or enflurane, maintained with 1 minimum alveolar anesthetic concentration. Normovolemia and normocapnea were maintained, but passive cooling was permitted. The occurrence of signif-

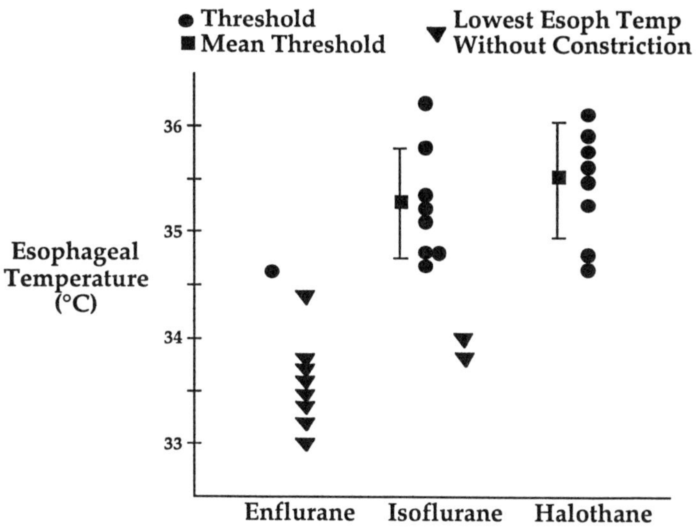

FIGURE 1.—The vasoconstriction thresholds were comparable in patients anesthetized with isoflurane and halothane: 35.2 ± 0.5 and 35.5 ± 0.6°C, respectively. In contrast, all but 1 of the patients given enflurane failed to vasoconstrict at a minimum core temperature of 33.6 ± 0.4°C ($P < .001$). (Courtesy of Nebbia SP, Bissonnette B, Sessler DI: Enflurane decreases the threshold for vasoconstriction more than isoflurane or halothane. *Anesth Analg* 83:595–599, 1996.)

icant vasoconstriction was signaled by a gradient of 4°C between the forearm and fingertip skin temperatures, and the core temperature at that time was regarded as the threshold triggering vasoconstriction.

Results.—The 3 anesthetic groups were similar in their morphometric characteristics, initial core temperatures, ambient operating room temperatures, and end-tidal anesthetic potencies. Core temperature at vasoconstriction was 35.5°C for all 8 patients in the halothane group. Vasoconstriction occurred at 35.2°C for 8 of the 10 patients receiving isoflurane, but did not occur at core temperatures as low as 33.8°C in the other 2 patients. In the enflurane group, 1 patient showed vasoconstriction at a core temperature of 34.6°C, whereas the other 6 showed no vasoconstriction despite core temperatures as low as 33.6°C (Fig 1).

Conclusions.—Enflurane causes profound inhibition of thermoregulatory responses in children undergoing abdominal surgery. If they are not actively warmed, children anesthetized with enflurane will become much colder than those anesthetized with halothane or isoflurane. The reason for this effect of enflurane is unknown—there is no apparent pharmacologic or physiologic explanation. In adults, there is evidence that enflurane and isoflurane cause similar vasoconstrictive responses.

► This paper is included because it is an elegant exposition of thermoregulatory physiology. I doubt that it has much clinical relevance because little anesthesia is done in children with enflurane.

J.H. Tinker, M.D.

Analgesic Site of Epidural Buprenorphine

Mode and Site of Analgesic Action of Epidural Buprenorphine in Humans

Inagaki Y, Mashimo T, Yoshiya I (Osaka Univ, Japan)
Anesth Analg 83:530–536, 1996 9–12

Background.—Buprenorphine is a mixed agonist-antagonist opioid that produces postoperative pain relief. Its ability to produce significant spinal segmental analgesia when administered epidurally and the primary site of its analgesic action have not been clarified. These questions were investigated in a randomized, placebo-controlled, prospective study that evaluated the analgesic intensity of buprenorphine in different doses and with different modes of administration.

Methods.—Fifty patients undergoing gastrectomy were randomly assigned postoperatively to receive 1 of 5 analgesic regimens: epidural normal saline; epidural injection of buprenorphine at doses of either 2 or 4 μg/kg plus IV injection of saline; or IV injection of buprenorphine at doses of either 2 or 4 μg/kg plus epidural injection of saline. Analgesic intensity was monitored using a visual analogue scale, and the pressure pain threshold (PPT) was determined using a coiled pressure algesimeter at 5 sites corresponding to different dermatomes. Adverse effects were recorded.

Results.—The onset of analgesia occurred more quickly in the IV than in the epidural group, but the duration of analgesia was longer in the epidural than in the IV group (Table 2). Although there were no significant differences in the changes of PPT at the forehead among the groups at any time, PPT near the surgical incision was significantly greater after epidural administration than after IV administration, with the changes in PPT exhibiting dose dependency. Visual analogue scale values also were dose-dependent and were significantly lower in the epidural group during the middle period than in the IV group at the same dose. The 4 groups did not

TABLE 2.—Onset Time and Duration of Analgesia Produced by Buprenorphine

Group	Onset time (min)	Duration (min)
Epidural buprenorphine		
2 μg/kg	33.0 ± 9.5†	769 ± 151†
4 μg/kg	28.5 ± 8.5*	883 ± 164†
Intravenous (IV) buprenorphine		
2 μg/kg	19.5 ± 7.2	283 ± 95
4 μg/kg	16.5 ± 4.7	547 ± 142‡

Note: Values are expressed as mean ± SD.
*P <.05, significantly different from both IV buprenorphine groups.
†P <.01, significantly different from both IV buprenorphine groups.
‡P <.01, significantly different from the IV buprenorphine 2-μg/kg group.
(Courtesy of Inagaki Y, Mashimo T, Yoshiya I: Mode and site of analgesic action of epidural buprenorphine in humans. *Anesth Analg* 83:530–536, 1996.)

differ significantly in the incidence of adverse effects, except that the larger dose of IV buprenorphine produced more drowsiness.

Conclusions.—Epidural buprenorphine does produce spinal segmental analgesia in a dose-dependent fashion. Its action can be described primarily as long-lasting supraspinal analgesia along with dose-related spinal analgesia.

▶ Neuraxial buprenorphine administration appears to have pharmacodynamic characteristics similar to those of other lipid-soluble opioids. There is relatively little difference between epidural and IV dose requirements for buprenorphine, there is evidence of supraspinal effects of epidurally administered drug, and there are modest segmental analgesic effects. Because buprenorphine has high receptor affinity, the segmental effects may last for many hours. For the same reason, accidental intrathecal injection may produce prolonged supraspinal side effects that may be difficult to reverse by opioid antagonists.

S.E. Abram, M.D.

Halothane Genetic Resistance

Halothane Resistance in *Drosophila melanogaster*: Development of a Model and Gene Localization Techniques

Dapkus D, Ramirez S, Murray MJ (Winona State Univ, Minnesota; John Marshall High School, Rochester, Minn; Mayo Clinic and Found, Rochester, Minn)

Anesth Analg 83:147–155, 1996 9–13

Background.—Previous studies have identified anesthetic resistance in genetically altered strains of *Drosophila melanogaster*. The molecular basis of anesthetic resistance was investigated in this animal model.

Methods.—Four *Drosophila* strains were studied: Canton-S (CS), a standard wild-type strain; brown scarlet (bw st), a strain with 1 gene for brown eyes on the second chromosome and 1 gene for scarlet eyes on the third chromosome; the dumpy black cinnabar brown strain, characterized by dumpy wings, black thorax, markers for cinnabar and brown eye color, and wings with veinlet markings; and 91R, a halothane-resistant strain. Groups of each strain were tested for halothane resistance in a closed chamber injected with liquid halothane. The effect of the X chromosome on resistance was investigated by crossing 91R females with CS males and examining resistance in the offspring. The 7 phenotypes in a third generation of test flies were separated and tested to determine associations between halothane resistance and genes on the second chromosome.

Results.—The 50% effective dose of halothane was 0.46% in 91R females, 0.27% in CS females, 0.40% in 91R males, and 0.27% in CS males. In the 91R strain, the relative resistance was 1.69 in females and 1.48 in males. In these flies, resistance was not influenced by either the X or the third chromosome, but was significantly linked to the second chromosome. There were significant differences between the 91R and CS resistance in flies with 5 genotypes, including wild, dumpy wings, brown eyes, black thoracic color and dumpy wings, and cinnabar eye color and brown eye color. However, there were no significant differences between the strains in flies with black thoracic color, cinnabar eye color, and brown eye color and in flies with dumpy wings, black thoracic color, and cinnabar eye color.

Conclusions.—The halothane-resistance gene or genes are likely to be located between the gene for black thoracic color and the gene for cinnabar eye color. Further analysis of the localization of the gene for halothane resistance in the 91R strain can lead to a better understanding of the molecular mechanisms involved in anesthetic action.

► Last year, there was considerable interest in the idea that our old friend, the old fruit fly *Drosophila*, whose genetic mapping is as complete as that of any animal, including us, in the universe, might be used to understand more about mechanisms of anesthesia. These authors were able to find a strain of *Drosophila* that did indeed show substantially increased resistance to halothane. The resistance was located on a particular chromosome, but they could not localize this resistance or determine how it worked. I could not resist including this article to take a few potshots at it. Once again, our molecular biology geneticists have promised us the moon and the stars, but in fact they can only tell us that the resistance phenomenon is located on a particular chromosome. That seems similar to developing a global-positioning system that tells you that you are somewhere in the state of Nebraska.

J.H. Tinker, M.D.

Magnesium Sulfate Affects Fetal Survival

Magnesium Sulfate Adversely Affects Fetal Lamb Survival and Blocks Fetal Cerebral Blood Flow Response During Maternal Hemorrhage

Reynolds JD, Chestnut DH, Dexter F, et al (Univ of Iowa, Iowa City; Univ of Alabama, Birmingham)

Anesth Analg 83:493–499, 1996 9–14

Background.—Magnesium sulfate is commonly used as a tocolytic agent in women at risk of preterm delivery and as prophylaxis against seizures in parturients with pregnancy-induced hypertension and/or preeclampsia. However, the actions of magnesium sulfate on the fetus during maternal/fetal stress are not well understood. Magnesium sulfate was hypothesized to alter the fetal cerebral blood flow response to hypoxemia produced during maternal hemorrhage.

Methods.—In instrumented, near-term fetal lambs, 123 days' gestation, maternal hemorrhage was induced for 60 minutes during fetal infusion of 0.25 g (in 5 fetuses) or 0.30 g (in 6) magnesium sulfate or during infusion of normal saline (in 11). Radiolabeled microspheres were used to determine the level of fetal cerebral blood flow.

Findings.—Maternal hemorrhage produced fetal hypoxemia and some fetal demise in all 3 groups. Nine percent of the fetuses in the saline group

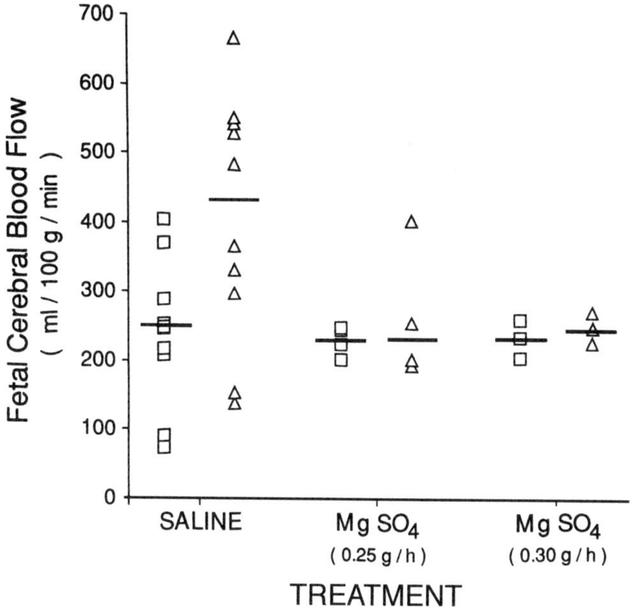

FIGURE 1.—Individual cerebral blood flow values of the surviving fetuses during fetal infusion of saline (n = 10), 0.25 g magnesium sulfate (*Mg* SO_4) per hour (n = 4), or 0.30 g $MgSO_4$ per hour (n = 3) before (*squares*) and after (*triangles*) maternal hemorrhage. The mean value within each group is denoted by the *dark line*. Fetal infusion of magnesium sulfate inhibits the increase in fetal cerebral blood produced by maternal hemorrhage ($P = 0.003$). (Courtesy of Reynolds JD, Chestnut DH, Dexter F, et al: Magnesium sulfate adversely affects fetal lamb survival and blocks fetal cerebral blood flow response during maternal hemorrhage. *Anesth Analg* 83:493–499, 1996.)

died as compared with 20% in the 0.25 g magnesium sulfate group and 50% in the 0.30 g magnesium sulfate group. Among survivors, hypoxemia induced by bleeding increased fetal cerebral blood flow during saline infusion. However, magnesium sulfate infusion inhibited this compensatory increase in fetal cerebral blood flow (Fig 1).

Conclusions.—In this fetal lamb model, magnesium sulfate increased fetal mortality and inhibited the compensatory increase in fetal cerebral blood flow during fetal hypoxemia induced by maternal bleeding. Thus the use of magnesium sulfate in women at risk for hemorrhage may need to be re-evaluated.

▶ Magnesium is widely believed to have little negative effect on hemodynamic measurements. Indeed, bolus IV infusion of $MgSO_4$ typically produces only a transient decrease in maternal systemic vascular resistance and mean arterial pressure. However, in an earlier study we demonstrated that hypermagnesemia worsens the maternal compensatory response to hemorrhage.[1] Magnesium readily crosses the human placenta. Thus we performed the present study to evaluate the effects of hypermagnesemia on the fetal compensatory response to maternal hemorrhage and hypotension. The present study does not warrant abandonment of the use of $MgSO_4$ tocolysis or seizure prophylaxis in pregnant women. Further, this study conflicts with other studies that have demonstrated that magnesium provides a protective effect on the brain. However, this study calls attention to the fact that hypermagnesemia may have an adverse effect on the compensatory response to hemorrhage in both the mother and the fetus.

D.H. Chestnut, M.D.

Reference

1. Chestnut DH, Thompson CS, McLaughlin GL, et al: Does the intravenous infusion of ritodrine or magnesium sulfate alter the hemodynamic response to hemorrhage in gravid ewes? *Am J Obstet Gynecol* 159:1467–1473, 1988.

Cross-linked Hemoglobin Studies

Diaspirin Cross-linked Hemoglobin Does Not Increase Brain Oxygen Consumption During Hypothermic Cardiopulmonary Bypass in Rabbits

Hindman BJ, Dexter F, Cutkomp J, et al (Univ of Iowa, Iowa City)
Anesthesiology 83:1302–1311, 1995 9–15

Introduction.—Cardiopulmonary bypass (CPB), hypothermia, or both may cause decreased erythrocyte permeability. This can lead to decreased erythrocyte transit in the brain capillary beds, and therefore to impaired brain oxygenation during CPB. Capillary plasma flow in the brain continues even without erythrocyte flow. This suggests that a non–erythrocyte-associated oxygen transport molecule might be used to increase brain oxygen uptake during hypothermic CPB and thus enhance plasma oxygen uptake; an hypothesis that was studied with diaspirin cross-linked hemoglobin in a rabbit model.

Methods.—New Zealand white rabbits were placed on CPB at 27° C and randomly assigned into 3 intervention groups. Those in group 1 received α-α diaspirin cross-linked hemoglobin to increase their plasma oxygen content; verapamil, 0.5 mg/kg, was given before treatment to prevent hypertension. Rabbits in group 2 received verapamil, but not α-α diaspirin cross-linked hemoglobin; those in group 3 received neither treatment. Bypass continued for 60 minutes, at which time cerebral blood flow was measured with microspheres and cerebral metabolic rate for oxygen was measured by the Fick method.

Results.—The 3 groups were similar in their systemic physiologic variables. All had a total arterial oxygen content equivalent to 12.1 mL O_2 dL. However, the proportion of total arterial oxygen content that was present in a non–erythrocyte-associated form was 29% in group 1 vs 6% in group 2 and 5% in group 3. There were no significant differences in cerebral blood flow or cerebral metabolic rate for oxygen. This meant no differences in the availability of oxygen to the brain, whether or not it was erythrocyte-associated oxygen.

Conclusions.—In hypothermic CPB, oxygen transfer from the blood to the brain is not limited by erythrocyte/capillary interactions. Administration of α-α diaspirin cross-linked hemoglobin causes a hypertensive response, most likely because of nitric oxide scavenging. The work performed so far in this rabbit model suggests that hypoperfusion and/or impaired brain aerobic metabolism during CPB are not responsible for postoperative neurologic dysfunction. Future research should concentrate on the way in which CPB modifies injuries that result from embolic events and how CPB affects the brain and its response to injury.

▶ This rabbit model of CPB is the only remotely validated animal model for the study of bypass-related cerebral physiology. In this study, the authors test Baxter's new stroma-free diaspirin cross-linked hemoglobin. The purpose of the cross-linkage is to try to keep the body from splitting stroma-free hemoglobin into α and β chains and thus filtering it more rapidly at the kidney. As we use these "artificial" hemoglobins more and more, we will find many fascinating responses. Those interested in cerebral physiology will want to explore this article in detail. My point is that this CPB model is valid to test all sorts of drugs, techniques, and different physiologic maintenance approaches. As most of our readers know, much of the current CPB is simply the product of "tradition," usually local. We do need scientific studies of the various things people do during CPB.

J.H. Tinker, M.D.

Can "Chip"-based Devices Keep Shrinking?

Can Chip Devices Keep Shrinking?
Service RF
Science 274:1834–1836, 1996 9–16

Can Chip Devices Keep Shrinking?—In 1965, the co-founder of Intel Corporation, Gordon Moore, predicted that the number of transistors on computer chips would double every 18 months. This prediction, called "Moore's Law," has turned out to be accurate. The techniques for carving features on silicon waters (lithography) have continued to develop.

Advances in optical lithography depend on shortening the wavelength of the light used to etch features. As lithography operations use ever shorter ultraviolet (UV) light waves, analysts expect that this shrinking, which has been driving the semiconductor industry, will continue for another 10 years. However, it is not known what will happen after that.

Researchers worldwide are working to find alternative chip-patterning techniques to use when lithographic tools are no longer useful. The main question is whether any of the new possibilities can be sealed up to pattern the billions of features per hour needed for a system to be economically viable. To pattern silicon wafers, current optical systems use a template, or "mask," made from a sheet of glass topped with a thin coating of a light-absorbing metal. An electron beam or laser is used to carve the desired features through the mask's metal coating to the transparent glass. The tiny patterns created are focused on a thin layer of light-sensitive "resist," which sits on top of a silicon wafer. The molecular structure of the resist changes where it is bombarded by photons.

Industry scientists expect to be able to mass-produce features of 0.18 μm by the year 2001. This will be achieved by reducing the wavelength of the UV light used to 193 nm. However, at wavelengths shorter than 193 nm, conventional quartz lenses absorb light rather than refract it. If new etching techniques are not found, the number of transistors on computer memory chips may top out at 4 billion. (The current standard is 16 million.)

X-ray lithography is a promising successor for lithography. Typical x-ray systems fire photons with 4 nm wavelengths. Several groups have recently developed x-ray systems that can pattern devices by the millions and build densely packed transistors on integrated circuits. Using this technique, a record 4 billion transistors may be crammed on a single DRAM chip, which is about 250 times the number on today's standard DRAMs.

▶ This is a fascinating article by Robert F. Service, who describes in lay terms why Moore's Law has held for 30 years and why it is likely to hold only for another 10 years. Moore's Law is that the number of transistors on a computer chip would double every 18 months, thanks largely to continuous advances in techniques for carving patterns into silicon wafers. Moore's prediction turned out to be unbelievably accurate for the last 30 years. In fact, the number of transistors on chips has doubled about every 18 months for the past 35 years, helping to propel semiconductor production into a $150 billion/yr industry. The limits of this are the limits of patterns that can be focused by visible and now UV light. The future is one of focusing with x-ray lithography. Whether this proves to be cost-effective or needed is unclear at this time, and thus, the limits of UV light etching and of lithographic improvements may well be reached by the year 2006.

M.F. Roizen, M.D.

Cerebral Metabolism Improvement

Amelioration of Impaired Cerebral Metabolism After Severe Acidotic Ischemia by Tirilazad Posttreatment in Dogs

Kim H, Koehler RC, Hurn PD, et al (Johns Hopkins Med Insts, Baltimore, Md; Upjohn Company, Kalamazoo, Mich)
Stroke 27:114–121, 1996 9–17

Introduction.—Neuronal injury is exacerbated by increasing the severity of lactic acidosis during global ischemia by hyperglycemia. Antioxidant tirilazad mesylate is a drug that inhibits lipid peroxidation in vitro by combining chemical radical scavenging and membrane stabilizing mechanisms. Tirilazad should be effective if administered at the time of reperfusion because lipid peroxidation is presumed to occur most intensely during the reoxygenation period after ischemia. Whether treatment with tirilazad improves metabolic and intracellular pH recovery and prevents delayed hypoperfusion if started early during reperfusion after 30 minutes of severe incomplete cerebral ischemia accompanied by hyperglycemia was investigated. An optimal dose of tirilazad was found for this effect. After hyperglycemic ischemia, it was determined whether the endogenous cytosolic antioxidant glutathion is depleted and whether tirilazad treatment increases this depletion.

Methods.—To reduce perfusion pressure to 10–12 mm Hg, arterial glucose concentration was increased to 500–600 mg/dL and global incomplete cerebral ischemia was produced for 30 minutes by ventricular fluid infusion in anesthetized dogs. Phosphorus MR spectroscopy was used to measure metabolic recovery and intracellular pH. At reperfusion in the first experiment, 4 groups of 8 dogs received either vehicle or 0.25, 1, or 2.5 mg of tirilazad mesylate per kilogram of body weight. Microspheres were used to measure cerebral blood flow. At reperfusion in the second experiment, 2 groups of 8 dogs each received either vehicle or 2.5 mg of tirilazad per kilogram. At 3 hours of reperfusion, cortical glutathione was measured.

Results.—In all groups, cerebral blood flow decreased to approximately 6 mL/min per 100 g and intracellular pH decreased to approximately 5.6 during ischemia. Adenosine triphosphate (ATP) recovery was transient in the vehicle group, and pH remained less than 6.0. By 3 hours, cerebral blood flow, O_2 consumption, and ATP eventually declined to near-zero levels. In a dose-dependent fashion, recovery was improved by tirilazad posttreatment. Cerebral blood flow and O_2 consumption were sustained near preischemic levels at the highest dose. Recovery of ATP greater than 50% and of pH greater than 6.7 was found in 5 of 8 dogs. By 17 minutes of reperfusion, recovery of ATP and phosphocreatine became significantly greater than in the vehicle group, despite similar levels of early hyperemia. This shows that the drug acts before the onset of hyperfusion. In the vehicle group, cortical glutathione concentration was 27% less than in the tirilazad group, and 34% less than in the nonischemic controls.

Conclusion.—Tirilazad acting as an antioxidant in vivo is consistent with decreased depletion of endogenous antioxidant glutathione. An early onset of a functionally significant oxygen radical injury is consistent with improvement in high-energy phosphate recovery 17 minutes after starting tirilazad infusion during reperfusion. Early ischemic injury seems to be affected by severe acidosis through an oxygen radical mechanism sufficient to block metabolic recovery.

▶ Experimental models continue to show a favorable effect of tirilazad in minimizing cerebral ischemia both as a pretreatment[1] and after neurologic insult.

D.M. Rothenberg, M.D.

Reference

1. 1995 Year Book of Anesthesiology, p. 353.

Pain Mechanisms After Spinal Injury

Central Dysesthesia Pain After Traumatic Spinal Cord Injury Is Dependent on N-Methyl-D-Aspartate Receptor Activation

Eide PK, Stubhaug A, Stenehjem AE (Ullevå Hosp, Oslo, Norway; Natl Hosp, Oslo, Norway; Univ of Oslo, Norway)
Neurosurgery 37:1080–1087, 1995 9–18

Background.—A major sequela of traumatic spinal cord injury, affecting approximately one third of patients, is central dysesthesia pain. The neurochemical basis of central pain after spinal cord injury—specifically, the role of the central *N*-methyl-D-aspartate (NMDA) receptors—was examined with the hypothesis that blocking of the NMDA receptors could decrease central pain by downregulating neuronal hyperactivity and hyperexcitability. The actions of the noncompetitive NMDA blocker ketamine were compared with those of saline and the μ-opioid receptor agonist alfentanil in a randomized, double-blind, crossover study.

Methods.—Nine patients with central dysesthesia after traumatic spinal cord injury were studied. Spontaneous continuous and intermittent pain and evoked pain were part of this central pain syndrome. Non-noxious stimulation of the skin (allodynia) and repeated pricking of the skin (wind-up like) evoked pain. Pain severity was measured before and after intravenous infusion of ketamine (a bolus of 60 μg/kg followed by infusion of 6 μg/kg/min), alfentanil (a bolus dose of 7 μg/kg followed by infusion of 0.6 μg/kg/min), or 0.9% sodium chloride as placebo.

Results.—Both the blockade of NMDA receptors by ketamine and the activation of μ-opioid receptors by alfentanil markedly reduced continuous and evoked pain. Threshold for sensation of heat pain was not changed significantly by either drug. Alfentanil administration resulted in only modest side effects; the only bothersome side effect reported from ketamine was dizziness in 1 patient.

Conclusions.—Clinical evidence suggests that central dysesthesia pain after traumatic spinal cord injury is dependent on the activation of NMDA receptors and is sensitive to the activation of μ-opioid receptors.

▶ Although this study demonstrates that both alfentanil and ketamine produce analgesia to both spontaneous and evoked pain in spinal cord injury patients, it may be inadvisible to assume that ketamine's analgesic effect is related to antagonism of the NMDA receptor. Unlike some of the more selective NMDA antagonists, ketamine produces profound analgesia to acute noxious stimuli (hence its success as an anesthetic/analgesic agent in surgical settings). We may, therefore, be observing analgesia related to other effects of the drug. It would be interesting to determine whether dextromethorphan, an NMDA antagonist that has little direct antinociceptive action, would provide the same effect. Our initial experience with that drug in a small number of spinal cord injury patients with chronic pain has been disappointing.

S.E. Abram, M.D.

Ketamine in Pain Studies

Effect of Systemic *N*-Methyl-D-Aspartate Receptor Antagonist (Ketamine) on Primary and Secondary Hyperalgesia in Humans

Ilkjaer S, Petersen KL, Brennum J, et al (Skejby Univ, Aarhus, Denmark; Glostrup Univ, Copenhagen)

Br J Anaesth 76:829–834, 1996 9–19

Background.—Previous studies have shown that the *N*-methyl-D-aspartate receptor plays an important role in spinal hypersensitivity. Ketamine exerts its antinociceptive action by binding to the phencyclidine site of the *N*-methyl-D-aspartate receptor-gated ion channel. The effects of systemic ketamine treatment on pain, primary hyperalgesia (thought to be caused by sensitization of peripheral receptors plus the central neurones), and secondary hyperalgesia (thought to be caused by sensitization of dorsal horn neurones) were evaluated.

Methods.—Nineteen healthy, unmedicated male volunteers were studied. First-degree burn injuries were induced on the dominant calf with a rectangular thermode at a temperature of 47°C applied for 7 minutes. The men continually rated their pain with an electronic visual analogue scale. A heat pain detection threshold (HPDT) was determined at the site of injury and on the contralateral calf to evaluate primary hyperalgesia. The border of hyperalgesia to punctuate and stroke stimuli was determined to evaluate secondary hyperalgesia. The side effects of drowsiness, discomfort, and hallucinations were assessed at varying doses of ketamine administered on 3 separate days, at least 1 week apart.

Results.—Without ketamine, pain increased quickly during the first 15–30 sec of heat application, then plateaued. The HPDT decreased at the burn injury site from 45.9°C to 41.6°C but was unchanged on the contralateral calf after injury. The borders of secondary hyperalgesia were easily detected. Ketamine treatment reduced pain in a dose-dependent fashion. Primary hyperalgesia was reduced only with high-dose ketamine. The HPDT on the contralateral calf was not affected by ketamine at any dose. High-dose ketamine reduced the areas of secondary hyperalgesia for both punctuate and stroke stimuli, whereas low-dose ketamine only reduced the area of secondary hyperalgesia for stroke stimuli.

Drowsiness occurred in a dose-dependent fashion. Discomfort also was related to the dose. No individuals experienced hallucinations, but most of them reported dizziness during ketamine administration.

Conclusions.—Ketamine therapy can reduce the pain of burn injuries as well as both primary and secondary hyperalgesia without affecting phasic heat pain perception in undamaged skin, which distinguishes its effects from the effects of local anesthetics and opioids. Frequent but clinically acceptable side effects occur.

► In both animal and human models, *N*-methyl-D-aspartate antagonists are capable of reducing spinal sensitization induced by a relatively brief noxious stimulus. It remains to be determined whether preemptive administration of such agents reduces pain sensitivity after surgery. The 2 agents in current clinical use with known *N*-methyl-D-aspartate receptor antagonist effects are ketamine and dextromethorphan, although there is evidence that amitriptyline may have such properties as well.

S.E. Abram, M.D.

Pain Studies Using Excitatory Amino Acid Antagonists

Treatment of a Chronic Allodynia-like Response in Spinally Injured Rats: Effects of Systemically Administered Excitatory Amino Acid Receptor Antagonists

Hao J-X, Xu X-J (Huddinge Univ, Sweden)
Pain 66:279–285, 1996 9–20

Background.—Neuropathic pain can occur after injury to the peripheral or central nervous system. It is frequently a chronic pain that is refractory to currently available analgesic regimens. Its mechanisms are poorly understood, but receptor antagonists for excitatory amino acids have been implicated in the underlying pathophysiology. An animal model of chronic pain after ischemic spinal cord injury has been developed, which mimics central pain and produces allodynia-like symptoms. This model was used to evaluate the efficacy of 4 antagonists of excitatory amino acid receptors, including 3 *N*-methyl-D-aspartate (NMDA) receptor antagonists and 1 α-amino-3-hydroxyl-5-methyl-4-isoxazolepropionic acid (AMPA) receptor antagonist.

Methods.—After the performance of a photochemically induced spinal cord ischemia injury, female rats were randomly assigned to treatment with either CGS 19755 (a competitive NMDA receptor antagonist), dextromethorphan hydrobromide (a noncompetitive NMDA antagonist), MK-801 (a noncompetitive NMDA antagonist), or NBQX (a competitive AMPA antagonist). Before and after treatment with varying doses of the study drug, the rats were tested for mechanical allodynia using graded mechanical pressure with calibrated von Frey hairs until consistent vocalization was induced. Motor performance, activity level, and sedation also were evaluated.

Results.—After the ischemic spinal cord injury, the vocalization threshold decreased by about 50%. A dose of 0.25 mg/kg of MK-801 was required to relieve the chronic allodynia. However, this dose also produced significantly impaired motor function, reduced activity levels, and stereotypical behavioral abnormalities. CGS 19755 abolished chronic allodynia at a dose of 10 mg/kg, which also produced severe motor dysfunction, hyperactivity, and stereotypical behavior. Dextromethorphan relieved allodynia at a dose of 20 mg/kg in 2 of 5 rats and at a dose of 40 mg/kg in all rats. These doses did not increase motor deficits or produce stereotypical behavior, and there was a moderate increase in activity only with the highest dose. NBQX, at a dose of 30 mg/kg, abolished allodynia, but induced motor deficits, reduced activity, and sedation.

Conclusions.—Analgesia for chronic pain in rats after spinal cord injury can be provided by systemic NMDA, but not AMPA, antagonists. However, the NMDA antagonists also induce significant side effects, including motor dysfunction and hyperactivity. Dextromethorphan produced the best results with the fewest side effects, suggesting that it may hold promise for treating chronic neuropathic pain.

► In addition to their ability to block the development of spinally mediated hyperalgesia, NMDA antagonists have been shown to block or reverse tolerance to opioids and to at least temporarily reduce the hyperalgesia and allodynia associated with experimental mononeuropathy. It is encouraging to find that this class of drugs may be helpful in controlling the pain and hyperalgesia associated with spinal cord injury. Although the side effects of clinically available NMDA antagonists are clearly problematic, low doses of these drugs combined with partially effective analgesic agents may be helpful for certain patients.

S.E. Abram, M.D.

Postoperative Pain: The Role of Magnesium Sulfate

Role of Magnesium Sulfate in Postoperative Analgesia
Tramèr MR, Schneider J, Marti R-A, et al (Univ Hosp of Geneva)
Anesthesiology 84:340–347, 1996 9–21

Background.—There is evidence that calcium channel blockers and *N*-methyl-D-aspartate (NMDA) antagonists might help in the prevention and treatment of pain. Magnesium, a physiologic NMDA antagonist, may have an antinociceptive effect in humans. The capability of perioperative magnesium sulfate ($MgSO_4$) administration to reduce postoperative pain was investigated.

Methods.—The randomized, double-blind trial included 44 American Society of Anesthesiologists class 1 or 2 patients undergoing elective abdominal hysterectomy for benign disease. They were randomized to receive either 20% $MgSO_4$ or physiologic saline. Magnesium sulfate was given IV in a 15 mL bolus after induction of anesthesia with thiopental and fentanyl. Thereafter, the patients received a continuous IV infusion of $MgSO_4$, 2.5 mL/hr over 20 hours with a syringe pump. The maximum dose of $MgSO_4$ was 13 g. After surgery, the patients were given a patient-controlled analgesia device containing morphine, 2 mg/dose. The $MgSO_4$ and placebo groups were compared in terms of analgesic requirements, pain, comfort, and quality of sleep postoperatively. They were also re-evaluated after 1 month to determine the long-term effects of surgery and $MgSO_4$ treatment.

Results.—The 2 groups were comparable in their demographic characteristics, duration of surgery, intraoperative fentanyl and vecuronium doses, and time from last fentanyl dose to the end of surgery. By 48 hours, the mean cumulative morphine dose was 65 mg in the patients receiving $MgSO_4$ vs. 91 mg in those receiving placebo. The difference in morphine consumption was significant only in the first 6 hours after surgery. Patients in the $MgSO_4$ group reported significantly less discomfort from 18 to 48 hours than those in the control group. Insomnia was the same preoperatively and postoperatively in the $MgSO_4$ group, whereas it increased significantly during the first and second postoperative nights for the control group. Respiratory depression occurred in 3 patients in the control group vs. none in the $MgSO_4$ group.

Conclusions.—Perioperative magnesium administration can reduce analgesic requirements, decrease discomfort, and improve sleep in the postoperative period. Magnesium treatment is associated with a 30% decrease in morphine consumption in this randomized trial. The reasons for the benefits of $MgSO_4$ therapy are unknown, but it may be that magnesium has a clinically significant antinociceptive effect, either a specific one via blockade of the NMDA receptor or a nonspecific one via prevention of hypomagnesemia.

▶ Intrathecal magnesium has been shown experimentally to be neurally protective to the spinal cord during aortic crossclamping. It would be interesting to speculate whether magnesium's NMDA antagonistic action would act similarly in an antinociceptive fashion, as was described in this study, if administered intrathecally.

D.M. Rothenberg, M.D.

Pain Perception: Volunteer Studies

The Effects of Electrical Stimulation at Different Frequencies on Perception and Pain in Human Volunteers: Epidural Versus Intravenous Administration of Fentanyl

Liu SS, Gerancher JC, Bainton BG, et al (Virginia Mason Med Ctr, Seattle; Wake Forest Univ, Winston-Salem, NC)
Anesth Analg 82:98–102, 1996 9–22

Objective.—Electrical stimulation at different frequencies produces different sensations. The ability of epidurally administered fentanyl to produce segmental sensory changes to perception and pain during transcutaneous electrical stimulation at 5,250, and 2,000 Hz was evaluated in a randomized, double-blind, crossover study.

Methods.—Moderate pain and perception thresholds were determined in 8 healthy volunteers (3 male), aged 31 to 46 years, by slowly increasing the current at each frequency delivered at the ipsilateral C2 and L2 dermatomes. Level of moderate pain (C_{mp}) and perception thresholds were measured at 5, 15, 30, 45, and 60 minutes after the injection of 10 mL of 1-µg /kg fentanyl delivered IV or epidurally.

Results.—Intravenous or epidural fentanyl did not significantly affect perceptions at 5,250, or 2,000 Hz. Intravenous fentanyl increased C_{mp} at both dermatomes at 5 and 250 Hz, whereas epidural fentanyl increased C_{mp} only at 5 Hz at the L2 dermatome.

Conclusion.—The administration of epidural fentanyl produces segmental spinal analgesia in response to electrical stimulation only at certain frequencies. The fact that the administration of IV and epidural fentanyl produces different analgesic results suggests that separate pain mechanisms operate at different frequencies.

▶ Transcutaneous sine-wave stimulation at 3 different frequencies is used diagnostically to determine sensory detection thresholds in patients with neuropathies. On the basis of indirect evidence, it appears likely that 5 Hz of stimulation produces predominantly C-fiber activation at detection threshold, 250 Hz of stimulation affects mainly A-delta fibers, and 2,000 Hz of stimulation is most specific for A-beta activation. Unfortunately, direct neurophysiologic correlation is lacking. If there is such selectivity of different frequencies in activating different fiber types, this would indicate that epidural fentanyl is capable of selective suppression of C-fiber–mediated pain, whereas systemic fentanyl suppresses both C-delta–and A-delta–mediated pain. Studies to characterize the effect of transcutaneous sine-wave stimulation on different fiber types are under way.

S.E. Abram, M.D.

Subject Index*

* *All entries refer to the year and page number(s) for data appearing in this and previous editions of the* Year Book.

B

C

E

F

G

H

I

J

K

M

N

O

Q

R

S

T

U

V

W

X

Z

Author Index

S

T

U

V

W

X

Y

Z